Handbook of Experimental Pharmacology

Volume 85

The Pharmacology of Lymphocytes

Contributors

S.S. Alkan · J.-F. Bach · R.R. Bartlett · T.W. Behrens · R. Benner
K. Brune · J.C. Cambier · L. Chedid · R.G. Coffey · M. Dardenne
C.A. Dinarello · J. Drews · W. Englberger · J.-F. Gauchat
C. Gaveriaux · D. Gemsa · S.C. Gilman · Th. Ginsberg
G. Goldstein · J.S. Goodwin · J. Gordon · H.U. Gubler · W. Haas
J. Hamuro · P.C. Hiestand · K. Hirai · M.M. Khan · J. Klein
S. Kotani · J.R. Lamb · A.J. Lewis · P.E. Lipsky · F. Loor
R.T. Maguire · K.L. Melmon · M. Parant · M.J. Parnham
S.S. Pathak · T. Payne · J.T. Ransom · M.J.H. Ratcliffe
N.R. Sabbele · H.F.J. Savelkoul · Y. Shiokawa · B.M. Stadler
T.B. Strom · H. Takada · M.A. Talle · J.M. Williams · G. Wolberg

Editors

M.A. Bray and J. Morley

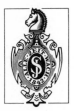

Springer-Verlag
Berlin Heidelberg New York
London Paris Tokyo

MICHAEL A. BRAY, Ph.D.
Research Department
CIBA-GEIGY AG
CH-4002 Basel

JOHN MORLEY, Ph.D., FRC Path.
Pharmaceutical Division
Preclinical Research
SANDOZ Ltd.
CH-4002 Basel

With 69 Figures

ISBN 3-540-18609-3 Springer-Verlag Berlin Heidelberg New York
ISBN 0-387-18609-3 Springer-Verlag New York Berlin Heidelberg

Library of Congress Cataloging-in-Publication Data. The Pharmacology of lymphocytes. (Handbook of experimental pharmacology; v. 85) Includes index. 1. Immunopharmacology. 2. Lymphocytes. I. Alkan, S.S. II. Bray, Michael A. III. Morley, J. (John), 1938– . IV. Series. [DNLM: 1. Lymphocytes – immunology. 2. Lymphocytes – physiology. W1 HA51L v.85/QW 568 P536] QP905.H3 vol. 85 [RM370]   615′.1 s   [615′.7]   88-3275 ISBN 0-387-18609-3 (U.S.)

Typesetting, printing and bookbinding: Brühlsche Universitätsdruckerei, Giessen
2122/3130-543210

List of Contributors

S. S. ALKAN, Research Department, Pharmaceuticals Division, CIBA-GEIGY AG, CH-4002 Basel

J.-F. BACH, INSERM U25-CNRS LA 122, Hôpital Necker, 161, rue de Sèvres, F-75743 Paris Cedex 15

R. R. BARTLETT, Pharmacological Research, Hoechst AG, Werk Albert, P.O. Box 129101, D-6200 Wiesbaden 12

T. W. BEHRENS, Medical College of Wisconsin, Department of Medicine, 8700 West Wisconsin Ave., Milwaukee, WI 53226, USA

R. BENNER, Department of Cell Biology, Immunology and Genetics, Erasmus University Rotterdam, Postbus 1738, NL-3000 DR Rotterdam

K. BRUNE, Institute of Pharmacology and Toxicology, University of Erlangen-Nürnberg, Universitätsstr. 22, D-8520 Erlangen

J. C. CAMBIER, Department of Medicine, National Jewish Center for Immunology and Respiratory Medicine, 1400 Jackson Street, Denver, CO 80206, USA

L. CHEDID, Immunothérapie Experimentale, Institut Pasteur, 28, rue du Dr. Roux, F-75015 Paris Cedex 15

R. G. COFFEY, University of South Florida Medical Center, College of Medicine, Department of Pharmacology and Therapeutics, 12901 North 30th Street, Box 9, Tampa, FL 33612, USA

M. DARDENNE, INSERM U25-CNRS LA 122, Hôpital Necker, 161, rue de Sèvres, F-75743 Paris Cedex 15

C. A. DINARELLO, Division of Geographic Medicine und Infectious Diseases, Tufts University, New England Medical Center Hospitals, 750 Washington Street, Box 68, Boston, MA 02111, USA

J. DREWS, Research Department, F. Hoffmann - La Roche & Co. Ltd., CH-4002 Basel

W. ENGLBERGER, Inflammation/Immunopharmacology, A. Nattermann & Cie. GmbH, P.O. Box 350120, D-5000 Köln 30

J.-F. GAUCHAT, Institut of Clinical Immunology, University of Bern, Inselspital, CH-3010 Bern

C. GAVERIAUX, Pharmaceutical Division, Preclinical Research, SANDOZ Ltd., CH-4002 Basel

D. GEMSA, Institute of Immunology, Medical Center of Hygiene and Medical Microbiology, University of Marburg, Robert-Koch-Str. 8, D-3550 Marburg/Lahn

S. C. GILMAN, Wyeth Laboratories, Inc., P.O. Box 8299, Philadelphia, PA 19101, USA

TH. GINSBERG, Newport Pharmaceuticals International, Inc., 897 West 16th Street, Newport Beach, CA 92663, USA

G. GOLDSTEIN, ORTHO Pharmaceutical Corporation, ORTHO-BIOTECH Division, Route 202, P.O. Box 300, Raritan, NJ 08869-0602, USA

J. S. GOODWIN, Medical College of Wisconsin, Department of Medicine, 8700 West Wisconsin Ave., Milwaukee, WI 53226, USA

J. GORDON, Chiron Ophthalmics, 15A Marconi, Irvine, CA 92718, USA

H. U. GUBLER, Pharmaceutical Division, Preclinical Research, SANDOZ Ltd., CH-4002 Basel

W. HAAS, Research Department, F. Hoffmann - La Roche & Co., Ltd., CH-4002 Basel

J. HAMURO, Division of Immunology, Department of Basic Research, Central Research Laboratories, Ajinomoto Co., Inc., 214 Maeda-cho, Tatsuka-ku, Yokohama, Kanagawa 244, Japan

P. C. HIESTAND, Pharmaceutical Division, Preclinical Research, SANDOZ Ltd., CH-4002 Basel

K. HIRAI, Institute of Clinical Immunology, University of Bern, Inselspital, CH-3010 Bern

M. M. KHAN, Departments of Medicine and Pharmacology, Stanford University School of Medicine, Room S-025, Stanford, CA 93205, USA

J. KLEIN, Max-Planck-Institute of Biology, Correnstr. 42, D-7400 Tübingen

S. KOTANI, Department of Oral Microbiolohy, Osaka University, Faculty of Dentistry, 1–8 Yamadaoka, Suita, Osaka 565, Japan

J. R. LAMB, MRC Tuberculosis and Related Infections Unit, Hammersmith Hospital, Ducane Road, London W12 OH5, Great Britain

A. J. LEWIS, Wyeth Laboratories, Inc., P.O. Box 8299, Philadelphia, PA 19101, USA

P. E. LIPSKY, Rheumatic Disease Division, Department of Internal Medicine, Harold C. Simmons Arthritis Research Center, University of Texas Health Science Center at Dallas, Dallas, TX 75235, USA

F. LOOR, Pharmaceutical Division, Preclinical Research, SANDOZ Ltd., CH-4002 Basel

R. T. MAGUIRE, Wyeth Laboratories, Inc., P.O. Box 8299, Philadelphia, PA 19101, USA

K. L. MELMON, Departments of Medicine and Pharmacology, Stanford University School of medicine, Room S-025, Stanford, CA 94305, USA

M. PARANT, Laboratoire Immunopharmacologie Experimentale, CNRS UA 579, Institut Biomédical des Cordeliers, 15, rue de l'École de Médecine, F-75270 Paris Cedex 06

M. J. PARNHAM, Inflammation/Immunopharmacology, A. Nattermann & Cie. GmbH, P.O. Box 350120, D-5000 Köln 30

S. S. PATHAK, Department of Cell Biology, Immunology and Genetics, Erasmus University Rotterdam, Postbus 1738, NL-3000 DR Rotterdam

T. PAYNE, Pharmaceutical Division, Preclinical Research, SANDOZ Ltd., CH-4002 Basel

J. T. RANSOM, DNAX Research Institute of Molecular and Cellular Biology, Inc., 901 California Ave., Palo Alto, CA 94304-1104, USA

M. J. H. RATCLIFFE, Imperial Cancer Research Fund, Tumour Immunologic Unit, Department of Zoology, University College London, London WC1E 6BT, Great Britain
Present Address: Department of Microbiology and Immunology, McGill University, 3775 University Str., Montreal, Quebec H3A ZB4, Canada

N. R. SABBELE, Department of Histology, Hasanuddin University, Ujang Pandang 8, Indonesia

H. F. J. SAVELKOUL, Department of Cell Biology, Immunology and Genetics, Erasmus University Rotterdam, Postbus 1738, NL-3000 DR Rotterdam

Y. SHIOKAWA, Department of Rheumatology, Juntendo University School of Medicine, Sengoku-4-37-14, Bunkyo-ku, Tokyo 112, Japan

B. M. STADLER, Institute of Clinical Immunology, University of Bern, Inselspital, CH-3010 Bern

T. B. STROM, Department of Medicine, Renval Division, Harvard Medical School, Beth Israel Hospital, 330 Brookline Ave., Boston, MA 02215, USA

H. TAKADA, Department of Oral Microbiology, Osaka University, Faculty of Dentistry, 1–8 Yamadaoka, Suita, Osaka 565, Japan

M. A. TALLE, ORTHO Pharmaceutical Corporation, ORTHO-BIOTECH Division, Route 202, P.O. Box 300, Raritan, NJ 08869-0602, USA

J. M. WILLIAMS, Department of Medicine, Renal Division, Harvard Medical School, Beth Israel Hospital, 330 Brookline Ave., Boston, MA 02215, USA

G. WOLBERG, Experimental Therapy Department, Burroughs Wellcome Co., 3030 Cornwallis Road, Research Triangle Park, NC 27709, USA

Preface

"Immunopharmacology",
why not "pharmacoimmunology"?
Professor H. O. Schild
University College London, 1962

An intact immune response is essential for survival, as is evidenced by the various innate immune deficiency syndromes and by the emergence of the acquired immune deficiency syndrome (AIDS) as a pandemic during the last decade. Substances which stimulate the immune response might contribute to the therapy of AIDS and its precursor, AIDS-related syndrome, as well as of other clinical conditions in which immune responses can be diminished, such as carcinoma and infections. In other circumstances, an intact or heightened immune response may pose clinical problems; hence there is need to suppress, or diminish, components of the immune response. For instance, it is necessary to impair cellular immunity in order to ensure lasting acceptance of heterografts and it is already established that agents effective in transplantation are therapeutically effective in an range of autoimmune diseases. More recently, experimental studies have indicated that aberrant manifestations of humoral immunity, as in allergies, may also be amenable to pharmacological intervention.

Extensive immunological research during the last decade has led to a good understanding of the regulation and expression of immune responses. Clarification of the cellular interactions during immune responses has led to considerable optimism; hence, there is a widely held belief that selection of potential therapeutic agents using high-capacity drug screening tests will be more easily achieved because of this knowledge. Moreover, it has been concluded that there is sufficient information available for the rational design of immunoreactive compounds. The practical utility of these approaches remains to be proven; nonetheless, existing models of the immune response have already provided a rationale for preparation and clinical evaluation of certain endogenous products of lymphocyte activation (i.e., interferons, interleukins, and colony stimulating factors) as potential therapeutic agents. It has been appropriate to build upon the precedent provided by these materials by outlining contemporary knowledge of lymphocyte physiology, as a prelude to discussing lymphocyte pharmacology.

Thus, the first section of this volume has been devoted to an overview of lymphocyte interactions during immune responses and to a description of existing knowledge of lymphocyte receptors, membrane events during activation, signal transduction mechanisms, and second messenger systems in lymphocytes. The second section describes the methodology employed for experimental studies on lymphocytes and products of lymphocyte activation, since familiarity with these techniques is necessary for the measurement of lymphocyte interactions and responses to various lymphocyte products. The third section has focused upon the capacity of endogenous autocoids to modify lymphocyte activation.

Amines and arachidonate products are discussed as immunoregulatory agents that have attracted considerable attention. The final section comprises a series of chapters, each devoted to a specific drug or drug category for which there is already evidence of clinical efficacy or for which experimental data indicates likelihood of clinical efficacy.

The study of lymphocyte interactions has led to the propagation of specific lymphocyte clones and to the characterization, purification, and synthesis of particular immunological mediators. The groundwork provided by these extensive immunological studies is now substantial, so that it is timely for industrial pharmacologists to effect the transition for immunopharmacology to pharmaco-immunology. In this way, it is to be hoped that the opportunities available to physicians for immunotherapy will achieve a range comparable to those already available for other major organ systems (e.g. cardiovascular, gastrointestinal, neuronal, central and peripheral airways). We hope that this volume will contribute to that objective.

We are pleased to acknowledge the efforts of the contributors who have provided the chapters that comprise this book and we are grateful for their willingness to revise contributions at a late stage, in order to offset the delays that inevitably arise when assembling a multi-author volume. A brief glossary of immunological terms had been included, for which we gratefully acknowledge the help and advice of Professor Sefik Alkan; we are also indebted to Dr. Jennifer M. Hanson for providing the index.

Basel   MICHAEL A. BRAY
                                                                   JOHN MORLEY

Contents

CHAPTER 4

Intracellular Events During Lymphocyte Activation
R. G. COFFEY. With 1 Figure 83

Part 2

CHAPTER 5

Generation and Measurement of Antibodies
H. F. J. SAVELKOUL, S. S. PATHAK, N. R. SABBELE, and R. BENNER
With 3 Figures 141

CHAPTER 6

**Monoclonal Antibodies to Lymphocyte Surface Molecules as Probes
for Lymphocyte Functions**

CHAPTER 7

**Interleukin 1 Production from Various Cells and Measurement of its Multiple
Biologic Activities**

CHAPTER 10

Factors Regulating IgE Synthesis
C. GAVERIAUX, T. PAYNE, and F. LOOR. With 2 Figures 275

CHAPTER 11

Generation, Biology, and Assay of Efferent Lymphokines
D. GEMSA 291

CHAPTER 12

Lymphocyte Purification, Growth, Cloning and Functional Assays

CHAPTER 13

Screening Strategies for Detecting Immunotherapeutic Agents
S. C. GILMAN, R. T. MAGUIRE, and A. J. LEWIS. With 1 Figure 345

Part 3

CHAPTER 14

Selected Autacoids as Modulators of Lymphocyte Function
M. M. KHAN and K. L. MELMON. With 7 Figures 363

CHAPTER 15

Lipid Mediators and Lymphocyte Function
M. J. PARNHAM and W. ENGLBERGER. With 2 Figures 385

CHAPTER 16

Thymic Hormones and Lymphocyte Functions
J.-F. Bach and M. Dardenne

Part 4

CHAPTER 17

Glucocorticosteroids
T. W. Behrens and J. S. Goodwin. With 6 Figures

Contents

CHAPTER 25

Bacterial and Fungal Products
H. TAKADA, J. HAMURO, and S. KOTANI. With 7 Figures 555

CHAPTER 26

Nonsteroidal Anti-inflammatory Drugs: Effects on Lymphocyte Function
K. BRUNE 577

CHAPTER 27

Future Prospects for Drugs Design of Lymphocyte Modulators
J. DREWS and W. HAAS. With 2 Figures 587

Glossary of Common Immunological Terms

Term	Abbreviation	Definition	Chapter
Accessory cell	AC	Cell (generally monocyte) involved in antigen processing and presentation, necessary for many immune responses (see also APC)	
Adjuvant		A substance which nonspecifically enhances an immune response to antigen	
Adoptive transfer		The transfer of the ability to mount an immune response via the transfer of immunocompetent cells into a host made immunoincompetent (usually by irradiation)	
Allele		One of two or more alternative forms of a gene occupying corresponding loci on homologous chromosomes	
Allogeneic		Having cell types that are antigenically distinct	
Allotype		Product of an allele which is not common to all members of a species and therefor can be recognized as an antigen within the same species	
Antibody	Ab	A molecule generated by plasmocytes in response to antigen, able specifically to recognize that antigen	1, 5
Antibody-dependent cell-mediated cytotoxicity	ADCC	Ability of nonsensitized cells to lyse target cells coated with specific antibody	
Antigen	Ag	A molecule which induces an immune response	
Antigen presenting cell	APC	A cell able to carry antigen on its surface in a form which can be recognized by lymphocytes	

Term	Abbreviation	Definition	Chapter
Autoantibody		Antibody which reacts with self-antigens (i.e. components of the host's own tissues)	
Autoantigen		Antigen that is a normal constituent of the hosts tissues. Also known as self-antigen	
Autoimmunity		Immune response directed against the host's own tissues	
Autologous		From the same individual	
B lymphocyte	B cell	Bone-marrow derived lymphocyte sub-population which produces antibodies. First defined in birds where these cells mature in the Bursa of Fabricius (a lymphoepithelial organ), hence the term B cell	
Bovine γ-globulin	BGG	A widely used antigen	
Bovine serum albumin	BSA	A widely used antigen also used as a carrier for low molecular weight antigens. Prepared from Cohn's fraction V of bovine serum	
Capping		Coordinated movement of cell membrane molecules to one part of the cell surface after binding of a multivalent ligand such as an antibody or antigen	
Carrier		An immunogenic molecule or part of a molecule recognized by T cells during an antibody response (cf. hapten)	
Cell-mediated immunity	CMI	Immune response mediated by cells (specifically T cells) rather than antibodies (cf. humoral immunity)	
Clone		A family of cells or organisms having a genetically identical constitution	12
Cluster determinant, clusters of differentiation	CD	General term recently adopted for cell surface antigens defined by cross-reactivity with various "clusters" of monoclonal antibodies. Initially used to identify lymphocytes and now extended to other haemopoetic cell types	6

Term	Abbreviation	Definition	Chapter
Complement	C	An enzymatic system of serum proteins involved in a variety of immune responses (e.g. hemolysis, cytolysis)	
Concanavalin A	Con A	A mitogen for T cells derived from the jack bean *Canavalia einsformis*	
Congenic, coisogenic		Animals with a single genetic variation at a particular defined locus	
Cortex		The peripheral region of a lymph node or the thymus	
Cytokine		Generic term for intercellular mediators produced by cells involved in an immune response (cf. lymphokine, monokine)	
Cytotoxic lymphocyte	Tc	T cell subset able to lyse specific target cells	
Delayed-type hypersensitivity	DTH	Cellular immune response defined by a "delayed"-type skin rection (maximal within hours or days). Also known as type IV hypersensitivity	
Determinant		That part of an antigen that binds to the antibody combining site (cf. epitope)	
Dinitrophenol	DNP	A widely used hapten	
Enzyme-linked immunoabsorbant assay	ELISA	An in vitro immunochemical technique utilizing enzyme labelled antibodies (usually monoclonal antibodies) to detect specific substances (antigens)	
Epitope		A single antigenic determinant	
Fc receptor	FcR	The site on a lymphocyte or monocyte surface able to bind the Fc portion of an immunoglobulin (usually IgG)	
Fluorescence activated cell sorter	FACS	Instrument designed to separate cells based on surface fluorescent markers (e.g. monoclonal antibodies)	
Fragment, antigen binding	Fab	The portion of an antibody molecule containing the variable (antigen binding) regions	5

Term	Abbreviation	Definition	Chapter
Fragment, crystallizable	Fc	The C-terminal portion of an antibody molecule which is responsible for binding to antibody receptors on cells and to the complement components	5
Freund's adjuvant	FIA, IFA, FCA, CFA	An emulsion of aqueous antigen in mineral oil (FIA, IFA) which may also contain *Mycobacterium tuberculosis* as antigen (FCA, CFA)	
Genotype		The genetic material inherited from parents	
Germinal center		A spherical agglomeration of lymphocytes (principally B cells) found in lymph nodes and spleen following antigen stimulation	
Hemagglutination		Agglutination of erythrocytes. Used as an in vitro readout for aggregation of specific antigen coated erythrocytes	
Haplotype		A set of genetic determinants located on a single chromosome	
Hapten		A small molecule which can act as an epitope if coupled to a carrier but which cannot alone induce an immune response	
Helper cell	Th	A subset of T lymphocytes involved in the generation of other T lymphocytes and, in cooperation with B lymphocytes, the production of antibodies	1
Heterologous		Having interspecies antigenic differences ($=$xenogeneic)	
Histocompatability		Ability to accept grafts between individuals	
Histocompatability 2	H-2	The mouse major histocompatability complex (MHC)	
Homologous		Of the same species	
Human leukocyte antigens	HLA	The human major histocompatability complex (MHC)	
Humoral immunity		Immune response mediated by antibodies (present in body fluids)	

Term	Abbre-viation	Definition	Chapter
Hybridoma		Cell line(s) created in vitro by the fusion of two different cell types (usually a normal lymphocyte and a lymphoid tumor cell line)	12
Hypervariable region		Extremely variable regions of antibody heavy and light chains making up the antigen binding site and determining the idiotype of an antibody	
Idiotype		The antigenic characteristic of the variable (V) region of an antibody	
Immune complex	IC	Product of an antigen-antibody reaction. May also include complement components. May be soluble or insoluble	
Immune-response associated	Ia	Histocompatability antigens associated with antigen presenting cells and coded for by the I region of the MHC	
Immune-response genes	Ir gene	Genes associated with the MHC (I region) which determine the intensity of an immune response against a particular antigen	1
Immunoglobulin	Ig	γ-Globulin molecules which act as antibodies. Constructed of two light chains and two heavy chains. Human Ig's are in five major classes, IgM, IgD, IgG, IgA, and IgE, based on variations in heavy chain structural type	5
Interleukin(s)	IL	Generic term for peptides involved in signalling between cells of the immune system (cf. cytokine, lymphokine)	
Isotype		The class or subclass of immunoglobulin common to all members of a species	
Keyhole limpet hemocyanin	KLH	A widely used T cell-dependent antigen generally serving as a carrier molecule	
Killer cell	K cell	Type of lymphocyte able to destroy target cells via antibody-dependent cell-mediated reaction	

Term	Abbre-viation	Definition	Chapter
Lipopoly-saccharide	LPS	Active component of endotoxin derived from bacterial cell walls, used as a B cell mitogen in mice	
Lymphocyte antigens	Ly, Lyt (1, 2, 3)	T cell surface antigens used to distinguish T cell subsets	
Lymphokine activated killer cells	LAK	Cell (lymphocyte or monocyte) activated by lymphokines to lyse target cells (e.g., tumor cells)	
Lymphokines	LK	Generic term for nonantibody lymphocyte products involved in signaling between immune cells (cf. cytokine, interleukin)	
Major histocompatability complex (classes I, II, III)	MHC	Region of mammalian genome controlling histocompatability (e.g., self/nonself). Known as H-2 in the mouse and HLA in man. Codes for three major molecular classes, viz.: Class 1, peptide associated with β_2-microglobulin; Class 2, two non-covalently associated (Ia) peptides; Class 3, complement components. Also codes for immune response genes (cf. Ir) and lymphocyte surface antigens	1
Medulla		The central region of a lymph node	
Memory		The ability of the immune system to mount a specific, accelerated secondary response to a previously introduced antigen	
Mitogen		Any agent which induces cell mitosis. In immunology, generally used for agents which induce polyclonal lymphocyte activation (e.g., Con A, PHA, LPS)	
Mixed leukocyte reaction	MLR, MLC	Culture of leukocytes (lymphocytes) from different donors to generate an immune response, measured as the appearance of transformed T lymphocytes (blast cells)	5
Monoclonal (antibody)	m (mAb)	Derived from a single clone (thus producing homogeneous antibodies)	6

Term	Abbreviation	Definition	Chapter
Monokine(s)		Generic term for monocyte (non-lymphocyte) products involved in signalling between immune cells	
Natural killer cell	NK cell	Type of lymphocyte or monocyte intrinsically able to destroy some virally infected cells and some tumor cells	
Nude mouse	*nu/nu*	Genetically athymic mouse strain (hairless) with no T cell-driven immune responses	
Null cell		A type of lymphocyte that bears neither T or B cell surface antigen markers	
OKT		A group of monoclonal antibodies used primarily as T cell surface markers. Developed by the Ortho Pharmaceutical Corporation. Term now largely replaced by CD (cluster determinant)	6
Opsonization		Enhancement of phagocytosis of a particle, microorganism, or cell by virtue of its being coated with antibody	
Ovalbumin	OA, OVA, EA	Egg white albumin widely used as an antigen	
Paratope		A part of an antibody which interacts with an epitope	
Phenotype		The expressed characteristics of an individual	
Phorbol myristate (-ic) acetate	TPA, PMA	Mutagenic phorbol ester used to stimulate T cells in vitro	
Phytohemagglutinin	PHA	Plant cell mitogen for T cells extracted from the red kidney bean *Phaseolus vulgaris*	
Plaque forming cell	PFC, AFC	An antibody-producing (-forming) cell identified by its ability to lyse antigen-coated erythrocytes in vitro	5
Plasma cell, plasmocyte		A fully differentiated antibody-producing B cell	
Pokeweed mitogen	PWM	A mitogen for human B cells	
Primary immune response		Response occurring upon first exposure to an immunogen (mainly IgM antibody isotype)	
Priming		Initial sensitization to an antigen	

Term	Abbreviation	Definition	Chapter
Reticuloendothelial system	RES	System of bone-marrow-derived phagocytic cells associated with connective tissue (e.g., macrophages). Now more commonly called the mononuclear phagocyte system	
Secondary immune response		Response occurring upon secondary and subsequent exposures to an immunogen (involving antibody isotypes other than IgM)	
Suppressor cell	Ts	A subset of T lymphocytes which act to reduce the immune responsiveness of other lymphocytes	
Syngeneic		Genetically identical. Generally refers to highly inbred animal strains or grafts between such	
T lymphocyte	T cell	Subpopulation of lymphocytes involved in cell-mediated immune responses; mature in the thymus hence the term T cell	
Theta	Thy-1 θ	An antigen on mouse T cells (other Thy antigen surface markers also exist)	
Tolerance		A state of specific immunological unresponsiveness	
Transformation		Morphological change (in lymphocytes) associated with the onset of mitosis	
Type I hypersensitivity reaction	Type I	Antigen/passive fixed antibody reaction; Synonyms are immediate hypersensitivity, anaphylaxis	
Type II hypersensitivity reaction	Type II	Antibody/surface antigen or hapten interaction involving complement	
Type III hypersensitivity reaction	Type III	Antigen/antibody complex mediated reaction (e.g., Arthus responses) generally involving immune complex deposition in tissues	
Type IV hypersensitivity reaction	Type IV	Cellular immune response involving T cells; Synonyms are DTH and CMI	
Variable region	V region, V_H, V_L	Variable regions of an immunoglobulin (V_H, heavy chain V region; V_L, light chain V region)	
Xenogeneic		Having interspecies antigenic differences (=heterologous)	

Part 1

CHAPTER 1

The Evolution, Ontogeny, and Physiologic Function of Lymphocytes

J. KLEIN

A. What is a Lymphocyte?

To a morphologist, a lymphocyte is a small spherical cell (7–12 μm diameter) with scanty cytoplasm and a round, slightly indented and somewhat eccentrically located nucleus, containing coarse masses of chromatin (Fig. 1; WEISS and GREEP 1977; KRSTIĆ 1984).[1] This definition is adequate in dealing with mouse or human cells, although even in these species one can never be sure that one is always dealing with the same cell. When one turns to other mammals and other vertebrates, one faces even more uncertainties, and as far as the investigation of other animal phyla is concerned, here one is completely lost. To be sure, one finds small round cells with round nuclei in most animal species, but then one always faces the question: are they all lymphocytes or do they just *look* like lymphocytes, while in reality they are other kinds of cell? Here, morphology alone cannot answer this question and one must look for other ways of unambiguously identifying lymphocytes. The best way is by using functional criteria.

Lymphocytes carry out many functions, but one of these is unmistakably lymphocytic and is unique to them. It is the lymphocyte's ability to reshuffle its genes in such a way that they can then produce receptors for antigens, and via this re-

---

[1] The references in this chapter are limited largely to review articles; original papers are cited only in cases where reviews are not available or where direct citation is required for other reasons.

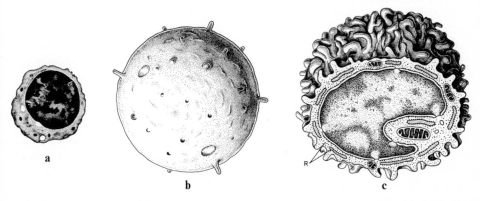

a

b   c

Fig. 1 a–c. Mammalian lymphocyte as seen with a light microscope (**a**) and an electron microscope (**b, c**). *R*, ribosomes. Two functional states of lymphocyte surface – smooth (**b**) and with microvilli (**c**) – are shown

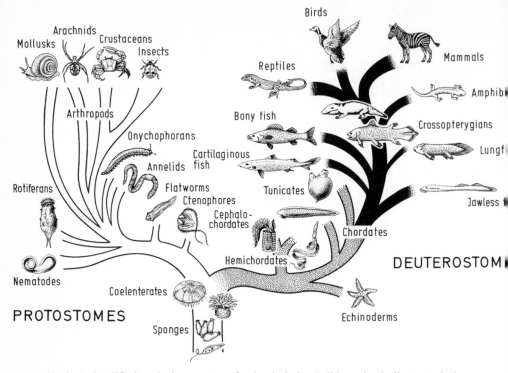

Fig. 2. A simplified evolutionary tree of animal phyla. *Full branches* indicate evolutionary lines in which true lymphocytes have been shown to be present; *stippled branches* lines in which lymphocytes may be present; *open branches* lines in which true lymphocytes are probably not present

ceptor, initiate a specific immune response. As far as we know, no other cell in the vertebrate body can do this and there is therefore no better way of defining a lymphocyte than according to this feature. The receptors also provide the basis for distinguishing two kinds of lymphocytes: T lymphocytes, differentiating largely in the thymus; and B lymphocytes, differentiating largely in the bone marrow (in mammals) or in the bursa of Fabricius (in birds). The receptor of the T lymphocyte, the T cell receptor (Tcr), is characterized by its ability to recognize two molecules or two molecular fragments at the same time – an antigen (nonself), and a molecule encoded in the genes of the major histocompatibility complex (Mhc; self in a physiologic situation; Fig. 2; see SCHWARTZ 1985; KLEIN 1986a). The receptor of the B lymphocyte, the immunoglobulin (Ig) molecule, on the other hand, recognizes one molecule only – the foreign antigen (nonself). The two kinds of receptor also differ in the form in which they are produced by their respective cells: the B cell receptor (Bcr) is secreted by the lymphocyte and the Tcr is not. This distinction is, however, not absolute: in certain stages of B cell development, the Bcr, like the Tcr, is integrated in the membrane and only acquires a secretory piece in the later phase (KINDT and CAPRA 1984). Similarly, there are indications that in a certain phase of T cell development, the Tcr may be released from the cell in a soluble form as an antigen-specific factor (WEBB et al. 1985; KLEIN 1986a). The exact composition of this form has not been determined and, to this date, no secretory segments have been identified in either the Tcr genes or the Tcr polypeptides. Furthermore, it cannot be ruled out that, in some animal groups, the Tcr is produced in a secreted, soluble form although, for reasons that will become clear later, it is most unlikely that all forms of Tcr could be secreted in any species.

The two kinds of receptor also differ in their structure, but this difference is in detail rather than in the overall design (HOOD et al. 1985; KRONENBERG et al. 1986). In fact, the extent to which Tcr and Bcr are similar in their general conception is quite remarkable. Both receptors consist of two kinds of chains (heavy and light in Bcr, α and β in Tcr); each chain is assembled from very similar basic modules (domains); the receptor genes are assembled from similar elements (the V, D, J, and C segments); the process of gene expression involves, in both instances, the silencing of one of two selected allelic elements (allelic exclusion); and the rearrangement of the elements probably occurs by the same principal mechanism. On the other hand, the Tcr and Bcr clearly have two different sets of genes in that they have different functions, different chromosomal localizations, and only a limited sequence homology. Because of the diverse ways in which they recognize antigens, there should also be some fundamental difference in the construction of the combining sites of the two receptors. All these features suggest that the Bcr and Tcr genes had a common ancestor a long time ago and that they have retained a similarity of organization because of similar functional constraints placed on them. The common origin of the receptors, in turn, suggests that the two kinds of lymphocyte, T and B, also evolved as two branches of a single evolutionary tree.

One other characteristic of a lymphocyte is its cyclic behavior (ZOLA 1985; STUTMAN 1986). Unlike most other cells in the body, lymphocytes (at least some of them) can pause in the middle of their differentiation and begin to cycle. Each cycle involves the transformation of the small, resting lymphocyte into a large, active blast cell, followed by several rounds of cell division and then a gradual return to the resting stage. This burst of activity can apparently be repeated a number (but apparently a finite number) of times. The periods between two consecutive bursts can be quite long for some of the lymphocytes (several years for T cells) and short for others (hours or days for some B cells). The process of cycling is not differentiation in the true sense of the word, despite the fact that the cell changes its phenotype in an orderly and predetermined manner; because of its reversibility, it must be regarded as an interruption in the differentiation process. Lymphocytes that have journeyed all the way along the differentiation pathway end up as dead-end, terminally differentiated cells.

B. Phylogenetic Origin of Lymphocytes

It is reasonably well established that all vertebrates, from cyclostomes to mammals, have true lymphocytes (COOPER 1976; MARCHALONIS 1977). This conclusion is based not so much on the morphological identification of lymphocytes in the different vertebrate classes as on the demonstration that even primitive vertebrates have immunoglobulin and Tcr genes (LITMAN et al. 1985). They probably also have Mhc genes, although this point has not been demonstrated unequivocally (KLEIN 1977, 1986a).

Many immunologists believe that the majority of invertebrates also have lymphocytes (RATCLIFFE et al. 1985). Indeed, this term is commonly used in reference to blood cells that resemble mammalian lymphocytes morphologically (RATCLIFFE and ROWLEY 1981).

Yet, to this day, no convincing evidence has been provided that any of these cells express Bcr- and Tcr-like molecules. In fact, all attempts to demonstrate immunoglobulins or Tcr in any phylum beyond the vertebrates has failed. The track along the evolutionary history of these molecules disappears below the cyclostomes (Fig. 2), but is it the true end or are we simply not in a position, as yet, to follow a fainter trail? There is no convincing answer to this question, but it would be surprising if the failure to detect such molecules did turn out to be merely a matter of sensitivity of the methodology. Probably no matter how hard one tries to detect Ig and Tcr among invertebrates, one will not find them.

There is no indication that invertebrates possess an immune system similar to that of vertebrates. Although they can distinguish self from nonself, this distinction in all those cases in which its mechanism has been elucidated, is not based on clonal distribution of a variety of antigen-specific receptors (RATCLIFFE et al. 1985). Invertebrates do not seem to have a single system for self-nonself discrimination as vertebrates do. Instead, they have a series of different systems, none of which approaches the Bcr-Tcr system of vertebrates in its degree of sophistication. The expectation is, therefore, that invertebrates (including annelids) either do not have Bcr- and Tcr-like genes at all, or if they do, that these genes carry out some function other than antigen recognition. In particular, I predict that these ancestral genes do not rearrange during the ontogeny of the cell as Bcr and Tcr genes do.

If these conclusions are correct, then it also follows that invertebrates do not have true lymphocytes. The blood elements that have been identified by some immunologists as "lymphocytes" are probably other cells that happen to resemble true lymphocytes morphologically. I propose that lymphocytes, Tcr, Bcr, and Mhc all evolved parallel to one another and that they all emerged, almost simultaneously, with the emergence of vertebrates. In vertebrates, a major revolution occurred in the mechanism of self-nonself discrimination – a revolution based on the invention of gene rearrangement for the purpose of generating a very large diversity of receptors. The diversity required clonal expression and hence a special cell capable of such expression – the lymphocyte. The revolution occurred more than 500 million years ago, just in time to provide a novel means of coping with the new demands on the defense mechanisms posed by the growing complexity of the emerging vertebrate body (ROMER 1959). According to this scenario, the origins of the lymphocyte must be sought in the introduction of clonal selection in immune responses at the time when the first vertebrates appeared on the scene.

Reshuffling of genes for the generation of diversity is, of course, not restricted to lymphocytes or to defense mechanisms. Some organisms, such as certain parasites, use it to achieve just the opposite of defense – the evasion of immune reactions (STEINERT and PAYS 1985; HAGBLOM et al. 1985; PLASTERK et al. 1985). All the other known cases of gene reshuffling, however, are based on different mechanisms and are clearly the result of separate events from those occurring in lymphocytes.

C. Ontogenetic Origin of Lymphocytes

The development of an embryo can be viewed as a series of steps which restrict gradually the differentiation potential of the individual cells (Fig. 3; DEUCHAR 1975). Up to the morula stage, all cells are totipotential, that is to say, if need be, each cell can give rise to an entire individual with all its complex organs and tissues. The first set of restrictions is imposed when the morula differentiates into the inner cell mass and the trophectoderm. Lymphocytes can eventually arise

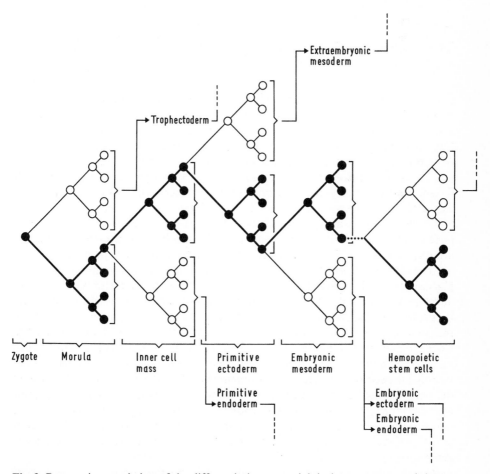

Fig. 3. Progressive restriction of the differentiation potential during ontogeny and the origin of lymphocytes. The line leading to lymphocytes is indicated by *full circles and segments*

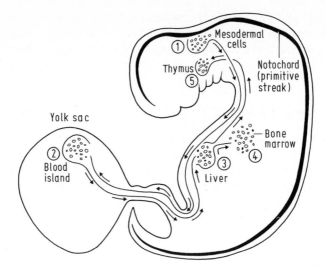

Fig. 4. Migrations of hemopoietic stem cells. Numbers indicate the sequence in which the stem cells migrate to the different sites in the developing embryo

from the former, but not from the latter cells (Hogan et al. 1986). In the mouse, in which lymphocyte origins have been studied most extensively (Owen and Jenkinson 1981), a second set of restrictions is imposed when the inner cell mass differentiates into the primitive ectoderm and the primitive endoderm. Here again, from this stage on, lymphocytes can derive from the former, but not from the latter. The third major set of restrictions is imposed when the primitive ectoderm differentiates into embryonic ectoderm, mesoderm, and endoderm. Lymphocytes can arise from mesoderm, but not from ectoderm or endoderm (Le Douarin 1977). Because they arise from cells of a specific region of the mesoderm, located beneath the primitive streak, some additional restrictions are apparently imposed after the emergence of the mesoderm, but these have not been identified.

The cells that eventually give rise to lymphocytes must then migrate to other places in the body, apparently for them to be able to interact with cells that have developed in these places in the meantime (Fig. 4). These interactions, whose nature is totally obscure, are necessary to stimulate the development of the cells in the right direction. The cells must first migrate to the yolk sac (which is derived from the extraembryonic mesoderm), then to the fetal liver (and spleen), and finally to the bone marrow. At each of these sites, the cells apparently find an environment conducive to their development. Whether the cells must pass through the yolk sac before they enter the fetal liver is uncertain; apparently, however, they do not need to pass through the bone marrow to become lymphocytes in the fetus; the passage through the liver suffices. After birth, most if not all the cells capable of giving rise to lymphocytes reside in the bone marrow. In addition to generating lymphocytes, the cells also produce erythrocytes, thrombocytes, granulocytes, and monocytes – they thus constitute the hemopoietic stem cells (Golde and Takaku 1985). The sequence of shifts of hemopoiesis from organ to organ in the developing embryo is similar to that observed in vertebrate phylogeny (TISCHENDORF 1985). In many adult fish, hemopoiesis occurs in the liver (but also in the kidneys and even the gonads), in many adult amphibians it occurs in the liver and spleen; and in adult frogs, birds, and mammals it occurs in the red bone marrow. This similarity may be a manifestation of Haeckel's law that ontogeny repeats phylogeny.

In the bone marrow, the hemopoietic tissue is organized around the network of venous sinuses, specifically in the meshes of the reticulum formed by adventitial cells on the external side of the sinuses (DE BRUYN 1981). During maturation, the hemopoietic cells pass through the walls of the sinus, between or through the endothelial cells, and enter the bloodstream. The immediate progenitors of the different blood cells appear to have different locations in the hemopoietic tissue whereby the less mature cells are further away from the sinus wall than the more mature cells. In adult mammals, all blood cells except T lymphocytes differentiate in the bone marrow and enter the circulation as mature or almost mature cells. The T lymphocytes complete most of their differentiation in the thymus. In birds, T lymphocytes differentiate in the thymus, B lymphocytes in the bursa of Fabricius, and other blood cells in the bone marrow.

The hemopoietic stem cells are pluripotent cells, which means that although they can no longer give rise to certain cells, they can still differentiate into a variety of different cell types. They cannot differentiate, say, into epidermal cells or neurons, but they can produce erythrocytes, thrombocytes, and all the other blood cells. Whether they can also produce other cells beside blood cells is uncertain. There is a mutation in the mouse (*Steel, Sl*) that affects blood cells, melanocytes, and male germ cells simultaneously (BANNERMAN et al. 1973), and this fact

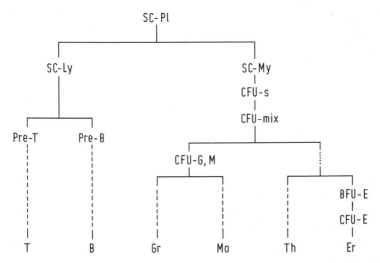

Fig. 5. Binary restriction model of hemopoiesis. *B*, B lymphocyte; *BFU-E*, burst-forming unit/erythroid; *CFU-E*, colony-forming unit/erythroid; *CFU-G,M*, colony-forming unit/ granulocyte, monocyte; *CFU-S-S*, colony-forming unit/spleen; *CFU-mix*, colony-forming unit/mixed; *Er*, erythrocyte; *Gr*, granulocyte (eosinophil, basophil, neutrophil); *Mo*, monocyte; *SC-Ly*, stem cell/lymphoid; *SC-My*, stem cell/myeloid; *SC-Pl*, stem cell/pluripotential; *T*, T lymphocyte; *Th*, thrombocyte

may indicate an ontogenetic relationship among all these cells, but there are also other explanations for the pleiotropic effect of the mutation.

All stem cells have two characteristics: self-renewal, i.e., the ability to generate new stem cells; and determination, i.e., the ability to commit themselves to a particular differentiation pathway. How stem cells manage to renew themselves continuously and at the same time continuously to replenish the differentiated cells remains a great puzzle. The two principal possibilities are: first, that every time a stem cell divides, one daughter cell commits itself to differentiate and the other returns into the self-renewing pool; and second, that in some divisions both daughter cells return to the self-renewing pool, whereas in other divisions, both cells commit themselves. In the latter case, a mechanism would have to exist to maintain the number of self-renewing divisions at 50%, otherwise the stem cell pool would soon be exhausted, or would produce an excess of stem cells.

How the committed cells differentiate into the individual lineages is also uncertain. Here, the two principal possibilities are: first, a binary sequence of events;

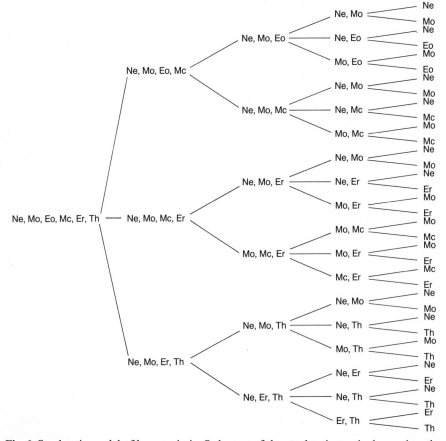

Fig. 6. Stochastic model of hemopoiesis. Only part of the stochastic tree is shown, i.e., that part demonstrated in an actual experiment. *Eo,* eosinophil; *Er,* erythrocyte; *Mc,* mast cell or basophil; *Mo,* monocyte; *Ne,* neutrophil; *Th,* thrombocyte. (Deduced from the data of Suda et al. 1983)

and second, a stochastic process (BURGESS and NICOLA 1983). In the binary model (Fig. 5; METCALFE and MOORE 1971), the committed cells make a series of binary (either or) decisions during their differentiation. The first decision is whether to become lymphoid or myeloid progenitors. The lymphoid progenitors (stem cells) then decide whether to embark on a pathway leading to a T lymphocyte or one leading to a B cell. The myeloid progenitors choose between committing themselves to the granulocyte-monocyte or thrombocyte-erythrocyte pathways, and so on. In the stochastic model of hemopoiesis (Fig. 6; SUDA et al. 1983), random restrictions in the potential for each lineage occur gradually as the cell differentiates. Some cells, for example, may lose the ability to differentiate into erythrocytes, while retaining the potential to differentiate into any other of the remaining blood cells. Some of progency of these cells may then gradually lose their potential to differentiate into monocytes and granulocytes, so that the only potential remaining is that of differentiating into thrombocytes. Other progeny might be left with the potential to differentiate into erythrocytes, others still to differentiate into monocytes, and so on. Even in this model, however, the progenitor of the lymphoid cells separates early in the differentiation from the rest of the cells (the myeloid cells). Some investigators also believe that there is not one, but two lymphoid progenitors, one for T lymphocytes and a separate one for B cells.

D. Generation of the B Cell Repertoire

There may be a difference between birds and mammals in the way in which the B cell progenitors develop. In birds, this may be connected with the existence of a special organ for B lymphocyte differentiation, the bursa of Fabricius (PINK 1986). The sign that the stem cell is committed to the B lymphocyte lineage is the rearrangement of the Ig heavy chain genes. In a particular stem cell, one V_H gene among many is selected at random and transposed to a randomly selected D gene segment, and the V-D segment may then be moved next to the selected J gene (HONJO 1983). The rearrangement is accompanied by the deletion of the intervening DNA and is thus irreversible. From here on, the cell can develop only into a B lymphocyte. In another stem cell, other V_H, D, and J genes are selected and brought together. The two cells will then be identical except for the rearrangement of their *Igh* genes and the Bcr to which these genes will eventually contribute one-half of the blueprint. By proliferation, the two cells will become two different *clones* of B lymphocytes. Since birds, or at least the domestic fowl, have only a few dozen different V_H genes, and a few D and J gene segments, the random combination of V-D-J segments in different cells generates perhaps a few hundred B progenitor cell clones.

The *Igh* gene rearrangement probably occurs in the embryonic mesoderm or the yolk sac at 7–8 days of embryonic development of the chicken (LE DOUARIN 1977). The cells then migrate via the blood to the bursa in the period between 8 and 14 days, with a peak between 10 and 12 days. The committed cells settle in the bursa, in groups of three or four, and begin to proliferate extensively. Each group gives rise to a separate cluster of lymphoid cells, the lymphoid follicles of the bursa. There are some 10000 follicles in the bursa of an individual bird, and each follicle contains, at the peak of its development (a few weeks after hatching), some 100000 lymphocytes. After hatching (day 21), the bursa begins to release cells into the blood which, according to all the criteria, are typical B lymphocytes. It continues sending B cells via the blood to peripheral lymphoid organs (spleen and lymph nodes) for a few weeks, and then gradually ceases this activity and involutes. But before it does so, it also sends out a few stem cells which are then responsible for the renewal of the B lymphocyte pool during the life of the bird.

In those few weeks of high bursal activity, the stem cells that seeded the organ differentiate into mature B cells, undergoing extensive proliferation. Not all the steps in this differentiation have been identified, but some have (ZOLA 1985; ALT et al. 1986; KINCADE 1981). The cells that arrive in the bursa have their *Igh* genes rearranged, but they do not express them. They are large cells which divide repeatedly. Sometimes during this phase, the cells begin to transcribe the *Igh* genes, that is, the *V-D-J* segment, together with the nearest C_H gene, the C_μ gene.

After splicing out all intervening sequences, the transcript is translated into a heavy chain polypeptide, the μ chain, which then begins to accumulate in the cytoplasm of the pre-B cell. Although the μ chain has a hydrophobic transmembrane region for insertion into the plasma membrane, without the light chain it cannot reach the cell surface. The next step in the differentiation of the pre-B cell is the rearrangement of the genes in one of the two light chain families, either κ or λ. The rearrangement proceeds in a similar manner to that of the *Igh* chain genes. One V_L gene is selected randomly and moved to the *J* gene segment (the light chain gene family lacks the *D* segments). The rearranged V_L-J_L segment is then transcribed, together with the C_L gene, and the transcript is translated into the light chain. The H and L chain genes join together and thus form the basic monomeric IgM molecule which is then integrated into the plasma membrane via the transmembrane region of the H chain. The cell which has, during this process, reduced its size, thus expresses its first B cell receptor and becomes a true B lymphocyte. The immature B lymphocyte leaves the bursa and moves via the bloodstream to the peripheral lymphoid organs.

What happens during the maturation of B lymphocytes in the peripheral lymphoid organs is not clear. It is thought that, after the initial expression of the IgM receptor, the virgin B cell must encounter antigen to differentiate further. If it does not encounter antigen, it dies after a few days and is replaced by another cell. If it does encounter antigen, and at the same time receives the necessary signals (help) from a T lymphocyte, it enlarges and begins to proliferate. During this proliferation, different cells in the expanding B cell clone may express other genes of the C_H cluster, and different Ig receptors on the cell surface. After the initial expression of the C_μ gene, most of the cells in the clone also begin to express the adjacent C_δ gene, together with the same *V-D-J* segment with which they express the C_μ gene. Such cells then display two kinds of Ig receptors on the cell surface, IgM and IgD, both carrying identical light chains and identical *V-D-J* regions, but different *C* regions. The expression of the δ chain is probably achieved by differential splicing of the same primary transcript used for the production of the μ chains. The B cell then contains two differently spliced mRNA species, one translated into the μ and the other into the δ chain. After maturing further, the B lymphocyte may express additional C_H genes: one of the γ genes, the ε or the

α gene. Correspondingly, it may display IgG, IgE, or IgA receptors on the surface. A single cell may express as many as three different Ig receptors simultaneously – for example, IgM, IgD, and IgG – in various combinations, always together with the same V-D-J segment.

How the maturing B cell accomplishes this heavy chain isotype switch (the different heavy chains are referred to as isotypes) is not known (CEBRA et al. 1984; HONJO 1983). According to one hypothesis, the switch occurs in two steps, first at the RNA and then at the DNA level. The V-D-J segment is transcribed with several of the C_H genes, and the large primary transcript is then spliced in such a way that an mRNA is generated for two of the three different H chains, for example, μ and δ, or μ and γ. The different chains are expressed in low amounts on the cell surface as Ig receptors. If these receptors encounter an antigen to which they can bind, the B lymphocyte is activated and during subsequent proliferation a cell is selected in which the expression of the particular C_H gene is fixed at the DNA level by a special kind of chromosome recombination.

The differentiating B lymphocyte appears to have two options as to its further fate. First, it can switch from the synthesis of membrane-bound Ig molecules to the secretion of antibodies. If it takes this option, it converts into a terminally differentiated plasma cell which continues to secrete antibodies at a high rate (several thousand molecules per second) for a while until, after 2–3 days, it dies. Second, the differentiating cell can convert into a small resting lymphocyte, the memory B cell, which is relatively long-lived. Memory B lymphocytes are more easily triggered on a subsequent encounter with the same antigen than the original virgin B cells, and they respond promptly to the encounter by a heightened antibody production. Most of the memory B lymphocytes eventually lose their surface IgD.

In mammals, which lack the bursa of Fabricius or its homolog, the entire process of B lymphocyte differentiation takes place in the fetal liver and then in the bone marrow. In the mouse, for example, pre-B cells with μ chains in their cytoplasm appear in the fetal liver at 12 days of gestation (OWEN and JENKINSON 1981; VOGLER and LAWTON 1985). At birth, B lymphocyte production shifts to the bone marrow; in adult animals, it occurs almost exclusively in the bone marrow. There may also be another difference between birds and mammals with regard to B cell differentiation (WEILL et al. 1986). While from a certain stage onward in birds, all the stem cells committed to the B lymphocyte lineage apparently have their H chain genes rearranged and no new committed cells are generated from the primitive hemopoietic stem cell after the involution of the bursa, in mammals the production of committed stem cells is believed to continue throughout life. In the bone marrow of a mammal, primitive hemopoietic cells may continuously give rise to low numbers of cells committed to the B cell lineage, which then rearrange their IgH genes in preparation for the differentiation into B lymphocytes. The reason for this differences between birds and mammals may lie in the number of V_H genes possessed by the two vertebrate classes. Birds apparently have a rather low number of V_H genes and, to generate a B cell repertoire of sufficient size, they rely heavily on somatic diversification of these few genes, in particular by somatic mutations (REYNAUD et al. 1985). Since mutations occur predominantly during DNA replication, the immune system in birds must provide enough opportunity, in terms of abundant, pre-B cell proliferation, for the mutations to accumulate. This proliferation occurs in the bursa, both during the generation of virgin B cells and during the self-renewing process of the committed stem cells. These latter cells have their *Igh* genes rearranged, with the result that the mutations which they accumulate in the bursa will be retained when they finally leave the bursa. In mammals, the high number of V_H genes (several hundred) provides a broader base on which to build the B cell repertoire. The need for somatic diversification (and hence for extensive proliferation in a special organ) is not as high as it is in birds.

The question whether or not the B lymphocyte repertoire is complete, in the sense that it also contains cells capable of recognizing self-antigens, has not been answered convincingly. On the one hand, the need to eliminate, or at least inactivate, self-reactive B cells has been an article of faith for many immunologists over the last two decades (Burnet 1959). On the other hand, evidence is growing that self-reactive B cells are present in normal individuals without, apparently, causing any harm (Cooke et al. 1983). Although it seems clear that B lymphocytes can be made unresponsive (tolerant) by certain artificial manipulations (Klinman et al. 1985), there is no convincing evidence that B cells are naturally tolerant. Furthermore, there does not seem to be any need for the majority of B lymphocytes to be naturally tolerant. Even if they do recognize a self-antigen, if they happen to carry a fitting combining site in their Bcrs, they will not be triggered unless T lymphocytes are stimulated by the same antigen and begin to secrete the factors necessary for B lymphocyte differentiation (Howard and Paul 1983). Hence, for those B cells that are dependent on T cell help, there does not seem to be any need to become tolerant of self-antigens; it seems to suffice that the T cells are tolerant of these antigens. There are, however, subpopulations of B cells that are largely independent of T cell help in their response to a special set of antigens (Sher 1982). Some of these cells might have to be inactivated, if a self-antigen happens to fall into the category that they are capable of recognizing. On the whole, however, the B lymphocyte repertoire might be larger than the T cell repertoire (see Sects. E and F).

E. Generation of the T Cell Repertoire

A large part of T lymphocyte differentiation takes place in the thymus (Scollay et al. 1986). In the mouse, the thymic primordium derives from the pharyngeal epithelium and is first colonized by blood-borne stem cells from the yolk sac or fetal liver at day 11 of gestation (Owen and Jenkinson 1981). The arriving cells settle in a region that will later become the thymic cortex, and begin to proliferate extensively. The cells produced by these divisions at first retain the characteristics of the colonizing stem cells; only later do they begin to diversify. This conclusion is based on the observation that the entire thymus can be repopulated and the T cell repertoire generated from a single stem cell placed into the thymus in vitro (Kingston et al. 1985). The diversification of the stem cells begins with the rearrangement of the Tcr β genes (Snodgrass et al. 1985; Raulet et al. 1985; Born et al. 1985). The rearrangement consists, first, of selecting one of several *D* gene segments and moving it to one of several J gene segments, and second, of moving one of the selected V_β genes to the vicinity of the D-J rearrangement. Because different segments are selected in different cells (there is variability in the sites at which the V_β, D_β, and J_β segments join) and because nucleotides may be added randomly to either side of a D_β gene segment while it is joined to the V_β and J_β segments, different cells will eventually express different Tcr β chains. The proliferating and differentiating T cells thus begin to diversify clonally. The first cells with rearranged β genes appear in the mouse thymus at 14 days of gestation.

The rearranged β genes are transcribed and the transcripts are translated into β chains which accumulate in the cytoplasm. The chains have a transmembrane region, but without the α chains they apparently cannot reach the cell surface. The rearrangement of Tcr α genes begins shortly afterward, so that at 16 days of gestation, surface Tcr can be detected (CHIEN et al. 1984; SAITO et al. 1984a). Shortly before birth, the first immunocompetent T lymphocytes appear in the thymus. These then leave the thymus and reach the peripheral lymphoid organs via the bloodstream. The cells that have already rearranged their β genes, but have not yet rearranged their α genes, probably proliferate extensively. This means that different α gene rearrangements occur in cells carrying the same β gene rearrangement. There are thus T cells produced that express the same β chain, but different α chains. Thus, the delayed rearrangement of α chains allows further diversification of the T cell repertoire. However, evidence for diversification of the Tcr genes by somatic mutations, which play an important role in the generation of the B cell repertoire (BALTIMORE 1981), has not been obtained.

In addition to Tcr α and β genes, another family of γ genes has been demonstrated (SAITO et al. 1984b). These genes also rearrange; in fact, they are probably the first Tcr genes to rearrange in the thymus (RAULET et al. 1985). In fetal mouse thymocytes, γ chain mRNA appears at about 14 days of gestation, reaches maximal levels at 15 days, and then declines rapidly. (The β chain mRNA levels remain relatively constant after day 16, and α chain mRNA levels reach a maximum at day 19.) There is, however, no evidence to date that the γ chains are needed for anything. Although it is apparently expressed, together with a largely hypothetical δ chain, on a small subpopulation of T lymphocytes (BRENNER et al. 1986; BANK et al. 1986), no function of this heterodimer has as yet been demonstrated. It is possible that in other vertebrate classes, the Tcr γ genes are functional but in mammals, exemplified by the mouse and the human, their activation seems to be an atavistic trait.

The studies on Tcr expression suggest that the thymus plays a similar role for the T lymphocytes as the avian bursa of Fabricius does for the B lymphocytes. It is the site where committed progenitor cells settle down, proliferate, and differentiate. These processes are probably driven by a set of hormone-like substances, the thymic hormones, several of which have been identified, isolated, and purified (TRAININ et al. 1983, Chap. 16). The vital question is: does the thymus provide more than just a conducive environment for T lymphocyte differentiation? Two extra functions have been proposed for the thymus, the induction of tolerance and the individualization of the T cell repertoire.

In contrast to B lymphocytes, T lymphocytes must be made unresponsive to self molecules with which they come in contact. If they were not tolerant of self, autoreactivity and autoimmunity would be rampant and would lead to the death of the individual. Before anything was known about the Tcr, the possibility that T cell tolerance is induced in the bone marrow was considered. But since it has been established that the Tcr is first expressed in the thymus, this possibility must be discounted. As it is difficult to envision a way in which lymphocytes might become tolerant without first expressing their antigen-specific receptor, it must be concluded that T cell tolerance is induced either in the thymus or post-thymically. Which of these two possibilities applies cannot be deduced from the available data. Even conceptually it is not easy to put forward arguments as to why it should be one and not the other site. Tolerance induction in the thymus would seem to make sense when viewed from the vantage point of T cell differentiation because one could argue that self-reactive lymphocytes should be eliminated as soon as they express their antigen-specific receptor, which, as already mentioned, happens in the thymus. On the other hand, if tolerance were induced in the thymus, it is difficult to explain how the emerging self-reactive cells manage to contact the various self molecules in this rather sequestered location, in particular, the tissue-specific antigens. Perhaps tolerance is induced both in the thymus and in the periphery.

Be that as it may, the T cell repertoire *is* altered by the process of tolerance induction. The actual repertoire becomes smaller than the potential repertoire encoded in the Tcr genes and generated by somatic mechanisms during T cell differentiation. *How* the reduction in the size of the repertoire occurs, in other words, what mechanism is responsible for the induction of tolerance, is not known (SCOTT 1984). The three principal possibilities are as follows (KLEIN 1986a). First, on encountering self-molecules, the T cells are either killed or die because of a lack of further differentiation. Second, the self-reactive cells persist in low numbers, but are inactivated and hence normally cannot expand. Third, the self-reactive cells are kept from responding by a set of suppressor cells. The first possibility, the original clonal deletion hypothesis of BURNET (1959), is least likely since the existence of autoimmune phenomena could be interpreted as attesting to the persistance of self-reactive T cells. (However, it has not been established convincingly that the targets of the autoimmune T cells are true self- rather than modified self-molecules.) Arguing against the third possibility is the finding that tolerance states have been demonstrated in which the involvement of suppressor T cells has been excluded (KLEIN 1986a). What has not been excluded, however, is the existence of a possible new form of unconventional inhibitory cell, distinct from the suppressor T cell detectable by the methods currently available. By exclusion, therefore, the second possibility seems to be the most attractive. An individual may, indeed, have a low number of self-reactive cells whose ability to proliferate has been blocked intrinsically by their exposure to self-molecules at a certain sensitive stage of their differentiation. If that is the mechanism underlying tolerance induction, then tolerance changes the T cell repertoire quantitatively rather than qualitatively.

Individualization of the repertoire refers to the dependence of T cells, in contrast to B cells, on the recognition not of the antigen alone, but together with (in the context of) molecules encoded in the genes of the Mhc (Fig. 7; ZINKERNAGEL and DOHERTY 1974). Thus, the Tcr is constructed in such a way that it normally

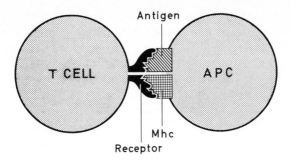

Fig. 7. Recognition of an antigen by the T cell receptor. The antigen is recognized in the context of Mhc molecules on the surface of the antigen-presenting cell

participates in T cell activation only when it is occupied simultaneously by the foreign antigen and by a portion of the Mhc molecule. Using a form of shorthand, we can express the specificity of a T lymphocyte by the symbol $T_A\!\!<^{\text{Mhc}^a}_{\ X}$ which means that in an individual A, foreign antigen X is recognized by T cells in the context of a self-Mhc molecule (Mhc^a). The genes coding for the functional Mhc molecules are, however, polymorphic so that different individuals express different molecules. Individual A expresses Mhc^a, individual B expresses Mhc^b, individual C expresses Mhc^c, and so on. The original (unselected) T cell repertoire of an individual A should, therefore, contain not only $T_A\!\!<^{\text{Mhc}^a}_{\ X}$ cells, but also $T_A\!\!<^{\text{Mhc}^b}_{\ X}$, $T_A\!\!<^{\text{Mhc}^c}_{\ X}$, and so on. Of course, since it normally possesses only Mhc^a molecules and not Mhc^b or Mhc^c molecules, it uses only the $T_A\!\!<^{\text{Mhc}^a}_{\ X}$ and not the $T_A\!\!<^{\text{Mhc}^c}_{\ X}$ cells. The question then arises: what does an individual A do with all the cells that could potentially recognize antigen X in the context of allogeneic Mhc (Mhc^b, Mhc^c, ...) molecules (the so-called allorestricted T cells)? The two possibilities are: first, that allorestricted cells are eliminated; and second, that the cells arise, but since they are never used, are overwhelmed by the self-restricted cells ($T_A\!\!<^{\text{Mhc}^a}_{\ X}$ in individual A). In both instances, the T cell repertoire would be individualized – tailored to the needs of the individual – in the first instance almost completely (qualitatively) and in the second instance only partially (quantitatively). In both cases, the T cell repertoire of an individual A would differ (qualitatively or quantitatively) from that of individuals B, or C (where each individual would express different forms of functional Mhc genes, i.e., Mhc^a, Mhc^b, and Mhc^c, respectively). Let us then consider these two possible forms of T cell repertoire individualization (qualitative and quantitative).

The hypothesis of qualitative individualization of the repertoire postulates that the allorestricted T cells are somehow prevented from emerging (ZINKERNA-

GEL et al. 1978; BEVAN 1977; ZINKERNAGEL and DOHERTY 1979). How could this be achieved? According to one specific form of this hypothesis (DROEGE 1981; SCHWARTZ 1982), emerging T cells are handled differently, depending on the affinity of their receptors for self-Mhc molecules. Three grades of affinity – high, intermediate, and low – result in three different ways of handling in two phases of development. In the first phase, T cells with high affinity for self-Mhc molecules alone or for self-Mhc and some other self-molecule are eliminated in the process of tolerance induction. In the second phase, cells with intermediate affinity for self-Mhc molecules – an affinity which normally is not high enough for stimulation – are brought over the threshold needed for activation in the special environment in which T cells differentiate. They divide repeatedly and the clones expand enormously. In the same phase, T cells with low affinity for self-Mhc molecules fail to be stimulated and they wither away. The T-cell repertoire therefore consists only of cells capable of recognizing self-Mhc molecules with intermediate affinities. Once out of the special environment, these cells cannot be activated by self-Mhc molecules alone, but if their receptors encounter the right antigen, the combined affinities for self-Mhc and antigen molecules once again cross the threshold and the cells are activated. The special environment is believed to be provided by the thymus (JERNE 1971), and the main function of this organ is, therefore, to expand clones of T cells with intermediate affinity for self-Mhc molecules – to "educate lymphocytes," to individualize the T cell repertoire. From the thymus of an individual A emerge only Mhc^a-restricted cells, from the thymus of an individual B emerge only Mhc^b-restricted cells, and so on. Although most hypotheses allow for a certain imperfection in the individualization process, allorestricted T lymphocytes are by and large not expected to be present in peripheral lymphoid organs.

According to the second hypothesis (KLEIN and NAGY 1982), the only positive selection to which T lymphocytes are exposed occurs in the periphery when the cells encounter foreign antigen in the context of self-Mhc molecules. In the encounter, activated clones expand and some of the lymphocytes turn into memory cells, which then continue to recirculate through the periphery. Since an immune response against some antigen or another occurs all the time in the body, self-restricted T cells accumulate gradually, and since allogeneic Mhc molecules are not available and allorestricted cells are therefore not used, self-restricted cells gradually gain the upper hand over allorestricted cells. It may seem that, through the continuous expansion of the self-restricted repertoire and the lack of any expansion whatsoever of the allorestricted repertoire, the former might eventually replace the latter entirely. This event, however, probably does not happen, for two reasons. First, some of the functional Mhc loci are highly polymorphic (KLEIN and FIGUEROA 1981), so that there may be hundreds of genetic forms of a given Mhc molecule (allomorphs) and each form may differ from the other by hundreds of determinants, recognized by different receptors and different T cell clones. The individual, therefore, starts off with a great preponderance of allorestricted cells, some of which are bound to persist, even after prolonged preferential selection of self-restricted clones. Second, it has been shown that some $T_A\!\!\begin{smallmatrix}\diagup \mathrm{Mhc}^a \\ \diagdown \mathrm{X}\end{smallmatrix}$ cells cross-react with $Mhc^b + Y$ (KLEIN 1986a). In other words, some cells are self-restricted when responding to one antigen but allorestricted when stimulated by another antigen – the allorestricted and self-restricted repertoire overlap to a certain degree. The expansion of the self-restricted repertoire should, therefore, lead to a concurrent, partial expansion of the allorestricted repertoire.

What do the data say in regard to these two hypotheses? A large number of experiments have been carried out to test whether the thymus educates T cells and shapes their repertoire (KLEIN and NAGY 1982; KLEIN 1986a), but the voluminous literature that has accumulated does not permit one to choose unreservedly between the hypotheses. The prevalent view seems to be that there is a difference in thymus involvement between the cells that use class I and those that use class II molecules as the context for antigen recognition (KRUISBEEK and LONGO 1985; LONGO et al. 1981). For the former, intrathymic events do not fully account for the generation of the self-restricted repertoire. Individualization also clearly occurs extrathymically, either by the encounter with foreign antigen or by a process similar to that postulated to occur in the thymus. On the other hand, restriction to self-class II molecules seems to be determined largely in the thymus. It must, however, be emphasized that these conclusions have been reached by using highly artificial experimental models, and that it is uncertain to what degree these models actually reflect physiologic situations. The question of individualization of the T cell repertoire by the thymus must, therefore, be considered for the most part as open. It appears likely, however, that expansion of T cell clones through an immune response in physiologic situations sways the repertoire toward the predominance of self-restricted cells.

Do allorestricted cells exist at all? Undoubtedly! They have been demonstrated in several laboratories, and clones have been isolated from them (KLEIN 1984). Hence, they are real and there is no excuse for the perpetuation of the myth that T cells can recognize foreign antigen only in the context of self-Mhc molecules. It is, of course, true that every T lymphocyte isolated from a given individual after immunization against a given antigen is self-restricted, that is to say, it cannot be restimulated by the same antigen presented on an allogeneic cell. But this observation has nothing to do with the individualization of the T cell repertoire or with the existence or nonexistence of allorestricted cells. It simply reflects the fact that, once you stimulate a T lymphocyte capable of recognizing foreign antigen in the context of Mhc^a, you cannot force this T cell to recognize the same antigen in the context of Mhc^b molecules (the cell is committed to expressing one particular Tcr and cannot normally express a different Tcr). By immunizing an individual A, no cells other than those using Mhc^a as context can be stimulated because no other Mhc molecules are present in this individual.

However, the question remains: with what frequency do allorestricted T cells occur? Only in one laboratory have investigators attempted to answer this question, and they have reached the conclusion that the self-restricted T cells are approximately six times more frequent than allorestricted cells (STOCKINGER et al. 1981). This answer would mean that the allorestricted repertoire is very large, a conclusion hardly consistent with the hypothesis that the thymus passes only, or largely, self-restricted T cells to the periphery. On the other hand, this result is fully in line with the notion that the predilection for self-restricted cells is the consequence of expansion of these cells by antigen stimulation in the periphery. It is, of course, possible that the method used in these studies (the limiting dilution assay) gives, for some reason, artificially inflated estimates of allorestricted cells. Also, until the degree of overlap between allorestricted and self-restricted repertoires has been determined, it is not possible to decide how many of the cells classified as allorestricted for the particular antigen might turn out to be self-restricted when some other antigen is used.

F. Genetically Controlled Nonresponsiveness

The main function of lymphocytes is to recognize foreign antigen in the first step of the specific immune response. One might therefore expect lymphocytes to be perfect in carrying out this function – that is to say that they should be able to recognize and respond to almost any antigen in the world. The truth is, however, that only B lymphocytes approach this ideal; T lymphocytes are far from it (KLEIN 1986b). Via their receptors, the B lymphocytes recognize perhaps not all antigens that they encounter, but *almost* all, regardless of whether they are borne by proteins, polysaccharides, lipids, or nucleic acids. Of course, to be antigenic for a B cell, the molecules must fulfill certain physicochemical requirements (KLEIN 1982), but if they do, there seems to be no limit to what the Bcrs will recognize specifically. Although one may occasionally find this or that individual genetically incapable of responding to a particular antigen because it happens to lack the particular structural *IgV* gene necessary for the recognition of this antigen, these instances are relatively rare. By and large, the B cell repertoire seems to be complete, without blind spots. Furthermore, on a large, complex molecule, antigenic determinants recognizable by Bcrs are distributed over most of the molecular surface (BENJAMIN et al. 1984). It is true that, in a physiologic situation, certain regions of the surface are "immunodominant" in that they activate B cell clones preferentially (ATASSI and YOUNG 1985). However, when one makes the effort, one finds that other portions of the surface can each stimulate a few B cell clones as well. In other words, B lymphocytes behave as one would expect a priori of a system designed to identify foreigners specifically. The T lymphocytes, on the other hand, behave quite differently (KLEIN 1986b). First of all, they seem to be able to recognize only protein antigens and not polysaccharides, lipids, or nucleic acids. Although now and then T cell responses to non-protein antigens, in particular polysaccharides, have been described, these seem to be exceptions. Polysaccharide-specific T cells, if they exist, are rare and much more difficult to stimulate than protein-specific cells. Furthermore, even on proteins, T lymphocytes seem to concentrate on a few regions of the molecular surface and to ignore the rest of the molecule. For example, the T lymphocyte response of mice to pig lactate dehydrogenase B (LDH-B) concentrates on a single antigenic determinant residing in the exposed loop formed by amino acid residues 211–222. T cell clones recognizing any other region of the LDH-B could not be obtained (SERVIS et al. 1986).

The most spectacular limitation in the ability of T lymphocytes to recognize foreign antigen is, however, imposed by the Mhc. The basic observation is that many antigenic determinants are recognized only in individuals expressing a particular allele at a particular Mhc locus; individuals expressing other alleles at this locus are nonresponders to these determinants (KLEIN 1986 b; SCHWARTZ 1986). In other words, the ability to respond to a particular determinant is genetically controlled by the Mhc. At first, it was thought that the control was exerted by a special set of immune response or *Ir* genes residing in the Mhc, but later it became clear that the Mhc *are* the *Ir* genes (KLEIN et al. 1981). Now we also know the mechanism by which the Mhc exerts its influence on the immune response. The explanation is in the dual specificity of the Tcr, i.e., in its necessity to recognize simultaneously foreign antigen and an Mhc molecule – to recognize antigen in the context of the Mhc molecule (ZINKERNAGEL and DOHERTY 1974). As it turns out, certain combinations of foreign antigens and particular Mhc allomorphs are not recognized by T lymphocytes, which means that an individual expressing these and no other Mhc allomorphs is a nonresponder to these antigens. Because different individuals express different functional Mhc alleles, some individuals are responders and others nonresponders to antigens, and in a genetic cross between responders and nonresponders, the ability to respond segregates with the Mhc.

The Mhc influence on the T cell response is exerted both by the class I and class II loci. Often, however, it is easier to detect in class II-controlled responses, simply because there are fewer nonresponders in class I-controlled responses. The effect of class II loci on the immune response was also historically the first to be documented (McDEVITT et al. 1972), and the *Ir* genes were originally mapped to the class II region of the Mhc which then began to be referred to as the *I* region. It is now firmly established, however, that some combinations of antigens and class I molecules are also not recognized by T cells so that class I genes can also behave as *Ir* genes (KLEIN et al. 1981). Hence, the designation *I* region, and all other designations derived from it, are anachronisms that should be abandoned.

The reason why nonresponders are more frequent in class II- than in class I-restricted responses is connected with the organization of the Mhc. The complex contains a few functional and a large number of nonfunctional loci. In the mammals that have been studied, most of the nonfunctional loci are in class I, although some nonfunctional class II loci also exist (KLEIN 1986 a). In the mouse, the functional class I loci are *H-2K* and *D* (*L*), and the nonfunctional loci are *Qa* and *Tla*. The functional class II loci are $A_{\alpha 1}A_{\beta 1}$ (=A) and $E_{\alpha 1}E_{\beta 1}$ (=E). It so happens (probably because of the different ways by which the class I and class II loci evolved) that the *H-2K* locus is genetically closely related to the *H-2D* locus, so much so that from their sequences it is difficult to tell which allele represents *H-2K* and which *H-2D*. In contrast to the class I loci, the *H-2A* loci are clearly distinct from the *H-2E* loci so that here differentiating alleles from loci poses no problem. This difference between class I and class II loci seems to reflect also on the function of these loci. Because the *H-2A* and *H-2E* loci are so different from each other, the Tcr uses either one or the other, but rarely both for the context of recognition of a particular antigenic determinant. [Some determinants are recognized in the context of *H-2A* and others in the context of *H-2E*, but rarely is a determinant recognized in the context of both *H-2A* and *H-2E*; see BAXEVANIS et al. (1980).] With the class I loci, the situation is different. Here, because the *H-2K* genes are so similar to *H-2D* genes, a particular antigenic determinant can be recognized in the context of either of these genes (molecules). Hence, if there happens to be, in a particular individual, a nonresponder allele present at the *H-2K* locus, the chances are that there will be a responder allele at the *H-2D* locus, and that the individual will be a responder. But if there is a nonresponder allele at the *H-2A* locus, the *H-2E* locus cannot stand in for it, and the individual is a nonresponder. Phenotypically, nonresponders are, therefore, more easily detected in class II- than in class I-restricted responses.

Why certain combinations of antigenic determinants and Mhc allomorphs fail to stimulate T lymphocytes remains unresolved. Two answers have been given to this question and to date it is not clear whether both are correct or only one; and if so, which (SCHWARTZ 1978; KLEIN 1984). The answers reflect the fact that the initiation of the immune response involves two different cells: T lymphocytes and antigen-presenting cells (APC). The T lymphocyte recognizes the antigen presented on the surface of the APC in the context of the APC's Mhc molecule. Soluble antigen is ignored by the T lymphocytes, presumably because of the need for simultaneous recognition of Mhc molecules. (B lymphocytes, which recognize antigen alone, can be activated by soluble antigen.) Under laboratory conditions, the APC can, apparently, be any cell that expresses the right Mhc molecules at sufficient concentration on the cell surface, or even a lipid vesicle containing only the antigen and Mhc molecules in the lipid bilayer. Of course, T cell activation requires more than just the recognition of the antigen in the correct Mhc context; these additional factors are then provided by specialized cells. In a physiologic situation, the APC could be a dendritic cell, another lymphocyte, a Langerhans cell, or a certain type of macrophage, as well as a host of other elements (UNANUE 1984; LANGNER 1985).

Because there are only two cells involved in the triggering of the immune response, the reason for nonresponsiveness must lie either in the T lymphocyte or in the APC. In the former case, there simply may not be any T lymphocyte present which can be activated in the repertoire of the nonresponder individual and which would be capable of recognizing the combination of the particular antigen and the nonresponder Mhc molecule. The individual thus may have a gap or a blind spot in the T cell repertoire (the blind spot hypothesis of nonresponsiveness; KLEIN 1984). The reason for the blind spot could be connected with tolerance induction – the inactivation or elimination of self-reactive T cell clones. If some of the clones that recognize a self-Mhc molecule, or self-Mhc plus another self-molecule with high affinity, also recognize foreign antigen and a self-Mhc molecule, then inactivation of these clones in the tolerance induction process will generate a blind spot for this antigen in the T cell repertoire, and the particular individual will become a nonresponder. In another individual, carrying a different functional Mhc molecule, the inactivated clones may not overlap with those recognizing the particular foreign antigen and this individual will then be a responder. Of course, because of overlap in other clones, the second individual might be a nonresponder to another foreign antigen.

The second possibility is that a nonresponder does contain T lymphocytes capable of recognizing the particular combination of the foreign antigen and Mhc molecules, but that the APC, for some reason, cannot present these two elements (SCHWARTZ 1978). One specific form of this explanation postulates that, to be recognized, the antigen and the Mhc molecule must interact physically in the membrane of the APC. If they fail to interact, the T cell cannot recognize them, and the individual is a nonresponder. In this hypothesis, the Mhc molecules function as crude receptors for foreign antigens, receptors with limited specificity and low binding affinity. Another version of the hypothesis postulates that antigen must be processed, i.e., broken down into fragments inside the APC, before it can be recognized by the T cell. If, for some reason, the APC fails to generate a fragment that can bind to the Mhc molecule, the individual again becomes a nonresponder. In this version, the APC selects determinants for the association with Mhc molecules and ultimate recognition by T lymphocytes (the determinant selection hypothesis of nonresponsiveness).

Strong evidence is now available in support of both hypotheses. To give an example of the evidence supporting the blind spot hypothesis: VIDOVIĆ et al. (1985) observed that DBA/2 mice are responders to the synthetic polypeptide of glutamic acid and tyrosine (GT), whereas BALB/c mice are nonresponders (both strains express the same $H-2^d$ haplotype, but differ at a number of other genetic loci). T lymphocytes derived from DBA/2 mice immunized against GT respond when restimulated in vitro by GT presented by either DBA/2 (responder) of BALB/c (nonresponder) APC. This result suggests that the BALB/c mice express a non-H-2 antigen lacking in the DBA/2 mice. By becoming tolerant of this self-antigen, the BALB/2 mice inactivate T cell clones which normally recognize GT + H-2^d; the DBA/2 mice, which lack this antigen, contain these T cell clones and therefore respond to GT normally.

The strongest evidence supporting the alternative hypothesis is the observation, reported by investigators from two laboratories, that antigen can associate, at low affinity, with Mhc molecules isolated from responder individuals, but does not associate with Mhc molecules extracted from nonresponder individuals (BABBITT et al. 1985; BUUS et al. 1986). Investigators from a third laboratory (PHILLIPS et al. 1986) have, however, reported that, although the antigen associates with Mhc molecules, it associated equally well with molecules from responder and nonresponder individuals. This discrepancy between the laboratories needs to be resolved. If, however, the reported difference in the association constants between responders and nonresponders were to be confirmed, it would mean that, in some nonresponders, the defect is caused by the lack of the necessary T cell clones, while in others it results from the failure of Mhc molecules to associate with the antigen. This solution to the controversy would be the least satisfactory intellectually.

G. Lymphocyte Function

The main physiologic function of vertebrate lymphocytes is to distinguish self from nonself and to mount a specific attack on nonself. The recognition occurs via three sets of molecules, the Tcr, Bcr, and Mhc molecules. The Tcr of the T lymphocyte recognizes proteins in the context of Mhc molecules, normally self-Mhc molecules. If the recognition occurs at a certain stage of development of the organism or a certain phase of T cell differentiation, in which only self-molecules are present, the recognizing cell is inactivated or eliminated. If it occurs outside this stage or phase, and involves nonself proteins, the T lymphocyte develops into an effector cell which can influence the development of other cells (other T lymphocytes, B lymphocytes, and other cells) or can kill the target cell with which it reacts specifically. The process that leads to the elimination or inactivation of self-reactive T cell clones has, as its consequence, an imperfection in the specific immune system: certain individuals are unable to recognize certain foreign antigens. This imperfection is probably overcome by the complexity of the antigen (the chances are that an individual that is genetically a nonresponder to one antigenic determinant of a complex molecule or of a pathogen is a responder to another determinant; see MARUSIĆ et al. 1982); and by natural selection (individuals that are nonresponders to certain critical antigenic determinants of a parasite die, and only the responders survive; see KLEIN 1979). It may be a small price that the vertebrates have to pay for the enormous advantage of being able to mount a specific immune response – the ability to distinguish self from nonself.

The B lymphocytes probably recognize self and nonself antigens indiscriminately and also recognize a larger spectrum of substances. They normally avoid a response against self by being dependent on signals from activated T cells for stimulation. Even when they bind a substance via their antigen receptors, most of them do not develop into effector cells (antibody-secreting plasma cells) until they have received the go-ahead from T lymphocytes which have encountered the same substances. The details of the transmission of messages between T and B lymphocytes (T-B collaboration) are obscure. The two principal hypotheses are: (a) that the T lymphocyte binds to one region of the antigen (carrier) and the B lymphocyte to another region (hapten) and that the message is transmitted via this "antigen bridge" between the two cells (MITCHISON 1971); and (b) that the B lymphocyte binds the antigen first, processes (fragments) it, redisplays the fragments on its cell surface in the context of its Mhc molecules, and the T cell then recognizes the complex of the antigen and Mhc molecule, thereby stimulating the B cell (LANZAVECCHIA 1985). Decisive experiments which would rule out one of these two hypotheses have not yet been carried out.

In addition to this main function (initiation of specific immune response) lymphocytes also carry out a host of other functions, largely through soluble substances (lymphokines) which they secrete. (These are described in Chaps. 8, 9, and 11.) Most of the lymphokines are produced only after activation of the lymphocyte, which normally occurs when the lymphocyte encounters an antigen. T lymphocytes, in particular, appear to produce a wide spectrum of lymphokines having a wide variety of effects. The production of some of these lymphokines might have preceded the acquisition of antigen-specific receptors in phylogeny and might have been the original function of the ancestral cells.

Acknowledgments. I thank Ms. Lynne Yakes for excellent editorial assistance.

References

Alt FW, Blackwell TK, DePinho RA, Reth MG, Yancopoulos GD (1986) Regulation of genome rearrangement events during lymphocyte differentiation. Immunol Rev 89:5–30

Atassi MH, Young CR (1985) Discovery and implications of the immunogenicity of free small synthetic peptides: powerful tools for manipulating the immune system and for the production of antibodies and T cells preselected submolecular specificities. CRC Crit Rev Immunol 5:387–411

Babbitt BP, Allen PM, Matsueda G, Haber E, Unanue ER (1985) Binding of immunogeneic peptides to Ia histocompatibility molecules. Nature 317:359–361

Baltimore D (1981) Somatic mutation gains its place among the generators of diversity. Cell 26:295–296

Bank I, DePinho RA, Brenner MB, Cassimeris J, Alt FW, Chess L (1986) A functional T3 molecule associated with a novel heterodimer on the surface of immature human thymocytes. Nature 309:757–762

Bannerman RM, Edwards JA, Pinkerton PH (1973) Hereditary disorders of the red cell in mammals. Prog Hematol 8:131–179

Baxevanis CN, Wernet D, Nagy ZA, Maurer PH, Klein J (1980) Genetic control of T-cell proliferative responses to poly(Glu^{40}Ala^{60}) and poly(Glu^{51}Lys^{34}Tyr^{15}): subregion-specific inhibition of the responses with monoclonal Ia antibodies. Immunogenetics 11:617–628

Benjamin DC, Berzofsky JA, East IJ, Gurd FRN, Hannum C, Leach SJ, Margoliash E et al. (1984) The antigenic structure of proteins: a reappraisal. Annu Rev Immunol 2:67–101

Bevan M (1977) In a radiation chimaera, host H-2 antigens determine immune responsiveness of donor cytotoxic cells. Nature 269:417–418

Born W, Yague J, Palmer E, Kappler J, Marrack P (1985) Rearrangement of T cell receptor β chain genes during T cell development. Proc Natl Acad Sci USA 82:2925–2929

Brenner MB, McLean J, Dialynas DP, Strominger JL, Smith JA, Owen FL, Seidman JG et al. (1986) Identification of a putative second T-cell receptor. Nature 322:145–149

Burgess A, Nicola N (1983) Growth factors and stem cells. Academic, Sydney

Burnet FM (1959) The clonal selection theory of acquired immunity. Vanderbilt University Press, Nashville

Buus S, Colon S, Smith C, Freed JH, Miles C, Grey HM (1986) Interaction between a "processed" ovalbumin peptide and Ia molecules. Proc Natl Acad Sci USA 83:3968–3971

Cebra JJ, Komisar JL, Schweitzer PA (1984) C_H Isotype "switching" during normal B lymphocyte development. Annu Rev Immunol 2:493–548

Chien Y-H, Becker DM, Lindsten T, Okamura M, Cohen DI, Davis MM (1984) A third type of murine T-cell receptor gene. Nature 312:31–35

Cooke A, Lydyard PM, Roitt IM (1983) Mechanisms of autoimmunity: a role for cross-reactive idiotypes. Immunol Today 4:170–175

Cooper EL (1976) Comparative immunology. Prentice-Hall, Englewood Cliffs

De Bruyn PPH (1981) Structural substrates of bone marrow function. Semin Hematol 18:179–193

Deuchar EM (1975) Cellular interactions in animal development. Chapman and Hall, London

Droege W (1981) A random repertoire of V genes for T-cell receptors? Theoretical implications of recent experimental observations on T-cell specificity and self-restriction. Cell Immunol 64:381–391

Golde DW, Takaku F (eds) (1985) Hemopoietic stem cells. Dekker, New York

Hagblom P, Segal E, Billyard E, So M (1985) Intragenic recombination leads to pilus antigenic variation in *Neisseria gonorrhoeae*. Nature 315:156–158

Hogan B, Costantini F, Lacy F (1986) Manipulating the mouse embryo. A laboratory manual. Cold Spring Harbor Laboratory, Cold Spring Harbor

Honjo T (1983) Immunoglobulin genes. Annu Rev Immunol 1:499–528

Hood L, Kronenberg M, Hunkapiller T (1985) T-cell antigen receptor and the immuno-
globulin supergene family. Cell 40:225–229
Howard M, Paul WE (1983) Regulation of B-cell growth and differentiation by soluble fac-
tors. Annu Rev Immunol 1:307–333
Jerne NK (1971) The somatic generation of immune recognition. Eur J Immunol 1:1–9
Kincade PW (1981) Formation of B lymphocytes in fetal and adult life. Adv Immunol
31:177–245
Kindt TJ, Capra JD (1984) The antibody enigma. Plenum, New York
Kingston R, Jenkinson EJ, Owen JJT (1985) A single stem cell can recolonize an embryonic
thymus producing phenotypically distinct T-cell populations. Nature 317:811–813
Klein J (1977) Evolution and function of the major histocompatibility system: facts and
speculations. In: Götze D(ed) The major histocompatibility system in man and ani-
mals. Springer, Berlin Heidelberg New York, pp 339–378
Klein J (1979) The major histocompatibility complex of the mouse. Science 203:516–521
Klein J (1982) Immunology. The science of self-nonself discrimination. Wiley, New York
Klein J (1984) What causes immunological nonresponsiveness? Immunol Rev 81:177–202
Klein J (1986 a) Natural history of the major histocompatibility complex. Wiley, New
York
Klein J (1986 b) Ag-Mhc-Tcr: inquiries into the immunological *ménage à trois*. Immunol
Res 5:173–190
Klein J, Figueroa F (1981) Polymorphism of the mouse *H-2* loci. Immunol Rev 60:23–57
Klein J, Nagy ZA (1982) Mhc restriction and *Ir* genes. Adv Cancer Res 37:233–317
Klein J, Juretić A, Baxevanis CN, Nagy ZA (1981) The traditional and the new version of
the mouse *H-2* complex. Nature 291:455–460
Klinman NR, Riley RL, Morrow PR, Jennerson RR, Teale JM (1985) Tolerance and B
cell repertoire establishment. Fed Proc 44:2488–2492
Kronenberg M, Siu G, Hood LE, Shastri N (1986) The molecular genetics of the T-cell
antigen receptor and T-cell antigen recognition. Annu Rev Immunol 4:526–591
Krstić RV (1984) Illustrated encyclopedia of human histology. Springer, Berlin Heidelberg
New York
Kruisbeck AM, Longo DL (1985) Acquisition of MHC-restriction specificities: role of
thymic stromal cells. Surv Immunol Res 4:110–119
Langner J (1985) Antigen processing und Antigenpräsentation durch akzessorische Zellen
des Immunsystems. Allerg Immunol (Leipz) 31:131–156
Lanzavecchia A (1985) Antigen-specific interaction between T and B cells. Nature 314:537–
539
Le Douarin NM (1977) Ontogeny of primary lymphoid organs. In: Loor F, Roelants GE
(eds) B and T cells in immune recognition. Wiley, New York, pp 1–19
Litman GW, Berger L, Murphy K, Litman R, Hinds K, Ericksoon BW (1985) Immunoglobulin V_H gene structure and diversity in *Heterodontus*, a phylogenetically primitive
shark. Proc Natl Acad Sci USA 82:2082–2086
Longo DL, Matis LA, Schwartz RH (1981) Insights into immune response gene function
from experiments with chimeric animals. CRC Crit Rev Immunol 2:83–132
Marchalonis JJ (1977) Immunity in evolution. Arnold, London
Marusić M, Nagy ZA, Koszinowski U, Klein J (1982) Involvement of Mhc loci in immune
responses that are not *Ir*-gene controlled. Immunogenetics 16:471–483
McDevitt HO, Deak BD, Shreffler DC, Klein J, Stimpfling JH, Snell GD (1972) Genetic
control of the immune response. Mapping of the *Ir-1* locus. J Exp Med 135:1259–
1278
Metcalf D, Moore MAS (1971) Haemopoietic cells. North-Holland, Amsterdam
Mitchison NA (1971) The carrier effect in the secondary response to hapten-protein conjugates. II. Cellular cooperation. Eur J Immunol 1:18–27
Owen JJT, Jenkinson EJ (1981) Embryology of the lymphoid system. Prog Allergy 29:1–
34
Phillips L, Naquet P, Delovitch TL (1986) Antigen associates with Ia molecules in antigen-
presenting B cells. AIP Immunol D137:309–312

Pink JRL (1986) Counting components of the chicken's B cell system. Immunol Rev 91:115–128

Plasterk RHA, Simon MI, Barbour AG (1985) Transposition of structural genes to an expression sequence on a linear plasmid causes antigenic variation in the bacterium *Borrelia hermsii*. Nature 318:257–263

Ratcliffe NA, Rowley AF (1981) Invertebrate blood cells, vols 1, 2. Academic, London

Ratcliffe NA, Rowley AF, Fitzgerald SW, Rhodes CP (1985) Invertebrate immunity: basic concepts and recent advances. Int Rev Cytol 97:183–350

Raulet DH, Garman DR, Saito H, Tonegawa S (1985) Developmental regulation of T cell receptor gene expression. Nature 314:103–107

Reynaud C-A, Anguez V, Dahan A, Weill J-C (1985) A single rearrangement event generates most of the chicken immunoglobulin light chain diversity. Cell 40:283–291

Romer AS (1959) The vertebrate story. University of Chicago Press, Chicago

Saito H, Kranz DM, Takagaki Y, Hayday AC, Eisen HN, Tonegawa D (1984a) A third rearranged and expressed gene in a clone of cytotoxic T lymphocytes. Nature 312:36–40

Saito H, Kranz DM, Takagaki Y, Hayday AC, Eisen HN, Tonegawa S (1984b) Complete primary structure of a heterodimeric T-cell receptor deduced from cDNA sequences. Nature 309:757–762

Schwartz RH (1978) A clonal deletion model for Ir gene control of the immune response. Scand J Immunol 7:3–10

Schwartz RH (1982) Functional properties of *I* region gene products and theories of immune response. In: Ferrone S, David CS (eds) Ia antigens: mice, vol 1. CRC, Boca Raton, pp 161–192

Schwartz RH (1985) T-lymphocyte recognition of antigen in association with gene products of the major histocompatibility complex. Annu Rev Immunol 3:237–261

Schwartz RH (1986) Immune response (*Ir*) genes of the murine major histocompatibility complex. Adv Immunol 38:31–201

Scollay R, Smith J, Stauffer V (1986) Dynamics of early T cells: prothymocyte migration and proliferation in the adult mouse thymus. Immunol Rev 91:129–157

Scott DW (1984) Mechanisms in immune tolerance. CRC Crit Rev Immunol 5:1–25

Servis C, Seckler R, Nagy ZA, Klein J (1986) Two adjacent epitopes on a synthetic dodecapeptide induce lactate dehydrogenase B-specific helper and suppressor cells. Proc R Soc Lond [Biol] 228:461–470

Sher I (1982) The CBA/N mouse strain: an experimental model illustrating the influence of the X-chromosome on immunity. Adv Immunol 33:2–71

Snodgrass HR, Kisielow P, Kiefer M, Steinmetz M, von Boehmer H (1985) Ontogeny of the T cell antigen receptor within the thymus. Nature 313:592–595

Steinert M, Pays E (1985) Genetic control of antigenic variation in trypanosomes. Br Med Bull 41:149–155

Stockinger H, Barlett R, Pfizenmaier K, Röllinghoff M, Wagner H (1981) H-2 restriction as a consequence of intentional priming. Frequency analysis of alloantigen-restricted, trinitrophenyl-specific cytotoxicity T lymphocyte precursors within thymocytes of normal mice. J Exp Med 153:1629–1639

Stutman O (1986) Postthymic T-cell development. Immunol Rev 91:159–194

Suda T, Suda J, Ogawa M (1983) Single-cell origin of mouse hemopoietic colonies expressing multiple lineages in invariable combination. Proc Natl Acad Sci USA 80:6689–6693

Tischendorf F (1985) On the evolution of the spleen. Experientia 41:145–252

Trainin N, Pecht M, Handzel ZT (1983) Thymic hormones: inducers and regulators of the T-cell system. Immunol Today 4:16–21

Unanue ER (1984) Antigen-presenting function of the macrophage. Annu Rev Immunol 2:395–428

Vidović D, Klein J, Nagy ZA (1985) Recessive T cell response to poly(Glu^{50}Tyr^{50}) possibly caused by self tolerance. J Immunol 134:3563–3568

Vogler LB, Lawton AR (1985) Ontogeny of B cells and humoral immune functions. In: Rosen FS (ed) Development Immunology. Saunders, London, pp 235–252 (Clinics in immunology and allergy, vol 5/2)

Webb DR, Kapp JA, Pierce CW (1985) Antigen-specific factors: an overview. Methods Enzymol 116:295–303

Weill JC, Reynaud CA, Lassila O, Pink JRL (1986) Rearrangement of chicken immunoglobulin genes is not an ongoing process in the embryonic bursa of Fabricius. Proc Natl Acad Sci USA 83:3336–3340

Weiss L, Greep RO (1977) Histology. McGraw-Hill, New York, p 440

Zinkernagel RM, Doherty PC (1974) Restriction of in vitro T-cell mediated cytotoxicity in lymphocytic choriomeningitis within a syngeneic or semi-allogeneic system. Nature 248:701–702

Zinkernagel RM, Doherty PC (1979) MHC-restricted cytotoxic T cells: studies on the biological role of the polymorphic major transplantation antigens determining T-cell restriction specificity, function, and responsiveness. Adv Immunol 27:51–177

Zinkernagel RM, Callahan GN, Althage A, Cooper S, Klein PA, Klein J (1978) On the thymus in the differentiation of "H-2 self-recognition" by T cells: evidence for dual recognition? J Exp Med 147:882–896

Zola H (1985) Differentiation and maturation of human B lymphocytes: a review. Pathology 17:365–381

CHAPTER 2

De Novo Expression of Receptors on T Cells

J. M. WILLIAMS and T. B. STROM

A. T Cell Activation and De Novo Expression of Receptors

The ability to effect selective and limited regulation of the vigor of the immune response is a potential therapeutic tool of almost unlimited promise. Since transition of T cells from the quiescent to the active state is a prerequisite for most immune functions, a detailed understanding of the T cell activation process is a logical first step toward achieving this goal of immunotherapy. Antigenic or mitogenic activation of lymphocytes initiates an ordered, complex sequences of entra- and intracellular events. Activated lymphocytes are phenotypically as well as functionally distinct from their progenitors (see Chap. 1). Cell surface antigens, often receptor proteins, that are induced to appear on T cells activated by the lectin phytohemagglutinin-P (PHA) can be classified both on the basis of the kinetics of their appearance and on their growth association properties. Seven distinct T cell activation antigens, defined by monoclonal antibodies (mAb), have been classified as early, intermediate, or late antigens based on their temporal appearance relative to DNA synthesis. Four antigens, the transferrin receptor, the T cell activation antigen Tac, the 4F2 antigen, and Tac antigen 49.9 are early antigens, whereas the OKT10 antigen appears at intermediate times, and both HLA-DR and antigen 19.2 appear late (COTNER et al. 1983). These findings are similar to the previously reported early expression of insulin-binding sites on activated lymphocytes (HELDERMANN and STROM 1979) and confirms the result of UCHIYAMA et al. (1981 a) that Tac, the $_p$55 subunit of the interleukin 2 (IL-2) receptor, is expressed before DNA synthesis. These same four early antigens are found on virtually all T cells by the time they reach the S phase of the cell cycle. Thus, when just the cells in the S, G_2, or M stages of the cell cycle were examined, T cells express each of the four early antigens (COTNER et al. 1983). As each early activation antigen is expressed before the onset of DNA synthesis, it is likely that subsequent cell cycle progression does not occur before the function of each of these early antigens has been executed. Although a cell surface protein whose function was required for T cell growth would be expected to appear on all T cells before their entering the proliferative phase of the cell cycle, mere expression (COTNER et al. 1983) does establish an obligatory role for these proteins in promoting cell growth. However, the fact that these antigens are induced to appear on activated T cells and are present on essentially all T cells before the initiation of DNA synthesis marks these proteins as excellent candidates for molecules causally related to cell growth. One general approach that might establish a causal link between expression of the early activation antigens and subsequent events in the cell cycle is to see what effect inhibiting the function of the activation antigen has on cell growth. Abrogation of the activation antigen function can be achieved by blocking with antibody to the antigen, or in the case of an antigen that is a known receptor, by depriving the receptor of appropriate agonist. Antibody to each of the four early activation antigens partially inhibits T cell proliferation (TROWBRIDGE and OMARY 1981; COTNER et al. 1982) whereas antibody to intermediate or late antigens, e.g., OKT10, anti-19.2, and anti-HLA-DR, does not inhibit proliferation (PALACIOS 1982). The failure to achieve complete inhibition may result from the fact that a given mAb defines such a restricted site on its target antigen that it may not completely compromise the function of the target molecule. For instance, four mAb to the transferrin receptor (5E9, OKT9, B3/25, CP200) fail to block the binding of transferrin (HAYNES et al. 1981a; TERHORST et al. 1981; COTNER et al. 1983, unpublished work), and the only instance in which an mAb successfully blocked transferrin binding was achieved by specifically selecting an antibody for that property (TROWBRIDGE and LOPEZ 1982).

It is interesting to correlate the role of the early activation antigens with what is known about the growth-promoting activity of their ligands. Sato and his coworkers (reviewed in BARNES and SATO 1980) have determined that transferrin (or lactoferrin) is a universal requirement for the long-term growth of all mammalian cell types. The requirement in serum-free media for insulin, whose receptor is an early activation antigen (HELDERMANN and STROM 1979), is not as stringent, but it, too, is a desirable component of all defined media. Of special interest is the fact that both transferrin and insulin are components of defined media that support the growth of B cells (ISCOVE and MELCHERAS 1978) and T cells responding in mixed leukocyte reactions (SNOW et al. 1981; STROM and BANGS 1981). It is now universally accepted that IL-2 supports T cell proliferation (MORGAN et al. 1976; GILLIS and SMITH 1977); for reviews see (SMITH 1980; RUSCETTI and GALLO 1981; Chap. 8). The IL-2 receptor itself is an activation antigen that appears rapidly, i.e., 4–8 h after mitogen activation (LARSSON and CONTINO 1979; STADLER 1982), and would be expected to have the same growth association property exhibited by the other early activation antigens. On examining the cellular distributions of the IL-2 receptor and the early activation antigens, it became apparent that Tac antigen, but not the 4F2 antigen, had cell distributions congruent with that of the IL-2 receptor, i.e., present on all IL-2-dependent cells and lines, but absent from most T and B lymphoblastoid cell lines. The IL-2 receptor had previously been shown to be present on three lines derived from cutaneous T cell lymphomas (GOOTENBERG et al. 1981) that are not dependent on exogenous IL-2. On two of these, HUT-78 and HUT-102, both Tac and the 49.9 antigen, which define overlapping epitopes on activated T cells, are strongly expressed on HUT-102 and detectable on Hut-78. Eventually it was learned that anti-Tac must recognize the IL-2 receptor because it competes with IL-2 for binding to IL-2-dependent cells (LEONARD et al. 1982).

The supposition that there is a causal link between expression of the early activation antigens and cell growth is based on their absolute expression on growing cells and the ability of antibodies to these antigens to inhibit, albeit incompletely, T cell proliferation. Until antibodies are produced that are more effective in blocking T cell growth, this hypothesis relies heavily on the previously demonstrated growth-promoting activity of their ligands, transferrin, IL-2, and insulin. Regardless of what the functional activities of the remaining early activation antigens turn out to be, it seems reasonable to speculate that their functions will be important in influencing G_1 transit and the stimulation of DNA synthesis.

Does antigen-specific stimulation of T cells result in similar ordered expression of activation proteins as noted for PHA? The human alloimmune response results from antigenic stimuli that are due in large part to major histocompatibility complex disparities between individuals, and the resultant clonal expansion and differentiation of small populations of antigen-specific effector cells is modulated by interactions with regulatory cells (TERMIZTELEN et al. 1982; ENGLEMAN et al. 1980). The mixed lymphocyte reaction (MLR) is an in vitro model for the study of these events. Since de novo expression of early cell surface activation proteins, e.g., Tac (RINNOOY et al. 1984) and 4F2 (HAYNES et al. 1981 b), on lectin-stimulated T cells precedes DNA synthesis (COTNER et al. 1983), we hypothesized that expression of these activation-associated markers may also herald traditional methods of ascertaining effector cell alloactivation in the MLR, i.e., proliferation or cytotoxicity. The Tac antigen is indeed expressed on functionally mature cytotoxic cells, suppressor cells, and at least some helper cells generated in the MLR (UCHIYAMA et al. 1981 b). Cytotoxic effector cells also express the 4F2 antigen (HELDERMANN and STROM 1979).

Dual parameter flow cytometry has been employed to estimate DNA content, providing information on cell cycle position, and simultaneously to analyze cell surface immunofluorescence with antibodies that define activation antigens or major T cell subsets (i.e., OKT4$^+$ or OKT8$^+$) following initiation of MLR cultures. This technique directly ascribes measurements of the state of activation, cell cycle position, and/or T cell phenotype to the same cell. Direct analysis of human T cell subset proliferative kinetics during the MLR, analysis of the expansion of alloantigen-stimulated responder cell populations, as well as the relationship of activation antigen expression to responder cell entry into the proliferation stages of the cell cycle can be assessed (WILLIAMS et al. 1984 a; YTHIER et al. 1985 a; YTHIER et al. 1985 b). By these techniques, small populations of activated responder lymphocytes can be reproducibly identified by virtue of activation antigen expression *before* bulk proliferation in the MLR. We concluded that:

1. The kinetics of expression of the blastogenic response to alloantigen is slower than that stimulated by PHA.
2. The relative size ($\sim 1\%$–2% of T cells) of the alloantigen-responsive clones (YTHIER et al. 1985 a; YTHIER et al. 1985 b) is remarkably smaller than the PHA-responsive pool. The size of the pool of Tac $^+$ cells observed 24–48 h after MLR initiation is in line with the predicted size of the alloreactive clone (YTHIER et al. 1985 b).

Since the presence of activation antigens appears to delineate alloactivated clones specifically, mAbs against activation antigens should be excellent tools for implementing selective immunotherapy. Briefly, noxious agents could be directed to inactivate or destroy only activation antigen-positive cells, thus thwarting unwanted immune reactions (i.e., graft rejection) or autoimmune disease. Meanwhile, the rest of the host's potential for other essential and beneficial immune responses would remain intact within the huge reservoir of activation antigen-negative (resting) T cells. To begin to test this hypothesis, we performed the following experiment. Mixed lymphocyte cultures were allowed to proceed for 3 days, at which time only modest responder cell proliferation had occurred, yet 15% of the responder cells had recognized and responded to alloantigen and expressed the 4F2 and Tac antigens (WILLIAMS et al. 1984a). These 4F2$^+$ cells were lysed with anti-4F2 mAb and complement (C), and the MLR culture was reestablished with the remaining responder cells (4F2$^-$) and fresh stimulator cells. The extent of proliferation observed on day 7 (normal time of maximal responder cell growth) of the cultures treated in this manner was significantly blunted when compared with parallel MLR cultures that were not depleted of 4F2$^+$ cells. Treatment of responder cells with 4F2 mAb plus C prior to MLR initiation (before alloantigen recognition) did not alter the proliferative outcome of subsequent MLR cultures, showing that the 4F2 plus C treatment was specific for activated, 4F2$^+$ cells, and did not merely inhibit the growth of all T cells. The results of these experiments indicate that activation antigens are useful probes for defining those cells that are predestined to, or have already entered S/G$_2$/M phases of the cell cycle in response to alloantigen. Indeed, T cell activation antigens appear literally to define the major, and perhaps the entire, alloactivated T cell populations. These data indicate that the extremely exciting possibility of achieving selective downregulation of an unwanted immune response through targeting activation antigen-positive cells is approachable.

Parallel studies were conducted to identify the requirements for T cell activation, as well as to further dissect and to map events of T cell blastogenesis. The absolute requirement for accessory cell (AC) presence for successful mitogen-induced or soluble antigen-induced T cell proliferation has been widely accepted (SEEGER and OPPENHEIM 1970; UNANUE 1972; ROSENSTREICH et al. 1976; HABU and RAFF 1977; THIELE et al. 1983; HUNIG et al. 1983; GERY and WAKEMAN 1972; LARSSON et al. 1980; PALACIOS 1982). However, questions remained concerning the mechanism or mechanisms by which AC support T cell proliferation. This problem was initially addressed by divorcing T cells and AC via stringent AC depletion, and by analyzing multiple pre-S phase indicators of T cell activation throughout the cell cycle 18–40 h after PHA stimulation (WILLIAMS et al. 1984b). AC-depleted, PHA-stimulated T cells exhibit minimal, if any: (a) increases in RNA content; (b) expression of activation-associated Tac proteins (IL-2 receptors), transferrin receptors, and 4F2 protein; (c) IL-2 production; or (d) increases in DNA content. These indicators of activation were assayed by dual parameter flow cytometry (COTNER et al. 1983; WILLIAMS et al. 1984b), and IL-2 production was determined by bioassay (GILLIS et al. 1978). The vigor of T cell activation can be completely restored when plastic-adherent cells are added to the isolated T cells. In contrast, and to our surprise, activation was only minimally restored on addition of IL-1-rich AC-conditioned supernatants or "purified" IL-1. Thus, IL-1 alone does not fully replace the requirement for AC during T cell activation by PHA. In contrast, resting murine T cells can be activated in a two-part process, where the first part is an AC-independent activation of T cells that results from direct contact between T cells and lectin (WILLIAMS et al. 1984a; LARSSON et al. 1980; PALACIOS 1982). Such directly lectin-activated T cells are believed to express IL-2 receptors. However, T cell proliferation was believed to await the second part of the process, the elaboration of IL-2 by activated T cells, which completes the autocrine requirements for T cell proliferation (WILLIAMS et al. 1984a; LARSSON et al. 1980; PALACIOS 1982). The production of IL-2 by activated T cells is totally AC dependent (LARSSON et al. 1980; MAIZEL et al. 1979; SMITH et al. 1980) and it has been reported that the soluble monokine IL-1 is able to replace the AC requirement for IL-2 production (WILLIAMS et al. 1984a; LARSSON et al. 1980; PALACIOS 1982). Thus, most studies (WILLIAMS et al. 1984a; SEEGER and OPPENHEIM 1970; UNANUE 1972; ROSENSTREICH et al. 1976; HABU and RAFF 1977; LARSSON et al. 1980; OPPENHEIM et al. 1968) indicate that AC-conditioned supernatants or IL-2 are capable of substituting for AC in supporting the late (proliferative) phase of T cell activation following lectin stimulation. Cloned T cell lines, i.e., previously activated T cells that are obviously devoid of AC, have provided evidence that antigen/mitogen alone is sufficient to induce the release of IL-2 in secondary T cell activation (SMITH et al. 1980). These previous results are in apparent contradiction to those presented in our analysis of primary T cell activation, in that we do not find direct activation of resting human T cells by PHA in the absence of AC. This disparity may be resolved by examining the degree of AC depletion obtained in the two experimental systems. Partial AC depletion by adherence techniques is sufficient to significantly inhibit production of IL-2 by lectin-stimulated T cells, as well as to inhibit T cell entry into the S phase of the cell cycle. Most reports in the literature rely on methods involving some type of AC adherence and/or immunoaffinity techniques for AC depletion. We also note that the production of IL-2 as well as S phase entry portions of partially AC-depleted T cell activation can be reconstituted with AC products, including highly purified IL-1, to a level rivaling that obtained by addition of AC themselves. Other investigators (HUNIG et al. 1983) have reported similar results, in that partially AC-depleted murine T cells failed to produce IL-2, but did proliferate when exogenous IL-2 was added, suggesting that more AC were required to support IL-2 production than were needed to induce IL-2 receptor expression and IL-2 responsiveness (HUNIG et al. 1983). The intensity of early activation antigen expression, including Tac/49-9 on partially AC-depleted, PHA-stimulated cells is less than that expressed by unseparated, PHA-stimulated peripheral blood mononuclear cells (PBMC), suggesting that although the density of these activation-associated proteins on PHA-stimulated T cells was not as great after partial AC depletion by adherence techniques as was found on PHA-stimulated, unseparated PBMC, functional IL-2 receptors are present. Further AC depletion, accomplished by the simultaneous application of two mAb (which bind AC, but not resting T cells) and C before culture initiation, was associated with a further, dramatic, reduction (if not ablation) of the number of PHA-stimulated cells that expressed 4F2, OKT9, or Tac/49-9 antigens, HUNIG et al. (1983) who utilized similar additional steps to further deplete AC have presented complementary results in that the addition of IL-2-containing supernatants failed to support lectin-stimulated T cell proliferation. Collectively, these data suggest that a certain "threshold" number of IL-2 receptors and/or other activation-associated proteins must be expressed for S phase entry, and that the full, not necessarily partial, expression of these proteins is AC dependent. Addition of unfractionated AC-conditioned supernatants to maximally AC-depleted, PHA-stimulated T cells only partially reconstitutes AC function in the early events of T cell activation, and these supernatants were noticeably less potent than AC in supporting activation antigen expression and increased RNA content. As neither AC supernatants nor IL-1 fully reconstituted T cell activation to levels achieved with AC, additional AC functions may be required during mitogenic induction.

In order specifically to address these questions further, we attempted to build an artificial, non-IL-1-secreting AC that could "present" mitogenic/antigenic signals. In this way, the role of antigenic signals could be separated from the effects of IL-1 during T cell activation. Stringent AC depletion was followed by CD3-Ti stimulation (Ti represents idiotypic T cell receptor for antigen) by one of two forms of anti-CD3 mAb, soluble or sepharose-linked, in the presence or absence of exogenous IL-1.

Study of AC-dependent events occurring primary activation of normal, resting T cells has been hampered by the small pool size antigen-reactive clones (WILLIAMS et al. 1984a; YTHIER et al. 1985a; YTHIER et al. 1985b), and by an inability to achieve sufficient AC depletion by conventional methods. Although lectin induces a large polyclonal T cell response, the actual T cell surface sites that are stimulated by lectins on the T cell membrane are incompletely defined. In addition, the relative role of AC membranes and monokines still cannot be disentangled, because lectin-induced T cell activation is not fully supported by IL-1 and requires the presence of AC (HUNIG et al. 1983; WILLIAMS et al. 1984b). Physical linkage of the CD3 protein with the T cell receptor for antigen on the T cell membrane provides a unique opportunity to study primary polyclonal activation of normal T cells in a fashion analogous to activation by specific antigen (HAYNES et al. 1981b; DINARELLO et al. 1977; KAMMER et al. 1984). Finally, CD3-specific antibodies can be "presented" on a solid support in the absence of monokines, giving us the chance to dissect the effects of these two, i.e., potential divalent or polyvalent, AC inputs.

Binding of anti-CD3 OKT3 in the presence of AC leads to modulation of the CD3 antigen-receptor complex (REINHERZ et al. 1982; RINNOOY et al. 1983). In contrast to a recent report (RINNOOY 1984), stringently AC-depleted T cells also evidence modulation of the CD3 complex after interaction with soluble anti-CD3 mAB 64.1. Thus, AC-mediated Fc receptor binding is not necessarily required for CD3 modulation, and the mAb 64.1 presumably can induce modulation on a significant fraction of T cells directly through divalent binding. Nonetheless, not all anti-CD3 complex mAb induce modulation of the CD3 complex in the absence of AC (REINHERZ et al. 1982; RINNOOY et al. 1984), most likely because of the epitopes recognized by each mAb. CD3 modulation is immediately followed by "very early" (~ 2 h) events of activation that include increased Ca^{2+} and glucose uptake (A WEISS et al. 1984; MJ WEISS et al. 1984). RNA synthesis and activation antigen expression, including the insulin receptor, are "early" events of activation, detectable 4–16 h after T cell stimulation (BRUSZEWSKI et al. 1984; COTNER et al. 1983; HELDERMAN and STROM 1979; Chaps. 3 and 4).

However, after interaction with mAb 64.1, AC-depleted T cells demonstrated minimal RNA synthesis, IL-2 production, or immunofluorescence-detected expression of two activation-associated antigens, including the Tac subunit of the

IL-2 receptor (IL-2R). These findings are interesting in view of recent reports describing calcium uptake, by anti-CD3-stimulated leukemic cell lines, which are of course, devoid of AC (A WEISS et al. 1984). This suggests that T cells rapidly undergo "very early" events of activation independently of AC, yet fail to progress to the RNA and expression of activation antigens stages, which we have shown to the AC dependent. These data also suggest that activation of the calcium channel is not in itself sufficient to drive the entire T cell activation cascade (see Chap. 3). The addition of AC to T cells with simultaneous stimulation by mAb 64.1 fully reconstitutes the T cell response, whereas the addition of highly purified IL-1 consistently failed to reconstitute these activation events when T cells were stimulated with soluble anti-CD3 mAb 64.1 (SOL-64.1). Although CD3 stimulation by SOL 64.1 induces some degree of T cell activation, we, unlike others using less drastic means of AC depletion (MEUER et al. 1984; KAYE et al. 1984; KAYE et al. 1983), concluded that this event does not in itself successfully induce IL-2R expression. Theoretically, the contribution of AC to the T cell response could include, but is not necessarily limited to, the processing of T cell-bound mAb 64.1 by the Fc receptors of AC and/or production of monokines, including IL-1. Fc receptors on AC are crucial in AC support of anti-CD3-induced T cell activation (VAN WAUWE 1980; LANDGREN et al. 1984; RINNOOY et al. 1984). Therefore, further dissection of the events of T cell activation was attempted by: (a) "presenting" mAb 64.1 cross-linked to sepharose (SEPH) beads in an attempt to mimic AC "processing" of the mAb via Fc receptors in the absence of IL-1; (b) adding exogenous IL-1 in the presence of SEPH-64.1 (providing both IL-1 and polyvalent anti-CD3); and (c) stimulating T cells with SOL-64.1 in the presence and absence of exogenous IL-1 (providing monokines with divalent anti-CD3).

AC-depleted normal human T cells bind to SEPH-64.1, but appear to fail to express immunofluorescence-detectable concentrations of Tac and 4F2 proteins, produce IL-2, or enter G_1, S, G_2, or M phases of the cell cycle (WILLIAMS et al. 1985). Provision of AC (10%–20% cell to cell) reconstitutes these responses to levels observed with mAb 64.1-stimulated unseparated PBMC. Furthermore, stimulation of T cells with SEPH-64.1, (but not SOL-64.1), primed the T cells for responsiveness to IL-1, because the addition of human IL-1 allowed expression of all indicators of activation, including the Tac subunit of the IL-2R, RNA synthesis, IL-2 production, and DNA synthesis. Although SEPH-64.1-stimulated T cells always expressed evidence of activation when supported by exogenous IL-1, full reconstitution to levels obtained with unfractionated PBMC is not always attained. This is especially evident in the IL-2 production experiments, and suggests that additional monokines may be required for maximal support of T cell activation. We were surprised to find that addition of exogenous IL-2 to SEPH-64.1-stimulated T cells also fully supported T cell growth (PALACIOS 1985; ISOUKAS et al. 1985; MEUER and MEYER ZUM BUSCHENFELDE 1986), despite low levels of Tac expression (WILLIAMS et al. 1985; PALACIOS 1985; TSOUKAS et al. 1985; MEUER and MEYER ZUM BUSCHENFELDE 1986). This result was not obtained when parallel aliquots of T cells were stimulated by SOL-64.1 and IL-2. Apparently, remarkably few Tac units are required for IL-2 responsiveness. The role of IL-1 during primary T cell activation appears to be the support of IL-2 release. At the time that our initial anti-CD3 experiments were performed, the Tac protein was regarded as synonymous with the IL-2R, but the Tac is a subunit of the IL-2R (Sharon et al. 1986; Teshigawara 1987). IL-2 binds simultaneously to Tac and a 70 kdalton peptide (Sharon et al. 1986; Teshigawara 1987). Hence, we believe that polyvalent anti-CD3 mAb (and nominal antigen) elicit full expression of the 70 kdalton IL-2-binding protein. Activation of this "receptor" leads to expression of Tac. If this proves correct, study of the sequential expression of T cell surface receptors will again prove most valuable in dissecting the stages of T cell activation.

Apparently, there is a fundamental difference in the AC requirements for the reactivation of antigen-primed T cell clones as compared with the primary activation of normal T cells by mAb 64.1. Activation of resting T cells requires CD3-mAb-64.1 complex "cross-linking" by AC-mediated "cross-linking" on a solid phase support system (SEPH beads), as well as a second AC-derived signal. In contrast, many T cell clones will generate IL-2, IL-2R, and proliferate on stimulation of the T cell antigen-receptor complex by mAb without apparent need for AC (Meuer et al. 1983). However, one human T cell leukemia (Jurkat) has been described (Oppenheim et al. 1968) that exhibits a two-signal requirement for IL-2 production, including anti-CD3 mAb and phorbol myristate acetate, which is reminiscent of the results obtained with resting PBMC. In addition, AC or IL-1 have been shown to enhance the expression of the Tac homolog on at least one mouse T cell clone (Kaye et al. 1984).

These studies provide evidence that stimulation of CD3-Ti is necessary, but not sufficient, to induce several early events of T cell activation. Agonists of the CD3-Ti complex, i.e., antigen or mAb, must be "presented" to the T cell in a cross-linked form. AC or IL-1 then supports the expression of IL-2 release. Apparently, cross-linked (presented) antigenic stimuli simultaneously induce low levels of Tac expression with full IL-2 responsiveness. Interaction of IL-2 with the IL-2R then drives T cell proliferation. These studies provide a basis for additional dissection of T cell activation at the molecular level, because discrete stages of early T cell activation owing to stimulation of CD3-Ti and IL-1 have been identified and may be used to study gene activation.

B. Therapeutic Implications

An ideal antirejection therapy should effectively control rejection. A perfect therapy should also selectively target only those T cells that are committed to participate in rejection. Conventional immunosuppressive drugs cause unwanted side effects upon nonlymphoid tissues. The introduction of mAb as pharmacologic tools has long been awaited as the therapeutic use of T cell-specific mAb can obviate these side effects by providing new opportunities for a more targeted form of immunosuppressive therapy (see Chap. 6). Nonetheless, the pan-T cell antibodies, used with considerable success in transplantation, react with all T cells while an ideal therapy would target only those lymphocytes capable of participating in the unwanted immune reaction.

The immune response to an allograft involves a complex series of events, including T cell activation. In theory, a perfect therapeutic solution would be obtained by developing antibodies that react with the antigen-combining site of the receptors for antigens on the donor graft. This approach has been confounded, at least temporarily, by the incredible genetic diversity of transplantation antigens and the T cell receptor for antigen.

Our simpler approach is based on the knowledge that activated T cells express a variety of plasma membrane receptors (COTNER et al. 1983; WILLIAMS et al. 1984a) that are absent from the surface of resting T cells, e.g., receptors for IL-2, insulin, and transferrin. The acquisition of membrane receptors for IL-2 marks a critical event in the course of T cell activation (LARSSON and CONTINO 1979; CANTRELL and SMITH 1984). The induction of IL-2R on T cells is dependent on activation with either specific antigen or mitogen (COTNER et al. 1983; WILLIAMS et al. 1984a); a 200-fold amplification of IL-2R is detectable within 24 h of stimulation. Whereas engagement of the T cell antigen receptor with antigen is the first step in T cell activation, the interaction of IL-2 with newly expressed IL-2R is a necessary step in the common pathway of activation of all T cells. Interaction of IL-2 with IL-2R-bearing cells initiates a cellular program that is a prerequisite for clonal expansion and continued viability of most, if not all, activated T cells (COTNER et al. 1983; MORGAN et al. 1976; LARSSON and CONTINO 1979; CANTRELL and SMITH 1984; KUPIEC-WEGLINSKI 1986).

I. Immunosuppressive Therapy with M7/20 IL-2 Receptor-Specific Antibody

We have examined the effect of administration of M7/20, an IL-2R-specific antibody (GAULTON et al. 1985), on allograft rejection in mice (KIRKMAN et al. 1985a; KIRKMAN et al. 1985b). Inbred male mice, C57BL/10, B10.BR, and B10.AKM were used as these strains are completely mismatched for the H-2 locus. Vascularized, heterotopic heart or full thickness tail skin allografts were also performed.

Untreated B10.AKM recipients of C57BL/10 heart allografts rejected their grafts with a median survival of 8 days (Table 1) (KIRKMAN et al. 1985a; KIRKMAN et al. 1985b). In contrast, intraperitoneal injection with M7/20 mAb at a dose of 5 µg per mouse per day for 10 days caused indefinite survival (>90 days) in four of six grafts, with the other two rejecting at 20 and 31 days – a highly significant prolongation ($P < 0.01$).

To confirm that these results were related to the specificity of M7/20 for IL-2R-bearing cells, a control group of recipients was treated with RA3-2C2, a rat mAb of the same class as M7/20, which binds pre-B cells, but not T cells. The survival times of RA3-2C2-treated hosts were not different from the untreated controls, but were significantly shorter than those observed in animals treated with M7/20 ($P < 0.05$).

The remarkable effects of M7/20 treatment were not unique to one strain combination. A second set of experiments was performed with C57BL/10 recipients of B10.BR heart grafts. Untreated control recipients rejected their grafts at 10–20 days; treatment with M7/20 prolonged survival to 20, 27, 34, and 38 days, with two grafts still functioning at >60 days ($P < 0.01$) (Table 1).

Table 1. The effect of M7/20 on survival of murine heart allografts

Recipient	Donor	Treatment	Allograft survival (days)
B10.AKM	C57BL/10	None	8, 8, 8, 8, 16, 29
B10.AKM	C57BL/10	M7/20	20, 31, >90, >90, >90, >90
B10.AKM	C57BL/10	RA3-2C2[a]	6, 9, 9, 10, >90
C57/BL/10	B10.BR	None	9, 10, 10, 10, 14, 16, 20, 20
C57/BL/10	B10.BR	M7/20[a]	20, 27, 34, 38, >60, >60
C57/BL/10	B10.BR	M7/20, day 3[b]	11, 15, 17, 18, 47, >60, >60, >60
C57/BL/10	B10.BR	M7/20, day 6[c]	7, 17, 19, 27[d], 27[d], 58, >60, >60

[a] 5 µg i.p. daily for 10 days.
[b] 5 µg i.p. daily beginning day 3.
[c] 5 µg i.p. daily for 10 days beginning day 6.
[d] Died of anesthetic complication with functioning allograft.

The effect of M7/20 on graft rejection was analyzed histologically in C57BL/
10 recipients of B10.BR heart allografts. By 3 days post-transplantation, control
grafts were heavily infiltrated by mononuclear cells. Treatment with M7/20 prevented this graft infiltration (KIRKMAN et al. 1985a; KIRKMAN et al. 1985b). The
experiments demonstrate the utility of M7/20 treatment in preventing graft rejection. The efficacy of M7/20 in reversing established rejection was then examined
in C57BL/10 recipients of B10.BR allografts (Table 1). In eight animals, the onset
of treatment was delayed until day 3, by which time rejection was ongoing, and
continued through day 12. Five grafts were rejected on days, 11, 15, 17, 18, and
47, while three were still functioning at >60 days. When treatment was given on
days 6–15, four grafts were rejected at 7, 17, 19, and 58 days, while two were still
functioning at >60 days. Two additional grafts were still functioning at 27 days
when the animals succumbed to an anesthetic overdose while being bled. In both
delayed treatment groups, overall graft survival was prolonged significantly
beyond that of the controls (P <0.05) (KIRKMAN et al. 1985a; KIRKMAN et al.
1985b).

M7/20 at a daily dose of 5 µg for 10 days significantly prolonged survival of
C57BL/10 skin placed onto B10.AKM recipients, when compared with controls
(P <0.01) (KIRKMAN et al. 1985a; KIRKMAN et al. 1985b). Several of these grafts
showed no evidence of rejection until 4–5 days after the therapy was discontinued.
However, none of the skin grafts survived indefinitely. Nonetheless, prolonged
skin graft survival was not observed in the combination B10.BR into C57BL1/10.
Insofar as delayed-type hypersensitivity (DTH) mechanisms are important in allograft rejection, it is not surprising that the M7/20 antibody blocks DTH in vivo
(KELLEY et al. 1986)

II. The Effect of ART 18 IL-2 Receptor-Specific
Antibody Treatment in Rat Cardiac Allografts

In light of the successful use of M7/20 mAb in mouse allograft models, we have
utilized ART 18 mAb, a mouse anti-rat IL-2R antibody (OSAWA and DIAMANT-
STEIN 1983), in an attempt to combat rejection of (LEW × BN) F1 to Lewis (LEW)

Table 2. The effect of ART 18 on survival of heart allografts

Donor	Recipient	ART 18 dose	Mean graft survival (days)
(LEW × BN) F1	LEW	None	8 ± 1
(LEW × BN) F1	LEW	$25 \,\mu g \, kg^{-1} \, day^{-1} \times 10$[a]	13 ± 1
(LEW × BN) F1	LEW	$100 \,\mu g \, kg^{-1} \, day^{-1} \times 10$[a]	14 ± 3
(LEW × BN) F1	LEW	$300 \,\mu g \, kg^{-1} \, day^{-1} \times 10$[a]	21 ± 1
(LEW × BN) F1	LEW	$300 \,\mu g \, kg^{-1} \, day^{-1} \times 5$[a]	14 ± 2
(LEW × BN) F1	LEW	$300 \,\mu g \, kg^{-1} \, day^{-1} \times 5$[b]	18 ± 4
LEW	WF	None	8 ± 2
LEW	WF	$300 \,\mu g \, kg^{-1} \, day^{-1} \times 10$[a]	16 ± 1

[a] i.v. daily for 10 days beginning day 0.
[b] i.v. daily for 5 days beginning day 5.

strain heterotopic cardiac allografts (KUPIEC-WEGLINSKI 1986). ART 18 mAb was highly successful in prolonging cardiac graft survival, although permanent engraftment was not seen following cessation of therapy when this agent was used in the absence of other immunosuppressives (Table 2). Furthermore, ART 18 plus very low dose cyclosporin therapy ($1.5 \, mg \, kg^{-1} \, day^{-1}$) yields synergistic prolongation of graft survival.

As in the case of rat anti-mouse M7/20 mAb, the efficacy of the ART 18 mouse anti-rat anti-IL-2R mAb therapy in reversing well-established allograft rejection was then tested. Treatment was initiated 5 days after transplantation, at which time the grafts were grossly enlarged and heavily infiltrated with lymphocytes. Interestingly, ART 18 mAb therapy, started on day 5 after transplantation and continued for 5 days at a dose of $300 \,\mu g \, kg^{-1} \, day^{-1}$, improved allograft survival to 18 ± 4 days (Table 2, $P < 0.001$), comparable to the effect produced by ten consecutive injections. The dense cellular infiltrate virtually disappeared after ART 18 mAb treatment. Intermittent ART 18 mAb administration (days 5–9 and 15–19) extended graft survival to 26–28 days; whereas lower doses of mAb were ineffectual in reversing ongoing rejection. To demonstrate that the results of anti-IL-2R mAb treatement were not unique to one strain combination, we treated WF rat recipients of LEW cardiac grafts with ART 18mAb ($300 \,\mu g \, kg^{-1} \, day^{-1}$) for 10 days, beginning on the day of transplantation. Allograft survival was prolonged to 16 ± 1 days (Table 2, $P < 0.001$). Thus, ART 18 mAb therapy can be used to prevent or treat acute rejection.

To confirm that these results were related to the specificity of ART 18 mAb for IL-2R, an additional control group of animals was treated with anti-asialo-GM1-specific antibody, recognizing a structure on the surface of rat natural killer (NK) cells. A single, or repeated intravenous administration of mAb following transplantation virtually eliminated host NK activity. However, cardiac allograft survival was not modified.

III. ART 18 mAb Therapy Spares Suppressor T Cells

Spleen cells were harvested on day 10 from heart-grafted hosts, after the dose regimen of ART 18 mAb had been completed, and were transferred intravenously $(40–50 \times 10^6$ cells) into normal recipients that received test cardiac allografts 24 h later. Such adoptive transfer prolonged donor-specific (LEW $\times$ BN) F_1, but not third party (WF) test graft survival (15 ± 1 days and 8 ± 1 days, respectively, $P < 0.001$).

In contrast, adoptive transfer of unseparated spleen cells from untreated recipients undergoing acute rejection accelerated donor-specific test graft rejection in a second-set manner. Thus, potent, antigen-specific suppressor activity, but not alloaggressive immune activity can be demonstrated in animals maintaining well-functioning cardiac allografts following ART 18 mAb therapy.

The precise mechanism by which a vascularized or skin allograft is rejected remains a subject of intense investigation, but the participation of T cells in the process is unquestioned. Our results provide important evidence that IL-2R-bearing cells are required for allograft rejection. Administration of anti-IL-2R mAbs (M7/20 or ART 18), significantly prolonged major histocompatibility complex-mismatched vascularized heart allograft survival in mice and rats. Indeed, several grafts survived indefinitely, although the antibody was administered only for the first 10 days after transplantation. Rejection of the remaining grafts may well reflect inadequate dosage of antibody; no dose-response studies have been performed to date. In addition to preventing rejection, delayed treatment with anti-IL-2R was shown to reverse ongoing rejection in other recipients of heart allografts. Such long-term engraftment following cessation of therapy makes it unlikely that M7/20 prolongs graft survival by pharmacologic blockade of IL-2R. Furthermore, exogenous IL-2 does not diminish the beneficial effects of anti-IL-2R mAb therapy. Whether or not such prolonged graft survival represents deletion of the responding T cell clones is a subject of current investigation. Passive transfer experiments clearly prove that anti-IL-2 mAb spares suppressor T cells.

Finally, the availability of mAb directed against the human IL-2R provides an opportunity to extend these principles to clinical transplantation. The presence of IL-2R on all recently activated T cells and their absence from the surface of resting or memory T cells makes it possible to target only the relevant responding clones following an allograft, raising the hope of specific immunosuppression. The attempt to utilize activation-associated de novo expression of IL-2R as a therapeutic target for immunotherapy thus derives from more basic inquiries into the essential mechanisms of T cell activation.

References

Barnes D, Sato G (1980) Growth of cultured cells in serum-free medium. Anal Biochem 102:255

Bruszewski WB, Bruszewski JA, Tonnu H, Ferezy SL, O'Brien RL, Parker JW (1984) Early mitogen-induced metabolic events essential to proliferation of human T lymphocytes: dependence of specific events on the influence of adherent accessory cells. J Immunol 132:2837

Cantrell DA, Smith K (1984) The interleukin-2 T-cell system: a new cell growth model. Science 224:1312

Cotner T, Williams JM, Strom TB, Strominger JL (1982) The relationship between early T cell activation antigens and T cell proliferation. In: Hadden JE (ed) Immunopharmacology. 2nd International Symposium, 1983. Pergamon, London, pp 63–68

Cotner T, Williams JM, Christenson L, Shapiro HM, Strom TB, Strominger JL (1983) Simultaneous flow cytometric analysis of human T cell activation antigen expression and DNA content. J Exp Med 157:461

Dinarello CA, Renfer L, Wolff S (1977) Human leukocyte pyrogen: purification and development of a radioimmunoassay. Proc Natl Acad Sci USA 74:4624

Engleman EG, Benike CJ, Charron EJ (1980) Ia antigen on peripheral blood mononuclear leukocytes in man. II. functional studies of HLA-DR-positive T cells activated in mixed lymphocyte reactions. J Exp Med 152:1145

Gaulton GN, Bangs J, Maddock S, Springer T, Eardley DD, Strom TB (1985) Characterization of a monoclonal rat anti-mouse interleukin 2 (IL-2) receptor antibody and its use in the biochemical characterization of the murine IL-2 receptor. Clin Immunol Immunopath 36:18

Gery L, Wakeman BH (1972) Potentiation of the T-lymphocyte response to mitogens. II. The cellular source of potentiating mediators. J Exp Med 136:143

Gillis S, Smith KA (1977) Long term culture of tumor-specific cytotoxic T cells. Nature 268:154

Gillis SM, Ferm M, Ou W et al. (1978) T cell growth factor: parameters of production and a quantitative microassay for activity. J Immunol 120:2077

Gootenberg JE, Ruscetti FW, Mier J, Gazdar A, Gallo RC (1981) Human cutaneous T cell lymphoma and leukemia lines produce and respond to TCGF. J Exp Med 154:1403

Habu S, Raff M (1977) Accessory cell dependence of lectin-induced proliferation of mouse T lymphocytes. Eur J Immunol 7:451

Haynes BF, Hemler M, Cotner T et al. (1981 a) Characterization of a monoclonal antibody (SE9) that defines a human cell surface antigen of cell activation. J Immunol 127:347

Haynes BF, Hemler ME, Mann DL et al. (1981 b) Characterization of a monoclonal antibody (4F2) that binds to human monocytes and to a subset of activated lymphocytes. J Immunol 126:1409

Helderman JH, Strom TB (1979) Role of protein and RNA synthesis in the development of insulin binding sites on activated thymus-derived lymphocytes. J Biol Chem 254:7203

Hunig T, Loos M, Schimpl S (1983) The role of accessory cells in polyclonal T cell activation. 1. Both induction of interleukin-2 production and interleukin-2 responsiveness by concanavalin A are accessory cell dependent. Eur J Immunol 13:1

Iscove N, Melcheras F (1978) Complete replacement of serums by albumin, transferrin, and soybean lipid in cultures of lipopolysaccharide-reactive B cells. J Exp Med 147:923

Kammer GM, Kurrasch R, Scillian JJ (1984) Capping of the surface OKT3 binding molecule prevents the T cell proliferative response to antigens: evidence that this molecule conveys the activation signal. Cell Immunol 87:284

Kaye J, Porcelli S, Tite J, Jones B, Janeway CA (1983) Both a monoclonal antibody and antisera specific for determinants unique to individual cloned helper T cell lines can substitute for antigen and antigen-presenting cells in the activation of T cells. J Exp Med 158:836

Kaye J, Gillis S, Mizel SB, Shevach EM, Malek TR, Dinarello CA, Lachman LB, Janeway CA (1984) Growth of a cloned helper T cell line induced by a monoclonal antibody specific for the antigen receptor: interleukin 1 is required for the expression of receptors for interleukin 2. J Immunol 133:1339

Kelley VE, Naor D, Tarcic N, Gaulton GN, Strom TB (1986) Anti-interleukin-2 receptor antibody suppresses delayed-type hypersensitivity to foreign and syngeneic antigens. J Immunol 137:2122

Kirkman RL, Barrett LV, Gaulton GN, Kelley VE, Koltun WA, Schoen FJ, Ythier A, Strom TB (1985a) The effect of anti-interleukin-2 receptor monoclonal antibody on allograft rejection. Transplantation 40:719

Kirkman RL, Barrett LV, Gaulton GN, Kelley VE, Ythier A, Strom TB (1985b) Administration of an anti-interleukin 2 receptor monoclonal antibody prolongs allograft survival in mice. J Exp Med 162:358

Kupiec-Weglinski JW, Diamantstein T, Tilney NL, Strom TB (1986) Anti-interleukin-2 receptor monoclonal antibody spares T suppressor cells and prevents or reverses acute allograft rejection. Proc Natl Acad Sci USA 83:2624

Landgren U, Anderson J, Wizzell H (1984) Mechanism of T lymphocyte activation by OKT3 antibodies. A general model for T cell induction. Am J Immunol 14:325

Larsson EL, Contino A (1979) The role of mitogenic lectins in T-cell triggering. Nature 280:239

Larsson EL, Iscove NN, Coutinho A (1980) Two distinct factors are required for induction of T-cell growth. Nature 283:664

Leonard WJ, Depper JM, Uchiyama T, Smith KA, Waldmann TA, Greene WC (1982) A monoclonal antibody that appears to recognize the receptor for human T-cell growth factor; partial characterization of the receptor. Nature 300:267

Maizel AL, Mehta S, Ford RJ (1979) T-lymphocyte/monocyte interaction in response to phytohemagglutinin. Cell Immunol 48:388

Meuer SC, Meyer zum Buschenfelde KH (1986) T cell receptor and triggering induces responsiveness to IL-1 and IL-2 but does not lead to T cell proliferation. J Immunol 136:4106

Meuer SC, Hogdon JC, Hussey RE, Protentis JP, Schlossman SF, Reinherz EL (1983) Antigen-like effects of monoclonal antibodies directed at receptors on human T cell clones. J Exp Med 158:988

Meuer SC, Hussey RE, Cantrell DA et al. (1984) Triggering of the T3-Ti antigen receptor complex results in a clonal T cell proliferation through an IL-2 dependent autocrine pathway. Proc Natl Acad Sci USA 81:1509

Miyawaki T, Yachie A, Uwadana N, Ohzeki S, Nagaoki T, Taniguchi N (1982) Functional significance of Tac antigen expressed on activated human lymphocytes: Tac antigen interacts with T cell growth factor in cellular proliferation. J Immunol 129:2474

Moretta A, Mingari MC, Haynes BF, Sekall RP, Moretta L, Fauci AS (1981) Phenotypic characterization of the allogeneic mixed lymphocyte reaction-generated specific cytotoxic human lymphocyte. J Exp Med 153:213

Morgan DA, Ruscetti FW, Gallo R (1976) Selective in vitro growth of T lymphocytes from normal human bone marrow. Science 193:1007

Oppenheim JJ, Leventhal BG, Hersh EM (1968) The transformation of column-purified lymphocytes with non-specific and specific antigenic stimuli. J Immunol 101:262

Osawa H, Diamantenstein T (1983) The characteristics of a monoclonal antibody that binds specifically to rat lymphoblasts and inhibits IL-2 receptor functions. J Immunol 130:51

Palacios R (1982) Concanavalin A triggers T lymphocytes by directly interacting with their receptors for activation. J Immunol 128:337

Palacios R (1985) Mechanisms by which accessory cells contribute in growth of resting T lymphocytes initiated by OKT3 antibody. Eur J Immunol 15:645

Reinherz EL, Meuer SC, Fitzgerald KA, Hussey RE, Levine H, Schlossman SF (1982) Antigen recognition by human T lymphocytes is linked to surface expression of the T3 molecular complex. Cell 30:735

Rinnooy Kan EA, Wang CY, Evans RL (1983) Noncovalently bonded subunits of 22 and 38 kd are rapidly internalized by T cells reacted with anti-Leu-4 antibody. J Immunol 131:536

Rinnooy Kan EA, Platzer E, Welte K, Wang CY (1984) Modulation induction of the T3 antigen by OKT3 antibody is monocyte dependent. J Immunol 133:2979

Rosenstreich DL, Farrar JJ, Dougherty B (1976) Absolute macrophage dependency of T lymphocyte activation by mitogens. J Immunol 116:131

Ruscetti FW, Gallo RC (1981) Human TCGF: regulation of growth and function of lymphocytes. Blood 57:379

Ruscetti FW, Morgan DA, Gallo RC (1977) Functional and morphologic characterization of human T cells continuously grown in vitro. J Immunol 119:131

Seeger RC, Oppenheim JJ (1970) Synergistic interactions of macrophages and lymphocytes in antigen-induced transformation of lymphocytes. J Exp Med 132:44

Sharon M, Klausner RD, Cullen BR, Chizzonite R, Leonard W (1986) Novel interleukin-2 receptor subunit detected by crosslinking under high affinity conditions. Science 234:859

Smith KA (1980) T cell growth factor. Immunol Rev 51:337

Smith KA, Gilbride KJ, Favata MF (1980) Lymphocyte-activating factor promotes T cell growth factor production by cloned murine lymphoma cells. Nature 287:853

Snow EC, Feldbush TL, Oaks JA (1981) The effect of growth hormone and insulin upon mixed leukocyte culture responses and the generation of cytotoxic T lymphocytes. J Immunol 126:161

Stadler BM, Dougherty SF, Farrar JJ, Oppenheim JJ (1982) Relationship of cell cycle to recovery of IL-2 activity from human mononuclear cells. J Immunol 127:1036

Strom TB, Bangs JD (1982) Human serum-free mixed lymphocyte response: the stereospecific effect of insulin and its potentiation by transferrin. J Immunol 126:1555

Terhorst C, Van Agthoven A, LeClair K, Snow P, Reinherz E, Schlossman S (1981) Biochemical studies of the human thymic differentiation antigens. T6, T9, and T10. Cell 23:771

Termiztelen A, Van Leuwen A, Van Rood JJ (1982) HLA-linked lymphocyte activating determinants. Immunol Rev 66:79

Teshigawara K, Wang H-M, Kato K, Smith KA (1987) Interleukin 2 high affinity receptor expression requires two distinct binding proteins. J Exp Med 165:223

Thiele DL, Kurosaka M, Lipsky PE (1983) Phenotype of the accessory cell necessary for mitogen-stimulated T and B cell responses in human peripheral blood: delineation by its sensitivity to the hyposomotropic agent, L-leucine methyl ester. J Immunol 131:2282

Trowbridge IS, Lopez F (1982) Monoclonal antibody to the transferrin receptor blocks transferrin binding and inhibits human tumor cell growth in vitro. Proc Natl Acad Sci USA 79:1175

Trowbridge IS, Omary MB (1981) Human cell surface glycoprotein related to cell proliferation is the receptor for transferrin. Proc Natl Acad Sci USA 78:4514

Tsoukas CD, Landgraf B, Bentin J, Valentine M, Lotz M, Vaughan JH, Carson DA (1985) Activation of resting T lymphocytes by anti-CD3 (T3) antibodies in the absence of monocytes. J Immunol 135:1719

Uchiyama T, Broder S, Waldmann TA (1981 a) A monoclonal antibody (anti-Tac) reactive with activated and functionally mature human T cells. J Immunol 126:1393

Uchiyama T, Nelson DL, Fleisher TA, Waldmann TA (1981 b) A monoclonal antibody (anti-Tac) reactive with activated and functionally mature human T cells II. Expression of Tac antigen on activated cytotoxic killer T cells, suppressor cells, and one of two types of helper cells. J Immunol 126:1398

Unanue ER (1972) The regulatory role of macrophages in antigenic stimulation. Adv Immunol 15:95

Van Wauwe JP, De Mey JR, Goossens JG (1980) OKT3: a monoclonal anti-human T lymphocyte antibody with potent mitogenic properties. J Immunol 124:2708

Weiss MJ, Daley JF, Hogdon JC, Reinherz EL (1984) Calcium dependency of antigen specific (T3-Ti) and alternative (T11) pathways of human T cell activation. Proc Natl Acad Sci USA 81:6836

Weiss A, Imboden J, Shoback D, Stobo J (1984) Role of T3 surface molecules in human T cell activation: T3 dependent activation results in an increase in cytoplasmic free calcium. Proc Natl Acad Sci USA 81:4169

Williams JM, Loertscher R, Cotner T, Shapiro HM, Reddish M, Carpenter CB, Strominger JL, Strom TB (1984 a) Dual parameter flow cytometric analysis of activation antigen expression and T cell subset proliferation in the human mixed lymphocyte reaction. J Immunol 132:2330

Williams JM, Ransil BJ, Shapiro HM, Strom TB (1984b) Accessory cell requirement for activation antigen expression and cell cycle progression by human T lymphocytes. J Immunol 133:2936

Williams JM, Deloria D, Hansen JA, Dinarello CA, Loertscher R, Shapiro HM, Strom TB (1985) The events of primary T cell activation can be staged by use of sepharose-bound anti-T3 (64.1) monoclonal antibody and purified IL-1. J Immunol 135:2249

Ythier A, Williams JM, Shapiro HM et al. (1985a) The early (18 hour) human mixed lymphocyte reaction: identification and isolation of activated T cell clones. Cell Immunol 91:215

Ythier A, Abbud-Filho M, Williams JM et al. (1985b) Interleukin-2 dependent interleukin-3 activity release by T4 positive human T cell clones. Proc Natl Acad Sci USA 82:7020

CHAPTER 3

Membrane Events During Lymphocyte Activation

J. T. RANSOM and J. C. CAMBIER

A. Introduction

Our understanding of the biochemical and biophysical events associated with lymphocyte activation and mitogenesis has grown with improvements in technology and with advances in our knowledge of the regulation of the immune system as a whole. Since receptors peculiar to the immune system apparently utilize signal transduction pathways common in other more extensively studied systems such as muscle and liver, it has been possible to apply techniques and concepts developed previously in other systems to the investigation of B and T cell signaling. As a result our understanding of signal transduction in lymphocytes has progressed rapidly. Indeed, it appears that some novel concepts such as the role of K^+ channels in mitogenesis and the interactions between Ca^{2+}, Na^+, H^+, and K^+ transport mechanisms in the regulation of mitogenesis are now being developed with lymphocytes as model systems. This chapter will focus on the ion transport mechanisms identified in lymphocytes and the changes in their transport properties observed on cell activation by a number of stimuli, e.g., ligand-receptor interaction, nonspecific mitogens, tumor promotors. As one signal transduction mechanism commonly observed in these cells involves turnover of membrane inositol and subsequent activation of protein kinase C, a survey of the literature concerning these phenoma is also included. However, it is clear that in lymphocytes, as in other systems, intracellular mediators interact in a complex and delicately regulated manner, and the reader is urged to read reviews in this volume and elsewhere which address other biochemical events associated with lymphocyte activation (Chaps. 2 and 4).

B. Phosphatidylinositol Turnover (see also Chap. 4)

It is well documented that one commonly shared mechanism of signal transduction involves the rapid degradation of plasma membrane phosphatidylinositol (PtdIns) and its less prevalent polyphosphorylated relatives, phosphatidylinositol 4-phosphate (PtdInsP) and phosphatidylinositol 4,5-bisphosphate (PtdInsP$_2$) (reviewed in BERRIDGE and IRVINE 1984). By an as yet undetermined mechanism, ligand-receptor interaction causes specific breakdown of PtdInsP$_2$, a very minor component of B lymphocyte membrane phospholipids ($\sim 0.05\%$), and inositol lipids ($\sim 1\%$) by intracellular phospholipase C, resulting in formation of diacylglycerol (DAG) and inositol 1,4,5-trisphosphate (InsP$_3$). DAG has been shown to activate the Ca^{2+}/phospholipid-dependent protein kinase C at resting intracellular Ca^{2+} levels, although increasing the Ca^{2+} level greatly enhances protein kinase C activation by DAG (reviewed in Nishizuka 1984). The effect of DAG on protein kinase C can be mimicked by biologically active phorbol esters (e.g., 12-O-tetradecanoylphorbol 13-acetate or TPA) (Castagna et al. 1982) and there is convincing evidence that protein kinase C is the receptor for the tumor-promoting phorbol esters (Niedel et al. 1983). Thus, the phorbol esters as well as lipophilic synthetic analogs of DAG such as diC_8 (LaPetina et al. 1985) have proven to be useful pharmacologic agonists of protein kinase C in investigating its role in signal transduction. The other product of $PtdInsP_2$ degradation, $InsP_3$, which is quickly hydrolyzed within the cell to the di- and monophosphoesters ($InsP$, $InsP_2$) (Storey et al. 1984; Connolly et al. 1985), can induce rapid release of Ca^{2+} ions which have been sequestered in the endoplasmic reticulum (Berridge and Irvine 1984). In vivo, the simultaneous formation of DAG and release of Ca^{2+} ions pursuant to ligand-receptor interaction would serve to activate T cell kinase C optimally. One common phenomenon observed in cells activated via this mechanism is translocation of protein kinase C activity from the cytosol to the membrane where the acidic phospholipids also required for activation are located (reviewed in Sect. C). In an erythrocyte ghost vesicle system it has been shown that protein kinase C translocation results from a synergistic action between TPA and Ca^{2+} ions (Wolf et al. 1985), thus supporting the notion that protein kinase C activation in vitro is optimized by DAG and Ca^{2+}. The PI cycle, or turnover of membrane phosphatidylinositides, has been implicated in transmembrane signaling by the antigen-specific receptors of both B and T cells and constitutes the first detectable event in signal transduction by these receptors.

I. B Cells

Cross-linking of surface immunoglobulin (mIg) with mIg-specific antibodies leads to increased cytosolic levels of $InsP_3$ and $InsP_2$ within seconds and formation of phosphatidic acid (a rapid phosphorylation product of DAG) within minutes (Coggeshall and Cambier 1984; Ransom et al. 1986a). These responses are dependent on mIg cross-linking and are inhibited by elevation of intracellular cAMP levels with theophylline and dibutyryl-cAMP (dbcAMP). The mechanism of inhibition of $PtdInsP_2$ turnover by cAMP is currently unknown, but it has been determined that adenylate cyclase and protein kinase C activities in the membrane of activated cells are inversely correlated, suggesting that cAMP formation inhibits protein kinase C activation in vitro (reviewed by Anderson et al. 1985). Evidence that subsequent B cell responses – Ca^{2+} mobilization, depolarization, increased class II major histocompatibility complex molecule (I-A) message and surface I-A expression – are blocked by elevation of intracellular cAMP levels and can be initiated by exogenously added phospholipase C indicates that subsequent events are dependent on initial $PtdInsP_2$ turnover (Coggeshall and Cambier 1985). In the pre-B lymphocyte cell line 70Z/3, the mitogen lipopolysaccharde (LPS) causes a substantial increase in DAG and $InsP_2$ levels with concomitant decreases in $PtdInsP$ and $PtdInsP_2$, suggesting that LPS promotes $PtdInsP_2$ turnover in these cells (Rosoff and Cantley 1985a). Conversely, TPA and a synthetic analog of DAG, 1-oleyl-2-acetylglycerol (OAG), reduces DAG and $InsP_3$ levels while increasing PtdInsP and $PtdInsP_2$ levels, suggesting that protein kinase C activation may cause increased formation of phosphatidylinositides. However, in splenic B cells, LPS and phorbol myristate acetate (PMA) have no significant effect on polyphosphoinositol formation or DAG levels (BIJSTERBOSCH et al. 1985). It should be noted that this apparent discrepancy, i.e., the occurrence of different biochemical responses with different cell subtypes to identical stimuli, is a frequently recurring observation and suggests that the mechanism of signal transduction may depend on the differentiative stage of the cell.

II. T Cells

In the human T cell line Jurkat, antibodies against the antigen receptor or the T3 complex associated with the receptor (WEISS et al. 1984) cause the rapid formation of inositol phosphates similar to that observed with anti-mIg stimulation of B cells (IMBODEN and STOBO 1985). The mitogenic lectin phytohemagglutinin (PHA) also causes enhanced degradation of $PtdInsP_2$ in both Jurkat cells (SASAKI and HASEGAWA-SASAKI 1985) and in the human T cell lymphoblastoid line CCRF-CEM (HASEGAWA-SASAKI and SASAKI 1983). Formation of $InsP_2$ and $InsP_3$ before InsP, as observed with anti-mIg stimulation of B cells (RANSOM et al. 1987 a), suggests that the PtdInsP and $PtdInsP_2$ are preferentially hydrolyzed in Jurkat cells stimulated with antibodies against the T cell antigen receptor-T3 complex. In murine thymocytes, it has been shown that $InsP_3$ formation occurs rapidly after the addition of concanavalin A (Con A) and the release can be blocked by 8-Br-cAMP, while neither TPA nor A23187 (Ca^{2+} ionophore) has any effect on $InsP_3$ formation (TAYLOR et al. 1984). In the case of PtdInsP and $PtdInsP_2$, Con A, TPA, and A23187 all cause an increase in steady state levels to a similar extent, although with Con A a transient initial decrease was observed owing to the initial breakdown of $PtdInsP_2$ caused by Con A. If the $PtdInsP_2$ turnover is taken into account, the rate of $PtdInsP_2$ synthesis stimulated by Con A is actually tenfold greater than the rates observed with TPA or A23187. These effects are similar to those of TPA and synthetic DAG on the intermediates of $PtdInsP_2$ turnover in the 70Z/3 pre-B cell line (ROSOFF and CANTLEY 1985 a). Further data from the thymocyte study indicate that the pathway (or pathways) responsible for increases in net polyphosphoinositide synthesis may be regulated by both Ca^{2+}-dependent and Ca^{2+}-independent mechanisms. This raises the possibility that both DAG and increased Ca^{2+} levels may activate synthesis of $PtdInsP_2$ by a feedback mechanism.

Finally, a recent study suggests that interleukin 2 (IL-2) does not transduce a signal by phosphatidylinositide hydrolysis (MILLS et al. 1986 b). It was found that addition of IL-2 to IL-2-sensitive human or murine cells affects neither $^{32}PO_4$ incorporation into any of the phosphatidylinositides nor release of any of the ^3H inositol-labeled phosphoinositols from prelabeled cells, although mitogenic lectins affected both parameters. These data suggest that IL-2 must utilize some mechanism of signal transduction other than protein kinase C, perhaps, as suggested by the authors, by direct activation of another protein kinase. It might be argued that the number of IL-2 receptors on these cells is too low to permit resolution of products formed by interaction of IL-2 with its receptor. However, flow cytometric analysis of Ca^{2+} mobilization in the IL-2-dependent cell line HT2 which expresses a high receptor copy number, indicates that IL-2 does not cause Ca^{2+} mobilization, regardless of whether the cells were grown in the presence of IL-2 or starved of IL-2 (J. T. Ransom and J. C. Cambier 1986, unpublished work). This observation supports the conclusion of Mills et al. (1986 a), that IL-2 does not utilize phosphatidylinositide hydrolysis.

C. Protein Kinase C Translocation

The involvement of protein kinase C has been implicated in the activation and proliferation of several cell types as well as in tumor promotion. Detectable protein kinase C activity at the membrane is increased in cells under low density, high growth conditions, in cells which have undergone viral transformation, and in cells exposed to TPA (Anderson et al. 1985). Conversely, under these conditions the activity detectable in the cytosol is decreased, suggesting that the C kinase is translocated from the cytosol to the membrane by an as yet poorly defined mechanism, although DAG and Ca^{2+} are directly involved. Thus, modification of endogenous membrane protein substrates by protein kinase C may be of critical importance to proliferation and tumorigenesis (May et al. 1985). In lymphocytes, the evidence that protein kinase C translocation to the membrane occurs during activation is quite strong.

I. T Cells

Exposure of EL4 thymoma cells to TPA causes a rapid, dose-dependent decrease in cytosolic protein kinase C activity (Kraft et al. 1982). With several different phorbol esters, the same order of potency for reduction of cytosolic protein kinase C was determined as for tumor promoting activity, and it was suggested that modulation of the cytosolic C kinase activity was the result of TPA binding to its receptor, presumably protein kinase C. More recently, it has been shown that IL-2 promotes association of C kinase activity with the membrane of IL-2-dependent murine CT6 cells, with simultaneous removal of activity from the cytosol (Farrar and Anderson 1985). Interleukin 3 produces similar translocation in FDC-P1 cells (Farrar et al. 1985). With each cell type, TPA also induced the translocation phenomenon, although the response was more protracted with TPA, presumably owing to the relatively greater stability of TPA in vivo. Protein phosphorylation studies with A23187, TPA, and PHA have been performed on intact human peripheral lymphocytes and with particulate fractions (Earp et al. 1985; Kaibuchi et al. 1985; Chaplin et al. 1980), and with murine particulate fractions (Harrison et al. 1984; Earp et al. 1984), but we are unaware of studies which have specifically investigated phosphorylation of only plasma membrane proteins in vivo. Although tyrosine-specific kinase activities were found and substrates identified, possible T cell membrane protein substrates for the C kinase remain undefined.

II. B Cells

Evidence indicating that protein kinase C plays a pivotal role in mIg-mediated activation and LPS-mediated mitogenesis of murine B cells is also strong (CAMBIER et al. 1985). Protein kinase C activity in resting B cells stimulated with monoclonal anti-μ, anti-δ, and anti-κ, or with LPS, A23187, or TPA is translocated from the cytosol to the membrane within minutes (CHEN et al. 1986, 1987; NEL et al. 1986). Subsequent to anti-Ig stimulation, (within 10–15 min) the activity is detectable primarily in a detergent-insoluble fraction before returning to the cytosol. These data suggest that protein kinase C is translocated from the cytosol to the plasma membrane and then to cytoskeletal or nuclear compartments of the cell. The anti-mIg-mediated translocation is inhibited by elevation of intracellular cAMP, indicating that PtdInsP$_2$ turnover is required for translocation to occur with these stimuli. Several substrates for tyrosine kinase activity were identified in vivo in human B lymphocytes stimulated with TPA (NEL et al. 1985), but these were found in a Triton-soluble fraction of the cells and could represent both cytosolic and membrane substrates. Phosphorylation of a major 29 kdalton plasma membrane substrate was later observed following stimulation of human B cells with TPA or anti-Ig (NEL 1986). The function of this species is unknown.

Finally, it should be noted that recent findings show that cross-linking of surface major histocompatibility complex class II molecules with monoclonal anti-I-A or anti-I-E causes translocation of protein kinase C activity directly from the cytosol to the detergent-insoluble nuclear component (CHEN and CAMBIER 1986). In addition, incubating B cells with class II-specific antibodies leads to association of a regulatory subunit of protein kinase A with the class II molecules, and increased levels of cAMP via preincubation with either dbcAMP or class II-specific antibodies blocks LPS induction of increased I-A expression (K. NEWELL, L. JUSTEMENT and J. C. CAMBIER 1985, unpublished work). These observations suggest that interaction of surface major histocompatibility complex class II molecules with a ligand simultaneously or prior to B cell stimulation with LPS may inhibit B cell activation by causing removal of the C kinase from the cytosol, thus preventing movement of protein kinase C to the plasma membrane following contact with mitogen. This effect may involve adenylate cyclase and cAMP-dependent protein kinase. Although the evidence is suggestive, at present the hypothesis merits further scrutiny.

In lymphocytes, activation of protein kinase C with either TPA or synthetic analogs of DAG leads to changes in membrane potential, intracellular pH, and intracellular Ca^{2+} levels (discussed in Sect. E). All of these parameters, which have implied roles in lymphocyte activation, are dependent to some degree on the action of a number of active or passive ion transport mechanisms in the plasma membrane. Thus, it would seem reasonable to hypothesize that protein kinase C can cause modification of the activity of these transport mechanisms, either by direct phosphorylation of the transport proteins or indirectly via a cascade of events initiated by the C kinase. To understand how the C kinase might affect various transport processes, it is first necessary to identify what transport mechanisms are present in the lymphocyte membrane. Then, the effects of activation of protein kinase C and other intracellular mediators are more easily interpreted.

D. Electrophysiologic Studies (see also Chap. 4)

The most accurate method of identification and characterization of ion channels in the plasma membrane of small cells is the gigaohm seal patch-clamp technique as described by Hamill et al. (1981). In contrast to earlier electrophysiologic techniques which require insertion of a recording electrode into the cell, this technique involves apposition of a small bore (1 μm) recording microelectrode (usually a drawn-out glass pipette) against the target cell. Gentle back-pressure within the electrode results in formation of a tight seal between the electrode tip and the cell membrane. A further increase in back-pressure causes rupture of the patch of membrane enclosed within the inner diameter of the electrode pipette, leaving the majority of the membrane undisturbed and the cell attached to the tip of the pipette. In this whole-cell recording conformation, as long as a tight seal is maintained between the rim of the pipette tip and the membrane, the cytosolic contents reach a diffusional equilibrium only with the solution originally in the pipette. Therefore, by altering the ionic constituents in the bathing medium or within the pipette, and by incrementally increasing (hyperpolarization) or decreasing (depolarization) the potential difference across the membrane, it is possible to identify voltage-dependent channels in the plasma membrane, evident as current fluctuations across the membrane. The channels can be characterized in terms of a number of parameters, including ion specificity, kinetics and voltage-dependent gating of opening and closing, peak conductance, and approximate number of channels per cell. Patch-clamp studies have clearly identified the presence of voltage-gated K^+ channels and Ca^{2+} channels in lymphocytes and thus aid in the interpretation of results obtained from experiments with radiolabeled ions and ion-sensitive fluorescent probes. Several other reviews which deal specifically with the electrophysiology of lymphocytes have recently been published (Chandy et al. 1985a, b; DeCoursey et al. 1986).

I. K^+ Channels (see also Chap. 4)

1. T Cells and T Cell Lines

Voltage-gated K^+ channels were first described in human peripheral T cells which had been rendered stationary by selective adhesion of a T11-positive subpopulation to solid surfaces with OKT11 monoclonal antibodies (Matteson and Deutsch 1984; Deutsch et al. 1985; Chap. 6) and in nonspecifically "slightly adherent" populations (DeCoursey et al. 1984b; Cahalan et al. 1985). The channels open on depolarization and carry an outward current when the solutions in the pipette and the bath approximate normal physiologic ion contents. At different extracellular K^+ concentrations, reversal potentials were experimentally determined which closely agreed with the K^+ equilibrium potential predicted by the Nernst equation, thereby indicating that the outward current is mediated by K^+ channels. Potassium channels have since been identified in a clonal murine cytotoxic T cell line (Fukushima et al. 1984a), murine helper T cell clone (Lee et al. 1986b), human natural killer (NK) cells (Schlicher et al. 1986), cultured murine macrophages (Ypey and Clapham 1984), human peripheral B cells (Chandy et al. 1985a), and most recently in human helper-inducer (T4$^+$), suppressor-cyto-

Table 1. Properties of K^+ channels in lymphoid cells as determined by the patch-clamp electrophysiologic technique

	CAHALAN et al. (1985)	MATTESON and DEUTSCH (1984)	FUKUSHIMA et al. (1984a)	SCHLICHTER et al. (1986)	YPEY and CAHALAN (1984)
Cell type	Human peripheral T cells ($SRBC^+$)	Human peripheral T cells ($T11^+$)	Clonal murine cytotoxic T cells	Human peripheral natural killer cells	Cultured murine macrophages
Maximum K^+ conductance (nS)	Fresh: 4.5±2.4 ($N=30$) Overnight: 3.9±1.6 ($N=35$)	11.8±2.8 ($N=9$)	3.6±2.9 ($N=36$)	2.3±0.3 ($N=36$)	ND
Single-channel conductances (pS)	9,16	ND	ND	ND	15.7±5.0 ($N=7$)
Current onset (mV) (holding potential)	−40 (−80)	−45 (−70)	−50 (−90)	−50 (−100)	−40 (−80)
Half-maximal conductance (mV)	−40	−36	−36 (est)	ND	ND
Half-maximal inactivation (mV)	−70	ND	ND	ND	ND
Estimated channel no. (density/μm^2)	400 (3)	ND	ND	ND	ND
Relative selectivity	$K^+ > Rb^+ > NH_4^+ > Cs^+ > Na^+$	ND	ND	ND	ND

ND = not done; est = estimated.

toxic (T8$^+$), and human alloreactive cytotoxic T cells (DeCoursey et al. 1986). A summary of some of the properties of the K$^+$ channel identified in the different cell types are shown in Table 1. Analysis of inactivation kinetics and properties are complex. However, it is generally concluded that inactivation is relatively slow and recovery from inactivation is also slow (Cahalan et al. 1985; Fukushima et al. 1984a; Schlichter et al. 1986; Ypey and Clapham 1984). Analysis of the channel properties (Cahalan et al. 1985; DeCoursey et al. 1984b; Fukushima et al. 1984a) strongly suggests that the channel is not a Ca^{2+}-activated K$^+$ channel, but is very similar to the delayed rectifier K$^+$ channel described in nerve and muscle cells (see Cahalan et al. 1985). Furthermore, despite the sensitivity of the K$^+$ current to quinine or quinidine, efforts to demonstrate the presence of a Ca^{2+}-activated K$^+$ channel by studying the effect of a range of intracellular Ca^{2+} concentrations on K$^+$ currents have failed (Cahalan et al. 1985; Fukushima et al. 1984a). Thus, despite data from nonelectrophysiologic studies which suggest that Ca^{2+}-activated K$^+$ channels might be present in lymphocytes (reviewed by Rink and Deutsch 1983), K$^+$ current recordings performed thus far do not support this possibility.

Table 2. Pharmacologic sensitivity of K$^+$ conductance as determined by patch-clamp recordings

	Chandy et al. (1984)	Matteson and Deutsch (1984)	Fukushima et al. (1984a)	Schlichter et al. (1986)	Ypey and Clapham (1984)
K_i (or blocking concentration tested)					
Tetraethyl-ammonium	8 mM	ND	14 mM	ND	+ (10 mM, intra-cellular)
Quinine	14 µM	+ (100 µM)	ND	ND	ND
Quinidine	ND	ND	23 µM	30 µM	ND
4-Aminopyridine	190 µM	ND	ND	368 µM	+ (5 mM)
Ni^{2+}	ND	+ (1 mM)	ND	ND	ND
Verapamil	6 µM	ND	ND	7 µM	ND
Diltiazem	60 µM	ND	ND	ND	ND
Cd^{2+}	ND	ND	ND	343 µM	ND
Ba^{2+} (intracellular)	ND	ND	ND	ND	+ (5 mM)
Cs$^+$ (intracellular)	ND	+ (140 mM)	ND	ND	+ (5 mM)
EGTA (pipette concentration)	ND	ND	− (50 mM)	ND	ND

ND = not done.

Pharmacologic data have helped to characterize the channel and to identify its role in T cell activation. The sensitivity of the channel to various K^+ channel blockers and organic Ca^{2+} channel blockers is summarized in Table 2. It is clear that several defined K^+ channel blockers (4-aminopyridine, quinine, quinidine, tetraethylammonium (TEA), intracellular Cs^+) block the K^+ current in T cells and T cell lines. The K^+ current is also sensitive to agents originally described as Ca^{2+} channel blockers (verapamil, diltiazem, Ni^{2+}, Cd^{2+}) although at concentrations greatly in excess of those required to block voltage-gated Ca^{2+} channels in cardiac tissue (LEE and TSIEN 1983). The results obtained with Ca^{2+} channel blockers suggest that the effect of these blockers on Ca^{2+} movements and mitogenesis may actually be due to a direct effect of the blockers on K^+ channels and membrane potential, and thus a secondary effect on Ca^{2+} influx. The role of the membrane potential on Ca^{2+} fluxes is described further in Sect. E.I.

It has been shown that resting T cells from MRL-n mice express two types of K^+ channels (DeCOURSEY et al. 1985 b). The n-type most resembles the channel expressed by human peripheral T cells while the l-type activates at 20–40 mV more positive potential, inactivates more slowly, and are 100-fold more sensitive to blockage by TEA. The MRL-n mice develop a disease resembling human systemic lupus erythematosus late in life, while MRL-l mice develop the disease early in life and express a large number of functionally abnormal T cells. The predominant channel in the MRL-l T cell is the l-type.

2. B Cells

There is no published electrophysiologic evidence for the existence of similar K^+ channels in B cells, although evidence which indicates the existence of such channels in human B cells has recently been alluded to (CHANDY et al. 1985a). Firm evidence for, and a thorough characterization of, such channels is eagerly anticipated.

3. Variation in K^+ Channel Properties and Density

It has been reported that the mitogens phytohemagglutinin (PHA) and succinyl concanavalin A (Con A) alter the gating properties of the human T cell K^+ channel within 1 min of stimulation, so that the channels open more rapidly and at more negative membrane potentials (DeCOURSEY et al. 1984b). Human T cells cultured for 20 h with Con A expressed a 1.9-fold increase in K^+ current (MATTESON and DEUTSCH 1984). However, human T cells exposed to TPA while in the recording conformation exhibited no immediate increase in K^+ conductance, but after 24–48 h in culture with TPA, the cells exhibited a 1.7-fold increased K^+ conductance (DEUTSCH et al. 1985). DEUTSCH et al. (1985) have proposed that the increases in K^+ conductance within 1 day of mitogen stimulation are due to increased synthesis and insertion of K^+ channels, while DeCOURSEY et al. (1986) have convincingly demonstrated that the immediate effect of lectins is to enhance opening. Thus, it is clear that in human T cells, changes in K^+ channel properties and density correlate with both the short- and long-term effects of mitogenic lectins. In addition, it has been determined that mouse T cells obtained from lymphoid organs express relatively small numbers of K$^+$ channels as compared with human peripheral T cells. However, activation of the murine cells with Con A for 16–54 h leads to a tenfold increase in channel density (DECOURSEY et al. 1985 a). This increase in channel density also appears to be the result of synthesis and insertion of new channels (M.D. CAHALAN 1985, personal communication).

That K$^+$ channels may play an important role in human T cell mitogenesis is suggested by evidence that agents which block the K$^+$ channel also inhibit mitogenesis, IL-2 secretion, and protein synthesis with identical dose potency sequences as for K$^+$ channel blockade (CHANDY et al. 1984; DEUTSCH et al. 1985). Although 4-aminopyridine (K$^+$ channel blocker) inhibits PHA-induced IL-2 production, it does not inhibit a PHA-induced increase in IL-2 receptor expression (GUPTA et al. 1985). Interestingly, it has recently been demonstrated that K$^+$ conductance of the murine IL-2-dependent, noncytolytic T cell line, L2, is increased fourfold within 8 h of addition of IL-2, and remains elevated for 72 h (LEE et al. 1986 b). As the cells leave the cell cycle, the conductance drops to almost the same level as observed before IL-2 addition. The K$^+$ channel blocker quinine inhibits passage of the cells through the cell cycle and reduces the rate of stimulated protein synthesis. Thus, although IL-2 receptor expression is independent of functional K$^+$ channels, IL-2-dependent proliferation apparently is dependent. A role for K$^+$ channels in cell-mediated cytotoxicity has also been implicated by evidence that K$^+$ channel blockers inhibit killing of target cells by human NK cells (SCHLICHTER et al. 1986). The channel blockers do not affect the target cells, but appear to interfere with the formation of effector-target cell conjugates and with the Ca^{2+}-dependent programming stage of lysis which leads to release of NK cytotoxic factor (SIDELL et al. 1986). Finally, in the MRL system, evidence suggests that the n-type (the type found in normal resting T cells; see Sect. D.I.1), but not the l-type K$^+$ channels are required for mitogenesis (DECOURSEY et al. 1985 b).

II. Ca^{2+} Channels (see also Chap. 4)

1. T Cells and T Cell Lines

Attempts to identify one or more voltage-gated Ca^{2+} channels in mouse or human T cells or from T cell lines have been unsuccessful (DECOURSEY et al. 1986; CAHALAN et al. 1985; MATTESON and DEUTSCH 1984; SCHLICHTER et al. 1986; FUKUSHIMA et al. 1984 a). This is somewhat perplexing in light of direct and circumstantial evidence that mitogenic and nonmitogenic stimulation leads to an influx of Ca^{2+} (HESKETH et al. 1985; WHITNEY and SUTHERLAND 1972, 1973; PARKER 1974). One hypothesis (CHANDY et al. 1985 a; DECOURSEY et al. 1986) developed to explain this discrepancy is based on observations that a similar relative potency sequence for agents which block K$^+$ channels is also observed for partial blockade of the mitogen-stimulated rise in intracellular free Ca^{2+}, and that voltage-gated K$^+$ channels also conduct a certain amount of Ca^{2+}. Thus, it has been suggested that the observed Ca^{2+} influx represents "leakage" of Ca^{2+} through the K$^+$ channels which are opened on mitogen binding. An important cautionary note has been made regarding this hypothesis (LEE et al. 1986 a). There is a substantial discrepancy between K_i (the concentration which gives 50% inhibition of the measured response) for channel block by these compounds and the K_i determined for inhibition of mitogenesis which cannot be attributed to serum binding of the compound during culture. In addition, inhibition of proliferation by the channel blockers cannot be overcome by elevation of extracellular Ca^{2+} or by the presence of the Ca^{2+} ionophore ionomycin. Clearly, the K^+ channel is implicated in regulation of Ca^{2+} levels within the cell, and in regulation of proliferation, but the exact nature of this involvement requires further investigation.

2. B Cells, Myelomas, B Cell Lines, and Hybridomas

Patch-clamp studies on the mouse myeloma cell lines S194/5.XXO and a hybridoma (MAb-7B) derived from the fusion of S194 cells with murine splenic B cells have permitted description of a voltage-gated Ca^{2+} channel in cells of B cell lineage (FUKUSHIMA and HAGIWARA 1983, 1985). In addition, flow cytometric analysis of resting murine splenic B cells loaded with the fluorescent Ca^{2+} indicators Quin2 or indo-1 have shown that stimulation with mIg-specific antibodies leads to an increased plasma membrane permeability to Ca^{2+} in less than 1 min (RANSOM et al. 1986a; see Sect. E.II). Characteristics of the Ca^{2+} channel (or increased membrane permeability) and the pharmacologic sensitivities are summarized together in Tables 3 and 4. The peak inward Ca^{2+} current increases as the extracellular Ca^{2+} is increased from 10–15 mM (FUKUSHIMA and HAGIWARA 1983) while decay of the current is due to voltage-dependent inactivation of the channel rather than Ca^{2+}-dependent inactivation (FUKUSHIMA and HAGIWARA 1985). When external Ca^{2+} or Mg^{2+} are reduced to the micromolar range, the channel will carry monovalent cations, and its ability to transport Ca^{2+} ions decreases (FUKUSHIMA and HAGIWARA 1985). The parmacologic sensitivity of the B cell lineage, voltage-dependent Ca^{2+} channel is much different from the L-type channel found in cardiac tissue which is sensitive to micromolar doses of D600 (LEE and TSIEN 1983). FUKUSHIMA et al. (1984b) determined the B cell Ca^{2+} current to be insensitive to 10 μM D600 (a methoxy derivative of the Ca^{2+} channel blocker verapamil) and a similar pharmacologic sensitivity range has been observed for the anti-mIg-induced increase in plasma membrane permeability (RANSOM et al. 1987b). The increased permeability is only sensitive to concentrations of verapamil, diltiazem, and nifedipine, which are approximately 100-fold greater than concentrations which block voltage-dependent Ca^{2+} channels in cardiac and nervous tissues.

3. Variation in Ca^{2+} Current Density

Ca^{2+} currents were studied in the nonsecreting S194 myeloma and in two immunoglobulin-secreting hybridomas (MAb2-1 and MAb-7B) (FUKUSHIMA et al. 1984b). It was determined that the density of Ca^{2+} current was greater in the secreting cells than in the nonsecreting cells, and that the density increased after the cells were transferred to fresh medium. The current density showed no correlation with the cell density, but an increased individual cell secretion level closely paralleled the increased Ca^{2+} current density. The authors concluded that the increase in Ca^{2+} current might be causally related to the increased individual secretion rate, but were cautious to note that the evidence was correlative and that a strong conclusion would require further investigation.

Table 3. Properties of calcium conductance and membrane permeability to calcium as determined by patch-clamp recordings or flow cytometric analysis

	FUKUSHIMA and HAGIWARA (1983)	FUKUSHIMA and HAGIWARA (1985)	FUKUSHIMA et al. (1984b)	RANSOM et al. (1986b, d)
Cell type	Mouse myeloma (S194/5.XXP)	Mouse hybridoma (MAb-7B)	Mouse hybridoma (MAb-7B, MAb2-1) Mouse myeloma (S194)	Mouse spleen (BDF$_1$)
Current onset (mV) (holding potential)	-50 (-90)	-65 (-108)	ND	ND
Current variable between cells	+	+	+	+
Selectivity	$Sr^{2+} > Ba^{2+} > Ca^{2+} > Mn^{2+}$	$Sr^{2+} > Ca^{2+} \sim Ba^{2+} > Mn^{2+} > Mg^{2+}$	ND	ND
Current dependent on [Ca$_o^{2+}$]	+	+	ND	+
Voltage-dependent inactivation	+	+	ND	ND

ND = not done.

Table 4. Pharmacologic sensitivity of B cell calcium conductance and membrane permeability to calcium

	FUKUSHIMA et al. (1984b)	RANSOM et al. (1986d)
K_i (or blocking concentration)		
D600	$+(100\,\mu M)$	ND
Verapamil	ND	$100\,\mu M$
Diltiazem	ND	$100\,\mu M$
Nifedipine	ND	$50\,\mu M$
4-Aminopyridine	ND	$10\,\text{m}M$
Tetraethylammonium	ND	$-(30\,\text{m}M)$
Tetramethylammonium	ND	$-(30\,\text{m}M)$

ND = not done; $-$ = no effect.

III. Na$^+$ Channels (see also Chap. 4)

Evidence against the existence of voltage-gated Na$^+$ channels and against the involvement of Na$^+$ channels in B cell activation is fairly strong. FUKUSHIMA and HAGIWARA (1983) determined that voltage-dependent inward current was independent of external Na$^+$ [Na$_o^+$]. Voltage-activated inward Na$^+$ currents have been detected in a small fraction of human (CAHALAN et al. 1985) and murine T cells (DECOURSEY et al. 1984a) which have properties and sensitivity to tetrodotoxin identical to Na$^+$ channels in excitable cells. A greater density of Na$^+$ channels has also been found in an NK cell line, but as tetrodotoxin has no effect on mitogenesis or on NK activity, it has been difficult to assign a specific role for these channels (CHANDY et al. 1985a).

E. Fluorescent Probe and Radioisotope Studies

Fluorescent probes which are sensitive to fluctuations in the plasma membrane potential (WAGGONER 1979), intracellular pH (RINK et al. 1982), and intracellular free Ca^{2+} concentration (TSIEN et al. 1982b; GRYNKIEWICZ et al. 1985) have greatly improved our ability to investigate alterations in the flux of various ions as mediated by transport complexes in the plasma membrane. Similarly, studies with radiolabeled ions permit investigation of changes in the regulation of specific ion fluxes by the plasma membrane of intact cells. These two techniques are complementary and are frequently utilized in the same report. Therefore, these techniques will be considered together when discussing the observed stimulus-induced shifts in membrane potential, intracellular pH (pH$_i$), and intracellular free Ca^{2+} concentration [Ca$_i^{2+}$]. Of course, these phenomena should also be considered in light of the electrophysiologic evidence which identifies individual ion channel types.

I. Membrane Potential

The membrane potential of murine spleen lymphocytes and B cell-enriched suspensions have been investigated with the carbocyanine dye, diS-C$_3$-(5), and an oxonol dye (Rink et al. 1980). It was concluded that the plasma membranes of both population have a higher permeability to K$^+$ than to Na$^+$, and that the resting membrane potential of approximately -62 mV is primarily dependent on the K$^+$ gradient. Na$^+$ and Cl$^-$ ions appear to make minor contributions to the resting potential. Removal of Ca^{2+} with EGTA or substitution of Ca$_0^{2+}$ with Mg$_0^{2+}$ apparently collapsed the membrane potential, perhaps by enhancing K$^+$ efflux and thus dissipating the K$^+$ gradient (Quastel et al. 1981). Mitogenic stimulation of mouse thymocytes with Con A caused hyperpolarization of the membrane within minutes from a potential of -50 to -70 mV (Tsien et al. 1982a). In this study, it was suggested that the hyperpolarization is a consequence of the rise in Ca$_i^{2+}$ (which may activate a putative Ca^{2+}-dependent K$^+$ channel) and is independent of stimulation of the ouabain-sensitive, electrogenic Na$^+$, K$^+$ pump. Enhanced K$^+$ efflux would tend to hyperpolarize the membrane, but electrophysiologic studies have been unable to identify a Ca^{2+}-activated K$^+$ channel in these cells (see Sect. D.I). Thus, enhanced K$^+$ efflux is probably due to activation of the voltage-gated K$^+$ channel, as observed by DeCoursey et al. (1984b).

T cell hyperpolarization is in contrast to the observation that nonmitogenic (mIg-specific antibodies, A23187, TPA) and mitogenic (LPS) stimulation of murine B cells leads to depolarization of the membrane. This effect, which commences within minutes, is not optimal until 1–2 h after stimulation, as determined with a carbocyanine dye (Monroe and Cambier 1983) or within 2–3 h, as determined by [^{3}H] tetraphenylphosphonium distribution (Kiefer et al. 1980). In the latter study, it was determined that Con A depolarizes T cells, although this event also required several hours to develop. The independent and synergistic induction of B cell depolarization by A23187 and TPA suggests that this event is mediated by protein kinase C activation (Monroe et al. 1984; Ransom and Cambier 1986).

A number of factors, such as the origin of the T cells, e.g., thymus (Tsien et al. 1982a) versus spleen (Kiefer et al. 1980) may contribute to the differing results obtained with T cells and B cells. The different isolation procedures may also affect the relative degree of activation of the populations. In light of evidence that resting T cells obtained from lymphoid organs can be induced by mitogens to increase the channel-mediated K$^+$ current across their membrane to a level similar to that detected in peripheral T cells (DeCoursey et al. 1986), it appears that the degree of activation on maturation of the cells may well be an important consideration. Furthermore, the oxonol technique used by Rink et al. (1980) more accurately reflects very early events (1–10 min) whereas [^{3}H] tetraphenylphosphonium used by Kiefer et al. (1980), which requires a 30-min equilibration time, may more accurately reflect later events. Thus, it is conceivable that T cells initially hyperpolarize and subsequently depolarize over several hours on mitogenic stimulation. The apparent difference between the two cell types following mitogenic stimulation may also be due to a relatively high density of K$^+$ channels on T cells as compared with B cells which have only recently been found to have K$^+$ channels (Chandy et al. 1985a). Unfortunately, a comparative study has not yet been published. However, as it has been shown that the B cell plasma membrane, like the T cell, is more permeable to K^+ than Na^+, and the B cell membrane potential also approximates the equilibrium potential for K^+ (RINK et al. 1980), it may be that an increase in T cell K^+ permeability following lectin stimulation is induced by an intracellular regulatory molecule (or molecules) not operative in the B cell stimulated by anti-mIg.

Evidence that mitogenic (PHA) stimulation of human T cells enhances both $^{42}K^+$ efflux and active transport of $^{42}K^+$ into the cell without any net change in the intracellular K^+ concentration also suggests that mitogens enhance T cell permeability to K^+ (SEGEL and LICHTMAN 1976). Increased efflux of K^+ would generate a diffusion potential and thus hyperpolarize the membrane. The increased K^+ transport into the cell is apparently the result of a PHA-induced increased permeability to Na^+ which in turn elevates the intracellular Na^+ concentration sufficiently to stimulate the Na^+, K^+ pump (SEGEL et al. 1979). Thus, activity of the electrogenic Na^+, K^+ pump would serve to compensate for K^+ loss due to the increased permeability and also hyperpolarize the membrane. An increased permeability to Na^+ would imply the existence of Na^+ channel. However, as patch-clamp studies have suggested that Na^+ channels are present in relatively small numbers, the Na^+ influx may be mediated primarily by other transport proteins such as the Na^+/H^+ exchanger (see Sect. E.III).

A possible role for the membrane potential in lymphocyte activation is suggested by the work of GELFAND et al. (1984a). Results of this study indicated that the magnitude of lectin-induced increases in cytoplasmic Ca^{2+} levels correlated with proliferation, and that extracellular ion substitutions which decreased the membrane potential also decreased lectin-induced Ca^{2+} fluxes. The requirement for a polarized membrane to observe optimal Ca^{2+} flux is similar to the inhibitory effect of K^+ channel blockade on Ca^{2+} influx in B cells (RANSOM et al. 1987b) and on proliferation in T cells (CHANDY et al. 1984) and tends to support the hypothesis that K^+ channels are involved in both Ca^{2+} regulation and proliferation. Another study aimed at investigating the role of membrane potential in lymphocyte activation was performed by DEUTSCH and PRICE (1982b). It was shown that isotonic replacement of K^+ for Na^+ neither stimulated mitogenesis nor inhibited lectin-stimulated mitogenesis in human peripheral blood lymphocytes. Other results showed that isotonic replacement of Na^+ with mannitol (which did not reduce membrane potential) inhibited PHA-induced mitogenesis, even if the replacement was for only 3 h (DEUTSCH et al. 1981). It was concluded that the membrane potential does not play a significant role in the initial stages of mitogenesis. This conclusion is inconsistent with the results of GELFAND et al. (1984a) and illustrates the difficulties encountered in attempting either to dissect mitogenesis into component biochemical and biophysical events or to assign specific roles for the individual events.

II. Intracellular Free Ca^{2+} Levels

A role for Ca^{2+} ions in lymphocyte mitogenesis has been suggested by a number of early studies which demonstrate that T cell mitogenesis is dependent on extracellular Ca^{2+} [Ca_0^{2+}] (WHITNEY and SUTHERLAND 1972) and that mitogens increase $^{45}Ca^{2+}$ uptake (Whitney and Sutherland 1973; Parker 1974). However, evidence that early responses to PHA are independent of $[Ca_0^{2+}]$ and are partially inhibited only by incubations of at least 30 min in Ca^{2+}-free EGTA media indicated that Ca^{2+} influx may be important during later stages of activation (Greene et al. 1976). Resolution of this apparent discrepancy has been aided by the recent development of fluorescent, Ca^{2+}-sensitive dyes, which have the primary advantage of indicating the unbound cytoplasmic Ca^{2+} concentration $[Ca_i^{2+}]$ rather than the total cell Ca^{2+} content as determined by flame photometry, plasma membrane Ca^{2+} fluxes as determined by $^{45}Ca^{2+}$, or current flow through specific channels in the plasma membrane as measured by the patch-clamp technique. Thus, it is now possible to correlate stimulus-induced changes in $[Ca_i^{2+}]$ with $^{45}Ca^{2+}$ flux studies, electrophysiologic channel studies, and total cell Ca^{2+} studies. This represents a tremendous advance since the important parameter in assessing the effect of Ca^{2+} on intracellular processes is $[Ca_i^{2+}]$, which is precisely regulated by a number of active and passive transport processes located in the plasma membrane, the endoplasmic reticulum, the mitochondria, and a vast milieu of membrane-bound and cytoplasmic proteins which tend to buffer $[Ca_i^{2+}]$ (Carafoli and Crompton 1978). Another recent advance in our understanding of $[Ca_i^{2+}]$ regulation is the demonstration that in many cell types, including lymphocytes (Sect. B), specific ligand-receptor interaction leads to the hydrolysis of membrane phosphatidylinositol 4,5-bisphosphate (PtdInsP$_2$). One product, diacylglycerol (DAG), serves to activate the Ca^{2+}/phospholipid-dependent protein kinase C while the other product inositol 1,4,5-trisphosphate (InsP$_3$) promotes release of Ca^{2+} which is stored in the endoplasmic reticulum. The phenomenon of protein kinase C translocation and its dependence on an increase in $[Ca_i^{2+}]$ and DAG levels was reviewed in Sect. C.

It is important to note that in B cells it has been shown that cross-linking of surface immunoglobulin (mIg) with mIg-specific antibodies induces the rapid release of InsP$_3$ (Bijsterbosch et al. 1985; Ransom et al. 1986a), release of intracellular Ca^{2+} stores as well as an influx of Ca^{2+} (Ransom et al. 1987a) and a rapid increase in $[Ca_i^{2+}]$ (Pozzan et al. 1982). Furthermore, it has recently been demonstrated that mIg cross-linking leads to an increased $[Ca_i^{2+}]$ in an entire mIg$^+$ mouse spleen cell population (Ransom et al. 1986b). These findings, coupled with evidence that exogenous addition of InsP$_3$ causes release of preaccumulated $^{45}Ca^{2+}$ from a nonmitochondrial store in permeabilized B cells (Ransom et al. 1986a), suggests that cross-linking of mIg promotes an increase in $[Ca_i^{2+}]$ by releasing endoplasmic reticular stores (via InsP$_3$) and by enhancing opening of Ca^{2+} channels in the plasma membrane by an as yet undetermined mechanism. Recent experiments with a "second generation" Ca^{2+} indicator dye indo-1 suggest that the Ca^{2+} mobilization response is characterized by a rapid $[Ca_i^{2+}]$ increase, presumably due to intracellular release and increased membrane permeability, followed by a rapid decline in $[Ca_i^{2+}]$ (Ransom et al. 1987a). The decline phase may be due to the rapid dephosphorylation of InsP$_3$ to its inactive di- and monophosphoesters (Sect. B) which would permit rapid ATP-dependent resequestration of cytosolic Ca^{2+} into the endoplasmic reticulum (Prentki et al. 1984; Ransom et al. 1986a) and potential-dependent inactivation of the channels (Fukushima and Hagiwara 1983). At present, the most likely candidate responsible for the decline phase is the Ca^{2+}-activated, Mg^{2+}-dependent ATPase described by LICHTMAN et al. (1981) in human peripheral lymphocyte membranes which has a Michaelis constant K_m for Ca^{2+} of 0.55 μM. It was determined that Mg^{2+}, ATP-dependent uptake into inside-out plasma membrane vesicles was stimulated by Ca^{2+}, with a K_m for free Ca^{2+} of 1 μM, and both the ATPase activity and Ca^{2+} uptake were stimulated by calmodulin. Values of $K_m = 1$ μM for Ca^{2+} uptake and 0.55 μM for Ca^{2+}-ATPase activity correlate well with determinations that $[Ca_i^{2+}]$ rises from resting levels of approximately 120 nM to >1 μM in stimulated B cells (POZZAN et al. 1982; RANSOM et al. 1986b). Unfortunately, the effects of TPA or purified protein kinase C on these two activities were not assessed in this study. Finally, it appears that a slight increase in plasma membrane permeability to Ca^{2+} is sustained for at least 30 min in anti-mIg-stimulated B cells (RANSOM et al. 1987a); thus, inactivation of the channels may be slower than activation or Mg^{2+} ATP-dependent Ca^{2+} extrusion may be decreased slightly.

The Ca^{2+} response of mIg[+] splenic B cells to mIg cross-linking is apparently quite different from the response of a transformed pre-B cell line (70Z/3) to the mitogen LPS which induces differentiation of the cells into an IgM (+) phenotype (ROSOFF and CANTLEY 1985a). In these cells, LPS causes a rapid increase of $[Ca_i^{2+}]$ which is independent of $[Ca_0^{2+}]$, enhanced levels of DAG and InsP$_3$, and a decrease in PtdInsP$_2$ and PrdInsP. These results indicate that Ca^{2+} is released from intracellular stores without enhancement of Ca^{2+} influx. Such effects have not been observed in mature B cells in which LPS does not stimulate Ca^{2+} mobilization (J.T. RANSOM, L.K. HARRIS and J.C. CAMBIER 1985, unpublished work) or PdtIns metabolism (GRUPP and HARMONY 1985). Thus, it appears that the mechanism of Ca^{2+} mobilization during B cell activation may be dependent on the type of stimulus used and the maturational state of the cell.

In T cells, there is also evidence that stimulation causes release of intracellular Ca^{2+} stores and an increased plasma membrane permeability to Ca^{2+}, although the majority of experiments have been done with nonspecific mitogens. Only recently have receptor-specific antibodies made it possible to study T3 or the heterodimeric T cell receptor-mediated Ca^{2+} mobilization events. As previously discussed, mitogens enhance $^{45}Ca^{2+}$ uptake yet several early events, but not later events, can occur in Ca^{2+}-deficient medium. It has also been demonstrated that mitogens induce a rapid increase in $[Ca_i^{2+}]$ in freshly isolated thymocytes (HESKETH et al. 1983) and in quiescent, rested thymocytes (HESKETH et al. 1985). It has been shown that a proportion of the response is derived from intracellular sources (HESKETH et al. 1985) while evidence that the response is severely reduced when $[Ca_i^{2+}]$ is decreased to <1 μM (TSIEN et al. 1982a; HESKETH et al. 1985) and restored by returning $[Ca_0^{2+}]$ to 1 mM (TSIEN et al. 1982a) suggests that the response is also partially due to an increased plasma membrane Ca^{2+} permeability. Evidence that reduction of extracellular Na[+] fails to alter the increase in cell Ca^{2+} following succinylCon A stimulation and does not affect resting Ca^{2+} levels (DEUTSCH and PRICE 1982a) argues against the existence of an Na[+]/Ca^{2+} exchange mechanism in T cells.

Recent studies of the effect of antibodies directed against the constant and variable regions of the human T cell receptor (OETTGEN et al. 1985; ROSOFF and

CANTLEY 1985 b) and the T3 complex associated with the receptor (IMBODEN and STOBO 1985; OETTGEN et al. 1985) have indicated that the T cell receptor also transduces signals by elevating $[Ca_i^{2+}]$. OETTGEN et al. (1985) demonstrated that stimulation of the cloned human T cell line HPB-ALL with antibodies against the receptor or the T3 complex initiated an increase in $[Ca_i^{2+}]$ which was dependent on $[Ca_0^{2+}]$ and could be blocked with La^{3+}. In contrast to anti-mIg stimulation of B cells (RANSOM and CAMBIER 1986) monovalent fragments of T3-specific antibodies also induced an increase $[Ca_i^{2+}]$, but with a five- to tenfold lower efficiency, suggesting that receptor cross-linking may not be essential in T cell receptor-mediated $[Ca_0^{2+}]$ mobilization. Hyperpolarization of the cell (with the K^+ ionophore valinomycin) blocked the anti-T3 response while depolarization (with isotonic KCl) blocked either anti-T3 or anti-receptor $[Ca_i^{2+}]$ responses, suggesting that this influx mechanism is sensitive to membrane potential. This result is consistent with that of GELFAND et al. (1984 a) who found that depolarization of peripheral human T cells with isotonic KCl reduced the PHA-induced $[Ca_i^{2+}]$ increase from greater than 100% to only 40%. IMBODEN and STOBO (1985) determined that antibodies against the antigen receptor of the human T cell line Jurkat caused a rapid increase in $[Ca_i^{2+}]$ which was partially independent of $[Ca_0^{2+}]$. Their evidence that T3-specific and receptor-specific antibodies increased cellular levels of the inositol phosphates, and that $InsP_3$ releases Ca^{2+} from permeabilized Jurkat cells indicates that ligation of either component of the T cell antigen-receptor complex mediates Ca^{2+} mobilization via intracellular release and influx mechanisms. However, it should be noted that WT-31, a mitogenic antibody directed against the constant region of the T cell receptor, failed to induce a Ca^{2+} response in normal human peripheral cells while three mitogenic antibodies against T3 increase $[Ca_i^{2+}]$. When assessed with the T cell clone HA1.7, neither WT-31 nor the specific antigen for HA1.7 elicit a Ca^{2+} response while anit-T3 (UCHT1) gives a response similar to that seen with T cells. Pretreatment of the clone with WT-31 led to an enhancement of the response to UCHT1, an effect not observed with peripheral cells. In purified murine spleen T cells, a panspecific rabbit anti-mouse T cell receptor antibody fails to elicit a Ca^{2+} response, just as KJ-16 (anti-constant region) fails to cause Ca^{2+} mobilization in the KJ-16(+) DO.11.10 cell line (M. BEKOFF and J. T. RANSOM 1985, unpublished work). As the latter studies were performed with flow cytometric analysis of cells loaded with indo-1, which permits detection of responsive subpopulations, it is doubtful that the percentage of responsive cells was low enough to escape detection. The role of antigen-presenting cells in these systems remains unclear at present.

It has been shown that monocytes, which appear to have an accessory role in the T cell proliferation response to antigens and mitogens, may also play a role in generation of a Ca^{2+} signal (LEDERMAN et al. 1984). Using E-rosette (+), i.e., T11 antigen-positive human peripheral blood cells and an E-rosette (−) fraction or the monocyte-like human cell line U-937, it was found that the proliferative response of E-rosette (+) cells to *Staphylococcus aureus* protein A was completely restored only by monocytes which had interacted with the protein A. Furthermore, only protein A-pretreated U-937 cells were capable of eliciting an increase in $[Ca_i^{2+}]$ or E-rosette (+) cells. Thus, the authors conclude that protein A activation of T cells requires T cell-monocyte interaction since supernatants of protein

A-treated monocytes had no effect and the activation may be dependent on the ability of the pretreated monocyte to increase plasma membrane Ca^{2+} permeability.

Although T cell mitogens such as PHA and Con A induce a rapid Ca^{2+} response and enhance phosphatidylinositol turnover (MAINO et al. 1975), several reports suggest that the mobilization of Ca_i^{2+} may represent one of at least two independent signal pathways leading to T cell activation. GELFAND et al. (1985) have demonstrated that pretreatment of human peripheral T cells with TPA, which serves as a comitogen with lectins and can replace the requirement for accessory cells, permits PHA-induced mitogenesis, even under conditions where a Ca^{2+} influx is prohibited on binding of lectin. As TPA alone is nonmitogenic, these results suggest that binding of PHA generates a calcium-independent signal as well as a calcium-dependent one which may explain the observation of GREEN et al. (1976) that early responses to PHA are independent of $[Ca_0^{2+}]$. These observations have been expanded with the demonstration that inhibition of a Ca^{2+} influx blocks PHA-induced IL-2 secretion, but will not inhibit IL-2 receptor expression (MILLS et al. 1985a). However, it has been shown that Ca^{2+} ionophores can induce expression of the IL-2 receptor (KORETZKY et al. 1983), although this may have been due to nonspecific activation of phospholipases or protein kinase C, as discussed by KAIBUCHI et al. (1985), in view of the large doses of ionphore used (approximately 1 μM). The proliferative response of IL-2 receptor-bearing T cells to IL-2 can proceed normally in the absence of extracellular Ca^{2+} while binding of IL-2 does not generate a Ca^{2+} response in IL-2 receptor-bearing cells (MILLS et al. 1985b; O'FLYNN et al. 1985; J.T. RANSOM and J.C. CAMBIER 1985, unpublished work). These results suggest that the Ca^{2+}-requiring step in lectin-induced mitogenesis of T cells is neither the induction of IL-2 receptor expression nor the generation of a signal when IL-2 binds to its receptor. Studies with suboptimal concentrations of PHA, which fail to evoke a Ca^{2+} response, in the presence or absence of exogenous IL-2, suggest that the poor mitogenic and IL-2 receptor expression responses at low PHA concentrations are due to the inability of the cells to increase production of IL-2 (MILLS et al. 1985d). Restoration of the proliferative response under these conditions by low concentration of Ca^{2+} ionophore or accessory cells indicates that the Ca^{2+} response is important for secretion of IL-2. Furthermore, inhibition by antibodies against IL-2 or its receptor of the proliferative response induced by a suboptimal PHA dose in combination with the Ca^{2+} ionophore or accessory cells indicates that restoration of the response is linked to the action of IL-2. Thus, the overall conclusions of these studies are that IL-2 secretion, but not IL-2 receptor expression or IL-2-dependent signaling, is dependent on a Ca^{2+} influx, and that mitogenic lectins may activate both Ca^{2+}-independent and Ca^{2+}-dependent pathways leading to expression of the IL-2 receptor.

Evidence that mitogen or anti-receptor stimulation causes an influx of Ca^{2+} in T cells is inconsistent with the electrophysiologic studies which have been unable to detect any depolarization or mitogen-induced Ca^{2+} movement across the plasma membrane. It has been proposed that T cell K^+ channels which have been demonstrated to be capable of also passing Ca^{2+} current, are actually the channel responsible for Ca^{2+} influx (DECOURSEY et al. 1986). Since it has been shown that several T cell responses to mitogen are blocked by these agents (see Sect. D.I.3) at doses which block K^+ channels, but greatly in excess of those which block classically studied Ca^{2+} channels, it has been suggested that K^+ channels are vital to T cell activation (CHANDY et al. 1984). Furthermore, evidence suggests that mitogen-induced Ca^{2+} mobilization is also inhibited by these agents, but only at doses which block K^+ current in patch-clamp studies (LEE et al. 1986a). It can also be shown that anti-mIg-indcued Ca^{2+} influx is blocked by the same agents in the identical dose range (RANSOM et al. 1987b). Thus, as Ca^{2+} channels and K^+ channels have both been identified in cells of the B cell lineage, two possibilities are apparent. Either K^+ channels in B and T cells pass Ca^{2+} ions as well as K^+, or T cells have Ca^{2+} channels at such low density that they have escaped detection and the gating of the putative Ca^{2+} channel is dependent on an unblocked, functional K^+ channel. Other alternatives are also possible and resolution of this question is a key issue in the understanding of the role of ion movements in regulation of lymphocyte activation.

III. Cytoplasmic Alkalinization

A membrane-mediated phenomenon receiving much attention recently is the activation of an Na^+/H^+ antiport system which results in the elevation of both the intracellular Na^+ level $[Na_i^+]$ and intracellular pH (pH_i). Using the weak acid $[^{14}C]$ DMO GERSON et al. (1982) first observed that Con A or LPS stimulation of mouse spleen lymphocytes induces elevation of pH_i from 7.2 to approximately 7.4 for 6–8 h, followed by a return to 7.2 and then a more prolonged yet also transient elevation of pH_i. As the initial increase correlated with increased metabolite, RNA, and protein synthesis, while the second rise correlated well with increased DNA synthesis, it was suggested that the increased pH_i might shift various kinase reaction kinetics to favor increased metabolism and mitotic activity. However, closer scrutiny of the cause of greater accumulation of $[^{14}C]$ DMO in actively cycling cells demonstrated that the weak acid was also partitioned into the mitochondrial compartment of the cells (GRINSTEIN et al. 1984). It was clearly demonstrated that actively cycling cells contained 2.5-fold more mitochondria per unit cell volume, which is sufficient to account for the increased $[^{14}C]$ DMO accumulation in such actively cycling cells. This does not, however, rule out the possibility that alkalinization occurs rapidly in activated, but not cycling cells. DEUTSCH et al. (1984) used a ^{19}F nuclear magnetic resonance technique to study intracellular pH and were unable to detect any indication of cytoplasmic alkalinization in mitogen-stimulated human peripheral blood lymphocytes. These findings support the observations of MILLS et al. (1986a) that inhibitors of Na^+/H^+ exchange fail to block lectin-induced mitogenesis.

It has been clearly demonstrated that both LPS and TPA cause an increase in pH_i within minutes in the pre-B cell line 70Z/3 (ROSOFF et al. 1984). Anti-mIg or TPA stimulation of mouse spleen B cells also induces cytoplasmic alkalinization (RANSOM and CAMBIER 1986). Both cytoplasmic alkalinization and elevation of $[Na_i^+]$ are dependent on $[Na_o^+]$ and can be blocked by amiloride while LPS induction of differentiation is inhibited by amiloride and can be mimicked by the Na^+/H^+ exchange ionophore monensin or the inhibitor of the Na^+/K^+-ATPase, ouabain (ROSOFF and CANTLEY 1983; ROSOFF et al. 1984). These results indicate that activation of Na^+/H^+ exchange accompanies stimulation of a pre-B cell line and resting normal B cells, and suggest that activation of the exchanger can be mediated by protein kinase C. However, it has not yet been clearly demonstrated whether an increase in either $[Na_i^+]$ or pH_i alone are necessary and/or sufficient for B cell activation.

A larger body of literature concerning the regulation and role of Na^+/H^+ exchange exists for T cells than for B cells. In T cells it has been shown that Na^+/H^+ exchange is activated by osmotic cell shrinking in rat thymocytes (a condition which initiates the regulatory volume increase response, Sect. E.IV) or by phorbol esters (GRINSTEIN et al. 1985b) and IL-2 (MILLS et al. 1985c). The extensive similarities between osmotic and TPA induction of Na^+/H^+ exchange and similar susceptibilities to inhibition under these conditions would suggest that the osmotic compensation may depend on activation of protein kinase C which in turn activates Na^+/H^+ exchange (GRINSTEIN et al. 1985b). However, recent data obtained from rat thymocytes which had been depleted of cytosolic and detergent-soluble protein kinase C activity by pretreatment with TPA shows that Na^+/H^+ exchange can still be induced by hypertonic treatment of these cells (GRINSTEIN et al. 1986). As TPA can no longer induce exchange activity in the pretreated cells, it is concluded that hypertonic activation of the exchange activity does not require protein kinase C. It has been shown that antibodies against T3 or the T cell receptor, as well as phorbol esters, can stimulate Na^+/H^+ exchange activity in the human T cell line HPB-ALL (ROSOFF and CANTLEY 1985b). Several interesting aspects of regulation of the exchange process were demonstrated in this study. The T3-mediated enhancement was dependent on $[Ca_0^{2+}]$ while the TPA-mediated effect was not. Furthermore, simultaneous addition of TPA and T3-specific antibodies (OKT3) led to an additive enhancement of Na^+/H^+ exchange, but preincubation with TPA abolished the response to OKT3. Hence, it is clear that protein kinase C plays a role in activation of the Na^+/H^+ exchange mechanism in lymphocytes, although an alternative activation pathway may also exist. It also appears that preactivation of the kinase serves to regulate receptor-mediated signal transduction by a feedback mechanism.

Activation of Na^+/H^+ exchange by either IL-2 or the cytoplasmic alkalinization observed on mitogenic lectin stimulation of T cells is apparently not required for proliferation of T cells (MILLS et al. 1985c, 1986a). To avoid the problem of the inhibitory effects of amiloride (a diuretic which blocks the proliferative response to growth factors) on protein kinase C, MILLS et al. (1985c) used amiloride analogs to block Na^+-dependent alkalinization and IL-2-induced alkalinization. Since the analogs failed to block IL-2-induced proliferation, it was concluded that alkalinization is not essential for IL-2-dependent proliferation. In another study, MILLS et al. (1986) demonstrated that, even at concentrations of amiloride analogs tenfold greater than those required to inhibit exchange activity, the drugs were unable to block either PHA-induced mitogenesis or increased IL-2 receptor expression in human peripheral lymphocytes. Nor could the analogs block the comitogenic effects of lectins with either IL-2 or TPA in human thymocytes. These results suggest that cytoplasmic alkalinization is not required for either T cell mitogenesis or T cell activation. Interesting data which sheds some light on a possible role for cytoplasmic alkalinization has been presented by Grinstein and Goetz (1986). It was found that elevation of the intracellular pH with monensin or NH_3, but not an increase in intracellular Na^+ with ouabain or gramicidin led to an increase in $[Ca_i^{2+}]$. These data indicate that intracellular pH may play an important role in regulating $[Ca_i^{2+}]$. It might be argued that TPA does not cause an increase in $[Ca_i^{2+}]$, even though it rapidly induces cytoplasmic alkalinization. However, TPA actually reduces $[Ca_i^{2+}]$, perhaps by increasing Mg^+, ATP-dependent Ca^{2+} extrusion (Ransom et al. 1987b), and this effect would prevent any increases in $[Ca_i^{2+}]$ that might otherwise be caused by TPA-mediated alkalinization. Further work should resolve whether the effect of alkalinization alone is mediated by an inhibition of Ca^{2+} extrusion at the plasma membrane or by an effect on the influx of Ca^{2+} across the plasma membrane. The observations of Deutsch and Price (1982a) that the increase in cell calcium, as measured by $^{45}Ca^{2+}$ accumulation, which follows succinylCon A stimulation of T cells is unaffected by a low extracellular Na^+ concentration (63 mM) would tend to suggest that $[Ca_i^{2+}]$ may be independent of extracellular Na^+. However, this study did not investigate Na^+/H^+ exchange under these conditions, and it is uncertain to what extent a partial reduction in extracellular Na^+ affects cytoplasmic alkalinization.

IV. Regulatory Volume Responses

Lymphocytes, along with many different cell types, compensate for the swelling or shrinking which initially occurs when they are subjected to hypotonic or hypertonic media by returning to nearly their original volume. The responses are apparent within minutes and complete within 30 min. Regulatory volume decrease (RVD) and regulatory volume increase (RVI) refer to the cellular responses observed in hypotonic and hypertonic media respectively. The two responses result from the redistribution of anions and cations, owing to changes in membrane permeability to specific ions, and result in adjustment of the osmolarity within the cell toward that of the medium. Near equilibration of the osmotic gradient across the plasma membrane results in the compensatory increase or decrease in cell water content which is apparent as an adjustment in cell volume. Although RVD and RVI have not been demonstrated to be directly involved in lymphocyte activation, the ionic basis for these changes provides a great deal of information regarding transport phenomena in lymphocytes. As it has been shown that RVI-activated Na^+/H^+ exchange in T cells (Grinstein et al. 1985a, b) and hypotonic treatment of T cells inhibits lectin-induced mitogenesis (Deutsch et al. 1982), it appears that the underlying mechanisms of RVD and RVI may be indirectly involved in lymphocyte activation. Again, the majority of the work to date has been performed on T cells. Indeed, the greatly reduced RVD response observed in cells of B cell lineage as compared with T cells can be used as a rapid diagnostic tool to determine the B cell or T cell lineage of lymphocytic leukemias (Gelfand et al. 1984b).

The ionic basis of RVD in human thymic, tonsillar, and peripheral blood lymphocytes was investigated by Cheung et al. (1982a) to determine why the tonsillar lymphocytes, in contrast to the peripheral cells, failed to restore their isotonic volume following the initial swelling in hypotonic media. It was shown that RVD in peripheral, thymic, and tonsillar T lymphocytes was characterized by a loss of $^{86}Rb^+$ (a radioisotope commonly used as a substitute for $^{42}K^+$) and a decrease in cellular K^+ content, suggesting that an increase in K^+ permeability occurs. It was also shown by CHEUNG et al. (1982 b) that ouabain-sensitive and ouabain-insensitive components of enhanced $^{86}Rb^+$ influx are induced by hypotonic stress while Na^+ content and Na^+ efflux are unaffected. Their evidence that high K^+ or high Rb^+ media blocked RVD and revealed a secondary swelling phase supports the proposal that K^+ efflux mediates RVD initially and indicates that a secondary ion permeability (discussed later in this section) is also present. The ensuing efflux of K^+ would reduce the intracellular osmolarity, and the passive redistribution of water then tends to restore the cell volume. In contrast, tonsillar B cells demonstrate only a minor increase in K^+ permeability during hypotonic stress and thus are only partially able to restore their original volume. CHEUNG et al. (1982 a) reported preliminary studies which indicate that an increase in anion conductance develops in hypotonically stressed T cells and B cells alike. This phenomenon was further investigated in tonsillar B cells by GRINSTEIN et al. (1983). It was demonstrated that, if the permeability to exogenous cations such as Na^+ is increased by the channel-forming ionophore gramicidin, then hypotonic swelling leads to a secondary volume increase in both T and B cells. As the effect was not observed when Cl^- in the media was replaced by large impermeant anions such as gluconate or SO_4^{2-}, the effect was presumed to be due to Cl^- influx resulting from an increased permeability to Cl^-. The direction of Cl^- movement is mediated by the electrochemical gradient of the permeant ions, in this case, the gradient is mediated by depolarization of the membrane (owing to the increased Na^+ permeability) which drives Cl^- in. When choline is substituted for Na^+, gramicidin transports K^+ out of the cell (resulting in hyperpolarization), the electrochemical gradient drives Cl^- out, and a volume decrease is observed. Consistent with an increased Cl^- permeability, it was shown that hypotonicity enhances $^{36}Cl^-$ efflux under normal conditions. Furthermore, it was shown that hypotonic stress depolarizes the cells and the equilibrium potential for Cl^- was calculated to be -38 mV, substantially less negative than the resting membrane potential of -60 mV. Thus, it could be concluded that enhanced Cl^- efflux was not due to an increase in membrane potential, but rather to an increased Cl^- permeability and resetting of the membrane potential toward the equilibrium potential for Cl^-. It should be noted that the secondary Cl^- conductance pathway has also been characterized in T cells by GRINSTEIN et al. (1982 a, b). Thus, it is clear that during hypotonic stress of T cells an increased K^+ permeability develops, resulting in K^+ efflux and reshrinking of the cell.

In B cells this permeability does not develop, and consequently no K^+-mediated shrinking can occur. In both cell types hypotonic stress enhances Cl^- permeability and Cl^- efflux increases, causing only a minor reshrinking in B cells, and perhaps some undetermined minor component of the RVD in T cells. Inhibition of the $^{86}Rb^+$ (K^+) efflux pathway in T cells by quinine (GRINSTEIN et al. 1982 b) is similar to the inhibition by quinine (and other K^+ channel blockers) of the voltage-gated K^+ channel described in Sect. D.I.1. The apparent lack of these channels in B cells and the absence of a statistically significant enhanced K^+ efflux in hypotonically stressed B cells would suggest that RVD in T cells may be mediated through activation of the K^+ channels described by the electrophysiologists. If this were indeed the case, then activation of these two efflux pathways during mitogen stimulation of T cells, and only the Cl^- efflux pathway during anti-mIg stimulation of B cells, could explain why T cells hyperpolarize initially (Tsien et al. 1982a), then become depolarized (Kiefer et al. 1980), while B cells have only been observed to depolarize (Monroe and Cambier 1983). Clearly, further work is required to verify the hypothesis, but currently it represents the most compatible explanation for apparently disparate events. Initial studies toward this end have been presented by Deutsch et al. (1986) who have shown that noncycling L2 cells (a noncytolytic T cell clone) exhibit no RVD. When the cells are provided with exogenous IL-2 they initiate DNA synthesis, exhibit fourfold increased K^+ conductance and demonstrate RVD. The RVD response is blocked by quinine and verapamil (see Sect. D.I.1) and by 90 mM KCl. These data suggest that the enhanced K^+ permeability of RVD is mediated by the voltage-gated K^+ channel detected in T cells.

An increased volume (RVI) in response to hypertonic shrinking is also apparent in human peripheral blood lymphocytes and rat thymocytes. An investigation into the mechanism of RVI has recently been presented by Grinstein et al. (1985a). Upon hypertonic shock, the Na^+/H^+ exchange system is shifted from a quiescent state to an active state. Alkalinization of the interior consequently leads to compensatory efflux of HCO_3^- via an HCO_3^-/Cl^- exchange system whose presence in lymphocytes has been indirectly indicated. The net result of enhanced activity of the two exchangers is the accumulation of NaCl, and hence an increased intracellular osmolarity. Data are presented which suggest that activation of the Na^+/H^+ exchanger is set by the interaction between protons and a kinetic modifier site. The threshold for activation is a function of the extent of protonation of the modifier site which is distinct from the substrate (H^+) binding site. On shrinking, the threshold for activation is shifted to more alkaline levels as the result of an alteration in sensitivity of the modifier to intracellular pH. Although the mechanism whereby shrinking alters pH sensitivity of the modifier is not addressed, the hypothesis is consistent with the observations. Further characterization of the interaction between HCO_3^-/Cl^- exchange, Na^+/H^+ exchange, osmotic shrinking, and intracellular pH should prove helpful in understanding how the different transport complexes interact and, ultimately, regulate lymphocyte activation.

References

Anderson WB, Estival A, Tapiovaara H, Gopalakrishna R (1985) Altered subcellular distribution of protein kinase C (a phorbol ester receptor). Possible role in tumor promotion and the regulation of cell growth: relationship to changes in adenylate cyclase activity. In: Cooper DMF, Seamon KB (eds) Advances in cyclic nucleotide and protein phosphorylation research, vol 9. Raven, New York, pp 287–306

Berridge MJ, Irvine RF (1984) Inositol trisphosphate, a novel second messenger in cellular signal transduction. Nature 312:315–321

Bijsterbosch MK, Meade JC, Turner GA, Klaus GGB (1985) B lymphocyte receptors and polyphosphoinositide degradation. Cell 41:999–1006

Cahalan MD, Chandy KG, De Coursey TE, Gupta S (1985) A voltage gated potassium channel in human lymphocytes. J Physiol (Lond) 358:197–237

Cambier JC, Monroe JG, Coggeshall KM, Ransom JT (1985) On the mechanisms of trans-membrane signaling by membrane immunoglobulin. Immunol Today 6:218–222

Carafoli E, Crompton M (1978) The regulation of intracellular calcium. In: Bronner F, Kleinzeller A (eds) Current topics in membranes and transport, vol 10. Academic, New York, pp 151–216

Castagna M, Takai Y, Kaibuchi K, Sano K, Kikkawa U, Nishizuka Y (1982) Direct activation of calcium-activated, phospholipid-dependent protein kinase by tumor-promoting phorbol esters. J Biol Chem 257:7847–7851

Chandy KG, DeCoursey TE, Cahalan MD, McLaughlin C, Gupta S (1984) Voltage-gated potassium channels are required for human lymphocyte activation. J Exp Med 160:369–385

Chandy KG, DeCoursey TE, Cahalan MD, Gupta S (1985a) Ion channels in lymphocytes. J Clin Immunol 5:1–6

Chandy KG, DeCoursey TE, Cahalan MD, Gupta S (1985b) Electroimmunology: the physiologic role of ion channels in the immune system. J Immunol 135:787s–791s

Chaplin DD, Wedner HJ, Parker CW (1980) Protein phosphorylation in human peripheral blood lymphocytes: mitogen-induced increases in protein phosphorylation in intact lymphocytes. J Immunol 124:2390–2398

Chen ZZ, Coggeshall KM, Cambier JC (1986) Translocation of protein kinase C during membrane immunoglobulin mediated transmembrane signaling in B lymphocytes. J Immunol 136:2300–2304

Chen ZZ, McGuire JC, Leach KL, Gambier JC (1987) Transmembrane signaling through B cell MHC class II molecules: anti-Ia antibodies induce protein kinase C translocation to the nuclear fraction. J Immunol 138:2345–2352

Cheung RK, Grinstein S, Dosch H-M, Gelfand EW (1982a) Volume regulation by human lymphocytes: Characterization of the ionic basis for regulatory volume decrease. J Cell Physiol 112:189–196

Cheung RK, Grinstein S, Gelfand EW (1982b) Volume regulation by human lymphocytes. Identification of differences between the two major lymphocyte subpopulations. J Clin Invest 70:632–638

Coggeshall KM, Cambier JC (1984) B cell activation. VIII. Membrane immunoglobulins transduce signals via activation of phosphatidylinositol hydrolysis. J Immunol 133:3382–3386

Coggeshall KM, Cambier JC (1985) B cell activation. VI. Studies of modulators of phospholipid metabolism suggest an essential role for diacylgercerol in transmembrane signalling by mIg. J Immunol 134:101–107

Connolly TM, Bross TE, Majerus PW (1985) Isolation of a phosphomonoesterase from human platelets that specifically hydrolyzes the 5-phosphate of inositol 1,4,5-trisphosphate. J Biol Chem 260:7868–7874

DeCoursey TE, Chandy KG, Fischbach M, Talal N, Cahalan MD, Gupta S (1984a) Differences in ion channel expression in T lymphocytes from MRL-lpr and MrL $-+/+$ mice. Fed Proc 43:1736

DeCoursey TE, Chandy KG, Gupta S, Cahalan MD (1984b) Voltage-gated K^+ channels in human T lymphocytes: a role in mitogenesis? Nature 307:465–468

DeCoursey TE, Chandy KG, Fischbach M, Talal N, Gupta S, Cahalan MD (1985a) Potassium channel expression in proliferating murine T lymphocytes. Fed Proc 44:1310

DeCoursey TE, Chandy KG, Fischbach M, Talal N, Gupta S, Cahalan MD (1985b) Two types of K channels in T lymphocytes from MRL mice. Biophys J 47:387A

DeCoursey TE, Chandy KG, Gupta S, Cahalan MD (1986) Voltage-dependent ion channels in T-lymphocytes. J Neuroimmunol 10:71–95

Deutsch C, Price M (1982a) Cell calcium in human peripheral blood lymphocytes and the effect of mitogen. Biochem Biophys Acta 687:211–218

Deutsch C, Price M (1982b) Role of extracellular Na and K in lymphocyte activation. J Cell Physiol 113:73–79

Deutsch C, Price MA, Johansson C (1981) A sodium requirement for mitogen-induced proliferation in human peripheral blood lymphocytes. Exp Cell Res 136:359–369

Deutsch C, Slater L, Goldstein P (1982) Volume regulation of human peripheral blood lymphocytes and stimulated proliferation of volume adapted cells. Biochem Biophys Acta 721:262–267

Deutsch C, Taylor JS, Price M (1984) pH homeostasis in human lymphocytes: modulation by ions and mitogen. J Cell Biol 98:885–893

Deutsch C, Krause D, Lee SC (1985) Votage-gated potassium conductance in human T lymphocytes stimulated with phorbol ester. J Physiol (Lond) 358:35

Deutsch C, Patterson J, Price M, Lee S, Prystowsky M (1986) Volume regulation in cloned T-lymphocytes. Biophys J 49:162 A

Earp HS, Austin KS, Buessow SC, Dy R, Gillespie GY (1984) Membrane from T and B lymphocytes have different patterns of tyrosine phosphorylation. Proc Natl Acad Sci USA 81:2347–2351

Earp HS, Austin KS, Gillespie GY, Buessow SC, Davies AA, Parker PJ (1985) Characterization of distinct tyrosine-specific protein kinase C in B and T lymphocytes. J Biol Chem 260:4351–4356

Farrar WL, Anderson WB (1985) Interleukin-2 stimulates association of protein kinase C with plasma membrane. Nature 315:233–235

Farrar WL, Thomas PT, Anderson WB (1985) Altered cytosol/membrane enzyme redistribution on interleukin-3 activation of protein kinase C. Nature 315:235–237

Fukushima Y, Hagiwara S (1983) Voltage-gated Ca^{2+} channel in mouse myeloma cells. Proc Natl Acad Sci USA 80:2240–2242

Fukushima Y, Hagiwara S (1985) Currents carried by monovalent cations through calcium channels in mouse neoplastic B lymphocytes. J Physiol (Lond) 358:255–284

Fukushima Y, Hagiwara S, Henkart M (1984a) Potassium current in clonal cytotoxic T lymphocytes from the mouse. J Physiol (Lond) 351:645–656

Fukushima Y, Hagiwara S, Saxton RE (1984b) Variation of calcium current during the cell growth cycle in mouse hybridoma lines secreting immunoglobulins. J Physiol (Lond) 355:313–321

Gelfand EW, Cheung RK, Grinstein S (1984a) Role of membrane potential in the regulation of lectin-induced calcium uptake. J Cell Physiol 121:533–539

Gelfand EW, Cheung RK, Ha K, Grinstein S (1984b) Volume regulation in lymphoid leukemia cells and assignment of cell lineage. N Engl J Med 311:939–944

Gelfand EW, Cheung RK, Mills GB, Grinstein S (1985) Mitogens trigger a calcium-independent signal for proliferation in phorbol-ester-treated lymphocytes. Nature 315:419–420

Gerson DF, Kiefer H, Eufe W (1982) Intracellular pH of mitogen-stimulated lymphocytes. Science 216:1009–1010

Greene WC, Parker CM, Parker CW (1976) Calcium and lymphocyte activation. Cell Immunol 25:74–89

Grinstein S, Goetz JD (1986) Control of free cytoplasmic calcium by intracellular pH in rat lymphocytes. Biochem Biophys Acta 819:267–270

Grinstein S, Clarke CA, DuPre A, Rothstein A (1982a) Volume-induced increase of anion permeability in human lymphocytes. J Gen Physiol 80:801–823

Grinstein S, DuPre A, Rothstein A (1982b) Volume regulation by human lymphocytes: role of calcium. J Gen Physiol 79:849–868

Grinstein S, Clarke CA, Rothstein A, Gelfand EW (1983) Volume-induced anion conductance in human B lymphocytes is cation independent. Am J Physiol 245:C160–163

Grinstein S, Cohen S, Lederman HM, Gelfand EW (1984) The intracellular pH of quiescent and proliferating human and rat thymic lymphocytes. J Cell Physiol 121:87–95

Grinstein S, Cohen S, Goetz JD, Rothstein A (1985a) Na^+/H^+ exchange in volume regulation and cytoplasmic pH homeostasis in lymphocytes. Fed Proc 44:2508–2512

Grinstein S, Cohen S, Goetz JD, Rothstein A (1985b) Osmotic and phorbol ester-induced activation of Na^+/H^+ exchange: possible role of protein phosphorylation in lymphocyte volume regulation. J Cell Biol 101:269–276

Grinstein S, Mack E, Mills GB (1986) osmotic activation of the Na^+/H^+ antiport in protein kinase C-depleted lymphocytes. Biochem Biophys Res Commun 134:8–13

Grupp SA, Harmony JAK (1985) Increased phosphatidylinositol metabolism is an important but not an obligatory early event in B lymphocyte activation. J Immunol 134:4087–4094

Grynkiewicz G, Poenie M, Tsien RY (1985) A new generation of Ca^{2+} indicators with greatly improved fluorescence properties. J Biol Chem 260:3440–3450

Gupta S, Chandy KG, Vayuvegula B, Ruhlig M, DeCoursey TE, Cahalan MD (1985) Role of potassium channels in interleukin-1 and interleukin-2 synthesis, and interleukin-2 receptor expression. Cell Mol Biol Lymphokines. Academic, New York, pp 39–44

Hamill OP, Marty A, Neher E, Sakmann B, Sigworth FJ (1981) Improved patch-clamp techniques for high resolution current recording from cells and cell-free membrane patches. Pflügers Arch 391:85–100

Harrison ML, Low PS, Geahlen RL (1984) T and B lymphocytes express distinct tyrosine protein kinases. J Biol Chem 259:9348–9350

Hasegawa-Sasaki H, Sasaki T (1983) Phytohemagglutinin induces rapid degradation of phosphatidylinositol-4,5-bisphosphate and transient accumulation of phosphatidic acid and diacylglycerol in a human T lymphoblastoid cell line CCRF-CEM. Biochim Biophys Acta 754:305–314

Hesketh TR, Smith GA, Moore JP, Taylor MV, Metcalfe JC (1983) Free cytoplasmic calcium concentration and the mitogenic stimulation of lymphocytes. J Biol Chem 258:4876–4882

Hesketh TR, Moore JP, Morris JDH, Taylor MV, Rogers J, Smith GA, Metcalfe JC (1985) A common sequence of calcium and pH signals in the mitogenic stimulation of eukaryotic cells. Nature 313:481–484

Imboden JB, Stobo JD (1985) Transmembrane signalling by the T cell antigen receptor. Perturbation of the T3-antigen receptor complex generates inositol phosphates and releases calcium ions from intracellular stores. J Exp Med 161:446–456

Kaibuchi K, Takai Y, Nishizuka Y (1985) Protein kinase C and calcium ion in mitogenic response of macrophage-depleted human peripheral lymphocytes. J Biol Chem 260:1366–1369

Kiefer H, Blume AJ, Kaback HR (1980) Membrane potential changes during mitogenic stimulation of mouse spleen lymphocytes. Proc Natl Acad Sci USA 77:2200–2204

Koretzky GA, Daniele RP, Green WC, Nowell PC (1983) Evidence for an interleukin-independent pathway for human lymphocyte activation. Proc Natl Acad Sci USA 80:3444–3447

Kraft AS, Anderson WB, Cooper HL, Sando JJ (1982) Decrease in cytosolic calcium/phospholipid-dependent protein kinase activity following phorbol ester treatment of EL4 thymoma cells. J Biol Chem 257:13193–13196

LaPetina EG, Reep B, Ganong BR, Bell RM (1985) Exogenous sn-1,2-diacylglycerols containing saturated fatty acids function as bioregulators of protein kinase C in human platelets. J Biol Chem 260:1358–1361

Lederman HM, Lee JWW, Cheung RK, Grinstein S, Gelfand EW (1984) Monocytes are required to trigger Ca^{2+} uptake in the proliferative response of human lymphocytes to Staphylococcus aureus protein A. Proc Natl Acad Sci USA 81:6827–6830

Lee KS, Tsien RW (1983) Mechanism of calcium channel blockade by verapamil D600, diltiazem and nitrendipine in single dialyzed heart cells. Nature 302:790–794

Lee SC, Price M, Deutsch C (1986a) K-channel blockers and T-lymphocyte proliferation. Biophys J 49:167A

Lee SC, Sabath DE, Deutsch C, Prystowsky MB (1986b) Increased voltage-gated potassium conductance during interleukin 2 stimulated proliferation of a mouse helper T-lymphocyte clone. J Cell Biol 102:1200–1208

Lichtman AH, Segel GB, Lichtman MA (1980) Total and exchangeable calcium in lymphocytes: effects of PHA and A23187. J Supramol Struct 14:65–75

Lichtman AH, Segel GB, Lichtman MA (1981) Calcium transport and calcium-ATPase activity in human lymphocyte plasma membrane vesicles. J Biol Chem 256:6148–6154

Maino VC, Hayman MJ, Crumpton MJ (1975) Relationship between enhanced turnover of phosphatidylinositol and lymphocyte activation by mitogens. Biochem J 146:247–252

Matteson DR, Deutsch C (1984) K channels in T lymphocytes: a patch-clamp study using monoclonal antibody adhesion. Nature 307:468–471

May WS, Sahyoun N, Wolf M, Cuatrecasas P (1985) Role of intracellular calcium mobilization in the regulation of protein kinase C-mediated membrane processes. Nature 317:549–551

Mills GB, Cheung RK, Grinstein S, Gelfand EW (1985a) Increase in cytosolic free calcium concentration is an intracellular messenger for the production of interleukin 2 but not for expression of the interleukin 2 receptor. J Immunol 134:1640–1643

Mills GB, Cheung RK, Grinstein S, Gelfand EW (1985b) Interleukin 2-induced lymphocyte proliferation is independent of increases in cytosolic-free calcium concentrations. J Immunol 134:2431–2435

Mills GB, Cragoe EJ, Gelfand EW, Grinstein S (1985c) Interleukin 2 induces a rapid increase in intracellular pH through activation of a Na^+/H^+ antiport. Cytoplasmic alkalinization is not required for lymphocyte proliferation. J Biol Chem 260:12500–12507

Mills GB, Lee JWW, Cheung RK, Gelfand EW (1985d) Characterization of the requirements for human T cell mitogenesis by using suboptimal concentration of phytohemagglutinin. J Immunol 135:3087–3093

Mills GB, Cheung RK, Cragoe EJ, Grinstein S, Gelfand EW (1986a) Activation of the Na^+/H^+ antiport is not required for lectin-induced proliferation of human T lymphocytes. J Immunol 136:1150–1154

Mills GB, Stewart DJ, Mellors A, Gelfand EW (1986b) Interleukin 2 does not induce phosphatidylinositide hydrolysis in T cells: evidence against signalling through phosphatidylinositide hydrolysis. J Immunol 136:3019–3024

Monroe JG, Cambier JC (1983) B cell activation. I. Receptor crosslinking by anti-immunoglobulin antibodies induces a rapid decrease in B cell plasma membrane potential. J Exp Med 157:2073–2086

Monroe JG, Niedel JE, Cambier JC (1984) B cell activation. VI. Induction of cell membrane depolarization and hyper I-A expression by phorbol diesters suggests a role for protein kinase C in murine B lymphocyte activation. J Immunol 132:1472–1478

Nel AE, Navailles M, Rosberger DF, Landreth GE, Goldschmidt-Clermont PJ, Baldwin GJ, Galbraith RM (1985) Phorbol ester induces tyrosine phosphorylation in normal and abnormal human B lymphocytes. J Immunol 135:3448–3453

Nel AE, Wooten MW, Landreth GE, Goldschmidt-Clermont PJ, Stevenson HC, Miller PJ, Calbraith RM (1986) Translocation of phospholipid/Ca^{2+}-dependent protein kinase in B lymphocytes activated by phorbol ester or crosslinking of membrane immunoglobulin. Biochem J 233:145–149

Niedel JE, Kuhn LJ, Vandenbark GR (1983) Phorbol diester receptor copurifies with protein kinase C. Proc Natl Acad Sci USA 80:36–40

Nishizuka Y (1984) The role of protein kinase C in cell surface signal transduction and tumor promotion. Nature 308:693–698

Oettgen HC, Terhorst C, Cantley LC, Rosoff PM (1985) Stimulation of the T3-T cell receptor complex induces a membrane potential sensitive calcium influx. Cell 40:583–590

O'Flynn K, Zanders ED, Lamb JR, Beverly PCL, Wallace DL, Tathan PER, Tax WJM, Linch DC (1985) Investigation of early T cell activation: analysis of the effect of specific antigen, interleukin 2 and monoclonal antibodies on intracellular free calcium concentration. Eur J Immunol 15:7–11

Parker CW (1974) Correlation between mitogenicity and stimulation of calcium uptake in human lymphocytes. Biochem Biophys Res Commun 61:1180–1186

Pozzan T, Arslan P, Tsien RY, Rink TJ (1982) Anti-immunoglobulin, cytoplasmic free calcium, and capping in B lymphocytes. J Cell Biol 94:335–340

Prentki M, Biden TJ, Janjic D, Irvine RF, Berridge MJ, Wallheim CB (1984) Rapid mobilization of Ca^{2+} from rat insulinoma microsomes by inositol-1,4,5-trisphosphate. Nature 309:562–564

Quastel MR, Segel GB, Lichtman MA (1981) The effect of chelation on lymphocyte monvalent cation permeability, transport and concentration. J Cell Physiol 107:165–170

Ransom JT, Cambier JC (1986) B cell activation. VII. Independent and synergistic effects of mobilized calcium and diacylglycerol on membrane potential and I-A expression. J Immunol 136:66–72

Ransom JT, Harris LK, Cambier JC (1986a) Anti-Ig induces release of inositol 1,4,5 trisphosphate which mediates mobilization of intracellular Ca^{2+} stores in B lymphocytes. J Immunol 137:708–714

Ransom JT, DiGiusto D, Cambier JC (1986b) Single cell analysis of calcium mobilization in anti-receptor antibody stimulated B lymphocytes. J Immunol 136:54–57

Ransom JT, Thorpe D, Cambier JC (1987a) Flow cytometric analysis of Ca^{2+} mobilization in anti-Ig stimulated B lymphocytes: evidence for release of intracellular stores and Ca^{2+} influx. J Biol Chem (submitted)

Ransom JT, DiGiusto D, Thorpe D, Cambier JC (1987b) Ca^{2+} influx in anti-Ig stimulated B lymphocytes is enhanced by a rapid K^+ efflux. J Biol Chem (submitted)

Rink TJ, Deutsch C (1983) Calcium-activated potassium channels in lymphocytes. Cell Calcium 4:463–473

Rink TJ, Montecucco C, Hesketh TR, Tsien RY (1980) Lymphocyte membrane potential assessed with fluorescent probes. Biochem Biophys Acta 595:15–30

Rink TJ, Tsien RY, Pozzan T (1982) Cytoplasmic pH and free Mg^{2+} in lymphocytes. J Cell Biol 95:189–196

Rosoff PM, Cantley LC (1983) Increasing the intracellular Na^+ concentration induces differentiation in a pre-B lymphocyte cell line. Proc Natl Acad Sci USA 80:7547–7550

Rosoff PM, Cantley LC (1985a) Lipopolysaccharide and phorbol esters induce differentiation but have opposite effects on phosphatidylinositol turnover and Ca^{2+} mobilization in 70Z/3 pre-B lymphocytes. J Biol Chem 260:9209–9215

Rosoff PM, Cantley LC (1985b) Stimulation of the T3-T cell receptor-associated Ca^{2+} influx enhances the activity of the Na^+/H^+ exchanger in a leukemic human T cell line. J Biol Chem 260:14053–14059

Rosoff PM, Stein LF, Cantley LC (1984) Phorbol esters induce differentiation in a pre-B lymphocytic cell line by enhancing Na^+/H^+ exchange. J Biol Chem 259:7056–7060

Sasaki T, Hasegawa-Sasaki H (1985) Molecular species of phosphatidylinositol, phosphatidic acid and diacylglycerol in a phytohemagglutinin stimulated T-cell leukemia line. Biochem Biophys Acta 833:316–322

Schlichter L, Sidell N, Hagiwara S (1986) Potassium channels mediate killing by human natural killer cells. Proc Natl Acad Sci USA 83:451–455

Segel GB, Lichtman MA (1976) Potassium transport in human blood lymphocytes treated with phytohemagglutinin. J Clin Invest 58:1358–1369

Segel GB, Simon W, Lichtman MA (1979) Regulation of sodium and potassium transport in phytohemagglutinin stimulated human blood lymphocytes. J Clin Invest 64:834–841

Sidell N, Schlichter LC, Wright SC, Hagiwara S, Golub SH (1986) Potassium channels in human NK cells are involved in discrete stages of the killing process. J Immunol 137:1650–1658

Storey DJ, Shears SB, Kirk CJ, Michell RH (1984) Stepwise enzymatic dephosphorylation of inositol 1,4,5-trisphosphate to inositol in liver. Nature 312:374–376

Taylor MV, Metcalfe JC, Hesketh TR, Smith GA, Moore JP (1984) Mitogens increase phosphorylation of phosphoinositides in thymocytes. Nature 312:462–465

Tsien RY, Pozzan T, Rink TJ (1982a) T-cell mitogens cause early changes in cytoplasmic free Ca^{2+} and membrane potential in lymphocytes. Nature 295:68–71

Tsien RY, Pozzan T, Rink TJ (1982b) Calcium homeostasis in intact lymphocytes: cytoplasmic free calcium monitored with a new intracellularly trapped fluorescent indicator. J Cell Biol 94:325–334

Waggoner AS (1979) The use of cyanine dyes for the determination of membrane potential in cells, organelles and vesicles. Methods Enzymol 55:689

Weiss A, Imboden J, Wiskocil R, Stobo J (1984) The role of T3 in the activation of human T cells. J Clin Immunol 4:165–173

Whitney RB, Sutherland RM (1972) Requirement for calcium ions in lymphocyte transformation stimulated by phytohemagglutinin. J Cell Physiol 80:329–337

Whitney RB, Sutherland RM (1973) Characteristics of calcium accumulation by lymphocytes and alterations in the process induced by phytohemagglutinin. J Cell Physiol
  82:9–20
Wolf M, LeVine H, May WS, Cuatrecasas P, Sahyoun N (1985) A model for intracellular
  translocation of protein kinase C involving synergism between Ca^{2+} and phorbol
  esters. Nature 317:546–549
Ypey DL, Clapham DE (1984) Development of a delayed outward-rectifying K^+ conductance in cultured mouse peritoneal macrophage. Proc Natl Acad Sci USA 81:3083–
  3087

CHAPTER 4

Intracellular Events
During Lymphocyte Activation

R. G. COFFEY

A. Introduction

The term "lymphocyte activation" has been used interchangeably with lymphocyte transformation, blastogenesis, and mitogenesis. Occasionally, the term indicates only early T lymphocyte events such as volume changes or lymphokine production, but usually it refers to induction of proliferation. In this chapter lymphocyte activation will be used to denote the process that begins with the binding of
mitogenic agents or antigens to lymphocyte surface receptors, stimulating the
cells to leave the quiescent G_0 stage and traverse the G_1 and S phases.

A survey of the literature on lymphocyte activation reveals two periods of exciting research. The first period began in the 1960s after Nowell published that
phytohemagglutinin (PHA)[1], a glycoprotein from the bean *Phaseolus vulgaris*,
triggered polyclonal blast transformation of lymphocytes (NOWELL 1960). In the
following 12 years, several laboratories reported discoveries of a host of biochemical changes in T lymphocytes stimulated with PHA or other agglutinins extracted
from plants, especially the jack bean lectin concanavalin A (Con A), and in B lymphocytes stimulated with the plant pokeweed mitogen or bacterial lipopolysaccharide (LPS). A period of time then elapsed which was notable for the abundance of studies confirming or refining the initial discoveries. These include early
increases in lipid metabolism, accelerated transport of ions and nutrients, enhanced glucose metabolism, and changes in cyclic nucleotide metabolism, and are
summarized in Table 1. Morphological changes involving enlargement of the nucleus with the appearance of prominent nucleoli, increase in cytoplasm and
numbers of cytoplasmic organelles, and production of cell surface processes accompany or follow the early metabolic changes. Extensive reviews of this literature have appeared (LING and KAY 1975; WEDNER and PARKER 1976; O'BRIEN et
al. 1978; HUME and WEIDEMANN 1980) and contain more detail about certain
events than is included here.

---

[1] Abbreviations used are: AA arachidonic acid; AIB α-aminoisobutyric acid; cAMP cyclic
AMP; cGMP cyclic GMP; Con A concanavalin A; DAG diacylglyceride; ETYA eicosatetraynoic acid; HETE hydroxyeicosatetraenoic acid, HPETE hydroperoxyeicosatetraenoic
acid; Ig immunoglobulin; IFN interferon; ITP inositol-1,4,5-trisphosphate; LPS lipopolysaccharide; LT leukotriene; MAF macrophage-activating factor; NDGA nordihydroguaiaretic acid; PA phosphatidic acid; PC phosphatidylcholine; PE phosphatidylethanolamine; PG prostaglandin; PHA phytohemagglutinin; PI phosphatidylinositol; PIP_2 phos-
phatidylinositol-4,5-bisphosphate; PMA phorbol-12-myristate-13-acetate; PS phosphatidylserine; PWM pokeweed mitogen.

Table 1. Intracellular events stimulated in T lymphocyte activation

0–1 min	2–4 h
Ligand-receptor binding	Translocation of cAMP-dependent protein
Polyphosphoinositide breakdown, release	kinases I and II
of DAG and ITP	Membrane Mg^{2+}- and Ca^{2+}-ATPases
Ca^{2+} mobilization from membranes	Krebs cycle activity
Protein kinase C activation and trans-	Membrane glycolipid metabolism
location to membranes	DNA template activity
Arachidonate release and metabolism by	Actin mRNA expression
lipoxygenase	

2–15 min	4–12 h
PE methylation, synthesis of PC, PI, PIP_2	IL-2 mRNA expression
Guanylate cyclase activity	Ornithine decarboxylase, polyamine levels
Na^+/H^+ antiport and intracellular pH	Carbamylphosphate synthetase
Uptake of Ca^{2+}, K^+, glucose, amino acids,	Adenosine deaminase activity and
nucleosides, phosphate	secretion[d]
Non-histone protein binding to chromatin	Poly-A-rich RNA
Transglutaminase[a]	Purine synthesis
mRNA for protooncogenes *c-fos* and *c-myc*	Glucocorticoid receptors

20–30 min	12–24 h
Histone kinase and acetylase	Transferrin receptors
ATP, ADP levels	RNA polymerase II activity
RNA polymerase I activity	Uridine and thymidine kinases
Phosphoribosylpyrophosphate synthetase	Activator of DNA replication[e]
Acyltransferase activity	DNA polymerase
Fluidity of plasma membranes[b]	Histone phosphorylation
Chromatin dispersion[c]	Cystathionine synthetase
	mRNA for protooncogenes *c-myb, N-ras,*
	and for $_p53$

1–2 h	24–48 h
Choline and fatty acid incorporation into	Tubulin
phospholipids	Aerobic glycolysis
Arginine-rich histone acetylation	cAMP
Nuclear acidic protein phosphorylation	cAMP and cGMP phosphodiesterases
Appearance of receptors for IL-2, insulin,	Aminopeptidase activities[f]
and acetylcholine	
Messenger RNA	
Protein synthesis	48–72 h
Microtubule, microfilament organization	Cyclic GMP
Cyclic GMP-dependent protein kinase	Mitosis
Transfer RNA methylation	

The indicated times are approximate and apply to the first observable increases. The order of events does not imply causal relationships, nor does it imply that this is the exact order of events. References are found in the text or in the reviews cited, with a few exceptions: [a] NOVOGRODSKY et al. (1978); [b] INBAR and SHINITZKY (1975); [c] POMPIDOU et al. (1984); [d] HOVI et al. (1976b); [e] GUTOWSKI et al. (1984); [f] KOHNO and KANNO (1985).

The second period of intense research began with the discovery of the interleukin (IL) system (MORGAN et al. 1976; GILLIS and SMITH 1977), the availability of homogeneous IL-2 (SMITH et al. 1983), the development of methods for separating subpopulations of mononuclear cells and for cloning a variety of lymphocytes with restricted capabilities (Chap. 12). The biochemical changes noted in Table 1 were assumed to take place in the cells which proceed to divide, but since most studies were performed with mixed mononuclear cells, they could have occurred in cell populations different from those that eventually proliferate. Elegant experiments with the new technologies have led to the general understanding that mitogenic activation involves the perception by the T lymphocyte of at least three distinct signals, reviewed by CANTRELL and SMITH (1984) and by CAMBIER et al. (1985) and described briefly here. 1. The first signal is delivered by the binding of mitogen to receptors on the cell surface, and causes the production of lymphokines including macrophage-activating factor (MAF), also known as gamma interferon (IFN-γ). A key response to the first signal is the stimulation of transcription of mRNA for IL-2 receptors, which begins at 2–4 h (YAMAMOTO et al. 1985; REED et al. 1986) or 6–8 h (LEONARD et al. 1985a). T lymphocytes perceiving the first signal exit from the G_0 phase. 2. The second signal is delivered by interleukin 1, produced by monocytes/macrophages after they have reacted directly or indirectly with mitogen and lymphokines, and results in the stimulation of IL-2 production by a subpopulation of T lymphocytes. 3. The third signal is delivered by IL-2, which stimulates the cells to proceed through G_1, S, G_2, and mitosis. All T lymphocytes with a sufficient density of IL-2 receptors respond in this way (CANTRELL and SMITH 1984). A critical event in late G_1 is the appearance of receptors for transferrin (NECKERS and COSSMAN 1983; NECKERS et al. 1984).

Responses of T lymphocytes to antigens, or to antibodies directed against certain cell surface proteins, appear to involve basically the same key events, culminating in IL-2-dependent progression through the cell cycle (ACUTO and REINHERZ 1985; PALACIOS 1985; ISAKOV et al. 1986; KRONENBERG et al. 1986). A key feature of antigen- or anti-T3-mediated activation is the modulation of the T3 receptor and its associated clonotypic heterodimer (antigen receptor Ti) prior to expression of IL-2 receptors (SCHWAB et al. 1985; ACUTO and REINHERZ 1985). Accessory cells are required for this modulation, for the expression of IL-2 receptors, and for the production of IL-2. B lymphocytes are activated by certain mitogens, antigens, or anti-surface IgM in similar, but not identical, ways (HOWARD and PAUL 1983; CAMBIER et al. 1985). After the initial step, B lymphocytes can respond to B cell growth factors (BCGF, also called B cell stimulatory factors, BSF) or differentiating factors (BCDF), by either proliferating or differentiating into immunoglobulin- (Ig)-producing cells (KISHIMOTO 1984; MULLER et al. 1985). The same cells may respond to lymphokines of both categories in sequence; they can even display receptors for IL-2 and proliferate in response to it (MINGARI et al. 1984; MURAGUCHI et al. 1985). B lymphocyte responses to LPS, on the other hand, may not involve cell surface recognition signals (HOWARD and PAUL 1983; GRUPP and HARMONY 1985).

Few experiments attempting to analyze biochemical events of lymphocyte activation in carefully separated mononuclear subpopulations have been reported as of this writing. The exponential rate of growth of studies employing the new technologies leaves no doubt that such experiments will soon be reported. For example, MURAGUCHI et al. (1985) found that normal human B lymphocytes carefully freed of other cell types had no IL-2 receptors, but when the cells were treated with the tumor promoter phorbol myristate acetate (PMA) or anti-μ, they developed such receptors. Exogenous IL-2 then stimulated the cells to proliferate. KAIBUCHI et al. (1985) showed that a mitogenic response could be induced in accessory cell-free human T lymphocytes by the combination of a calcium ionophore and PMA. IL-2 is almost certainly involved, as the next example attests. ALBERT et al. (1985) employed alloreactive T cell clones to show that a calcium ionophore and PMA could induce the entire spectrum of responses leading to proliferation – if the clones were capable of producing IL-2. An interesting example of IL-2-independent T cell proliferation involves the use of a monoclonal antibody against PHA receptors (ISAKOV and ALTMAN 1986).

Such experiments demonstrate that it is possible to separate the myriad of biochemical changes, occurring when mononuclear cells are activated, into the stages during which they occur. In the following pages, special attention will be directed toward those studies that employed well-defined mononuclear cell populations. In the remainder of the studies, it is tacitly assumed that the reported changes occur in the cells that proceed to proliferate. Events thought to involve signaling mechanisms have been selected for this chapter. Space does not permit consideration of the many other interesting changes such as intermediary metabolism (STERNHOLM and FALOR 1970; ROOS et al. 1970) and macromolecular synthesis (CROSS and ORD 1971; COOPER and BRAVERMAN 1981; COOPER and LESTER 1982).

B. Cytoskeletal Changes

The cytoskeletal contractile structures include microfilaments and microtubules. Microfilaments (diameter 50–70 Å) consist mainly of actin, which interacts with myosin, ATP, and calcium in a way that enhances the ATPase activity of myosin and provides the contractile force for microfilament-regulated shape change and cell motility (STARK et al. 1982; FECHHEIMER and CEBRA 1982). Mitogens induce a conversion from the monomeric G form of actin to the polymerized F form in lymphocytes within 10 min. At about 30 min, a reorganization of actin and the development of a prominent fibrous process, termed the uropod, take place (SUNDQUIST et al. 1980). At 1–2 days actin-containing microvilli and ridges or ruffles appear on the cell surface. This is followed at 3 days by the loss of microvilli and the development of an actin-containing protuberance (OTTESKOG et al. 1983).

The actin-specific fungal metabolite cytochalasin B inhibits each of these changes. This drug also inhibited mitogen stimulation of DNA synthesis at high concentrations, but potentiated it at low doses (BERNARD et al. 1975; GREENE et al. 1976c; GERY and EIDINGER 1977; HOFFMAN et al. 1977). HUME et al. (1978) concluded that cytochalasin B inhibits thymocyte DNA synthesis by virtue of its effects on glucose uptake and not on microfilaments. Other studies (BELMONT and RICH 1981) indicated that effective inhibition of Con A-stimulated DNA synthesis by cytochalasin B required its continued presence, while a 4-h pulse with Con

A had little effect. Cytochalasins bind to three types of receptors, one cytosolic, and two on the membrane (MOOKERJEE and JUNG 1982). Perhaps the membrane receptors are involved in the unexpected augmentation by cytochalasins B, E, and A of mitogen-induced calcium and amino acid uptake, of cyclic AMP levels (GREENE and PARKER 1975), and of the metabolism of phosphatidylinositol (PI, also referred to as PtdInsP) (SASAKI and HASEGAWA-SASAKI 1981).

Microtubules (diameter 240 Å), which consist largely of the protein tubulin, form part of the cytoskeleton and participate in cell motility. Colchicine inhibits polymerization and is often used to determine the importance of these structures in biologic events. D_2O has the opposite effect. Only a few small lymphocytes have parallel tubular structures; most of these are T lymphocytes (SMIT et al. 1983). Murine spleen cells develop an extensive microtubule network several hours after Con A stimulation (WATERHOUSE et al. 1983). At 24 h, tubulin is increased by 50%, and at 48 h the number of microtubule fibers which radiate from the centrosome has increased fivefold (KECSKEMETHY and SCHAFER 1982). The early increases in tubulin (and actin) are due to post-transcriptional processing steps such as polyadenylation and methylation of RNA, which double in the first 2 h, while later increases are probably due to mRNA synthesis which begins to increase after 6 h (DEGEN et al. 1983; KECSKEMETHY and SCHAFER 1982).

EDELMAN (1976) and MCCLAIN and EDELMAN (1976) conducted many elegant experiments on cell surface changes induced by antibody and Con A, resulting in the "surface modulating assembly" hypothesis. The assembly was proposed to consist of submembranous arrays of microtubules, microfilaments, and associated contractile and membrane proteins. EDELMAN's (1976) notions of Ig and Con A receptor mobility (evidenced by the capping phenomenon), the capacity of Con A at high doses to inhibit, and the capacity of colchicine to augment receptor capping have been amply confirmed (SCHREINER and UNANUE 1975; OLIVER et al. 1980). In certain situations, both actin (TOH and HARD 1977) and adenylate cyclase (EARP et al. 1977) co-cap with Con A receptors. Cyclic AMP is thought to have a positive influence on capping since its levels are elevated during capping (BUTMAN et al. 1981; BOURGUIGNON and HSING 1983). Cyclic AMP is in turn elevated by colchicine in lymphocytes. Since succinylated Con A induces proliferation without causing capping, this phenomenon appears to be irrelevant to initiation of lymphocyte activation (GUNTHER et al. 1976).

Several workers (BETEL and MARTIJNSE 1976; GREENE et al. 1976d; SHERLINE and MUNDY 1977; RESCH et al. 1977, 1981; RUDD et al. 1979; BELMONT and RICH 1981; CUTHBERT and SHAY 1983) have concluded that microtubules play no significant role in the early events of lymphocyte activation. GREENE et al. (1976d) observed no inhibition by colchicine of mitogen-induced calcium uptake. RESCH et al. (1977, 1981) found that colchicine did not inhibit early processes such as phosphatidylcholine turnover, lymphotoxin synthesis, and RNA synthesis. SASAKI and HASEGAWA-SASAKI (1981) also showed that disruption of microtubules by colchicine or vinblastine did not prevent the receptor-stimulated changes in phosphatidylinositol metabolism. Finally, CUTHBERT and SHAY (1983) were unable to note an effect of colchicine on the mitogen-induced volume increase at 24 h. SCHELLENBERG and GILLESPIE (1980) observed paradoxical effects of colchicine and D_2O: both agents, which have opposing effects on microtubules, inhibited phosphatidylinositol labeling (having no effect on breakdown). They concluded that colchicine may act on a system not related to microtubules. In a definitive study, HALL et al. (1982) showed that colchicine did not inhibit commitment of stimulated lymphocytes to enter the cell cycle, but it decreased the rate of entry into S phase.

To summarize this section, there is no convincing evidence for important roles of either microfilaments or microtubules in the early events of lymphocyte activation. Observations relating microtubules to receptor patching and capping are of interest, but apparently these phenomena are not critical events. The importance of microtubules in mitosis and of both elements of the cytoskeleton in cell motility remain unquestioned.

C. Lipid Changes

I. Phosphatidylinositol Metabolism (see also Chap. 3)

FISHER and MUELLER (1968) first reported that PHA stimulated within 10 min a 10-fold increase in the labeling of membrane PI by [^{32}P] phosphate in human lymphocytes. Later, FISHER and MUELLER (1971 b) observed an 18-fold increase in [^{3}H] inositol labeling of PI. Interestingly, in the first 3 min of PHA addition, the labeling of phosphatidic acid (PA) by [^{32}P] phosphate exceeded that of PI, and other phospholipids showed only minor changes. Glycerol incorporation was slight, indicating that PA was synthesized by phosphorylation of 1,2-diacylglycerides (DAG) rather than by acylation of glycerol phosphate. In a detailed study, SUGIURA and WAKU (1984) determined that the resynthesized PI was preferentially labeled with tetraenes (82%), while the resynthesized PA contained more monoenes and dienes than tetraenes. LUCAS et al. (1971) separated the stimulated cells on gradients, and succeeded in showing that the cells which responded to PHA with enhanced PI labeling were the same ones that synthesized DNA after 3 days. These data strongly support the mitogen stimulation of the PI-DAG-PA-PI cycle (Fig. 1) as originally proposed by HOKIN and HOKIN (1953) for pancreatic responses to acetylcholine.

MASUZAWA et al. (1973) provided further confirmation of the specificity of the response by showing that several T cell mitogens stimulated labeling of PI in human T lymphocytes. Phosphatidylcholine (PC) and other phospholipids were not labeled significantly until after 3 h. MAINO et al. (1975) observed good correlations between the ascending part of the mitogen dose-response curves for both the phosphate uptake and DNA synthesis in pig lymph node lymphocytes. Many workers have confirmed all these essential findings concerning PI labeling in T lymphocytes (BETEL et al. 1974; SCHUMM et al. 1974; SCHELLENBERG and GILLESPIE 1977, 1980; MILLER 1979; SASAKI and HASEGAWA-SASAKI 1981; HASEGAWA-SASAKI and SASAKI 1981; KAIBUCHI et al. 1982; RODE et al. 1982; TAYLOR et al. 1984). CRUMPTON et al. (1976) found that inositol labeling of PI was prevented by calcium chelators, suggesting a dependency of PI turnover on calcium uptake. HUI and HARMONY (1980c) reported a very specific effect of low density lipoproteins to inhibit the early changes in PHA-induced PI labeling, calcium uptake, and cyclic GMP increase, in a coordinated fashion. The PI labeling response to mitogens is apparently limited to T cells. Neither MASUZAWA et al. (1983), BETEL et al. (1974), nor MAINO et al. (1975) observed labeling of PI in B cells, using either B or T cell mitogens. The importance of PI labeling in the initiation of lymphocyte activation is now in question because of the report of MELLORS et al. (1985) that it is inhibited by comitogenic phorbol esters in mouse spleen and human tonsil T lymphocytes stimulated by PHA (see also Chap. 3).

PI breakdown has been shown in a variety of stimulated cell systems to occur before PI synthesis, prompting MITCHELL (1975) to elaborate the hypothesis known as the "PI response." The first step in this response is the activation of phospholipase C which hydrolyzes PI to form DAG and inositol 1-phosphate. In many cases this is coupled to or followed by calcium influx and cyclic GMP increases (MITCHELL 1975, 1982; MITCHELL et al. 1981). The DAG can then be phosphorylated by a specific kinase to form PA, or deacylated by DAG lipase to form arachidonic acid (AA) and monoglyceride, as shown in Fig. 1a. A cycle is formed when PA interacts with CTP to form a complex which then reacts with inositol to form PI and CMP. Changes in the components of the cycle have been followed by prelabeling with phosphate, glycerol, inositol, and AA. FISHER and MUELLER (1971b) concluded from their human blood lymphocyte data, comparing [^{32}P] phosphate and [^{3}H] glycerol labeling, that PA was synthesized by phosphorylation of DAG rather than acylation of glycerol phosphate. PARKER et al. (1979a) allowed human blood T lymphocytes to incorporate [^{14}C] AA, then added PHA and observed the release of labeled AA as early as 1 min. It reached a peak in 10 min and accounted for nearly half of the cellular PI. Most of the AA is incorporated into PC of resting lymphocyte membranes, but after stimulation most of the AA is released from PI, indicating roles for phospholipase C and DAG lipase rather than phospholipase A$_2$ (PARKER et al. 1979a; HOMA et al. 1984). HASEGAWA-SASAKI and SASAKI (1982) measured Con A-induced changes in eight phospholipids of rat lymph node cells prelabeled with AA. Increases in PA and decreases in PI occurred as early as 0.5 min; DAG increased significantly at 2 min. After 5 min, PI increased again. No changes occurred during the first 15 min in PC, phosphatidylethanolamine (PE), phosphatidylserine (PS), triglycerides, or fatty acids. The authors concluded that PI breakdown precedes PI synthesis and may be the initial step in the T lymphocyte response to Con A.

B lymphocytes are again contrasted to T lymphocytes: whereas IgM-specific antibodies stimulate PI metabolism in B cells (COGGESHALL and CAMBIER 1985), LPS does not (GRUPP and HARMONY 1985). This indicates that the PI response may occur, but is not always essential for mitogenesis of lymphocytes. To evaluate these data in terms of MICHELL's (1975) hypothesis, that the PI response is somehow linked to calcium uptake, it is notable that MAINO et al. (1974) obtained data with the calcium ionophore A23187 suggesting that a rise in cytoplasmic calcium triggered PI turnover. In contrast inhibition of PI breakdown prevented calcium uptake (HUI and HARMONY 1980a). On the other hand, HUI and HARMONY (1980c) reported that PHA stimulated PI hydrolysis in a calcium-free medium. It is apparent that extracellular calcium is not required for lectin mitogen stimulation of the PI response, whereas the PI response may be essential for calcium uptake (see also Chap. 3). One possibility consistent with the data is that newly formed PA, unique among several phospholipids in its calcium ionophore activity, may function to transport calcium into the cell (RITTENHOUSE-SIMMONS 1980; SERHAN et al. 1982).

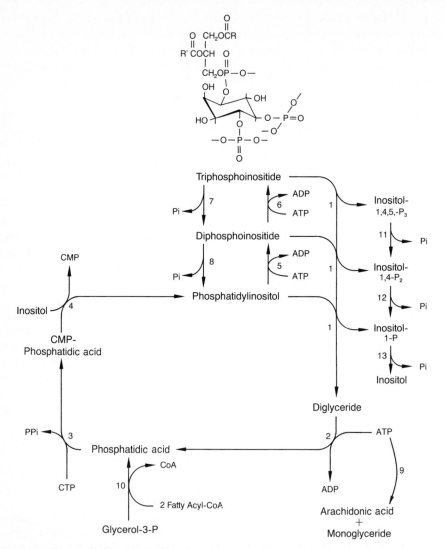

Fig. 1a,b. Phospholipid and arachidonic acid metabolism. **a** Enzymes catalyzing the reactions of the PI and poly-PI cycles are: *1*, phospholipases C; *2*, diacylglyceride kinase; *3*, phosphatidic acid: CTP cytidyltransferase; *4*, CMP-phosphatidic acid inositol phosphatidyltransferase; *5*, phosphatidylinositol kinase; *6*, phosphatidylinositol 5-phosphate 4-kinase; *7*, phosphatidylinositol 4,5-bisphosphate phosphatase; *8*, phosphatidylinositol 4-phosphate phosphatase; *9*, diacylglyceride lipase; *10*, de novo pathway for PA synthesis; *11*, inositol 1,4,5-triphosphatase; *12*, inositol 4,5-bisphosphatase; *13*, inositol 1-phosphatase

Inositol 1,4,5-trisphosphate (ITP) presently occupies center stage as a calcium mobilizer (BERRIDGE 1984). This compound and DAG are important intracellular messengers, formed from PI 4,5-bisphosphate (PIP$_2$), a minor component of cell membranes, by the action of a phospholipase C. The specific effects of DAG and

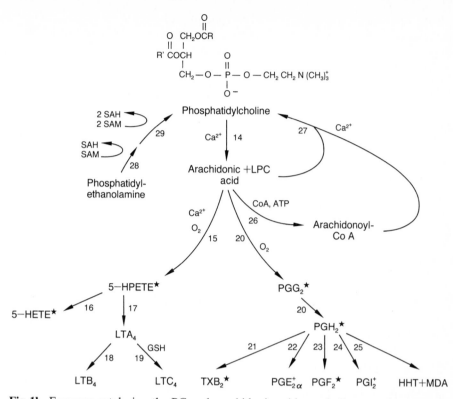

Fig. 1b. Enzymes catalyzing the PC and arachidonic acid metabolism reactions are: *14*, phospholipase A_2; *15*, 5-lipoxygenase; *16*, HPETE peroxidase (also occurs nonenzymatically); *17*, HPETE dehydrase; *18*; leukotriene A_4 hydrolase; *19*, glutathione *S*-transferase; *20*, cyclooxygenase; *21*, thromboxane synthetase; *22*, PG endoperoxide isomerase; *23*, PG endoperoxide reductase; *24*, prostacyclin synthetase; *25*, nonenzymatic hydrolysis; *26*, acyl-CoA synthetase; *27*, acyl-CoA: lysolecithin acyltransferase; *28*, phospholipid methyltransferase I; *29*, phospholipid methyltransferase II.
Compound marked with asterisks stimulate cGMP increases; compounds marked with pluses stimulate cAMP accumulation. Abbreviations are: *CoA* coenzyme A; *GSH* glutathione; *HETE* hydroxyeicosatetraenoic acid; *HPETE* hydroxyperoxyeicosatetraenoic acid; *HHT* 12-hydroxyheptadecatrienoic acid; *LPC* lysophosphatidylcholine; *LT* leukotriene; *MDA* malondialdehyde; *PG* prostaglandin; *SAH* *S*-adenosylhomocysteine; *SAM* *S*-adenosylmethionine; *TX* thromboxane

Ca^{2+} on the phospholipid-dependent protein kinase C are discussed in Sect. E III. HUI and HARMONY (1980a) found that inositol bisphosphate and trisphosphate are released along with inositol 1-phosphate after adding PHA to human lymphocytes. In a human T lymphocyte cell line, ITP was released within 10 s after PHA addition (HASAGAWA-SASAKI and SASAKI 1983). The breakdown of PIP_2 preceded that of PI in lymphocytes, and the consequences are consistent with a large amount of recent evidence that ITP acts rapidly to release Ca^{2+} from various nonmitochondrial membranes in liver and other tissues in response to a multitude of activating agents (BURGESS et al. 1984; DAWSON and IRVINE 1984; JOSEPH et al.

1984; NISHIZUKA 1984). Whether or not the phospholipase C that acts on PIP_2 is identical with the enzyme that degrades PI is controversial (FARESE et al. 1985). It is apparent that PIP_2 hydrolysis requires a GTP-binding protein that is separate from the N_s and N_i involved with adenylate cyclase regulation (LAD et al. 1985). Phosphorylation of PI to form the polyphosphoinositides is being investigated and the results suggest that the T lymphocyte mitogens Con A, A23187, and the comitogen PMA stimulate this event in thymocytes (TAYLOR et al. 1984), and splenocytes (BOON et al. 1985). Con A, but not PMA or the ionophore, stimulated ITP production. The question of whether a second increase in PI or PIP_2 breakdown occurs as a result of IL-2 was answered in the negative by the detailed experiments of MILLS et al. (1986). However, others have observed IL-2 activation of phospholipase C in a cytotoxic T cell line (FARRAR and RUSCETTI 1986).

The consensus at this time is that polyphosphoinositide breakdown (and possibly resynthesis as well) is an essential and very early event in T lymphocyte activation, but B lymphocytes may not require these reactions (GRUPP and HARMONY 1985; Chap. 3). Some years ago, FISHER and MUELLER (1971a) reported that an inhibitor of inositol reactions (γ-hexachlorocyclohexane) prevented mitogen-induced PI labeling and also the synthesis of RNA and DNA. This was interpreted to indicate the importance of PI labeling, but it will be interesting to learn whether this inositol-like inhibitor will also block the actions of ITP on Ca^{2+} mobilization.

II. Phosphatidylcholine Metabolism

In addition to PI metabolism, mitogen-induced PC changes have also received considerable attention. PC is synthesized by different routes, as shown in Fig. 1 b. T cell mitogens stimulate PC synthesis when measured by incorporation of choline (KAY 1968; FISHER and MUELLER 1969; RESCH and FERBER 1972; CHEN 1979; NATHANIEL and MELLORS 1983), of unsaturated fatty acids (RESCH et al. 1971, 1972, 1976, 1978, 1981; NORTHOFF et al. 1978), and by methylation of PE (FISHER and MUELLER 1969; HIRATA and AXELROD 1980; TOYOSHIMA et al. 1982a, b; BOUGNOUX et al. 1983). Incorporation of choline into PC is first noticeable in T cells 1 h after addition of mitogen (RESCH and FERBER 1972; CHEN 1979), and in B cells at 16 h (CHIEN and ASHMAN 1983; ASHMAN 1984). In contrast, fatty acid incorporation has been observed as early as 10 min (RESCH et al. 1983), but is progressive with time and therefore usually measured after 1–3 h (RESCH et al. 1971, 1978). Oleic acid prefers position 1 and AA position 2 of PC. T lymphocyte mitogens did not enchance the incorporation of AA into PC of human lymphocytes (PARKER et al. 1979a), but were very effective in rabbit thymocytes (RODE et al. 1982). The preference of PC for AA compared with other fatty acids increases with time, becoming absolute by 4 h (RODE et al. 1982). This effect contributes to the increasing fluidity of the plasma membrane. The importance of PC synthesis to the early events of mitogen action is questionable, since the incorporation of both choline and AA can be inhibited by dapsone without blocking subsequent DNA synthesis (NATHANIEL and MELLORS 1983).

The conversion of PE to PC by transmethylation reactions is perhaps more relevant; it occurs within 2 min after exposure of mouse spleen T cells to Con A or PHA (HIRATA et al. 1980; TOYOSHIMA et al. 1982a, b). The increase reached a peak at 10 min, when AA release was just beginning, and the magnitude of methylation was found to be proportional to that of DNA synthesis. Both events were inhibited by high concentrations of Con A and by specific S-adenosylinme-thionine antagonists. PE methylation, which is independent of Ca^{2+}, preceded activation of calcium uptake (TOYOSHIMA et al. 1982a). Since non-lectin mitogens such as the calcium ionophore A23187 and PMA did not stimulate PE methylation (HIRATA et al. 1980), the general importance of these reactions in lymphocyte activation is questionable. The initial enthusiasm for the importance of PE methylation has been further dampened by the reports of MOORE et al. (1982) and ASHMAN (1984), who were unable to detect PE methylation during the first 60 min of mitogen addition to T lymphocytes. Explanations for the effects of the trans-methylation inhibitors on calcium ion flux and DNA synthesis may be found in the effects of these compounds in inhibiting other important transmethylation reactions, or to increase cyclic AMP levels (ZIMMERMAN et al. 1980).

III. Arachidonic Acid Metabolism (see also Chaps. 14, 15)

AA may be produced by the action of position-specific phospholipase A_2 acting on PC or by the sequential actions of PI-specific phospholipase and DAG lipase, as shown in Fig. 1. Most of the AA arising from membranes of T lymphocytes arises from PI, not PC (PARKER et al. 1979a; HOMA et al. 1984). This is in agreement with the positive demonstration of phospholipase C (ALLAN and MICHELL 1974) and the failure to demonstrate a phospholipase A_2 (TROTTER and FERBER 1981; RESCH et al. 1984) in lymphocytes that have been freed of macrophages. It is important to note that the latter enzyme does occur in chronic lymphocyte leukemia B cells (SUZUKI et al. 1980), macrophages (RESCH et al. 1984), and natural killer cells (HOFFMAN et al. 1981).

Despite the lack of phospholipase A_2 in normal lymphocytes, TROTTER and FERBER (1981) and TROTTER et al. (1982) believe that AA can arise from PC in activated lymphocytes by the action of acyl-CoA: lysophosphatide acyltrans-ferase operating in reverse. For example, lysophosphatidylethanolamine and acyl-CoA appeared when ConA was added to PC in the presence of mouse thymocytes (TROTTER and FERBER 1981). In a second reaction lysophosphatidyl-ethanolamine plus acyl-CoA produced PE and CoA. A key step to produce free AA was thought to involve an acyl-CoA hydrolase acting on acyl-CoA. Thus AA could be derived by combining PC, CoA, the acyltransferase, and the hydrolase. Evidence for the release of AA in lymphocytes as well as macrophages by this mechanism was presented by TROTTER et al. (1982). In support of this pathway, RESCH et al. (1983, 1984) have reported that the acyltransferase is stimulated up to fourfold soon after adding Con A to intact cells. The stimulation does not require energy since it occurred in intact cells or in isolated membranes incubated with Con A at 37° or 0 °C. Both Na^+, K^+-ATPase and acyltransferase could be activated by AA, thought to be derived from triglycerides. The observations form the basis of a proposal for the activation of lymphocytes in which a "supramolecular complex" of the two enzymes and their lipid matrix would be altered in parallel by mitogens or inhibitors (RESCH et al. 1984). This proposal is attractive for several reasons, but a few problems present themselves. For example, the proposal requires that free AA be present in lymphocytes, contrary to published data, to initiate the release of more AA, and most of the mitogen-stimulated AA is derived not from PC but from PI, which was not a donor of acyltransferase-mediated AA release (TROTTER and FERBER 1981). Also, acyltransferase was found by others (DOBSON and MELLORS 1980) to be inhibited, not stimulated by Con A. Despite these drawbacks, mitogens do induce a small amount of AA release from PC (PARKER et al. 1979 a), and acyltransferase operating "in reverse" could well account for a portion of the increase in the percentage of polyenoic fatty acids found in lipids of stimulated cells (FERBER et al. 1975; RODE et al. 1982).

AA release occurs soon after addition of mitogen (PARKER et al. 1979 a; HIRATA et al. 1980; HOMA et al. 1984) and inhibition of its release is associated with inhibition of several events, including activation of guanylate cyclase (COFFEY et al. 1981), production of IL-2 (NAMIUCHI et al. 1984), and finally synthesis of DNA (HIRATA et al. 1980; PARKER 1982; COFFEY and HADDEN 1981 b; NAMIUCHI et al. 1984). Some of the inhibitors used in these experiments have now been shown to inhibit both phospholipase A_2 and C. Once liberated, AA may serve as a source of energy or it may be metabolized by three pathways, as shown in Fig. 1. It may be reincorporated into phospholipids, converted by cyclooxygenase to endoperoxides which are then converted to prostaglandins (PG), thromboxanes or prostacyclin, or converted by lipoxygenase to hydroperoxy derivatives (HPETE) which are further metabolized to hydroxy derivatives (HETE) or leukotrienes (LT) (SAMUELSSON et al. 1978; SAMUELSSON 1982; LANDS 1984).

Cyclooxygenase is specifically inhibited by low concentrations (0.1–1 μM) of indomethacin, which does not inhibit and sometimes augments mitogen activation of lymphocytes (GOODWIN et al. 1977; TOMAR et al. 1981). These results are consistent with data from many laboratories that PGs of the E series inhibit lymphocyte proliferation (see Chaps. 14, 15). Specifically, PGE_2 was shown to block the progression of lymphocytes from G_{1a} to G_{1b} (WALKER et al. 1983), by inhibiting the production of IL-2 (CHOUAIB et al. 1985). It had no effect on IL-2 receptor expression, but greatly reduced the expression of transferrin receptors.

It was therefore intriguing that BRAY et al. (1981) and GOLDYNE and STOBO (1982) found no PGs in either resting or activated lymphocytes, although TOMAR et al. (1981) found a small production of PGs in stimulated cells. Most workers now suspect that nearly all the PGs found in immune systems are synthesized by monocytes and/or macrophages (HUMES et al. 1977; BRAY et al. 1981; LOW et al. 1984). However, PGs may be produced by suppressor T lymphocytes (GOODWIN et al. 1977) in a way that requires participation of macrophages (WEBB and NOWOWIEJSKI 1981), and, in a positive feedback fashion, may be required for the generation of suppressor T cells (ORME and SHAND 1981). New light has been shed on the mechanism of suppression by the discovery of a population of human T lymphocytes, purified by virtue of its ability to bind PGE_2, that may evolve into suppressor cells upon exposure to PGE_2 (FISCHER et al. 1985). The actual suppression mediated by these cells does not require the continued presence of PG.

Thromboxane synthesis has been suggested as important in T lymphocyte activation (KELLY et al. 1979; UDEY and PARKER 1982). However, a comparison of several chemically unrelated and very potent inhibitors of thromboxane synthesis revealed no correlation between this inhibition and that of DNA synthesis in a study involving human blood lymphocytes and four T cell mitogens (GORDON et al. 1981). At this time one may conclude that no cyclooxygenase product is critical for triggering T lymphocyte activation, while a PG may be important in differentiative steps leading to suppressor cells.

The presence of lipoxygenase in lymphocytes is controversial. PARKER et al. (1979 b) reported the rapid increase of 5-HETE and 12-HETE in lymphocytes freed of platelets, and GOETZL (1981) reported fivefold increases in 5-, 11-, and 15-mono-HETEs as well as 5, 12-di-HETE (LTB$_4$) in mitogen-stimulated human T lymphocytes freed of monocytes. However, GOLDYNE et al. (1984) presented evidence that E-rosetted lymphocytes make no lipoxygenase products, while contaminating monocytes may convert AA, released from lymphocytes, into HETEs (GOLDYNE and STOBO 1982). It is possible that some lymphocytes not collected by the E-rosetting method can produce the products described. For example, J. Y. DJEU and J. Y. VANDERHOEK (1985, personal communication) found 5-HETE in large granular lymphocytes that were totally devoid of monocytes or platelets. A resolution of the controversy may lie in the data of ATLURU et al. (1986), who showed that human T cells (not prelabeled with AA) produce 10^{-9} M LTB$_4$ in response to PHA. They found that AA actually inhibited the synthesis of LTB$_4$ in lymphocytes (but not neutrophils). The practice of adding labeled AA to measure lipoxygenase activities would thus prevent the formation of LTB$_4$.

Lipoxygenase inhibitors were found to inhibit activation of human lymphocytes by PHA, pokeweed mitogen (PWM), and the calcium ionophore A23187 in the initial studies of KELLY et al. (1979 b) and this has been confirmed by many other workers in other lymphoid systems (reviewed by BAILEY et al. 1986; Chap. 15). Nordihydroguaiaretic acid (NDGA) blocks all lipoxygenases (being most potent on the 5-lipoxygenase; SALARI et al. 1984), but does not inhibit cyclooxygenase, and the inhibitors eicosatetraynoic acid (ETYA) and BW755c have been reported to block both cyclooxygenase and certain lipoxygenases. Both NDGA and ETYA were found to block mitogen activation of guanylate cyclase as well as DNA synthesis in human lymphocytes (COFFEY and HADDEN 1981 b). 15-HETE, a potent inhibitor of 5-lipoxygenase (VANDERHOEK et al. 1980), inhibited the actions of PHA and PMA in mouse spleen cells (BAILEY et al. 1982 a, b) and human T lymphocytes (PAYAN and GOETZL 1981). It also prevented the activation of lymphocyte guanylate cyclase by 5-HETE or by mitogens (COFFEY and HADDEN 1985 b).

The effects of exogenous AA are interesting. KELLY and PARKER (1979) showed that it augmented PHA stimulation of human lymphocytes at 0.5–1 μM, but inhibited it at higher doses. It inhibits PMA activation progressively from 0.01 to 10 μM (R. G. COFFEY 1985, unpublished work). Some of these effects may be mediated by the metabolic products of AA, although neither indomethacin, NDGA, nor ETYA prevented the inhibition of the effects of PMA. A reasonable interpretation is the direct inhibition of LTB$_4$ formation by AA (ATLURU et al. 1986). Some of the effects of exogenous AA may be due to cell surface actions of AA to provoke intracellular release and metabolism of AA from membrane phospholipids (HOMA et al. 1984). At physiologic AA levels, the affinity of 5-lipoxygenase for substrate exceeds that of 15-lipoxygenase, while at 10 μM AA, the

15-lipoxygenase is enhanced and 5-lipoxygenase is consequently inhibited (DELA-
CLOS et al. 1984). In addition, AA can act directly to stimulate protein kinase C
substituting for PS in neutrophils (MCPHAIL et al. 1984; HANSSON et al. 1986) and
lymphocytes (R. G. COFFEY 1986, unpublished work). These effects could account
for the enhancement and inhibition of PHA stimulation by low and high levels
of AA, respectively.

Several studies have indicated the importance of lipoxygenase in distinct steps
of lymphocyte activation. DINARELLO et al. (1984) reported that IL-1 production
was inhibited by ETYA and BW755c, but not by ibuprofen (specific for cyclooxygenase). BAILEY et al. (1986) found that 15-HETE prevented the production of IL-
2 in mouse and human lymphocytes, and KATO and MURATO (1985) reported inhibition of IL-2 production and action (but apparently not inhibition of IL-2 receptor appearance) in murine splenocytes by caffeic acid and AA861. These compounds, like 15-HETE, are quite specific inhibitors of 5-lipoxygenase. Using 15-
HETE and other lipoxygenase inhibitors with T lymphocyte cell lines, each capable of limited responses, FARRAR and HUMES (1985) determined that lipoxygenase activity is essential for at least three distinct steps in lymphocyte activation:
(a) IL-2 production in EL4 cells, stimulated by IL-1 or PMA; (b) lymphokine
(IFN-γ) secretion in BFS cells, stimulated by IL-2 or PMA; and (c) proliferation
of CT6 cells, stimulated by IL-2. Partial restoration of the responses to IL-2 was
obtained by adding 5-HETE in the experiments of FARRAR and HUMES (1985) and
by adding LTC$_4$ in the studies of PUPILLO (1985). Complete restoration of T cell
proliferation was obtained with 10^{-10} M LTB$_4$ in T cells treated with either lipoxygenase or phospholipase inhibitors (GOODWIN 1986). This suggests that
LTB$_4$ is the only AA metabolite required for signaling T cell proliferation.

GUALDE et al. (1983) postulated that 15-HPETE is a product of macrophages
rather than lymphocytes, and that it functions to limit lymphocyte function or activation. Since HPETEs are rapidly converted to HETEs, it is possible that 15-
HETE contributes to the inhibition by 15-HPETE. This is supported by the finding that 15-HETE induces the generation of immunosuppressive cells (ALDIGIER
et al. 1984). Interestingly, 15-HPETE (but not 15-HETE) causes a loss in Fcγ receptors on the surface of human T lymphocytes and monocytes (GOODWIN et al.
1984). 15-HPETE may be a precursor to a newly described series of 14-peptido-
leukotrienes which appear to be involved in the mitogen-induced proliferation of
suppressor T cells (BRYANT et al. 1985). It will be fascinating to watch the unveil-
ing of new lipoxygenase products and the description of their selective effects on
the many aspects of lymphocyte activation.

Natural killer cytotoxicity, attributed to large granular lymphocytes, is inhibited by noncytotoxic concentrations of NDGA and other inhibitors of lipoxygenase (ROSSI et al. 1985). LTB$_4$ was able to reconstitute activity at picomolar
levels. Others (ROLA-PLESZCZYNSKI et al. 1984) also found that leukotrienes
(A$_4$,B$_4$,D$_4$) enhanced natural killer activity. Some disagreement is apparent regarding the effects of stereoisomers of LTB$_4$.

In a few instances, relative affinities of site-specific lipoxygenase for substrates, and inhibition by products, have been reported. The comparison between
5- and 15-lipoxygenases (DELACLOS et al. 1984) has been mentioned. As a further
contribution to the diversity of the lipoxygenase control systems, LOW et al.

(1984) found that the inhibitory potencies of HETEs in the serum-free PHA mouse spleen system varied considerably, the most potent being the HETEs with the hydroxyl group at position 9 or 11, followed by intermediate effects with 12-, 15-, or 8-HETE, and no inhibition by 5-HETE. The effect of 11-HETE could be quite meaningful since vascular smooth muscle produces high amounts of this (as well as 15-HETE) after exposure to thrombin (Low et al. 1984). Both products can be derived via the cyclooxygenase pathway (Bailey et al. 1986), in contrast to other HETEs. Gualde et al. (1985a) confirmed the effect of 15-HPETE to inhibit DNA synthesis in unfractionated human T lymphocytes. These workers and Payan et al. (1984) observed that LTB_4 also inhibits synthesis, in contrast to the data of Goodwin (1986); other leukotrienes did not inhibit synthesis (Payan and Goetzl 1983). However, when the cells were separated further, both of these lipoxygenase products enhanced the induction, proliferation, and functions in the fraction enriched for cytotoxic suppressor cells, and inhibited proliferation in the fraction enriched for helper-inducer phenotype (Payan et al. 1984; Gualde et al. 1985a, b). Such detailed studies help one to interpret the diverse data that have emerged from unseparated mixtures of cells.

IV. Summary of Lipid Changes

In summarizing the discussions of lipid changes, it is apparent that breakdown of polyphosphoinositides occurs before the other changes and may in fact be the only critical lipid event for the mitogen-induced stimulation of T lymphocytes to exit from G_0. PI breakdown follows that of PIP_2 and both give rise to DAG which may then stimulate protein kinase C (see Sect. III.3). Only the breakdown of PIP_2 gives rise to ITP, which then causes liberation of Ca^{2+} from membrane stores. The status of the resynthesis of PI and PC is undecided; such reactions are of course important in the later events of cell enlargement and division. AA release and metabolism by the lipoxygenase pathway has been shown to be absolutely essential for at least three activation events in experiments utilizing carefully separated subcellular fractions and cloned T cell lines. The critical effector molecules may be HPETEs, HETEs, or LTs, with exacting specificity for the position on AA that is oxidized. The responses of T cells vary from inhibition to augmentation of induced function, and appear to depend to some extent on cell surface receptors. From the differential effects of glucocorticoids, it appears that B cells require arachidonate release for proliferation, but not for differentiation (Cupps et al. 1985).

D. Transport Changes (see also Chap. 3)

Increased movements of ions and nutrients across the plasma membrane are among the earliest changes observed after stimulation of lymphocytes. Various carriers or mediators of transport are involved, and enzyme activities have been identified with some. The transport of K^+, Na^+, H^+, Ca^{2+}, amino acids, glucose, nucleosides, and iron are discussed here. Uptake of fatty acids, phosphate, choline, and inositol are considered in Sect. C.

I. Ions

1. Potassium

The Na^+, K^+-ATPase spans the plasma membrane and accounts for the Na^+, K^+ pump which transports K^+ inward and Na^+ outward against gradients by means of the energy derived from hydrolysis of ATP (Schwartz et al. 1971). Ouabain binds to K^+ sites on the outer surface of the cell and inhibits the enzyme and the pump activity; K^+ reverses the inhibition. The stimulation of this system by T cell mitogens has been reported in over 50 papers among which only a few can be discussed here.

Quastel and Kaplan (1968) reported the first observation that ouabain inhibited PHA stimulation of RNA and DNA synthesis (assayed at 24 and 72 h, respectively) in lymphocytes. The effect was very specific, with an IC_{50} of 50 nM, and it was reversible by K^+. Kay (1972) found that ouabain did not affect uridine incorporation at 1 h, and concluded that the early stimulation of uridine uptake did not depend on the pump. PHA stimulates both uptake and efflux of K^+; ouabain inhibits only the uptake (Quastel and Kaplan 1975). Using $^{86}Rb^+$ as a K^+ analog, Averdunk (1972) measured an increase in uptake within 30 s of addition of PHA. The mechanism involved an increase in V_{max}. Kay (1972) considered that the capacity of ouabain to inhibit later protein and RNA synthesis might reflect the importance of maintaining K^+ levels. The PHA-induced increase in K^+ influx might be a homeostatic mechanism to reverse a more primary effect of the mitogen to induce membrane permeability and K^+ depletion.

Mitogen-induced K^+ permeability (sometimes called leak flux) was confirmed by several workers to occur in minutes (Averdunk and Lauf 1975; Segel et al. 1975; Negendank and Collier 1976). In addition to K^+, increased permeability to Mg^{2+}, Na^+, and Ca^{2+} was observed. Careful measurements of K^+ levels in human lymphocytes stimulated with PHA revealed no net change over 24 h, as the influx increase from 20 to 38 nmol was balanced by the efflux increase from 19 to 38 nmol per liter cell water (Segel et al. 1976; Segel and Lichtman 1976). Negendank and Shaller (1979) confirmed these results and determined that when K^+ levels appeared to decline after mitogen addition, this was an artifact of cell washing and resuspension. Exacting studies have shown that Con A causes a net intracellular K^+ increase, from 14 to 16 fmol per cell, owing to a slightly greater stimulation of active transport than of leak (Owens and Kaplan 1980; Kaplan and Owens 1982). When cell water expands proportionately, there is no change in K^+ concentration.

Potassium ions are now thought to be exported from cells by specific channels and the names for these will likely replace the terms "permeability" and "leak flux." Two types of Ca^+-activated K^+ channels have been discovered in other cells (Peterson and Maruyama 1984). Rink and Deutsch (1983) published evidence for activation of these channels as a consequence of A23187-induced Ca^{2+} influx, and also described a new patch-clamp technique which revealed the presence of voltage-gated K^+ channels in lymphocytes (see Chap. 3).

Using patch-clamp techniques, Gupta and co-workers (DeCoursey et al. 1984; Chandy et al. 1984) determined that voltage-gated K^+ channels were the predominant ion channels in human T lymphocytes. The channels open with sigmoid kinetics during depolarizing voltage steps, a feature that distinguishes them from Ca^{2+}-gated channels. However, subsequent studies (TATHAM et al. 1986) showed that Ca^{2+}-activated K^+ channels are stimulated within 10 min in association with increases of cellular ionized calcium. CHANDY et al. (1984) found that PHA affected K^+ channels within 1 min, causing them to open more rapidly and at more negative membrane potentials. Correlations were found between inhibition of K^+ current with tetraethylammonium or 4-aminopyridine and reduction of PHA-stimulated synthesis of RNA and DNA. Also effective were the Ca^{2+} channel blockers verapamil and diltiazem, and the Ca^{2+} blocker quinine. However, CHANDY et al. (1984) presented evidence that these inhibitors also act on the voltage-gated K^+ channels. It is believed that the Ca^{2+}-independent K^+ channels may participate in early events and are critical for protein and DNA synthesis. However, the inhibitors did not block the new expression of IL-2 receptors on T cells, and since they blocked DNA synthesis, even when added 20 h after mitogen, another interpretation would be that these channels are important for proliferation, but not for initial signal transmission.

Membrane potential changes accompany ion fluxes in innervated tissues and several studies indicate that slowly developing potential changes also occur in mitogen-activated lymphocytes (SHAPIRO et al. 1979; KIEFER et al. 1980; FELBER and BRAND 1983). Mouse spleen T lymphocytes have a normal surface charge of -65 mV; depolarization occurred 2–3 h after addition of Con A. Repolarization occurred over the next 7 h, and hyperpolarization was observed in the 48 h preceding mitosis. In the human T lymphocyte studies of GELFAND et al. (1984), PHA caused changes in potential at 1 h (becoming more negative). These changes paralleled the magnitude of subsequent DNA synthesis. The specificity of these changes in murine splenic and human peripheral T cells for T cell mitogens, and for similar changes in B cells for LPS, attest to their importance in the later events of mitogen action in these cells. TATHAM et al. (1986) also showed a small hyperpolarization in human T cells, maximal 1–2 min after addition of PHA or Con A. In murine thymocytes, T cell mitogens induced hyperpolarization, possibly as a result of Ca^{2+}-gated K^+ channel activation (TSIEN et al. 1982; FELBER and BRAND 1983). RINK and DEUTSCH (1983) stated that membrane potential plays no critical role in the response to mitogens for the first 2–3 h, while GELFAND et al. (1984) concluded that changes in potential are necessary for changes in Ca^{2+} uptake.

The data of QUASTEL and KAPLAN (1968, 1970) indicated that the Na^+,K^+-ATPase enzyme would be stimulated by mitogens. AVERDUNK and LAUF (1975) and POMMIER et al. (1975) did observe such increases in Na^+,K^+-ATPase of lymphocytes of human, mouse, and sheep if the intact cells were preincubated with mitogen prior to measurement of activity. Some controversy has developed regarding the ability of mitogens to stimulate the Na^+,K^+-ATPase by direct addition to isolated membranes, The effect was observed in thymocytes by RESCH et al. (1983), in human lymphocytes by AVERDUNK et al. (1976), and murine plasmacytoma (MOPC) cells by AUBRY et al. (1979), but has not been confirmed in human (SEGEL et al. 1979) or other lymphocytes (NOVOGRODSKY 1972; DORNAND et al. 1978). Stimulation of Na^+,K^+-ATPase by mitogens acting on intact cells has been documented in calf thymocytes (SZAMEL et al. 1981; RESCH et al. 1983) and in rabbit thymocytes (TANDON et al. 1983).

Inhibition of Na^+,K^+-ATPase by ouabain is associated with inhibition of several aspects of mitogen action: uridine uptake (QUASTEL and KAPLAN 1968; KAY 1972; SZAMEL et al. 1981), acyltransferase activation and oleate incorporation (SZAMEL et al. 1981), production of IL-2 (STOECK et al. 1983); and eventually of DNA synthesis (QUASTEL and KAPLAN 1968). Curiously, washing of cells was found to reverse ouabain inhibition of mitogen-induced, but not antigen-induced DNA synthesis (WRIGHT et al. 1973). Ouabain binds to specific high affinity sites on cells, and PHA increases this binding to human blood lymphocytes (QUASTEL et al. 1974; QUASTEL and KAPLAN 1975). The effect, which occurs within minutes after PHA addition in parallel with increases in active K^+ transport, is due to an increased number rather than affinity of the binding sites on Na^+,K^+-ATPase. Addition of K^+ reverses ouabain binding and also the inhibition of transport and RNA synthesis. It is suspected that ouabain may act at some point in addition to the ATPase since the concentration required for inhibiting activation of acyltransferase (0.1–0.1 mM) and of IL-2 production (1 mM) are much greater than the concentrations (1–10 μM) that inhibit the ATPase (STOECK et al. 1983; RESCH et al. 1984). It is not known if all these effects of ouabain are reversible by excess K^+.

FRIEDMAN and KATELEY (1974) noticed that immunization caused a large increase in mouse spleen Mg^{2+}-ATPase activity. In contrast to the Na^+,K^+-ATPase, most of the Mg^{2+}-ATPase activity is apparently on the outer surface of lymphocytes (POMMIER et al. 1975). AVERDUNK and LAUF (1975) and AVERDUNK et al. (1976) found that, in addition to the fivefold increase in human lymphocyte Na^+,K^+-ATPase, Con A also stimulated a two-fold increase in Mg^{2+}-ATPase activity. Several others have reported similar findings (NOVOGRODSKY 1972; KRISHNARAJ and TALWAR 1973; POMMIER et al. 1975; TANDON et al. 1983). In contrast, RESCH et al. (1983) observed a decrease in Mg^{2+}-ATPase after Con A treatment, possibly due to different methods of membrane preparation.

To conclude this section, mitogens activate several systems for maintaining homeostasis of K^+. One cannot be certain whether the active transport (Na^+,K^+-ATPase) or the voltage-gated (or Ca^{2+}-gated) channel is activated first, or whether there is some permeability not accounted for by the gated channels described to date. Since both hyperpolarization and depolarization have been reported to result from mitogen stimulation of different T lymphocytes, and since the effects are often delayed for hours, it is difficult to claim that changes in transmembrane potential are crucial for initiating lymphocyte activation. RANSOM and CAMBIER (Chap. 3; see also MONROE et al. 1984) discuss this in greater detail, especially in reference to B lymphocyte activation. Although the regulatory roles of the K^+ flux systems have not been thoroughly explored, it is evident that K^+ efflux through the channels is essential to the initial activation process, and that normal functioning of the Na^+,K^+-ATPase is essential for lymphocyte proliferation, as well as for viability.

2. Sodium and Hydrogen (see also Chap. 3)

Three new technologies have made intracellular pH (pH_i) measurements possible:
1. DEUTSCH et al. (1982) used a new application of nuclear magnetic resonance to measure a pH_i of 7.17 in human lymphocytes. They showed that lymphocytes

use energy for close regulation of their pH, which changes very little while the pH of the medium is varied from 6.8 to 7.4, and found that mitogenesis proceeds best when cells are in this range. 2. GERSON and KIEFER (1982) used the pH-dependent fluorochrome, 4-methylumbelliferone, to measure a gradual increase in pH_i, from 7.15 to 7.45, after activation of mouse spenic lymphocytes by Con A or LPS. This technique was used to show that three cell lines, transformed by virus, had a pH_i about 0.5 units higher than normal cells. ROGERS et al. (1983) employed the quene 1 fluorescence method to measure a pH_i of 7.15 in thymocytes. They saw no change within the first 3 min after adding mitogen, and in contrast to the results of DEUTSCH et al. (1982), they saw no change when the pH of the medium was increased to 8.0. 3. GERSON et al. (1982) used ^{14}C-labeled 5.5-dimethyloxazoline-2,4-dione distribution to measure a resting pH_i of 7.17 in mouse splenocytes. Two increases in pH_i were observed after mitogen addition: during the first 1–6 h pH_i increased by about 0.2 units, declined to the control value at 20 h, then increased slowly to 7.5 over the next 50 h. The second increase in pH_i appeared to be proportional to DNA synthesis, while the final decline occurred at mitosis.

A mechanism for increasing pH_i and Na^+ simultaneously is the Na^+/H^+ antiport, and this has now been described in human peripheral blood lymphocytes (GRINSTEIN et al. 1984). This Na^+/H^+ exchange system functions in the opposite direction from the Na^+,K^+-ATPase, bringing Na^+ into the cell, while transporting protons out. This antiport is rapidly stimulated by lectin mitogens and, again, by IL-2 (MILLS et al. 1985c). The system is one of many that are activated by protein kinase C (BESTERMAN et al. 1985), which is in turn activated by mitogens (see Sect. E.III). The antiport is potently inhibited by amiloride and this drug has become popular for investigating the mechanism of mitogen action. One role for the antiport system is to maintain constant $[Na_i^+]$ which would otherwise be lowered by the action of the Na^+,K^+-ATPase. Another important function is to activate enzymes with optima near 7.5. GRINSTEIN et al. (1984) found that the apparent increases in the pH_i of actively cycling thymocytes were caused by increases in the number of mitochondria per unit cell volume, thus raising some doubts about the interpretation of the data of GERSON et al. (1982). In agreement with DEUTSCH et al. (1982), GRINSTEIN et al. (1984) found that some pH indicators distribute preferentially in mitochondria, which have a higher pH than the cytoplasm. However, HESKETH et al. (1985) found that several mitogens caused increases in the pH_i of mouse thymocytes within 30 min, in a way that was dependent on a transient increase in $[Ca_i^{2+}]$. It is difficult to imagine an increase in mitochondria in so short a time. GRINSTEIN et al. (1985a, b) produced considerable data supporting the mitogen activation of the antiport. They measured concomitant increases in pH_i, increases in $[Na_i^+]$, and decreases in the pH of the medium after incubating rat thymic lymphocytes with PMA. One important aspect of these changes is that HCO_3^- and Cl^- would accumulate along with Na^+ and cause osmotic swelling. An increase in cell volume has long been observed as one morphological change caused by mitogens (see Chap. 3).

It is not possible to state at this time whether the changes in pH_i are critical early events in lymphocyte activation, because of the controversy concerning the timing. The changes are possibly important in mid to late cycle events, and are considered vital in the mitogen activation of other types of cells (MOOLENAAR et al. 1984). No area of investigation escapes controversy, and the data of MILLS et al. (1985c) were interpreted to indicate that cytoplasmic alkalinization caused by IL-2 stimulation of the antiport was not critical for lymphocyte proliferation. Also, results with an analog of amiloride, MK 685, have cast doubts on the importance of Na^+/H^+ exchange in mitogen activation of fibroblasts (BESTERMAN et al. 1984). This analog is more potent than amiloride for inhibiting the exchange, but while amiloride also inhibits proliferation, MK 685 does not inhibit mitogen activation of RNA, protein, or DNA synthesis. The effects of amiloride may act uniquely on other systems such as the growth factor receptor tyrosine kinase (DAVIS and CZECH 1985).

3. Calcium (see also Chap. 3)

The role of Ca^{2+} in lymphocyte activation has been extensively reviewed (LICHT-MAN et al. 1983). ALLWOOD et al. (1971) first showed that PHA caused rapid increases in cellular Ca^{2+} $[Ca_i^{2+}]$. In the ensuing years, a long list of mitogenic agents, including Con A, PWM, periodate, zinc, mercury, and trypsin have been shown to increase $[Ca_i^{2+}]$ in a variety of human and rodent lymphocytes (WHITNEY and SUTHERLAND 1972a; NEGENDANK and COLLIER 1976; PARKER 1974; FREEDMAN et al. 1975; HUI and HARMONY 1980a; TSIEN et al. 1982; TOYOSHIMA et al. 1982b; DEUTSCH and PRICE 1982; HESKETH et al. 1983b; O'FLYNN et al. 1984). Mitogenic lectins caused uptake of Ca^{2+} while nonmitogenic lectins did not (PARKER 1974; TSIEN et al. 1982). Neither did phorbol esters (GELFAND et al. 1985), which reduce the requirement of protein kinase C for Ca^{2+} (NISHIZUKA 1984). Ca^{2+} chelators such as EDTA and EGTA inhibited transformation in a way that could be reversed by adding more calcium (ALFORD 1970; WHITNEY and SUTHERLAND 1972b). The chelators also inhibited early events, including RNA synthesis (KAY 1971), uptake of inositol (CRUMPTON et al. 1976) and oleate (RESCH et al. 1976) into membrane phospholipids, and activation of guanylate cyclase (COFFEY et al. 1981).

Antigens also cause increases in $[Ca_i^{2+}]$ in T cell lines exposed simultaneously to antigen-presenting cells in a genetically restricted way that corresponds to stimulation of proliferation (NISBET-BROWN et al. 1985; IMBODEN et al. 1985). Further substantiating the importance of Ca^{2+} in early events of lymphocyte activation, calcium ionophores (A23187, ionomycin) have been employed as mitogens or comitogens by a number of investigators (LUCKASEN et al. 1974; MAINO et al. 1974; FREEDMAN et al. 1975, 1981; HADDEN et al. 1975; GREENE et al. 1976a; WHITESELL et al. 1977; LICHTMAN et al. 1979, 1983; OTANI et al. 1980; TSIEN et al. 1982).

The mechanism by which mitogens induce Ca^{2+} uptake may be through increased affinity of the transport sites (PHA studies: WHITNEY and SUTHERLAND 1973) or through increases in the number of transport sites (Con A studies: OZATO et al. 1977). Recent experiments by GELFAND et al. (1984) suggest that membrane potential is important in regulating Ca^{2+} uptake. Controversy over the magnitude and kinetics of Ca^{2+} influx has been considerable, owing to technical difficulties concerning filtering and washing procedures. The introduction of the fluorescent Ca^{2+} indicator quin2 has resolved many of these problems and has made it possible to measure $[Ca_i^{2+}]$ accurately without overly perturbing the cells (TSIEN et al. 1982). Resting $[Ca_i^{2+}]$ was estimated by O'FLYNN et al. (1984) as 107 nM in unfractionated mononuclear cells, 150 nM in non-T cells, and 67 nM in T cells; similar values were reported by TSIEN et al. (1982) and HESKETH et al. (1983 a, b). These and other studies (FREEDMAN 1979; GELFAND et al. 1984) indicate that Ca^{2+} uptake begins as early as 0.5 min and, in the early time period, reaches a maximum at 2–5 min after addition of PHA (2- to 4-fold over control) or Con A (1.5- to 2-fold over control). In long-term studies (WOLFF et al. 1985) $[Ca_i^{2+}]$ was found to peak at 24 h after addition of Con A to human T lymphocytes. The level reached at this time correlated well with subsequent DNA synthesis. Different kinetics were observed when *Staphylococcus aureus* protein A was used to stimulate transformation (GELFAND et al. 1985). This substance caused an increase in $[Ca_i^{2+}]$ at 2–3 h, compared with a few minutes for PHA. The delay was thought to be due to the requirement for a monocyte – T cell interaction for protein A to trigger Ca^{2+} uptake.

Exactly which steps of lymphocyte activation require Ca^{2+}, or increased $[Ca_i^{2+}]$, is controversial and under active investigation. Some of the results were derived from cloned cell lines with reduced medium Ca^{2+} requirements, and may not apply to normal lymphocytes in circulation. The earliest lipid change known, the breakdown of PIP_2, was found to be independent of Ca^{2+} mobilization when PHA was added to the JURKAT T cell leukemia line (SASAKI and HASEGAWA-SASAKI 1985). However, production of IL-2 by this line does appear to require Ca^{2+} (WEISS et al. 1984). In fact, it has been shown that the mitogenic capacity of A23187 is due to its stimulation of IL-2 production (JOSIMOVITZ et al. 1985).

The stimulation of Tac antigen appearance by Con A was prevented by three Ca^{2+} channel blockers, as was the influx of $^{45}Ca^{2+}$ and the proliferation of lymphocytes in response to either Con A or IL-2 (BIRX et al. 1984). In contrast, MILLS et al. (1985 a) found that PHA-induced increases in IL-2 receptor expression in human E-rosetted T lymphocytes does not require increased $[Ca_i^{2+}]$, while IL-2 production does. Using human and murine IL-2-sensitive cell lines, MILLS et al. (1985 b) could not detect a requirement for Ca^{2+} in IL-2-stimulated proliferation. On the contrary, highly purified recombinant IL-2 induced the influx of $^{45}Ca^{2+}$ into freshly isolated human T cells (FLEISHER and BIRX 1985). This might account for the increase in $[Ca_i^{2+}]$, at 24 h after addition of mitogen, found by WOLFF et al. (1985).

Inhibition of both Ca^{2+} influx and DNA synthesis by the Ca^{2+} channel antagonists verapamil, nifedipine, and diltiazem (CHEUNG et al. 1983), and also by a monoclonal antibody to the IL-2 receptor, confirmed the importance of Ca_i^{2+} in the effects of IL-2 in freshly isolated lymphocytes. JOHNSON et al. (1985) also measured the induction of Ca^{2+} influx by IL-2, and, with the intracellular Ca^{2+} antagonist chlorpromazine, demonstrated that the IL-2 stimulation of IFN-γ is similarly dependent on Ca^{2+}. In this connection it is useful to recall the early observations of WHITFIELD et al. (1969) that very high levels of Ca^{2+} could provoke rat thymocytes to move from a restricted G_1 phase into S phase. This observation and several subsequent ones (reviewed by WHITFIELD et al. 1976) probably relate to the actions of IL-2. Events that take place in peripheral blood lymphocytes more than 24 h after mitogen addition are apparently not dependent on Ca^{2+}.

This is evident from the results of timed addition of EGTA (Diamantstein and Ulmer 1975), of chlorpromazine (Ferguson et al. 1975), and of verapamil (Blitstein-Willinger and Diamantstein 1978). None of these agents which block calcium entry or its actions were effective in inhibiting DNA synthesis if added at 24 h or later.

Among the several intracellular actions of Ca^{2+}, important effects to stimulate the phospholipid-dependent protein kinase C and to combine with calmodulin are probably critical both for initiating lymphocyte activation and for mid and late cycle events (Ku et al. 1981; Kaibuchi et al. 1985). Lichtman et al. (1982) showed that trifluorperazine, a potent inhibitor of both Ca^{2+}-dependent proteins, inhibited mitogen-induced Ca^{2+} transport and Ca^{2+} export ATPase in human lymphocytes. Transformation of these cells is equally sensitive to the drug (Bachvaroff et al. 1984). The systems affected by these proteins are discussed in Sect. E.III.

4. Iron

The roles of iron and transferrin in lymphocyte activation now appear to be firmly established. The data reviewed by Brock and Mainou-Fowler (1983) indicate that activated lymphocytes have an increased need for iron, and possibly for its transport protein transferrin. Iron is a structural part of heme, which is found in the cytochromes, cyclooxygenase, guanylate cyclase, cytochrome P-450, tryptophan oxygenase, and many other enzymes of diverse function. Ribonucleotide reductase, a key enzyme in DNA synthesis, also requires iron. Transferrin partly saturated with iron markedly enhanced the responses of mouse lymph node cells, suspended in serum-free media, to Con A or LPS (Brock 1981). Significant iron uptake occurred only after about 20 h following addition of mitogen (Brock and Rankin 1981).

Larrick and Creswell (1979) first showed PHA- and Con A-induced increases in the binding of transferrin to its receptors on human lymphocytes. It is now established that transferrin receptors are present intracellularly in resting lymphocytes, but they increase by a factor of five and appear to a great extent on the surface after mitogen activation (Weiel and Hamilton 1984; Chap. 2). The increase occurs only after IL-2 receptors appear and, in experiments involving separation of the activation steps, only after IL-2 is added (Hamilton 1982, 1983; Neckers and Cossman 1983). Monocytes, or phorbol esters which replace some monocyte functions, are required for transferrin receptor expression after exposure to mitogen (Neckers and Cossman 1983; Neckers et al. 1984; Chouaib et al. 1985). Iron is made available to the cell only after the transferrin-receptor complex has been internalized, a step that is promoted by phosphorylation mediated by protein kinase C (May et al. 1984). Recycling of the receptors to the surface occurs after dephosphorylation.

Two groups (Mendelsohn et al. 1983; Neckers and Cossman 1983) have reported that monoclonal antibody against the transferrin receptor prevented mitogen- or IL-2-induced DNA synthesis in human lymphocytes. In the experiments of Mendelsohn et al. (1983), the inhibition could be reversed by removing the antibody after 48 h incubation. One might conclude that transferrin (and/or iron) is needed only in the latter stages of the cell cycle. The fact that inhibition was also partially reversed by iron nitrilotriacetate, bypassing the blocked receptor, suggests that the transferrin receptor is unimportant per se, but simply functions to increase cellular levels of iron. It can also function to bring zinc into the cell (PHILLIPS and AZAIR 1974). Several observations, including the fact that zinc, rather than iron, was found to augment mitogen action, support an important role for zinc in mitogen activation of lymphocytes (WILLIAMS and LOEB 1973; BERGER and SKINNER 1974).

II. Nutrients

1. Amino Acids

Over 20 papers report that the transport of many amino acids in lymphocytes is enhanced by mitogens. The earliest reports of amino acid uptake in mitogen-stimulated lymphocytes were those of KAY (1968) and HAUSEN et al. (1969) who found that uptake of leucine doubled in 4–6 h. This amino acid belongs to a group whose uptake is independent of Na^+ (YUNIS et al. 1963). Many workers prefer to use 2-aminoisobutyric acid (AIB) because it is nonmetabolizable. AIB belongs to a group that requires Na^+, is stimulated by Ca^{2+}, and is inhibited by ouabain. Activation of AIB uptake begins at about 5 min (VAN DEN BERG and BETEL 1971, 1973 a,b; MENDELSOHN et al. 1971; AVERDUNK 1972). Ouabain and a host of inhibitors of oxidative phosphorylation, glycolysis, and protein synthesis inhibited this uptake, whereas inhibitors of RNA and DNA synthesis did not (VAN DEN BERG and BETEL 1974 b). These authors also stated that Con A stimulated only the transport of those amino acids in the Na^+-dependent group (VAN DEN BERG and BETEL 1973 b).

Different conclusions were reached by BORGHETTI et al. (1979) and SEGEL and LICHTMAN (1981), who subdivided amino acid transport into three systems. The A and the ASC systems require Na^+, but only the A system, which involves AIB, increases as an adaptive response to amino acid deprivation. The L system is Na^+ independent. Of the three systems, A was the most rapidly and markedly increased by PHA in pig lymphocytes (BORGHETTI et al. 1979). The A and ASC systems were equally stimulated by T cell mitogens in human lymphocytes (SEGEL and LICHTMAN 1981). The L system was increased to a much smaller extent and several hours later than the others.

Kinetic studies indicated that AIB transport increases owing to an effect on V_{max} rather than on K_m, reaching a sixfold elevation at 9 h (MENDELSOHN et al. 1971; GREENE et al. 1976 a). The increased transport was further enhanced by cytochalasins, and was inhibited by colchicine (GREENE et al. 1976 d; RESCH et al. 1981). It was not affected by inhibitors of protein synthesis (MENDELSOHN et al. 1971), but was inhibited by cycloheximide in rat lymph node cells (VAN DEN BERG and BETEL 1974b) and in human leukemic lymphocytes (BARAN et al. 1972). Neither actinomycin D nor mitomycin D inhibited Con A-stimulated transport of the amino acids AIB, asparagine, and glycine (all in the A group) (VAN DEN BERG and BETEL 1974 b). It may be concluded that, depending on the species, stimulation of this system requires protein synthesis and energy, but not DNA or RNA synthesis.

The degree to which the early increase in amino acid transport is essential for lymphocyte activation is difficult to establish. Whereas Van den Berg and Betel (1973a, 1974a) found good correlations between AIB uptake stimulation and lectin mitogenicity in rodent lymphocytes, Udey et al. (1980) observed stimulation by the nonmitogen wheat germ agglutinin in human blood lymphocytes, and Greene et al. (1976c) found that this agglutinin inhibited Con A stimulation of AIB uptake. Since DNA synthesis requires cysteine and glutamine, it is possible that only the later period of amino acid uptake is crucial for proliferation.

2. Glucose

Glucose and its nonmetabolizable analogs (3-O-methylglucose and 2-deoxyglucose) are incorporated into T lymphocytes at accelerated rates within minutes of addition of mitogen (Hadden et al. 1971; Peters and Hausen 1971b; Averdunk 1972; Reeves 1975; Whitesell et al. 1977; Yasmeen et al. 1977; Hume et al. 1978). The effect of PHA is due to increased V_{max} of the facilitated diffusion system (Peters and Hausen 1971b).

Mitogen stimulation of glucose transport may represent a direct effect on the cell membrane since it is not inhibited by macromolecular synthesis inhibitors. Energy-linked processes are suggested by the inhibition by oligomycin and dinitrophenol of A23187-stimulated (but not control) uptake of glucose (Reeves 1975). Calcium was found to be necessary for the stimulation of glucose uptake, but not for its maintenance (Yasmeen et al. 1977; Nordenberg et al. 1983). Cyclic AMP inhibits glucose uptake (May et al. 1970), apparently by preventing the uptake of Ca^{2+} (Whitesell et al. 1977). Hydrocortisone inhibits glucose transport (Munck 1971), possibly through a mechanism involving its inhibition (through lipomodulin) of phospholipase since other inhibitors (p-bromophenacylbromide, Nordenberg et al. 1983; quercetin, Hume et al. 1979) of this Ca^{2+}-activated enzyme also block uptake of glucose. A more specific inhibitor of mitogen-activated glucose uptake is cytochalasin B (Hume et al. 1978). The mechanism of this effect is likely to be on the glucose carrier itself since Mookerjee and Jung (1982) showed that, of the three cytochalasin binding sites, one was specifically displaced by glucose.

This discussion of glucose reveals several interesting features about lymphocyte physiology and the pharmacologic regulation of it. The impingement of Ca^{2+} and phospholipid metabolism on this system is intriguing. The work reviewed in Sect. B suggests that inhibition of glucose uptake by cytochalasins has little effect on lymphocyte activation if the cells are exposed to the drugs for only a few hours. It may be fair to conclude that certain necessary early events are crucial for mitogen activation of glucose uptake, but that the latter is important only for later energy-requiring and synthetic events as the cells progress through the cycle.

3. Nucleosides

Uridine uptake is increased almost immediately after addition of PHA to human peripheral blood lymphocytes (Lucas 1967; Hausen and Stein 1968; Kay 1968; Quastel and Kaplan 1968). The effect is on V_{max}, like so many of the other transport systems. The increase reaches a maximum rate at about 8 h. It was proposed (HAUSEN and STEIN 1968) that uridine kinase was rate limiting since its activity rises in parallel. Others (LUCAS 1967; KAY and HANDMAKER 1970) measured uridine uptake hours before increases in the kinase were detectable, and suggested that neither the uptake nor its incorporation into RNA was limited by the kinase.

The possible importance of uridine uptake in the early events of lymphocyte activation was ruled out by the lack of effect of ouabain (which did inhibit uptake at 26 h; KAY 1972), and the lack of effect of dipyridamole, a general inhibitor of uptake of several nucleosides, on lymphocyte transformation (PETERS and HAUSEN 1971 a). The importance of the uptake of nucleosides in later events is, like that of amino acids and glucose, unquestioned.

E. Changes in Cyclic Nucleotides and Protein Phosphorylation

I. Cyclic AMP

Cyclic AMP (cAMP) is formed from ATP by the action of adenylate cyclase, an enzyme intrinsic to the plasma membranes of eukaryotic cells. Activation of the enzyme by hormones such as glucagon or PGE_2 requires GTP which binds to N_s, a regulatory protein that moves freely in the plasma membrane and may bind to hormonal receptors or to adenylate cyclase (ROSS and GILMAN 1980). Inhibition of adenylate cyclase is also mediated by a GTP-binding protein N_i, now identified in several mammalian cells (UI 1984). Many hormones can activate both reactions, depending on which receptor they bind. For example, epinephrine binding to β-receptors or adenosine binding to α_2-receptors activates the N_s unit, increasing cAMP. Epinephrine binding to α_2-receptors or adenosine binding to α_1-receptors activates the N_i unit, decreasing cAMP. The multitude of effects of mitogens, antigens, and hormones on these systems, and the effects of cAMP on lymphocyte activation, have been amply reviewed (PARKER et al. 1974; WEDNER and PARKER 1976; HADDEN 1977; STROM et al. 1977; ROBINS 1982), and will only be presented in outline here.

The first report of mitogen-induced changes in lymphocyte cAMP was that of SMITH et al. (1971). They observed small increases in cAMP in human lymphocytes 2 min after exposure to PHA. Confirmation of these early increases has been reported by some workers using Con A (WEBB et al. 1973; LYLE and PARKER 1974; WHITFIELD et al. 1974; WATSON 1975) or A23187 (ATKINSON et al. 1978; STOLC 1980). Most laboratories were unable to detect early increases in cAMP using optimal concentrations of mitogens (NOVOGRODSKY and KATCHALSKI 1970; DERUBERTIS et al. 1974; SMITH et al. 1974; MONAHAN et al. 1975; GLASGOW et al. 1975; HADDOX et al. 1976; COFFEY et al. 1977; WANG et al. 1978; CARPENTIERI et al. 1980 a,b; HUI and HARMONY 1980 b; ROCHETTE-EGLY and KEMPF 1981; TAKIGAWA and WAKSMAN 1980; GOODMAN and WEIGLE 1983; LARGEN and VOTTA 1983). When highly agglutinating preparations of PHA (HADDEN et al. 1972) or supramitogenic concentrations of PHA (GLASGOW et al. 1975) or Con A (COFFEY et al. 1977) were used, increases in cAMP were measurable. Such increases were greatly magnified if the cells were centrifuged prior to fixation by acid or other means (COFFEY et al. 1977). Interestingly, succinylated Con A did not cause increases in cAMP at any concentration, even if the cells were centrifuged (HADDEN et al. 1976; TAKIGAWA and WAKSMAN 1980). The mitogenic capacity of this substance is equal to that of native Con A, but unlike Con A, it does not cause receptor capping and does not inhibit proliferation at high (250 mg/ml) doses. The non-lectin mitogen periodate (HADDOX et al. 1976) also caused no change in splenic lymphocyte cAMP. Wheat germ agglutinin is a potent stimulant of cAMP in human lymphocytes (GREENE et al. 1976 b; R. G. COFFEY and E. M. HADDEN 1976, unpublished work), but this lectin is not mitogenic – in fact, it inhibits mitogenesis induced by other agents. PMA, selectively mitogenic for a subpopulation of human T lymphocytes (TOURAINE et al. 1977) actually caused a 50% decrease in adenylate cyclase activity of human lymphocytes (COFFEY and HADDEN 1983 a).

The collected observations have been interpreted (PARKER et al. 1974; WEDNER and PARKER 1976; ATKINSON et al. 1978) to indicate a role for cAMP perhaps in a small compartment of the lymphocyte, in promoting early events of T lymphocyte activation. In support of this notion, BLOOM et al. (1973) used fluorescent antibody techniques to demonstrate the increase in cAMP in the plasma membranes of lymphocytes incubated with PHA. Others (HADDEN 1977; STROM et al. 1977; ROBINS 1982) have interpreted the data to mean that cAMP is not increased by mitogens unless conditions are used which reduce mitogenicity.

Consistent with this interpretation are many reports that, if added at the same time as mitogen, cAMP or its lipophylic analogs (dibutyryl-cAMP and 8-Br-cAMP), and agents which stimulate increases in intracellular cAMP prevent subsequent events in lymphocyte activation (for reviews see PARKER et al. 1974; HADDEN 1977; COFFEY and HADDEN 1985 a). Among these agents are epinephrine and isoproterenol (acting on the β_2-receptor), histamine (acting on the H_2receptor), adenosine (acting on the A_2-receptor), cholera toxin and pertussis toxin (which activate and inhibit the functions of N_s and N_i, respectively), PGE_1 and PGE_2, phosphodiesterase inhibitors such as theophylline, and a unique T cell protein (or proteins) known as "inhibitor of DNA synthesis" or IDS (WAGSHAL et al. 1978). Using an innovative technique whereby antibodies are introduced into lymphocytes via resealed red cell ghosts, OHARA and WATANABE (1982) showed that cAMP-specific antibodies enhanced DNA synthesis in lymphocytes treated with Con A, while cGMP-specific antibodies inhibited synthesis. This technique may be extremely useful in probing the functions of several intracellular enzymes with the abundance of monoclonal antibodies now available.

In contrast to the inhibition of early events of activation, cAMP may be important at later times. WANG et al. (1978) observed an increase in cAMP 30–36 h after adding Con A to mouse spleen lymphocytes, and this was confirmed using both Con A and succinylated Con A by TAKIGAWA and WAKSMAN (1980). The increase may have been PG dependent since it was inhibited by indomethacin. ROCHETTE-EGLY and KEMPF (1981) also observed increases in cAMP at later times in human peripheral lymphocytes using four T lymphocyte mitogens: PHA,

Con A, A23187, and PMA. The rat thymic lymphoblast experiments of WHIT-FIELD et al. (1976) are considered to involve midcycle events in lymphocyte activation. In these experiments, a number of agents that stimulate cAMP increases were shown to stimulate the cells to pass from a G_1 boundary and undergo DNA synthesis. These experiments strongly suggest a role for cAMP at this time; however, WAGSHAL et al. (1978) produced evidence that IDS is produced during this period and inhibits DNA synthesis in T lymphocytes by virtue of its ability to elevate cAMP at this time. Three important late G_1 effects of cAMP are: (a) inhibition of IL-2 production (CHOUAIB et al. 1985); (b) prevention of transcription of the transferrin gene (TUIL et al. 1985); and (c) inhibition of the appearance of transferrin receptors (CHOUAIB et al. 1985). A mechanism for preventing these negative effects of cAMP exists; BECKNER and FARRAR (1986) found that IL-2 causes inhibition of adenylate cyclase and of the stimulation by PG of cAMP increase. The mechanism was thought to involve protein kinase C, and is mimicked by PMA (COFFEY and HADDEN 1983a).

In B lymphocytes, data of GILBERT and HOFFMANN (1985) suggest that cAMP is an essential signal for induction of antibody production: dibutyryl-cAMP and IL-1 together stimulated polyclonal Ab production in highly purified B cells. The effect was antigen specific, but did not involve IL-2; rather complex data were interpreted to indicate that cAMP acts to prevent the production of an inhibitor of BCGF. In contrast to activation for Ab production, MURAGUCHI et al. (1984) found that human B cell activation for proliferation by μ-specific antibodies plus BCGF was inhibited by forskolin, a diterpene which causes a strong and sustained increase in cAMP. This occurred when forskolin was added at any time up 36 h, and seems to rule out a positive role for cAMP during the G_1-S transition events of B cell activation.

The effects of cAMP at very late times (72 h) are suspected to be inhibitory since its levels rise at a time when T lymphocyte DNA synthesis begins to decline (MONAHAN et al. 1975; CARPENTIERI et al. 1981). It is not known whether these late increases represent nutritional deprivation or some other more specific effect. In our experiments with a T lymphoblastoid cell line (CEM) grown in suspension cultures, we have observed increasing basal levels of cAMP occurring with increasing cell density, and these rises were associated with decreasing responsiveness to hormonal stimulation (R. G. COFFEY and R. A. OLSSON 1987, unpublished work).

II. Cyclic GMP

Guanylate cyclase, the enzyme that converts GTP to cGMP, is found in membrane and cytosolic fractions of lymphocytes (WATSON et al. 1976; HADDOX et al. 1978; COFFEY et al. 1981). Activity is stimulated by a wide variety of oxidizing agents, including the HPETEs, nitrosoamines, and dehydroascorbic acid (GOLD-BERG and HADDOX 1977; HIDAKA and ASANO 1977; GRAFF et al. 1978; HADDOX et al. 1978). Stimulated levels of lymphocyte cGMP are quickly reduced by phosphodiesterase activities which, like cAMP phosphodiesterases, may exist in more than one form (WEDNER et al. 1979; COFFEY and HADDEN 1983a; COFFEY et al. 1984).

The first observations of mitogens inducing brisk increases of intracellular levels of cGMP involved the T cell mitogens PHA and Con A in human peripheral blood lymphocytes (HADDEN et al. 1972). These results have been confirmed by at least 20 laboratories (reviewed in COFFEY and HADDEN 1983b). Some laboratories (WEDNER et al. 1975; BURLESON and SAGE 1976; DERUBERTIS and ZENSER 1976; ATKINSON et al. 1978; KAEVER and RESCH 1985) have been unable to measure mitogen-induced cGMP increases in lymphocytes for reasons that may relate to differences in methodology (COFFEY 1977). The positive cGMP observations include the actions of both B and T lymphocyte mitogens to stimulate two- to ten-old increases in cGMP within 2–10 min in mouse and rat thymocytes (WHITFIELD et al. 1974; WESS and ARCHER 1981), splenocytes (HEIDRICK 1973; WATSON 1975; HADDOX et al. 1976; KATAGIRI et al. 1976; TAM and WALFORD 1978; SHENKER and GRAY 1979; BOMBOY and GRABER 1980; LARGEN and VOTTA 1983), and lymph nodes (WAKSMAN et al. 1980) in addition to peripheral blood lymphocytes of rat (SCHUMM et al. 1974) and human subjects (DEVILLER et al. 1975; OHARA et al. 1978; TAKEMOTO et al. 1979, 1982; CARPENTIERI et al. 1980a, b; HUI and HARMONY 1980b; ROCHETTE-EGLY and KEMPF 1981). The calcium ionophore A23187, mitogenic for T lymphocytes (MAINO et al. 1974; HOVI et al. 1976a), and the tumor promoter PMA, mitogenic for a subpopulation of T lymphocytes (TOURAINE et al. 1977) increase human lymphocyte cGMP within minutes (COFFEY et al. 1977; ROCHETTE-EGLY and KEMPF 1981; COFFEY and HADDEN 1983a). The effects of the mitogenic lectins and A23187 were dependent on extracellular Ca^{2+}, while those of PMA apparently required only intracellular Ca^{2+}.

Antigenic stimuli, represented by sheep red blood cells, also increase cGMP rapidly in splenocytes of mouse (YAMAMOTO and WEBB 1975) and rat (SPACH and ASCHKENASY 1979). At least two thymic hormones (see Chap. 16) which augment proliferation of T lymphocytes have been shown to cause increases in cGMP within minutes: thymopoietin (SUNSHINE et al. 1978) and thymosin fraction 5 (NAYLOR et al. 1979). A second increase in cGMP was found to occur in late G_1 or early S phase in human lymphocytes stimulated with four different T cell mitogens (ROCHETTE-EGLY and KEMPF 1981). This late increase may result from the increase in $[Ca_i^{2+}]$ caused by IL-2 (FLEISHER and BIRX 1985).

The mechanism by which lectin mitogens increase cGMP is unknown, but is considered to involve calcium-dependent and oxidative steps (COFFEY et al. 1977, 1981; HUI and HARMONY 1980a,b; ROCHETTE-EGLY and KEMPF 1981; LARGEN and VOTTA 1985). It is due to activation of guanylate cyclase rather than inhibition of phosphodiesterase, and is thought to be indirect, since it is only observed by incubating intact lymphocytes with mitogens and measuring enzyme activity in subsequently isolated membranes (COFFEY et al. 1981) or cytosol (DEVILLER et al. 1975). It was proposed that one or more HPETEs, formed in intact lymphocytes by Ca^{2+}-dependent phospholipases and lipoxygenases, would function as the proximal stimulants (COFFEY et al. 1981). Support for this mechanism, known to occur in broken cell preparations (HIDAKA and ASANO 1977; GOLDBERG et al. 1978; GRAFF et al. 1978) derived from observations that inhibitors of phospholipases (cAMP, quinacrine, p-bromophenacylbromide, and Rosenthal's inhibitor) and inhibitors of lipoxygenases (NDGA, ETYA, 15-HETE) prevented the activation by PHA of both guanylate cyclase and DNA synthesis (COFFEY et al. 1981;

COFFEY and HADDEN 1985b). Indomethacin did not inhibit the effects of PHA, but rather enhanced them, indicating the lack of a requirement for PGs or thromboxanes (see also Chap. 15).

Preliminary data suggest that more than one mechanism may be involved. For example, PMA (but not PHA) is able to stimulate guanylate cyclase in broken cells by the direct addition of PMA with PS (COFFEY 1986). Inhibitors of lipoxygenase do not interfere with this stimulation, but protein kinase C and calmodulin inhibitors do attenuate it in parallel with reduced stimulation of the kinase. Difficulties were encountered in that the inhibitors (phenothiazines, calmidazolium, palmitoylcarnitine) begin to inhibit basal guanylate cyclase at concentrations which prevent its activation by 50%–70%. Despite this, the mechanism is attractive because the phosphorylation and stimulation of guanylate cyclase by protein kinase C has been demonstrated with enzymes purified from other tissues (ZWILLER et al. 1985). Since lectin mitogens cause the release of DAG (reviewed in Sect. C), and both DAG and PMA stimulate protein kinase C, this mechanism may contribute to the stimulation of guanylate cyclase. It is reasonable to expect that mitogen stimulation of phospholipid breakdown leads to the stimulation via both the lipoxygenase-HPETE pathway and the DAG–protein kinase C route. In addition, arachidonate stimulates soluble guanylate cyclase directly, in the absence of oxidative reactions (GERZER et al. 1986; R. G. COFFEY 1986, unpublished work). Inhibitor data should be interpreted with caution since most inhibitors have more than one action, and a final determination of the intact cellular mechanisms may require isolation and reconstitution of purified components that contribute to the stimulation of guanylate cyclase.

Multiple effects of lipoxygenase products on cGMP have been noted. In addition to the direct stimulation of HPETEs, indirect stimulation of guanylate cyclase by concentrations of 5-HETE between 1 nM and 1 μM (and, to a lesser extent, by other HETEs) occurs in intact lymphocytes (COFFEY and HADDEN 1981b, 1985b). This may be receptor mediated, as it does not occur in broken cell preparations. By separation of murine lymphocyte subpopulations, MEXMAIN et al. (1985) showed that 15-HETE and LTB$_4$ stimulated up to threefold increases in cGMP of PNA$^+$ (peanut agglutinin-binding) immature thymocytes. Smaller increases occurred in mixed populations, and still smaller increases in the mature PNA$^-$ (non-peanut agglutinin-binding) thymocytes. Small decreases in cAMP levels were noted. The increases in cGMP were shown by inhibitor studies to depend on the lipoxygenase pathway and occurred in association with generation of Lyt–2$^+$ suppressor cells. Effects on DNA synthesis depend, correspondingly, on the cell type: it is stimulated by 15-HETE and LTB$_4$ in the immature cells, but may appear to be inhibited in mixtures in which mature cells predominate.

Cyclic GMP has several effects relative to activation in lymphocytes, as revealed by studies in which 8-Br-cGMP or agents inducing increases in intracellular cGMP were added. Cyclic GMP promotes Ca^{2+} uptake and reverses the inhibition of uptake caused by cAMP (FREEDMAN 1979; HUI and HARMONY 1980a). Cyclic GMP or its lipophilic derivatives induce B cell proliferation (WEINSTEIN et al. 1975; DIAMANTSTEIN and ULMER 1975), but the effect requires millimolar concentrations and is reproduced by other guanosine derivatives (GOODMAN and WEIGLE 1983). This suggests a lack of selectivity for cGMP, which in any case never exceeds micromolar levels intracellularly. It is important to note that these agents do not cause stimulation of T lymphocyte proliferation, although cGMP may, at physiologic doses, augment mitogen-induced DNA synthesis (reviewed in HADDEN and COFFEY 1982). Some specific effects of cGMP that are likely related to proliferation are the increases in phosphoribosylpyrophosphate synthetase, a key enzyme in purine and pyrimidine synthesis (CHAMBERS et al. 1974), and increases in RNA polymerase I and III activities (ANANTHAKRISHNAN et al. 1981). Of potential importance are the effects of cGMP to limit the influence of cAMP by two mechanisms: (a) inhibition of cAMP-dependent protein kinase; and (b) stimulation of a cAMP-specific phosphodiesterase (GOLDBERG et al. 1973; FARAGO et al. 1978).

An extensive literature (reviewed by STROM et al. 1977) documents the augmentation by cGMP (and inhibition by cAMP) of several lymphocyte functions beside that of proliferation. These include lymphocyte-mediated cytotoxicity, erythrocyte rosette formation, lymphocyte motility, and production of certain lymphokines. A specific effect of cGMP to replace the IL-2 requirement for IFN-γ synthesis in soybean agglutinin-stimulated murine splenocytes was observed by JOHNSON et al. (1982). Cyclic GMP could replace the IL-2 requirement for DNA synthesis in the same system. The effect is limited in terms of the stimulant; 8-Br-cGMP did not replace IL-2 in the stimulation of IFN-γ production in LPS-primed splenocytes (D. K. BLANCHARD, R. G. COFFEY and J. Y. DJEU 1985, unpublished work).

Cyclic GMP appears to participate in the lymphokine-generating actions of IL-1. SVENSON and BENDTZEN (1985) observed the augmentation of IL-1-induced production of leukocyte inhibitory factor by lipid-soluble cGMP analogs and by agents that increase cGMP intracellularly. These agents also reversed the inhibition of production exerted by cyclosporin. Another function of cGMP independent of proliferation may be the stimulation of receptor display on helper T cells (GUPTA 1979). Very high levels of cGMP may activate cAMP-dependent protein kinases, and thus some agents such as the nitrosoamines that stimulate such high levels may inhibit proliferation. It is of considerable interest that PMA stimulates early increases in human lymphocyte cGMP phosphodiesterase (COFFEY and HADDEN 1983a) and lectin mitogens stimulate increases in both cAMP and cGMP phosphodiesterases at 24–48 h (EPSTEIN et al. 1977; SHENKER and GRAY 1979). The significance of increased phosphodiesterases is uncertain, but the effect may protect the cells from inhibitory actions of the nucleotides in S phase.

III. Protein Phosphorylation

1. Cyclic AMP-Dependent Protein Kinases

WEDNER and PARKER (1975) observed stimulation of phosphorylation of several proteins derived from both cytoplasm and plasma membranes after 5 min exposure of human lymphocytes to PHA. Dibutyryl-cAMP also stimulated increases in phosphorylation of proteins, including some that were phosphorylated after PHA. More definitive studies by this group (CHAPLIN et al. 1979, 1980) indicated that the phosphorylation induced by cAMP did not mimic that induced by mitogens. Furthermore, PGE_2 stimulated intracellular increases in cAMP and prevented mitogen-induced changes in phosphorylation, suggesting that the mitogen-induced changes were not mediated by cAMP. In studies that analyzed the individual kinases, some workers (CARPENTIERI et al. 1981; LARGEN and VOTTA 1983) observed no changes in either of the two cAMP-dependent protein kinases within 1 h of mitogen addition. Others (BYUS et al. 1977, 1978) reported that type I, but not type II cAMP-dependent protein kinase was increased by PHA and Con A during the first hour. This group (KLIMPEL et al. 1979) subsequently obtained data suggesting that the change occurred between 1 and 6 h. They related this change to the increase in ornithine decarboxylase, an enzyme known to be induced by cAMP. The induction of ornithine decarboxylase by mitogens, however, was found to be inhibited by cAMP and augmented by cGMP when the nucleotides were added at the same time as the mitogens (KLIMPEL et al. 1979; MIZO-GUCHI et al. 1975).

An interesting examination of the compartmentalization of the two kinases revealed that Con A induced a translocation of type I kinase from the nucleus to the cytoplasm and movement of type II kinase in the opposite direction (MED-NIEKS and JUNGMANN 1982). The biologic sequelae of these translocations are not known, but may be envisioned to involve aspects of gene regulation. Midcycle events of lymphocyte activation may involve cAMP as discussed above. In relation to this possibility, it is notable that IYER et al. (1984), using a very sensitive technique for resolution of phosphorylated protein bands, found the phosphorylation of 25 proteins to be increased 24 h after Con A addition; cAMP was able to increase the phosphorylation of 10 of these. A reasonable conclusion of the studies to date is that early increases in mitogen-induced protein phosphorylation are mediated by kinases other than those that are stimulated by cAMP, while later events may involve cAMP-dependent kinases.

2. Cyclic GMP-Dependent Protein Kinase

Even less information is available regarding cGMP-dependent protein kinase in lymphocyte activation. Some of the actions of cGMP mentioned above may be mediated by such activities, but, with the exception of certain nuclear acidic proteins (JOHNSON and HADDEN 1975), no cGMP-specific substrates for phosphorylation have yet been identified in lymphocytes. Using exogenous substrates, CAR-PENTIERI et al. (1980a,b) showed that cGMP-dependent kinase activity of human lymphocytes was stimulated nearly fourfold following the PHA-induced increase in cGMP. The activity reached a peak at about 3 h and declined to control values at 8 h. This was confirmed with Con A in mouse spleen by LARGEN and VOTTA (1983) using specific antibody to cGMP-dependent kinase and histochemical staining techniques. These findings suggest that new enzyme is synthesized. It will be most interesting to learn whether any of the many proteins phosphorylated in response to mitogens are specifically phosphorylated by the cGMP-dependent kinases.

3. Protein Kinase C

Other protein kinases play important roles in lymphocyte activation. Protein kinase C requires phospholipid, preferably PS, is stimulated by Ca^{2+} and by DAG, and is considered to play a key role in several models of cellular activation (Nishizuka 1984; Nishizuka et al. 1984). Ku et al. (1981) found that protein kinase C was quite active in the cytosol of lymphocytes, and suggested, on the basis of the known actions of mitogens to stimulate PI breakdown and DAG formation, that this kinase would be activated by mitogens. Other routes of activation of the kinase have been suggested by the observation that AA and lipoxins (trihydroxy metabolites of AA) can replace PS (McPhail et al. 1984; Hansson et al. 1986). It is now thought that protein kinase C is important in activation of B lymphocytes (Monroe et al. 1984) as well as T lymphocytes (Farrar et al. 1986).

Castagna et al. (1982) found that PMA bound specifically to protein kinase C, substituting for DAG in the stimulation of the enzyme. One aspect of this stimulation is the sharp drop in K_a for Ca^{2+}, with no apparent change in the phospholipid requirement. Utilizing these findings, Kaibuchi et al. (1985) tested 1-oleoyl-2-acetylglycerol for its mitogenic capacity. This lipid, which activates protein kinase C and penetrates cells more readily than most DAGs, was found to mimic PMA in its ability to act synergistically with A23187 to stimulate DNA synthesis in human peripheral lymphocytes which had been depleted of monocytes. These data point to the powerful initiating nature of increased Ca^{2+} and protein kinase C in lymphocyte proliferation. However, a very small concentration of PHA was required for a full response, indicating the need for a third type of initiating signal. Others (Albert et al. 1985; Isakov et al. 1986) demonstrated the ability of phorbol esters and calcium ionophores, when combined but not singly, to stimulate IL-2 production.

A fascinating translocation of protein kinase C from the cytosol to the plasma membrane occurs in T lymphocytes exposed to the mitogen PHA and OKT3-specific antibody as well as to PMA (Farrar and Ruscetti 1986; Mire et al. 1986). The membrane association caused by PMA lasts more than 60 min compared with a brief 10–20 min association caused by PHA and the antibody. Cytosol protein kinase C activity was elevated threefold at 5 min in the PHA experiments of Mire et al. (1986), returned to control levels at 10 min, and was again elevated to twice control levels at 20 min. A much different pattern was seen with Con A (Averdunk and Gunther 1986). This T cell mitogen caused slowly developing increases in protein kinase C activity in both membrane (2 h) and cytosol (90 min and 12–48 h). B cell mitogens cause the association of protein kinase C with membranes (30 min) and, equally important, effect the proteolytic cleavage to a permanently active form which then migrates back into the cytosol (Guy et al. 1986). A second protein kinase C activation and translocation event is thought to occur in T lymphocytes since IL-2, which had no effect on resting cells, stimulated the temporal translocation of protein kinase C in 5-day-preactivated T cells (Farrar and Ruscetti 1986). This effect resembles that seen in IL-2-dependent T cell lines (Farrar and Anderson 1985; Farrar and Taguchi 1985). However, there is some controversy about the occurrence of this effect in normal human or murine lymphocytes (Mills et al. 1986).

The many effects pursuant to activating protein kinase C are just beginning to be understood. Several proteins are known to be phosphorylated by the enzyme, or by phorbol esters which stimulate only the protein kinase C, and among them certain ones are probably important in the activation of lymphocytes while others may mediate inhibition of growth and/or promotion of differentiation (FEUERSTEIN et al. 1984; KISS and STEINBERG 1985). The stimulation of guanylate cyclase has already been mentioned, and the activation of the Na^+/H^+ exchange and the consequent increase in pH_i and volume have been discussed in Sect. D.I.2. The expression of IL-2 receptors is stimulated by phorbol esters, as well as by antibody against cell surface antigens (anti-T3; FARRAR and RUSCETTI 1986). The IL-2 receptors are themselves phosphorylated in activated blood lymphocytes and cloned T cells (SHACKELFORD and TROWBRIDGE 1984). The phosphorylation of IL-2 receptors appears to occur following the translocation of protein kinase C from the cytosol to the plasma membrane (FARRAR and ANDERSON 1985; FARRAR and TAGUCHI 1985). It is not known if phosphorylation of IL-2 receptors alters their function (ISAKOV and ALTMAN 1986).

The production of IL-2 itself does not normally ensue from protein kinase C activation alone, although PMA enhances the production. A lymphoma cell line (EL4), however, does respond to PMA with increased IL-2 production (KRAFT and ANDERSON 1983). Another important effect of protein kinase C is to cause the inhibition of adenylate cyclase (BECKNER and FARRAR 1986). This would account for the frequent observation of reduced adenylate cyclase activity in mitogen-activated lymphocytes (COFFEY and HADDEN 1983a). Furthermore, both PMA and IL-2 are able to reverse the effects of PGE_2 to stimulate cAMP and to inhibit DNA synthesis.

Transferrin receptors are also phosphorylated by protein kinase C (MAY et al. 1985). This does not alter the affinity of the receptors for transferrin, but is followed by rapid internalization of the receptors. This may represent either a positive signal for iron delivery, or a negative feedback signal limiting surface receptors. It is interesting that hemin, a powerful stimulant of guanylate cyclase, also promotes phosphorylation of transferrin receptors, but inhibits their internalization in certain nonlymphocytic cells (COX et al. 1985). The phosphorylation of PI to form polyphosphoinositides is stimulated by Con A, PMA, and A23187 (TAYLOR et al. 1984). This is of uncertain significance for the very early events of activation. It is mimicked by cAMP (ENYEDI et al. 1983) which, curiously, inhibits production of inositol phosphates (TAYLOR et al. 1984). Another interplay between cAMP and PMA is evident from the data of TAYLOR et al. (1984) who showed that PMA inhibits the cAMP-stimulated phosphorylation of some proteins in bovine lymph node. Histones H2B and H4 are phosphorylated by phorbol esters in murine lymphocytes (PATSKAU and BAXTER 1985), and this was interpreted as relating more to tumor promotion than to proliferation. Other protein kinase C substrates that may not be directly involved in proliferation are the class 1 human leukocyte antigens (HLA). They are transmembrane proteins which interact with cytoskeletal elements and coprecipitate with myosin light chain when phosphorylated by protein kinase C (FEUERSTEIN et al. 1985).

4. Tyrosine Kinases

All the kinases mentioned so far phosphorylate serine or threonine residues. Tyrosine protein kinases are unique in the substrates phosphorylated, and have attracted much interest recently because of their activation in many mitogenic and oncogenic systems (HUNTER and COOPER 1985). These kinases are quite active in membranes of normal peripheral blood lymphocytes (TREVILLYAN et al. 1985). Four membrane substrates were found in the 55–64 kdalton range in lymphocytes (EARP et al. 1984). Proteins of 58–64 kdalton were more characteristic of T cells and the 55–61 kdalton proteins were specifically associated with B lymphocytes. Similar results were obtained by HARRISON et al. (1984). The membrane fractions of T and B lymphocytes were found to have at least two distinct protein kinases (EARP et al. 1985).

FISCHER et al. (1984) found a large stimulation of tyrosine protein kinase activity and of tyrosine phosphorylation in human lymphocytes 1–5 days after addition of PHA. In contrast, PIGA et al. (1985) found that particulate tyrosine protein kinase activity did not change for 24 h after PHA stimulation of human lymphocytes. After 24 h, it began to decline, reaching a minimum at the time of maximal DNA synthesis. Soluble activity also declined, starting at a later time. Endogenous proteins phosphorylated by the enzymes were characterized; interesting changes occurred which await interpretation. A 38 kdalton band was less intensely labeled 24 h after PHA addition, and it disappeared by 72 h. No changes were perceived in the labeling of the proteins in the 55–60 kdalton range for at least 96 h, at which time a new 32 kdalton band, phosphorylated on tyrosine residues, appeared. The pattern of phosphorylated proteins at 96 h resembled that of a malignant T lymphoblastic cell line. PIGA et al. (1985) concluded that tyrosine protein kinases are part of a mechanism which transduces external growth signals to the lymphocyte interior.

One well-characterized substrate for tyrosine protein kinases is lipomodulin. HIRATA et al. (1984) observed a marked increase of ^{32}P incorporation into its tyrosine residues after incubating murine thymocytes with either Con A, A23187, or PMA. This phosphorylation is associated with a decreased capacity of lipomodulin to inhibit phospholipases. It was thought to be due to a tyrosine-specific kinase which in turn is activated by protein kinase C and inhibited by cAMP-dependent protein kinase. CASNELLIE and LAMBERTS (1986) also observed the phosphorylation of a tyrosine protein kinase substrate, $_{pp}56^{T-cell}$. This was associated with the appearance of higher molecular weight forms of the substrate kinase. This fascinating regulation of one type of kinase by another outlines the complexity of the pleiotropic nature of lymphocyte activation and the need for caution in interpretations of limited data.

5. Other Protein Kinases

Still other lymphocyte protein kinases are found to be affected by mitogens. For example, GEAHLEN and HARRISON (1984) found that a nucleolar substrate protein of 112 kdalton was phosphorylated on serine residues by a casein kinase type II. This effect became pronounced at about 20 h, and may relate to important events in late G_1 or early S phase. Several other reports of protein phosphorylation have appeared recently, but have not yet been ascribed to specific kinases. For example, DASCH and STAVITSKY (1985) identified two cytosolic proteins (58 and 90 kdalton) whose phosphorylation was sharply increased after exposing rabbit B lymphocytes to anti-Ig for just 1.5 min. Three others (60, 65, and 95 kdalton) appeared later; some of these also appeared in rabbit T cells incubated with Con A. KOSTKA and SCHWEIGER (1985) observed biphasic increases in phosphorylation of an acid-soluble nuclear protein of 110 kdalton following Con A addition to rat lymph node lymphocytes. They found that the level of phosphorylation correlated with the synthesis of mRNA and suggested that this protein may be the same as identified by others in growth models including hepatoma. A membrane protein (20 kdalton) associated with the T cell antigen receptor is phosphorylated within minutes after adding Con A or antigen plus B cells bearing Ia molecules (SAMELSON et al. 1985). The results were interpreted as possibly involving the clonotypic heterodimer associated with T3 (which itself was not phosphorylated) and may therefore represent a counterpart to the well-known phosphorylation of growth factor receptors in other systems.

F. Conclusions

A careful study of the many excellent publications on intracellular events of T lymphocyte activation suggests that among the very early changes (0–15 min), only a few may be considered as critical trigger signals. The following early lectin mitogen-mediated changes appear essential for initiation of proliferation: PIP_2 (and possibly PI) breakdown, ITP release and mobilization of Ca^{2+}, uptake of Ca^{2+} and K^+, DAG release and activation (together with PS and Ca^{2+}) of protein kinase C, translocation of protein kinase C to the plasma membrane and phosphorylation of membrane proteins of receptor, transport or other functions, arachidonate release and metabolism to 5-HPETE by lipoxygenases, LTB_4 synthesis, and activation of guanylate cyclase both by protein kinase C and by HPETEs. It is quite likely that the rapid pace of research will soon render this list obsolete. Several membrane transport, permeability, and potential changes are of apparent importance, yet selective inhibition of some of these does not result in ablation of later events. In B lymphocytes, most of these events appear to be important, but the emphasis may shift, depending on whether activation is mediated by IL-2 or BCGF, and whether the result is proliferation or Ig synthesis. Some early events such as cAMP increases and formation of receptor micropatches and caps were once thought to be important, but are now considered as epiphenomena or as negative modulators.

Many of the later events are consequences of the early events, including altered synthesis and post-translational modification of proteins (DEPPER et al. 1984; LESTER and COOPER 1985). With very few exceptions, the steps linking the trigger signals to these later events are poorly understood. Critical changes in gene activation are exemplified by the cell cycle-dependent appearance of mRNA for the protooncogenes c-fos and c-myc within 10 min, and for c-myb, p53, and N-ras at about 14 h (REED et al. 1986), mRNA for IL-2 receptors at 1–2 h and for IL-2 at 4–12 h (DEPPER et al. 1984; EFRAT and KAEMPFER 1984; YAMAMOTO et al. 1985;

REED et al. 1986), and by increases in membrane receptors for transferrin at 12–24 h (DEPPER et al. 1984; NECKERS and COSSMAN 1983; KRONKE et al. 1985; REED et al. 1986). Other later changes have long been considered critical, but new evidence casts doubt on the generality of such conclusions. For example, the enhanced synthesis of ornithine decarboxylase, which occurs at 4–6 h (FILLINGAME and MORRIS 1973) is now known to be inhibited by retinoic acid (VERMA 1985), a substance that actually enhances PHA- or PMA-stimulated human T lymphocyte proliferation (VALONE and PAYAN 1985). A rare dissection of the mechanisms of activation of T and B lymphocytes is represented by the finding that retinoic acid inhibited the latter.

Many exciting discoveries are being reported which will add a new dimension to future research. Libraries of mRNA derived from normal, activated, and malignant lymphocytes (ARYA et al. 1984) are being examined to pinpoint exactly which proteins are transcribed and how these will influence progression through the cell cycle. Some genes will be found to be activated as a consequence of IL-1 action, mimicked by PMA, and others by IL-2 action. For example, an intracellular protein called "activator of DNA replication" (ADR, 100 kdalton; GUTOWSKI et al. 1984) appears to be synthesized as a specific response to IL-2. It could be considered as a second or perhaps a third messenger: purified ADR added to isolated nuclei stimulates DNA synthesis, thus reproducing the effect of mitogens on intact cells. The prospects of a much more detailed understanding of the intimate molecular nature of events in lymphocyte activation are rich indeed, as the powerful new tools of molecular biology, monoclonal antibody production and microinjection, and separation and cloning of lymphocytes are merged.

References

Acuto O, Reinherz EL (1985) The human T-cell receptor. N Engl J Med 312:1100–1111

Albert F, Hua C, Truneh A, Pierres M, Schmitt-Verhulst A-M (1985) Distinction between antigen receptor and IL 2 receptor triggering events in the activation of alloreactive T cell clones with calcium ionophore and phorbol ester. J Immunol 134:3649–3655

Aldigier JC, Gualde N, Mexmain S, Chable-Rabinovitch H, Ratinaud MH, Rigaud M (1984) Immunosuppression induced in vivo by 15 hydroxyeicosatetraenoic acid (15 HETE). Prostaglandins Leukotrienes Med 13:99–107

Alford RH (1970) Metal cation requirements for phytohemagglutinin-induced transformation of human peripheral blood lymphocytes. J Immunol 104:698–703

Allan D, Michell RH (1974) Phosphatidylinositol cleavage catalyzed by the soluble fraction from lymphocytes. Biochem J 142:591–597

Allwood G, Asherson GL, Davey MJ, Goodford PJ (1971) The early uptake of radioactive calcium by human lymphocytes treated with phytohemagglutinin. Immunology 21:509–516

Ananthakrishnan R, Coffey RG, Hadden JW (1981) Cyclic GMP and calcium in lymphocyte activation by phytohemagglutinin. Lymphocyte Diff 1:183–196

Arya SK, Wong-Staal F, Gallo RC (1984) Transcriptional regulation of a tumor promoter and mitogen-inducible gene in human lymphocytes. Mol Cell Biol 4:2540–2542

Ashman RF (1984) The influence of cell interactions on early biochemical activation events in human mononuclear cells. Prog Immunol 5:339–348

Atkinson JP, Kelly JP, Weiss A, Wedner JH, Parker CW (1978) Enhanced intracellular cGMP concentrations and lectin-induced lymphocyte transformation. J Immunol 121:2282–2291

Atluru D, Lianos EA, Goodwin JS (1986) Arachidonic acid inhibits 5-lipoxygenase in human T cells. Biochem Biophys Res Commun 135:670–676

Aubry J, Zachowski A, Paraf A, Colombani J (1979) Modulation of membrane-bound enzyme activity by binding of antibodies to major histocompatibility complex antigens. Ann Immunol (Paris) 130C:17–27

Averdunk A, Lauf PK (1975) Effects of mitogens on sodium-potassium transport, ^{3}H-ouabain binding and adenosine triphosphatase activity in lymphocytes. Exp Cell Res 93:331–342

Averdunk R (1972) Über die Wirkung von Phytohemagglutinin und Antilymphozytenserum auf den Kalium-, Glucose- und Aminosäure-Transport bei menschlichen Lymphozyten. Hoppe Seylers Z Physiol Chem 353:79–87

Averdunk R, Gunther T (1986) Protein kinase C in cytosol and cell membrane of concanavalin A-stimulated rat thymocytes. FEBS Lett 195:357–361

Averdunk R, Mueller J, Wenzel B (1976) Studies on the mechanism of activation of lymphocyte membrane ATPase by concanavalin A. J Clin Chem Clin Biochem 14:339–344

Bachvaroff RJ, Miller F, Rapoport FT (1984) The role of calmodulin in the regulation of human lymphocyte activation. Cell Immunol 85:135–153

Bailey JM, Bryant RW, Low CE, Pupillo MB, Vanderhoek JY (1982a) Regulation of T-lymphocyte mitogenesis by the leukocyte product 15-hydroxy-eicosatetraenoic acid (15-HETE). Cell Immunol 67:112–120

Bailey JM, Bryant RW, Low CE, Pupillo MB, Vanderhoek JY (1982b) Role of lipoxygenases in regulation of PHA and phorbol ester-induced mitogenesis. Adv Prostaglandin Thromboxane Leukotriene Res 9:341–353

Bailey JM, Coffey RG, Merritt WD, Hadden JW (1986) Role of eicosanoids in lymphocyte activation: a review. In: Chedid L, Hadden JW, Spreafico F, Dukor P, Willoughby D (eds) Advances in immunopharmacology. vol 3. Pergamon, Oxford, pp 177–188

Baran DT, Lichtman MA, Peck WA (1972) Alpha-aminoisobutyric acid transport in human leukemic lymphocytes: in vitro characteristics and inhibition by cortisol and cycloheximide. J Clin Invest 51:2181–2189

Beckner SK, Farrar WL (1986) Interleukin 2 modulation of adenylate cyclase. Potential role of protein kinase C. J Biol Chem 261:3043–3047

Belmont JW, Rich RR (1981) Role of calcium and magnesium and of cytochalasin-sensitive processes in lectin-stimulated lymphocyte activation. Cell Immunol 59:276–288

Berger NA, Skinner AM (1974) Characterization of lymphocyte transformation induced by zinc ions. J Cell Biol 61:45–55

Bernard DP, Carboni JM, Waksman BH (1975) Regulation of lymphocyte responses in vitro. VI. Potentiation of the response to phytohemagglutinin by cytochalasin B. Ann Immunol (Paris) 126:107–120

Berridge MJ (1984) Inositol triphosphate and diacylglycerol as second messengers. Biochem J 220:345–360

Besterman JM, Tyrey SJ, Cragoe EJ Jr, Cuatrecasas P (1984) Inhibition of epidermal growth factor induced mitogenesis by amiloride and an analog: evidence against a requirement for Na^+/H^+ exchange. Proc Natl Acad Sci USA 81:6762–6766

Besterman JM, May WS, Levine H, Cragoe EJ, Cuatrecasas P (1985) Amiloride inhibits phorbol ester-stimulated Na^+/H^+ exchange and protein kinase C. J Biol Chem 260:1155–1159

Betel I, Martijnse J (1976) Drugs that disrupt microtubuli do not inhibit lymphocyte activation. Nature 261:318–319

Betel I, Martijnse J, van den Berg KJ (1974) Absence of an early increase of phospholipid-phosphate turnover in mitogen stimulated B lymphocytes. Cell Immunol 14:429–434

Birx DL, Berger M, Fleisher TA (1984) The interference of T cell activation by calcium blocking agents. J Immunol 133:2904–2909

Blitstein-Willinger E, Diamantstein T (1978) Inhibition by isoptin (a calcium antagonist) of the mitogenic stimulation of lymphocytes prior to the S-phase. Immunology 34:303–308

Bloom FE, Wedner H, Parker CW (1973) The use of antibodies to study cell structure and metabolism. Pharmacol Rev 25:343–358

Bomboy JD Jr, Graber SE (1980) Stimulation of cyclic 3':5'-guanosine monophosphate levels in rat spleen cells by lipopolysaccharide preparations. J Lab Clin Med 95:654–659

Boon AM, Beresford BJ, Mellors A (1985) A tumor promoter enhances the phosphorylation of polyphosphoinositides while decreasing phosphatidylinositol labeling in lymphocytes. Biochem Biophys Res Commun 129:431–438

Borghetti AF, Kay JE, Wheeler KP (1979) Enhanced transport of natural amino acids after activation of pig lymphocytes. Biochem J 182:27–32

Bougnoux P, Bonvini E, Chang ZL, Hoffman T (1983) Effect of interferon on phospholipid methylation by peripheral blood mononuclear cells. J Cell Biochem 20:215–224

Bourguignon LYW, Hsing Y-C (1983) The participation of adenylate cyclase in lymphocyte capping. Biochem Biophys Acta 728:186–190

Bray MA, Powell RG, Lydyard PM (1981) Prostaglandin generation by separated human blood mononuclear cell fractions. Int J Immunopharmacol 3:377–381

Brock JH (1981) The effect of iron and transferrin on the response of serum-free cultures of mouse lymphocytes to concanavalin A and LPS. Immunology 43:387–392

Brock JH, Rankin C (1981) Transferrin binding and iron uptake by mouse lymph node cells during transformation in response to concanavalin A. Immunology 43:393–398

Brock JH, Mainou-Fowler T (1983) The role of iron and transferrin in lymphocyte transformation. Immunol Today 4:347–351

Bryant RW, Schewe T, Rapoport SM, Bailey JM (1985) Leukotriene formation by a purified reticulocyte lipoxygenase enzyme. J Biol Chem 260:3548–3555

Burgess GM, Godfrey PP, McKinney JS, Berridge MJ, Irvine RF, Putney JW Jr (1984) The second messenger linking receptor activation to internal Ca release in liver. Nature 309:63–65

Burleson DG, Sage HJ (1976) Effect of lectins on the levels of cAMP and cGMP in guinea pig lymphocytes: early responses of lymph node cells to mitogenic and non-mitogenic lectins. J Immunol 116:696–703

Butman BT, Jacobsen T, Cabatu OG, Bourguignon LYW (1981) The involvement of cAMP in lymphocyte capping. Cell Immunol 61:397–403

Byus CV, Klimpel GR, Lucas DO, Russell DH (1977) Type I and type II cyclic AMP-dependent protein kinase as opposite effectors of lymphocyte mitogenesis. Nature 268:63–64

Byus CV, Klimpel GR, Lucas DO, Russell DH (1978) Ornithine decarboxylase induction in mitogen-stimulated lymphocytes is related to the specific activation of type I adenosine cyclic 3',5'-monophosphate-dependent protein kinase. Mol Pharmacol 14:431–441

Cambier J, Monroe JG, Coggeshall KM, Ransom JT (1985) The biochemical basis of transmembrane signalling by lymphocyte-B surface immunoglobulin. Immunol Today 6:218–222

Cantrell DA, Smith KA (1984) The interleukin-2 T-cell system: a new cell growth model. Science 224:1312–1316

Carpentieri U, Minguell JJ, Haggard ME (1980a) Variation of activity of protein kinase in unstimulated and phytohemagglutinin-stimulated normal and leukemic human lymphocytes. Cancer Res 40:2714–2718

Carpentieri U, Monahan TM, Gustavson LP (1980b) Observations on the level of cyclic nucleotides in three populations of human lymphocytes in culture. J Cyclic Nucleotide Res 6:253–260

Carpentieri U, Minguell JL, Gardner FH (1981) Adenylate cyclase and guanylate cyclase activity in normal and leukemic human lymphocytes. Blood 57:975–978

Casnellie JE, Lamberts RJ (1986) Tumor promoters cause changes in the state of phosphorylation and apparent molecular weight of a tyrosine protein kinase in T lymphocytes. J Biol Chem 261:4921–4925

Castagna M, Takai Y, Kaibuchi K, Sano K, Kikkawa U, Nishizuka Y (1982) Direct activation of calcium-activated, phospholipid-dependent protein kinase by tumor-promoting phorbol esters. J Biol Chem 257:7847–7851

Chambers DA, Martin DW Jr, Weinstein Y (1974) The effect of cyclic nucleotides on purine biosynthesis and the induction of PRPP synthetase during lymphocyte activation. Cell 3:375–380

Chandy KG, DeCoursey TE, Cahalan MD, McLaughlin C, Gupta S (1984) Voltage-gated potassium channels are required for human T lymphocyte activation. J Exp Med 160:369–385

Chaplin DD, Wedner HJ, Parker CW (1979) Protein phosphorylation in human peripheral blood lymphocytes. Phosphorylation of endogenous plasma membrane and cytoplasmic proteins. Biochem J 182:537–546

Chaplin DD, Wedner HJ, Parker CW (1980) Protein phosphorylation in human peripheral blood lymphocytes: mitogen-induced increases in protein phosphorylation in intact lymphocytes. J Immunol 124:2390–2398

Chen S-HS (1979) Relationship between phosphatidylcholine biosynthesis and cellular commitment in concanavalin A-stimulated lymphocytes. Exp Cell Res 121:283–290

Cheung RK, Grinstein S, Gelfand EW (1983) Permissive role of calcium in the inhibition of T cell mitogenesis by calmodulin antagonists. J Immunol 131:2291–2294

Chien MM, Ashman RF (1983) Phospholipid synthesis by activated human B lymphocytes. J Immunol 130:2568–2573

Chouaib S, Welte K, Mertelsmann R, Dupont B (1985) Prostaglandin E_2 acts at two distinct pathways of T lymphocyte activation: inhibition of interleukin 2 production and down-regulation of transferrin receptor expression. J Immunol 135:1172–1179

Coffey RG (1977) Assays for cyclic nucleotides including clinical applications. In: Hadden J, Coffey R, Spreafico F (eds) Immunopharmacology. Plenum, New York, pp 389–412

Coffey RG (1986) Phosphatidylserine and phorbol myristate acetate stimulation of human lymphocyte guanylate cyclase. Int J Biochem 18:665–670

Coffey RG, Hadden JW (1981 a) Phorbol myristate acetate stimulation of lymphocyte guanylate cyclase. Biochem Biophys Res Commun 101:584–590

Coffey RG, Hadden JW (1981 b) Arachidonate and metabolites in mitogen activation of lymphocyte guanylate cyclase. In: Hadden J, Chedid L, Spreafico R, Mullen P (eds) Advances in immunopharmacology. Pergamon, Oxford, pp 365–373

Coffey RG, Hadden JW (1983 a) Phorbol myristate acetate stimulation of lymphocyte guanylate cyclase and cyclic guanosine 3′,5′-monophosphate phosphodiesterase and reduction of adenylate cyclase. Cancer Res 43:150–158

Coffey RG, Hadden JW (1983 b) Calcium and guanylate cyclase in lymphocyte activation. In: Chedid L, Hadden J, Willoughby A (eds) Advances in Immunopharmacology, vol 2. Pergamon, Oxford, pp 87–94

Coffey RG, Hadden JW (1985 a) Neurotransmitters, hormones, and cyclic nucleotides in lymphocyte regulation. Fed Proc 44:112–117

Coffey RG, Hadden JW (1985 b) Stimulation of lymphocyte guanylate cyclase by HETEs. In: Bailey JM (ed) Prostaglandins, leukotrienes, and lipoxins: biochemistry, mechanism of action, and clinical applications. Plenum, New York, pp 501–509

Coffey RG, Hadden EM, Hadden JW (1977) Evidence for cyclic GMP and calcium mediation of lymphocyte activation by mitogens. J Immunol 119:1387–1394

Coffey RG, Hadden EM, Hadden JW (1981) Phytohemagglutinin stimulation of guanylate cyclase in human lymphocytes. J Biol Chem 256:4418–4424

Coffey RG, Hartley L, Polson JB, Krzanowski JJ, Hadden JW (1984) Selective inhibition by NPT 15392 of lymphocyte cyclic GMP phosphodiesterase. Biochem Pharmacol 33:3411–3417

Coggeshall KM, Cambier JC (1985) B cell activation. VI. Effects of exogenous diglyceride and modulators of phospholipid metabolism suggest a central role for diacylglycerol generation in transmembrane signaling by mIg. J Immunol 134:101–107

Cooper HL, Braverman R (1981) Close correlation between initiator methionyl-tRNA level and rate of protein synthesis during human lymphocyte growth cycle. J Biol Chem 256:7461–7467

Cooper HL, Lester EP (1982) Nuclear activation and regulation of lymphocyte protein synthesis. In: Hadden J, Chedid L, Dukor P, Willoughby P (eds) Advances in immunopharmacology, vol 2, Pergamon, New York, pp 95–100

Cox TM, O'Donnell MW, Aisen P, London IM (1985) Hemin inhibits internalization of transferrin by reticulocytes and promotes phosphorylation of the membrane transferrin receptor. Proc Natl Acad Sci USA 82:5170–5174

Cross ME, Ord MG (1971) Changes in histone phosphorylation and associated early metabolic events in pig lymphocyte cultures transformed by phytohaemagglutinin or 6-N,2'-O-dibutyryladenosine 3',5'-cyclic monophosphate. Biochem J 124:241–248

Crumpton MJ, Auger J, Green NM, Maino VC (1976) Surface membrane events following activation by lectins and calcium ionophore. In: Oppenheim JJ, Rosenstreich DL (eds) Mitogens in immunobiology. Academic, New York, pp 85–101

Cupps TR, Gerrard TL, Falkoff RJM, Whalen G, Fauci AS (1985) Effects of in vitro corticosteroids on B cell activation, proliferation, and differentiation. J Clin Invest 75:754–761

Cuthbert JA, Shay JW (1983) Microtubules and lymphocyte responses: effects of colchicine and taxol on mitogen-induced human lymphocyte activation and proliferation. J Cell Physiol 116:127–134

Dasch JR, Stavitsky AB (1985) Mitogen-induced phosphorylation of cytosolic proteins in rabbit T- and B-lymphocytes. Mol Immunol 22:379–390

Davis RJ, Czech MP (1985) Amiloride directly inhibits growth factor receptor tyrosine kinase activity. J Biol Chem 260:2543–2551

Dawson AP, Irvine RF (1984) Inositol (1,4,5) triphosphate-promoted Ca^{2+} release from microsomal fractions of rat liver. Biochem Biophys Res Commun 120:858–864

DeCoursey TE, Chandy KG, Gupta S, Cahalan MD (1984) Voltage gated K^+ channels in human T lymphocytes: a role in mitogenesis? Nature 307:465–468

Degen JL, Neubauer MG, Degen SJF, Seyfrie CE, Morris DR (1983) Regulation of protein synthesis in mitogen-activated bovine lymphocytes. Analysis of active-specific and total mRNA accumulation and utilization. J Biol Chem 258:12153–12162

DeLaclos BF, Braquet P, Borgeat P (1984) Characteristics of leukotriene and HETE synthesis in human leukocytes in vitro. Effect of arachidonic acid concentration. Prostaglandins Leukotrienes Med 13:47–52

Depper JM, Leonard WJ, Kronke M, Noguchi PD, Cunningham RE, Waldmann TA, Greene WC (1984) Regulation of interleukin 2 receptor expression: effects of phorbol diester, phospholipase C, and reexposure to lectin or antigen. J Immunol 133:3054–3060

DeRubertis FR, Zenser T (1976) Activation of murine lymphocytes by cyclic guanosine 3',5'-monophosphate: specificity and role in mitogen action. Biochim Biophys Acta 428:91–103

DeRubertis FR, Zenser TV, Adler WH, Hudson T (1974) Role of cyclic adenosine 3',5'-monophosphate in lymphocyte mitogenesis. J Immunol 113:151–161

Deutsch C, Price MA (1982) Cell calcium in human peripheral blood lymphocytes and the effect of mitogen. Biochim Biophys Acta 687:211–218

Deutsch C, Taylor JS, Wilson DF (1982) Regulation of intracellular pH by human peripheral blood lymphocytes as measured by ^{19}F NMR. Proc Natl Acad Sci USA 79:7944–7948

Deviller P, Cille Y, Betuel J (1975) Guanyl cyclase activity of human blood lymphocytes. Enzyme 19:300–313

Diamantstein T, Ulmer A (1975) Regulation of DNA synthesis by guanosine-5'-diphosphate, cyclic guanosine-3',5'-monophosphate, and cyclic adenosine-3',5'-monophosphate in mouse lymphoid cells. Exp Cell Res 93:309–314

Dinarello CA, Bishai I, Rosenwasser LJ, Coceani F (1984) The influence of lipoxygenase inhibitors on the in vitro production of human leukocytic pyrogen and lymphocyte activating factor (interleukin-1). Int J Immunopharmacol 6:43–50

Dobson P, Mellors A (1980) Inhibition of acyltransferase in lymphocytes by concanavalin A. Biochim Biophys Acta 629:305–316

Dornand J, Reminiac C, Mani J-C (1978) Studies of $(Na^+ + K^+)$ sensitive ATPase activity in pig lymphocytes. Effects of concanavalin A. Biochim Biophys Acta 509:194–200

Earp HS, Utsinger PD, Yount WJ, Logue M, Steiner AL (1977) Lymphocyte surface modulation and cyclic nucleotides. J Exp Med 145:1087–1092

Earp HS, Austin KS, Buessow SC, Dy R, Gillespie GY (1984) Membranes from T and B lymphocytes have different patterns of tyrosine phosphorylation. Proc Natl Acad Sci USA 81:2347–2351

Earp HS, Austin KS, Gillespie GY, Buessow SC, Davies AA, Parker PJ (1985) Characterization of distinct tyrosine-specific protein kinases in B and T lymphocytes. J Biol Chem 260:4351–4356

Edelman GM (1976) Surface modulation in cell recognition and cell growth. Science 194:218–226

Efrat S, Kaempfer R (1984) Control of biologically active interleukin 2 messenger RNA formation in induced human lymphocytes. Proc Natl Acad Sci USA 81:2601–2605

Enyedi A, Farago A, Sarkadi B, Szasz I, Gardos G (1983) Cyclic AMP-dependent protein kinase stimulates the formation of polyphosphoinositides in the plasma membrane of different blood cells. FEBS Lett 161:158–162

Epstein P, Mills J, Ross C, Strada S, Hersh E, Thompson W (1977) Increased cyclic nucleotide phosphodiesterase activity associated with proliferation and cancer in human and murine lymphoid cells. Cancer Res 37:4016–4023

Farago A, Hasznos P, Antoni F, Romhanji T (1978) Two types of cyclic GMP binding site associated with the cyclic AMP-dependent protein kinase from lymphocytes. Biochim Biophys Acta 538:493–504

Farese RV, Orchard JL, Larson RE, Sabir MA, Davis JS (1985) Phosphatidylinositol hydrolysis and phosphatidylinositol-4,5-bisphosphate hydrolysis are separable responses during secretagogue action in the rat pancreas. Biochim Biophys Acta 846:296–304

Farrar WL, Anderson WB (1985) Interleukin-2 stimulates association of protein kinase C with plasma membranes. Nature 315:233–235

Farrar WL, Humes JL (1985) The role of arachidonic acid metabolism in the activities of interleukin 1 and 2. J Immunol 135:1153–1159

Farrar WL, Taguchi M (1985) Interleukin-2 stimulation of protein kinase C membrane association: evidence for IL-2 receptor phosphorylation. Lymphokine Res 4:87–94

Farrar WL, Ruscetti FW (1986) Association of protein kinase C activation with IL 2 receptor expression. J Immunol 136:1266–1273

Farrar WL, Cleveland JL, Beckner SK, Bonvini E, Evans SW (1986) Biochemical and molecular events associated with interleukin 2 regulation of lymphocyte proliferation. Immunol Rev 92:67–80

Fechheimer M, Cebra JJ (1982) Phosphorylation of lymphocyte myosin catalyzed in vitro and in intact cells. J Cell Biol 93:261–268

Felber SM, Brand MD (1983) Early plasma-membrane potential changes during stimulation of lymphocytes by concanavalin A. Biochem J 210:885–891

Ferber E, DePasquale GG, Resch K (1975) Phospholipid metabolism of stimulated lymphocytes: composition of phospholipid fatty acids. Biochim Biophys Acta 398:364–376

Ferguson RM, Schmidtke JR, Simmons RL (1975) Concurrent inhibition by chlorpromazine of concanavalin A-induced lymphocyte aggregation and mitogenesis. Nature 256:744–745

Feuerstein N, Sahai A, Anderson WB, Salomon DS, Cooper HL (1984) Differential phosphorylation events associated with phorbol ester effects on acceleration versus inhibition of cell growth. Cancer Res 44:5227–5233

Feuerstein N, Monod D, Cooper HL (1985) Phorbol ester effect in platelets, lymphocytes, and leukemic cells (HL-60) is associated with enhanced phosphorylation of class 1 HLA antigens: coprecipitation of myosin light chain. Biochem Biophys Res Commun 126:206–213

Fillingame RH, Morris DR (1973) Accumulation of polyamines and its inhibition by methyl glyoxol bis-(guanylhydrazone) during lymphocyte transformation. In: Russell DH (ed) Polyamines in normal and neoplastic growth. Raven, New York, pp 249–260

Fischer A, LeDeist F, Durandy A, Griscelli C (1985) Separation of a population of human T lymphocytes that bind prostaglandin E_2 and exert a suppressor activity. J Immunol 134:815–819

Fischer S, Fagard R, Gacon G, Genetet N, Piau JP, Blaineau C (1984) Stimulation of tyrosine phosphorylation in lectin-treated human lymphocytes. Biochem Biophys Res Commun 124:682–689

Fisher DB, Mueller GC (1968) An early alteration in the phospholipid metabolism of lymphocytes by PHA. Proc Natl Acad Sci USA 60:1396–1402

Fisher DB, Mueller GC (1969) The stepwise acceleration of phosphatidylcholine synthesis in PHA-treated lymphocytes. Biochim Biophys Acta 176:316–323

Fisher DB, Mueller GC (1971 a) Gamma-hexachlorocyclohexane inhibits the initiation of lymphocyte growth by phytohaemagglutinin. Biochem Pharmacol 20:2515–2518

Fisher DB, Mueller GC (1971 b) Studies on the mechanism by which phytohemagglutinin rapidly stimulates phospholipid metabolism of human lymphocytes. Biochim Biophys Acta 248:434–448

Fleisher TA, Birx DL (1985) The role of calcium in IL-2 dependent proliferation. Fed Proc 44:1309

Freedman MH (1979) Early biochemical events in lymphocyte activation. Cell Immunol 44:290–313

Freedman MH, Raff MC, Gomperts B (1975) Induction of increased calcium uptake in mouse T-lymphocytes by concanavalin-A and its modulation by cyclic nucleotides. Nature 255:378–382

Freedman MH, Khan NR, Frew-Marshall BJ, Cupples CG, Mely-Goubert B (1981) Early biochemical events in lymphocyte activation. Cell Immunol 58:134–146

Friedman H, Kateley JR (1974) Enhanced splenic ATPase activity in immunized mice. Proc Soc Exp Biol Med 147:460–463

Geahlen RL, Harrison ML (1984) Induction of a substrate for casein kinase II during lymphocyte mitogenesis. Biochim Biophys Acta 804:169–175

Gelfand EW, Cheung RK, Grinstein S (1984) Role of membrane potential in the regulation of lectin-induced calcium uptake. J Cell Physiol 121:533–539

Gelfand EW, Cheung RK, Mills GB, Grinstein S (1985) Mitogens trigger a calcium-independent signal for proliferation in phorbol-ester-treated lymphocytes. Nature 315:419–420

Gerson DF, Kiefer H (1982) High intracellular pH accompanies mitotic activity in murine lymphocytes. J Cell Physiol 112:1–4

Gerson DF, Kiefer H, Eufe W (1982) Intracellular pH of mitogen-stimulated lymphocytes. Science 216:1009–1010

Gery I, Eidinger D (1977) Selective opposing effects of cytochalasin B and other drugs on lymphocyte responses to different doses of mitogens. Cell Immunol 30:147–155

Gerzer R, Brash AR, Hardman JG (1986) Activation of a soluble guanylate cyclase by arachidonic acid and 15-lipoxygenase products. Biochim Biophys Acta 886:383–389

Gilbert KM, Hoffmann MK (1985) cAMP is an essential signal in the induction of antibody production by B cells but inhibits helper function of T cells. J Immunol 135:2084–2089

Gillis S, Smith KA (1977) Long term culture of tumor-specific cytotoxic T cells. Nature 268:154–156

Glasgow A, Polgar P, Saporoschetq I, Kim H, Rutenberg AM, Mannick JA, Cooperband SR (1975) Phytohemagglutinin stimulation of human lymphocytes: failure to detect an early increase in cyclic AMP concentration. Clin Immunol Immunopathol 3:353–362

Goetzl EJ (1981) Selective feed-back inhibition of the 5-lipoxygenation of arachidonic acid in human T-lymphocytes. Biochem Biophys Res Commun 101:344–350

Goldberg ND, Haddox MK (1977) Cyclic GMP metabolism and involvement in biological regulation. Annu Rev Biochem 46:823–896

Goldberg ND, O'Dea RF, Haddox MK (1973) Cyclic GMP. Adv Cyclic Nucleotide Res 3:155–223

Goldberg ND, Graff G, Haddox MK, Stephenson JH, Glass DB, Moser ME (1978) Redox modulation of splenic cell soluble guanylate cyclase activity: activation by hydrophilic and hydrophobic oxidants represented by ascorbic and dehydroascorbic acids, fatty acid hydroperoxides and prostaglandin endoperoxides. Adv Cyclic Nucleotide Res 9:101–130

Goldyne ME, Stobo JD (1982) Human monocytes synthesize eicosanoids from T lymphocyte-derived arachidonic acid. Prostaglandins 24:623–630

Goldyne ME, Burrish GF, Poubelle P, Borgeat P (1984) Arachidonic acid metabolism among human mononuclear leukocytes. Lipoxygenase-related pathways. J Biol Chem 259:8815–8819

Goodman MG, Weigle WO (1983) T cell-replacing activity of C8-derivatized guanine ribonucleosides. J Immunol 130:2042–2044

Goodwin JS (1986) Role of leukotriene B_4 in T cell activation. Transplant Proc [Suppl 4] 18:49–51

Goodwin JS, Bankhurst AD, Messner RP (1977) Suppression of human T-cell mitogenesis by prostaglandin. Existence of a prostaglandin-producing suppressor cell. J Exp Med 146:1719–1734

Goodwin JS, Gualde N, Aldigier J, Rigaud M, Vanderhoek JY (1984) Modulation of Fcγ receptors on T cells and monocytes by 15-hydroperoxyeicosatetraenoic acids. Prostaglandins Leukotrienes Med 13:109–112

Gordon D, Nouri AME, Thomas RU (1981) Selective inhibition of thromboxane biosynthesis in human blood mononuclear cells and the effects on mitogen-stimulated lymphocyte proliferation. Eur J Pharmacol 74:469–476

Graff G, Stephenson JH, Glass DB, Haddox MK, Goldberg D (1978) Activation of soluble splenic cell guanylate cyclase by prostaglandin endoperoxides and fatty acid hydroperoxides. J Biol Chem 253:7662–7676

Greene WC, Parker CW (1975) A role for cytochalasin-sensitive proteins in the regulation of calcium transport in activated human lymphocytes. Biochem Biophys Res Commun 65:456–463

Greene WC, Parker CM, Parker CW (1976a) Calcium and lymphocyte activation. Cell Immunol 25:74–89

Greene WC, Parker CM, Parker CW (1976b) Opposing effects of mitogenic and nonmitogenic lectins on lymphocyte activation. J Biol Chem 251:4017–4025

Greene WC, Parker CM, Parker CW (1976c) Cytochalasin sensitive structures and lymphocyte activation. Exp Cell Res 103:109–118

Greene WC, Parker CM, Parker CW (1976d) Colchicine-sensitive structures and lymphocyte activation. J Immunol 117:1015–1022

Grinstein S, Cohen S, Lederman HM, Gelfand EW (1984) The intracellular pH of quiescent and proliferating human and rat thymic lymphocytes. J Cell Physiol 121:87–95

Grinstein S, Cohen S, Goetz JD, Rothstein A (1985a) Osmotic and phorbol ester-induced activation of Na^+/H^+ exchange: possible role of protein phosphorylation in lymphocyte volume regulation. J Cell Biol 101:269–276

Grinstein S, Cohen S, Goetz JD, Rothstein A, Gelfand EW (1985b) Characterization of the activation of Na^+/H^+ exchange in lymphocytes by phorbol esters: change in cytoplasmic pH dependence of the antiport. Proc Natl Acad Sci USA 82:1429–1433

Grupp SA, Harmony JAK (1985) Increased phosphatidylinositol metabolism is an important but not an obligatory early event in B lymphocyte activation. J Immunol 134:4087–4094

Gualde N, Chabel-Rabinovitch H, Motta C, Durand J, Beneytout JL, Rigaud M (1983) Hydroperoxyeicosatetraenoic acids: potent inhibitors of lymphocyte responses. Biochim Biophys Acta 750:429–433

Gualde N, Atluru D, Goodwin JS (1985a) Effect of lipoxygenase metabolites of arachidonic acid on proliferation of human T cells and T cell subsets. J Immunol 134:1125–1128

Gualde N, Rigaud M, Goodwin JS (1985b) Induction of suppressor cells from peripheral blood T cells by 15-hydroperoxyeicosatetraenoic acid (15-HPETE). J Immunol 135:3424–3429

Gunther GR, Wang JL, Edelman GM (1976) Kinetics of colchicine inhibition of mitogenesis in individual lymphocytes. Exp Cell Res 98:15–22

Gupta S (1979) Subpopulations of human T lymphocytes. XII. In vitro effects of agents modifying intracellular levels of cyclic nucleotides on T cells with receptors for IgM (Tμ), IgG (Tγ), or IgA (Tα). J Immunol 123:2664–2668

Gutowski JK, Mukherji B, Cohen S (1984) The role of cytoplasmic intermediates in IL-2-induced T cell growth. J Immunol 133:3068–3074

Guy GR, Gordan J, Walker L, Michell RH, Brown G (1986) Redistribution of protein kin-
ase C during mitogenesis of human B lymphocytes. Biochem Biophys Res Commun
135:146–153
Hadden JW (1977) Cyclic nucleotides in lymphocyte proliferation and differentiation. In:
Hadden JW, Coffey RG, Spreafico F (eds) Immunopharmacology. Plenum, New
York, pp 1–28
Hadden JW, Coffey RC (1982) Cyclic nucleotides in mitogen induced lymphocyte proliferation. Immunol Today 3:299–304
Hadden JW, Hadden EM, Good RA (1971) Alpha adrenergic stimulation of glucose up-
take in the human erythrocyte, lymphocyte, and lymphoblast. Exp Cell Res 68:217–
219
Hadden JW, Hadden EM, Haddox MK, Goldberg ND (1972) Guanosine 3′,5′-cyclic
monophosphate: a possible intracellular mediator of mitogen influences in lympho-
cytes. Proc Natl Acad Sci USA 69:3024–3027
Hadden JW, Johnson EM, Hadden EM, Coffey RG, Johnson LD (1975) Cyclic GMP and
lymphocyte activation. In: Rosenthal A (ed) Immune recognition. Academic, New
York, pp 359–389
Hadden JW, Hadden EM, Sadlik JR, Coffey RG (1976) Effects of concanavalin A and a
succinylated derivative on lymphocyte proliferation and cyclic nucleotide levels. Proc
Natl Acad Sci USA 73:1717–1721
Haddox MK, Furcht LT, Gentry SR, Moser ME, Stephenson JH, Goldberg ND (1976)
Periodate-induced increase in cyclic GMP in mouse and guinea pig splenic cells in as-
sociation with mitogenesis. Nature 262:146–148
Haddox MK, Stephenson JH, Moser ME, Goldberg ND (1978) Oxidative-reductive
modulation of guinea pig splenic cell guanylate cyclase activity. J Biol Chem 253:3143–
3152
Hall DJ, O'Leary JJ, Rosenberg A (1982) Commitment and proliferation kinetics of human
lymphocytes stimulated in vitro: effects of colchicine on mitogen response. J Cell
Physiol 112:157–161
Hamilton TA (1982) Regulation of transferrin receptor expression in concanavalin A stimulated and gross virus transformed rat lymphoblasts. J Cell Physiol 113:40–46
Hamilton TA (1983) Receptor-mediated endocytosis and exocytosis of transferrin in concanavalin A-stimulated rat lymphocytes. J Cell Physiol 114:222–228
Hansson A, Serhan CN, Haeggstrom J, Ingelman-Sundberg M, Samuelsson B, Morris J
(1986) Activation of protein kinase C by lipoxin A and other eicosanoids: intracellular
action of oxygenation products of arachidonic acid. Biochem Biophys Res Commun
134:1215–1222
Harrison ML, Low PS, Geahlen RL (1984) T and B lymphocytes express distinct tyrosine
protein kinases. J Biol Chem 259:9348–9350
Hasegawa-Sasaki H, Sasaki T (1981) Phytomitogen-induced stimulation of synthesis de
novo of PtdIns, phosphatidic acid and diacylglycerol in rat and human lymphocytes.
Biochim Biophys Acta 666:252–258
Hasegawa-Sasaki H, Sasaki T (1982) Rapid breakdown of PtdIns accompanied by accumulation of phosphatidic acid and diacylglycerol in rat lymphocytes. J Biochem
91:463–468
Hasegawa-Sasaki H, Sasaki T (1983) Phytohemagglutinin induces rapid degradation of
phosphatidyl-inositol-4,5-bis-phosphate and transient accumulation of phosphatidic
acid and diacylglycerol in a human T-lymphoblastoid cell line, CCRF-CEM. Biochim
Biophys Acta 754:305–314
Hausen P, Stein H (1968) On the synthesis of RNA in lymphocytes stimulated by phytohemagglutinin. Eur J Biochem 4:401–406
Hausen P, Stein H, Peters H (1969) On the synthesis of RNA in lymphocytes stimulated
by phytohemagglutinin. Eur J Biochem 9:542–549
Heidrick ML (1973) Imbalanced cyclic-AMP and cyclic-GMP levels in concanavalin-A
stimulated spleen cells from aged mice. J Cell Biol 59:139a
Hesketh TR, Smith GA, Moore JP, Taylor MV, Metcalfe JC (1983a) Limits to the early
increase in free cytoplasmic calcium concentrations during the mitogenic stimulation
of lymphocytes. Biochem J 212:685–690

Hesketh TR, Smith GA, Moore JP, Taylor MV, Metcalfe JC (1983 b) Free cytoplasmic calcium concentration and the mitogenic stimulation of lymphocytes. J Biol Chem 258:4876–4882

Hesketh TR, Moore JP, Morris DH, Taylor MV, Rogers J, Smith GA, Metcalfe JC (1985) A common sequence of calcium and pH signals in the mitogenic stimulation of eukaryotic cells. Nature 313:481–484

Hidaka H, Asano T (1977) Stimulation of human platelet guanylate cyclase by unsaturated fatty acid peroxides. Proc Natl Acad Sci USA 74:3657–3661

Hirata F, Axelrod J (1980) Phospholipid methylation and biological signal transmission. Science 209:1082–1090

Hirata F, Toyoshima S, Axelrod J, Waxdal MJ (1980) Phospholipid methylation: A biochemical signal modulating lymphocyte mitogenesis. Proc Natl Acad Sci USA 77:862–865

Hirata F, Matsuda K, Notsu Y, Hattori T, del Carmine R (1984) Phosphorylation at a tyrosine residue of lipomodulin in mitogen-stimulated murine thymocytes. Proc Natl Acad Sci USA 81:4717–4721

Hoffman R, Ferguson R, Simmons RL (1977) Effect of cytochalasin B on human lymphocyte responses to mitogens. Time and concentration dependence. J Immunol 118:1472–1479

Hoffman T, Hirata F, Bougnoux P, Fraser BA, Goldfarb RH, Haberman RB, Axelrod J (1981) Phospholipid methylation and phospholipase A_2 activation in cytotoxicity by human natural killer cells. Proc Natl Acad Sci USA 78:3839–3843

Hokin MR, Hokin LE (1953) Enzyme secretion and the incorporation of P^{32} into phospholipides of pancreas slices. J Biol Chem 203:967–977

Homa ST, Conroy DM, Smith AD (1984) Unsaturated fatty acids stimulate the formation of lipoxygenase and cyclooxygenase products in rat spleen lymphocytes. Prostaglandins Leukotrienes Med 14:417–427

Hovi T, Allison AC, Williams SC (1976 a) Proliferation of human peripheral blood lymphocytes induced by A23187, a streptomyces antibiotic. Exp Cell Res 97:92–100

Hovi T, Smyth JF, Allison AC, Williams SC (1976 b) Role of adenosine deaminase in lymphocyte proliferation. Clin Exp Immunol 23:395–403

Howard M, Paul WE (1983) Regulation of B cell growth and differentiation by soluble factors. Annu Rev Immunol 1:307–333

Hui DY, Harmony JAK (1980 a) Inhibition of Ca^{2+} accumulation in mitogen-activated lymphocytes: role of membrane-bound plasma lipoproteins. Proc Natl Acad Sci USA 77:4764–4768

Hui DY, Harmony JAK (1980 b) Inhibition by low density lipoproteins of mitogen-stimulated cyclic nucleotide production by lymphocytes. J Biol Chem 255:1413–1419

Hui DY, Harmony JAK (1980 c) Phosphatidylinositol turnover in mitogen-activated lymphocytes. Biochem J 192:91–98

Hume DA, Weidemann MJ (1980) Intracellular second messengers in mitogenic lymphocyte transformation. Res Monogr Immunol 2:183–225

Hume DA, Hansen K, Weidemann MJ, Ferber E (1978) Cytochalasin B inhibits lymphocyte transformation through its effects on glucose transport. Nature 272:359–362

Hume DA, Weidemann MJ, Ferber E (1979) Preferential inhibition by quercetin of mitogen-stimulated thymocyte glucose transport. JNCI 62:1243–1246

Humes JL, Bonney RJ, Pelus L, Dahlgren ME, Sadowski SJ, Kuehl FA Jr, Davies P (1977) Macrophage synthesis and release of prostaglandins in response to inflammatory stimuli. Nature 269:149–151

Hunter T, Cooper JA (1985) Protein-tyrosine kinases. Annu Rev Biochem 54:897–930

Imboden J, Weiss A, Stobo J (1985) The antigen receptor on a human T cell line initiates activation by increasing cytoplasmic free calcium. J Immunol 134:663–665

Inbar M, Shinitzky M (1975) Decrease in microviscosity in lymphocyte surface membrane associated with stimulation induced by concanavalin A. Eur J Immunol 5:166–170

Isakov N, Altman A (1986) Lymphocyte activation and immune regulation. Immunol Today 7:155–157

Isakov N, Scholz W, Altman A (1986) Signal transduction and intracellular events in T-lymphocyte activation. Immunol Today 7:271–277

Iyer AP, Pishak SA, Sniezek MJ, Mastro AM (1984) Visualization of protein kinases in lymphocytes stimulated to proliferate with concanavalin A or inhibited with a phorbol ester. Biochem Biophys Res Commun 121:392–399

Johnson EM, Hadden JW (1975) Phosphorylation of lymphocyte nuclear acidic proteins: regulation by cyclic nucleotides. Science 1807:1198–1200

Johnson HM, Archer DL, Torres BA (1982) Cyclic GMP as the second messenger on helper cell requirement for gamma-interferon production. J Immunol 129:2570–2572

Johnson HM, Vassallo T, Torres BA (1985) Interleukin 2-mediated events in γ-interferon production are calcium dependent at more than one site. J Immunol 134:967–970

Joseph SK, Thomas AP, Williams RJ, Irvine RF, Williamson JR (1984) Myo-inositol 1,4,5-triphosphate, a second messenger for the hormonal mobilization of intracellular Ca^{2+} in liver. J Biol Chem 259:3077–3081

Josimovitz O, Osawa H, Diamantstein T (1985) The mode of action of the calcium ionophore A23187 on T-cell proliferation. I. The ionophore does not replace lymphokines but acts via induction of IL-2 production on IL-2 responsive cells. Immunobiology 170:164–174

Kaever V, Resch K (1985) Are cyclic nucleotides involved in the initiation of mitogenic activation of human lymphocytes? Biochim Biophys Acta 846:216–225

Kaibuchi K, Takai Y, Ogawa Y, Kimura S, Nishizuka Y, Nakamura T, Tonomura A, Ichihara A (1982) Inibitory action of adenosine 3',5'-monophosphate on phosphatidylinositol turnover. Biochem Biophys Res Commun 104:105–112

Kaibuchi K, Takai Y, Nishizuka Y (1985) Protein kinase C and calcium ion in mitogenic response of macrophage-depleted human peripheral lymphocytes. J Biol Chem 260:1366–1369

Kaplan JG, Owens T (1982) The cation pump as a switch mechanism controlling proliferation and differentiation in lymphocytes. Biosci Rep 2:577–581

Katagiri T, Terao T, Osawa T (1976) Activation of mouse splenic lymphocyte guanylate cyclase by calcium ion. J Biochem 79:849–852

Kato K, Murota S (1985) Lipoxygenase specific inhibitors inhibit murine lymphocyte reactivity to Con A by reducing IL-2 production and its action. Prostaglandins Leukotrienes Med 18:39–52

Kay JE (1968) Early effects of phytohaemagglutinin on lymphocyte RNA synthesis. Eur J Biochem 4:225–232

Kay JE (1971) Interaction of lymphocytes and phytohaemagglutinin: inhibition by chelating agents. Exp Cell Res 68:11–16

Kay JE (1972) Lymphocyte stimulation by phytohaemagglutinin: role of the early stimulation of potassium uptake. Exp Cell Res 71:245–247

Kay JE, Handmaker SD (1970) Uridine incorporation and RNA in normal and phytohaemagglutinin-stimulated human lymphocytes. Biochim Biophys Acta 186:62–84

Kecskemethy N, Schafer KP (1982) Lectin induced changes among polyadenylated and non-polyadenylated mRNA in lymphocytes. Eur J Biochem 126:573–582

Kelly JP, Parker CW (1979) Effects of arachidonic acid and other unsaturated fatty acids on mitogenesis in human lymphocytes. J Immunol 122:1556–1562

Kelly JP, Johnson MC, Parker CW (1979) Effect of inhibitors of arachidonic acid metabolism on mitogenesis in human lymphocytes: possible role of thromboxanes and products of the lipoxygenase pathway. J Immunol 122:1563–1571

Kiefer M, Blume AJ, Kaback HR (1980) Membrane potential changes during mitogenic stimulation of mouse spleen lymphocytes. Proc Natl Acad Sci USA 77:2200–2204

Kishimoto T (1984) Signals for B-cell activation and mechanism of transmembrane signaling. Prog Immunol 5:691–698

Kiss Z, Steinberg RA (1985) Phorbol ester-mediated protein phosphorylation in S49 mouse lymphoma cells. Cancer Res 45:2732–2740

Klimpel GR, Byers CV, Russell DH, Lucas DO (1979) Cyclic AMP-dependent protein kinase activation and the induction of ornithine decarboxylase during lymphocyte mitogenesis. J Immunol 123:817–824

Kohno H, Kanno T (1985) Properties and activities of aminopeptidases in normal and mitogen-stimulated human lymphocytes. Biochem J 226:59–66

Kostka G, Schweiger A (1985) Biphasic increase in the in vivo phosphorylation of nuclear 110-KDa protein during early lymphocyte transformation. Eur J Biochem 148:437–440

Krishnaraj R, Talwar GP (1973) Role of cyclic AMP in mitogen induced transformation of human peripheral leukocytes. J Immunol 111:1010–1017

Kronenberg M, Siu G, Hood LE, Shastri N (1986) The molecular genetics of the T-cell antigen receptor and T-cell antigen recognition. Annu Rev Immunol 4:529–592

Kronke M, Leonard WJ, Depper JM, Greene WC (1985) Sequential expression of genes involved in human T lymphocyte growth and differentiation. J Exp Med 161:1593–1599

Ku Y, Kishimoto A, Takai Y, Ogawa Y, Kimura S, Nishizuka Y (1981) A new possible regulatory system for protein phosphorylation in human peripheral lymphocytes. II. Possible relation to phosphatidylinositol turnover induced by mitogens. J Immunol 127:1375–1379

Lad PM, Olson CV, Smiley RA (1985) Association of the N-formyl-Met-Leu-Phe receptor in human neutrophils with a GTP-binding protein sensitive to pertussis toxin. Proc Natl Acad Sci USA 82:869–873

Lands W (1984) Biological consequences of fatty acid oxygenase reaction mechanisms. Prostaglandins Leukotrienes Med 13:35–46

Largen MT, Votta B (1983) Immunocytochemical evidence for 3',5'-cGMP and 3',5'-cGMP-dependent protein kinase involvement in lymphocyte proliferation. J Cyclic Nucleotide Protein Phosphor Res 9:231–244

Larrick JW, Creswell P (1979) Modulation of cell surface iron transferrin receptors by cellular density and state of activation. J Supramol Struct 11:579–586

Leonard WJ, Kronke M, Peffer NJ, Depper JM, Greene WC (1985 a) Interleukin 2 receptor gene expression in normal human T lymphocytes. Proc Natl Acad Sci USA 82:6281–6285

Leonard WJ, Depper JM, Kronke M, Robb RJ, Waldmann TA, Greene WC (1985 b) The human receptor for T-cell growth factor. Evidence for variable post-translational processing, phosphorylation, sulfation, and the ability of precursor forms of the receptor to bind T-cell growth factor. J Biol Chem 260:1872–1880

Lester EP, Cooper HL (1985) lymphocyte blastogenesis. Post-transcriptional controls of protein synthesis. Biochim Biophys Acta 824:365–373

Lichtman AH, Segel GB, Lichman MA (1979) Total and exchangeable calcium in mitogen-treated lymphocytes. In: Kaplan JG (ed) The molecular basis of immune cell function. Elsevier/North-Holland, Amsterdam, pp 417–419

Lichtman AH, Segel GB, Lichtman MA (1982) Effects of trifluorperazine and mitogenic lectins on calcium ATPase activity and calcium transport by human lymphocyte plasma membrane vesicles. J Cell Physiol 111:213–217

Lichtman AH, Segel GB, Lichtman MA (1983) The role of calcium in lymphocyte proliferation. Blood 61:413–422

Ling NR, Kay JE (1975) Lymphocyte stimulation. North Holland, Amsterdam

Low CE, Pupillo MB, Bryant RW, Bailey JM (1984) Inhibition of phytohemagglutinin-induced lymphocyte mitogenesis by lipoxygenase metabolites of arachidonic acid: structure-activity relationships. J Lipid Res 25:1090–1095

Lucas DO, Shohet SB, Merler E (1971) Changes in phospholipid metabolism which occur as a consequence of mitogenic stimulation of lymphocytes. J Immunol 106:768–772

Lucas ZJ (1967) Pyrimidine nucleotide synthesis: regulatory control during transformation of lymphocytes in vitro. Science 156:1237–1240

Luckasen JR, White JG, Kersey JH (1974) Mitogenic properties of a calcium ionophore, A23187. Proc Natl Acad Sci USA 71:5088–5090

Lyle LR, Parker CW (1974) Cyclic adenosine 3',5'-monophosphate responses to concanavalin A in human lymphocytes. Evidence that the response involves specific carbohydrate receptors on the cell surface. Biochemistry 13:5416–5420

Maino VC, Green NM, Crumpton MJ (1974) The role of calcium ions in initiating transformation of lymphocytes. Nature 251:324–327

Maino VC, Hayman MJ, Crumpton MJ (1975) Relationship between enhanced turnover of phosphatidylinositol and lymphocyte activation by mitogens. Biochem J 146:247–252

Masuzawa Y, Osawa T, Inoue K, Nojima S (1973) Effects of various mitogens on the phospholipid metabolism of human peripheral lymphocytes. Biochim Biophys Acta 326:339–344

May CD, Lyman M, Alberto R (1970) Effects of compounds which inhibit lymphocyte stimulation on the utilization of glucose by leukocytes. J Allergy 46:21–28

May WS, Jacobs S, Cuatrecasas P (1984) Association of phorbol ester-induced hyperphosphorylation and reversible regulation of transferrin membrane receptors in HL60 cells. Proc Natl Acad Sci USA 81:2016–2020

May WS, Sahyoun N, Jacobs S, Wolf M, Cuatrecasas P (1985) Mechanism of phorbol diester-induced regulation of surface transferrin receptor involves the action of activated protein kinase C and an intact cytoskeleton. J Biol Chem 260:9419–9426

McClain DA, Edelman GM (1976) Analysis of the stimulation-inhibition paradox exhibited by lymphocytes. J Exp Med 144:1494–1508

McPhail LC, Clayton CC, Snyderman R (1984) A potential second messenger role for unsaturated fatty acids: activation of Ca^{2+}-dependent protein kinase. Science 224:622–625

Mednieks MI, Jungmann RA (1982) Selective expression of type I and type II cyclic AMP-dependent protein kinases in subcellular fractions of concanavalin A-stimulated rat thymocytes. Arch Biochem Biophys 213:127–138

Mellors A, Stalmach ME, Cohen A (1985) Co-mitogenic tumor promoters suppress the phosphatidylinositol response in lymphocytes during early mitogenesis. Biochim Biophys Acta 833:181–188

Mendelsohn J, Skinner A, Kornfeld S (1971) The rapid induction by phytohemagglutinin of increased alpha-aminoisobutyric acid uptake by lymphocytes. J Clin Invest 50:818–826

Mendelsohn J, Trowbridge I, Castagnola J (1983) Inhibition of human lymphocyte proliferation by monoclonal antibody to transferrin receptor. Blood 62:821–826

Mexmain S, Cook J, Aldigier J-C, Gualde N, Rigaud M (1985) Thymocyte cyclic AMP and cyclic GMP response to treatment with metabolites issued from the lipoxygenase pathway. J Immunol 135:1361–1365

Michell RH (1975) Inositol phospholipids and cell surface receptor function. Biochim Biophys Acta 415:81–147

Michell RH (1982) Inositol lipid metabolism in dividing and differentiating cells. Cell Calcium 3:429–440

Michell RH, Kirk CJ, Jones LM, Downes CP, Creba JA (1981) The stimulation of inositol lipid metabolism that accompanies calcium mobilization in stimulated cells. Defined characteristics and unanswered questions. Philos Trans R Soc Lond [Biol] 296:123–137

Miller J (1979) Oncodazole (R 17934) an inhibitor of the turnover of phosphatidyl inositol in concanavalin A induced lymphocytes. Biochem Pharmacol 28:2967–2968

Mills GB, Cheung RK, Grinstein S, Gelfand EW (1985a) Increase in cytosolic free calcium concentration is an intracellular messenger for the production of interleukin 2 but not for expression of the interleukin 2 receptor. J Immunol 134:1640–1643

Mills GB, Cheung RK, Grinstein S, Gelfand EW (1985b) Interleukin 2-induced lymphocyte proliferation is independent of increases in cytosolic-free calcium concentrations. J Immunol 134:2431–2435

Mills GB, Cragoe EJ Jr, Gelfand EW, Grinstein S (1985c) Interleukin 2 induces a rapid increase in intracellular pH through activation of a Na^+/H^+ antiport. Cytoplasmic alkalinization is not required for lymphocyte proliferation. J Biol Chem 260:12500–12507

Mills GB, Stewart DJ, Mellors A, Gelfand EW (1986) Interleukin 2 does not induce phosphatidylinositol hydrolysis in activated T cells. J Immunol 136:3019–3024

Mingari MC, Gerosa F, Carra G, Accola RS, Moretta A, Zubler RH, Waldmann TA, Moretta L (1984) Human interleukin 2 promotes proliferation of activated B cells via surface receptors similar to those of activated T cells. Nature 312:641–642

Mire AR, Wickramasinghe RG, Hoffbrand AV (1986) Phytohemagglutinin treatment of T lymphocytes stimulates rapid increases in activity of both particulate and cytosolic protein kinase C. Biochem Biophys Res Commun 137:128–134

Mizoguchi Y, Otani S, Matsui I, Morisawa S (1975) Control of ornithine decarboxylase activity by cyclic nucleotides in the phytohemagglutinin induced lymphocyte transformation. Biochem Biophys Res Commun 66:328–335

Monahan TM, Marchand NW, Fritz RR, Abell CW (1975) Cyclic adenosine 3':5'-monophosphate levels and activities of related enzymes in normal and leukemic lymphocytes. Cancer Res 35:2540–2547

Monroe JG, Niedel JS, Cambier JC (1984) B cell activation. IV. Induction of cell membrane depolarization and hyper-IA expression by phorbol diesters suggests a role for protein kinase C in murine B lymphocyte activation. J Immunol 132:1472–1478

Mookerjee BK, Jung CY (1982) The effects of cytochalasins on lymphocytes: mechanism of action of cytochalasin A on responses to phytomitogens. J Immunol 128:2153–2159

Moolenaar WH, Tertoolen LGJ, deLaat SW (1984) Phorbol ester and diacylglycerol mimic growth factors in raising cytoplasmic pH. Nature 312:371–374

Moore JP, Smith GA, Hesketh TR, Metcalfe JC (1982) Early increases in phospholipid methylation are not necessary for the mitogenic stimulation of lymphocytes. J Biol Chem 257:8183–8189

Morgan DA, Ruscetti RW, Gallo RC (1976) Selective in vitro growth of T lymphocytes from normal human bone marrows. Science 193:1007–1008

Muller W, Kuhn R, Goldmann W, Tesch H, Smith FI, Radbruch A, Rajewsky K (1985) Signal requirements for growth and differentiation of activated murine B lymphocytes. J Immunol 135:1213–1219

Munck A (1971) Glucocorticoid inhibition of glucose uptake by peripheral tissues: old and new evidence, molecular mechanisms, and physiological significance. Perspect Biol Med 14:265–289

Muraguchi A, Miyazaki K, Kehrl JH, Fauci AS (1984) Inhibition of human B cell activation by diterpine forskolin. J Immunol 133:1283–1287

Muraguchi A, Kehrl JH. Longo DL, Volkmann DJ, Smith KA, Fauci AS (1985) Interleukin 2 receptors on human B cells. J Exp Med 161:181–197

Namiuchi S, Kumagai S, Imura H, Suginoshita T, Hattori T, Hirata F (1984) Quinacrine inhibits the primary but not secondary proliferative response of human cytotoxic T cells to allogeneic non-T cell antigens. J Immunol 132:1456–1461

Nathaniel D, Mellors A (1983) Mitogen effects on lipid metabolism during lymphocyte activation. Mol Immunol 20:1259–1266

Naylor PH, Thurman GB, Goldstein AL (1979) Effect of calcium on the cyclic GMP elevation induced by thymosin fraction 5. Biochem Biophys Res Commun 90:810–818

Neckers LM, Cossman J (1983) Transferrin receptor induction in mitogen-stimulated human T lymphocytes is required for DNA synthesis and cell division and is regulated by interleukin 2. Proc Natl Acad Sci USA 80:3494–3498

Neckers LM, Yenokida G, James SP (1984) The role of the transferrin receptor in human B lymphocyte activation. J Immunol 133:2437–2441

Negendank WG, Collier CR (1976) Ion contents of human lymphocytes. Exp Cell Res 101:31–40

Negendank W, Shaller C (1979) Potassium-sodium distribution in human lymphocytes: description by the association-induction hypothesis. J Cell Physiol 98:95–105

Nisbet-Brown E, Cheung RK, Lee JWW, Gelfand EW (1985) Antigen-dependent increase in cytosolic free calcium in specific human T-lymphocyte clones. Nature 316:545–547

Nishizuka Y (1984) The role of protein kinase C in cell surface transduction and tumor promotion. Nature 308:693–698

Nishizuka Y, Takai Y, Kishimoto A, Kikkawa U, Kaibuchi K (1984) Phospholipid turnover in hormone action. Recent Prog Horm Res 40:301–345

Nordenberg J, Stenzel KH, Novogrodsky A (1983) 12-O-tetradecanoylphorbol-13-acetate and concanavalin A enhanced glucose uptake in thymocytes by different mechanisms. J Cell Physiol 117:183–188

Northoff H, Dorken B, Resch K (1978) Ligand-dependent modulation of membrane phospholipid metabolism in Con A-stimulated lymphocytes. Exp Cell Res 113:189–196

Novogrodsky A (1972) Concanavalin A stimulation of rat lymphocyte ATPase. Biochim Biophys Acta 266:343–349

Novogrodsky A, Katchalski E (1970) Effect of phytohemagglutinin and prostaglandins on cyclic AMP synthesis in rat lymph node lymphocytes. Biochim Biophys Acta 215:291–296

Novogrodsky A, Quittner S, Rubin AL, Stenzel K (1978) Transglutaminase activation in human lymphocytes: early activation by phytomitogens. Proc Natl Acad Sci USA 75:1157–1161

Novogrodsky A, Ravid A, Rubin AL, Stenzel KH (1982) Hydroxyl radical scavengers inhibit lymphocyte mitogenesis. Proc Natl Acad Sci 79:1171–1174

Nowell PC (1960) Phytohemagglutinin: an initiator of mitosis in cultures of normal human leukocytes. Cancer Res 20:462–466

O'Brien RL, Parker JW, Dixon JFP (1978) Mechanisms of lymphocyte transformation. Prog Mol Subcell Biol 6:201–270

O'Flynn K, Linch DC, Tatham PER (1984) The effect of mitogenic lectins and monoclonal antibodies on intracellular free calcium concentration in human T-lymphocytes. Biochem J 219:661–666

Ohara J, Watanabe T (1982) Microinjection of macromolecules into normal murine lymphocytes by cell fusion technique. I. Quantitative microinjection of antibodies into normal splenic lymphocytes. J Immunol 128:1090–1096

Ohara J, Kishimoto T, Yamomura Y (1978) In vitro immune response of human peripheral lymphocytes. J Immunol 121:2088–2096

Oliver JM, Gelfand EW, Pearson CB, Pfeiffer JR, Dosch H-M (1980) Microtubule assembly and concanavalin A capping in lymphocytes: reappraisal using normal and abnormal human peripheral blood cells. Proc Natl Acad Sci USA 77:3499–3503

Orme M, Shand FL (1981) Inhibitors of prostaglandin synthetase block the generation of suppressor T cells induced by concanavalin A. Int J Immunopharmacol 3:15–19

Otani S, Matsui I, Morisawa S, Masutani M, Mizoguchi Y, Morisawa S (1980) Induction of ornithine decarboxylase in guinea pig lymphocytes by the divalent cation ionophore A23187 and phytohemagglutinin. J Biochem 88:77–85

Otteskog P, Wanger L, Sunquist KG (1983) Cytochalasins distinguish by their action resting human T lymphocytes from activated T cell blast. Eur Cell Res 144:443–454

Owens T, Kaplan JG (1980) Increased cationic fluxes in stimulated lymphocytes of the mouse: response of enriched B- and T-cell subpopulations to B- and T-cell mitogens. Can J Biochem 58:831–839

Ozato K, Huang L, Ebert JD (1977) Accelerated calcium ion uptake in murine thymocytes induced by concanavalin-A. J Cell Physiol 93:153–160

Palacios R (1985) Mechanisms by which accessory cells contribute in growth of resting T lymphocytes initiated by OKT3 antibody. Eur J Immunol 15:645–651

Parker CW (1974) Correlations between mitogenicity and stimulation of calcium uptake in human lymphocytes. Biochem Biophys Res Commun 61:1180–1186

Parker CW (1982) Pharmacologic modulation of release of arachidonic acid from human mononuclear cells and lymphocytes by mitogenic lectins. J Immunol 128:393–397

Parker CW, Sullivan TJ, Wedner HJ (1974) Cyclic AMP and the immune response. Adv Cyclic Nucleotide Res 4:1–80

Parker CW, Kelly JP, Falkenhein SF, Huber MG (1979a) Release of arachidonic acid from human lymphocytes in response to mitogenic lectins. J Exp Med 149:1487–1503

Parker CW, Stenson WF, Huber MG, Kelly JP (1979b) Formation of thromboxane B_2 and hydroxy arachidonic acids in purified human lymphocytes in the presence and absence of PHA. J Immunol 122:1572–1577

Patskau GJ, Baxter CS (1985) Specific stimulation by phorbol esters of the phosphorylation of histones H2B and H4 in murine lymphocytes. Cancer Res 45:667–672

Payan DG, Goetzle EJ (1981) The dependence of human T-lymphocyte migration on the 5-lipoxygenation of endogenous arachidonic acid. J Clin Immunol 1:266–270

Payan DG, Goetzl EJ (1983) Specific suppression of human T lymphocyte function by leukotriene B_4. J Immunol 131:551–553

Payan DG, Missirian-Bastian A, Goetzl EJ (1984) Human T lymphocyte subset specificity of the regulatory effects of leukotriene B_4. Proc Natl Acad Sci USA 81:3501–3505

Peters JH, Hausen P (1971a) Effect of PHA on lymphocyte membrane transport. I. Stimulation of uridine uptake. Eur J Biochem 19:502–508

Peters JH, Hausen P (1971 b) Effect of PHA on lymphocyte membrane transport. II. Stimulation of "facilitated diffusion" of 3-O-methyl-glucose. Eur J Biochem 19:509–513

Peterson OH, Maruyama Y (1984) Calcium-activated potassium channels and their role in secretion. Nature 307:693–696

Phillips JL, Azair P (1974) Zinc transferrin enhancement of nucleic acid synthesis in phytohemagglutinin-stimulated human lymphocytes. Cell Immunol 10:31–37

Piga A, Wickremasinghe MR, Taheri MR, Yaxley JC, Hoffbrand AV (1985) Phytohemagglutinin-induced changes in tyrosine protein kinase and its endogenous substrates in human lymphocytes. Exp Cell Res 159:103–112

Pommier G, Ripert G, Azoulay E, Depieds R (1975) Effects of concanavalin A on membrane-bound enzymes from mouse lymphocytes. Biochim Biophys Acta 389:483–494

Pompidou A, Rousset S, Mace B, Michel P, Esnous D, Renard N (1984) Chromatin structure and nucleic acid synthesis in human lymphocyte activation by phytohemagglutinin. Exp Cell Res 150:213–225

Quastel MR, Kaplan JG (1968) Inhibition by ouabain of human lymphocyte transformation induced by phytohemagglutinin in vitro. Nature 219:198–200

Quastel MR, Kaplan JG (1970) Early stimulation of potassium uptake in lymphocytes treated with PHA. Exp Cell Res 63:230–233

Quastel MR, Kaplan JG (1975) Ouabain binding to intact lymphocytes: enhancement by phytohemagglutinin and leucoagglutinin. Exp Cell Res 94:351–362

Quastel MR, Milthorpe P, Kaplan JG, Vogelfanger IJ (1974) Further studies on M-ATPase in lymphocytes and plaque-forming cells: possible species and functional differences between lymphocyte subclasses. In: Lindahl-Kiessling K, Osoba D (eds) Lymphocyte recognition and effector mechanisms. Academic, New York, pp 493–500

Reed JC, Alpers JD, Nowell PC, Hoover RG (1986) Sequential expression of protooncogenes during lectin-stimulated mitogenesis of normal human lymphocytes. Proc Natl Acad Sci USA 83:3982–3986

Reeves JP (1975) Calcium-dependent stimulation of 3-O-methylglucose uptake in rat thymocytes by the divalent cation ionophore A23187. J Biol Chem 250:9428–9430

Resch K, Ferber E (1972) Phospholipid metabolism of stimulated lymphocytes. Effects of phytohemagglutinin, concanavalin A and antiimmunoglobulin serum. Eur J Biochem 27:153–161

Resch K, Ferber E, Odenthal J, Fischer H (1971) Early changes in the phospholipid metabolism of lymphocytes following stimulation with phytohemagglutinin and with lysolecithin. Eur J Immunol 1:162–165

Resch K, Gelfand EW, Hansen K, Ferber E (1972) Lymphocyte activation: rapid changes in the phospholipid metabolism of plasma membranes during stimulation. Eur J Immunol 2:598–601

Resch K, Prester M, Ferber E, Gelfand EW (1976) The inhibition of initial steps of lymphocyte transformation by cytochalasin B. J Immunol 117:1705–1710

Resch K, Bovillon D, Gemsa D, Averdunk R (1977) Drugs which disrupt microtubules do not inhibit the initiation of lymphocyte activation. Nature 265:349–351

Resch K, Bovillon D, Gemsa D (1978) The activation of lymphocytes by the ionophore A23187. J Immunol 120:1514–1520

Resch K, Wood T, Northoff H, Cooper HL (1981) Microtubules: are they involved in the initiation of lymphocyte activation? Eur J Biochem 115:659–664

Resch K, Schneider S, Szamel M (1983) Characterization of functional domains of the lymphocyte plasma membrane. Biochim Biophys Acta 733:142–153

Resch K, Brennecke M, Goppelt M, Kaever V, Szamel M (1984) The role of phospholipids in the signal transmission of activated lymphocytes-T. Prog Immunol 5:349–360

Rink TJ, Deutsch C (1983) Calcium-activated potassium channels in lymphocytes. Cell Calcium 4:463–474

Rittenhouse-Simmons S (1980) Indomethacin-induced accumulation of diglyceride in activated human platelets. J Biol Chem 255:2259–2262

Robins RK (1982) Purine nucleoside 3',5'-cyclic monophosphates as hormonal modulators of cellular proliferation, metastases and lymphocyte response. Nucleosides Nucleotides 1:205–231

Rochette-Egly C, Kempf J (1981) Cyclic nucleotides and calcium in human lymphocytes induced to divide. J Physiol (Paris) 77:721–725

Rode HN, Szamel M, Schneider S, Resch K (1982) Phospholipid metabolism of stimulated lymphocytes. Preferential incorporation of polyunsaturated fatty acids into plasma membrane phospholipid upon stimulation with concanavalin A. Biochim Biophys Acta 688:66–74

Rogers J, Hesketh TR, Smith GA, Metcalfe JC (1983) Intracellular pH of stimulated thymocytes measured with a new fluorescent indicator. J Biol Chem 258:5994–5997

Rola-Pleszczynski M, Gagnon L, Rudzinska M, Borgeat P, Sirois P (1984) Human natural cytotoxic cell activity: enhancement by leukotriene A_4, B_4, and D_4 but not by stereoisomers of LTB_4 or HETEs. Prostaglandins Leukotrienes Med 13:113–117

Roos D, Loos JA, Bloom AJ, Scholte BM (1970) Changes in the carbohydrate metabolism of mitogenically stimulated human peripheral lymphocytes. I. Stimulation by phytohemagglutinin. Biochim Biophys Acta 222:565–582

Ross EM, Gilman AG (1980) Biochemical properties of hormone-sensitive adenylate cyclase. Annu Rev Biochem 49:533–564

Rossi P, Lindgren JA, Kullman C, Jondal M (1985) Products of the lipoxygenase pathway in human natural killer cell cytotoxicity. Cell Immunol 93:1–8

Rudd CE, Rogers KA, Brown DL, Kaplan JG (1979) Microtubules, colchicine, and lymphocyte blastogenesis. Can J Biochem 57:673–683

Salari H, Braquet P, Borgeat P (1984) Comparative effects of indomethacin, acetylenic acids, 15 HETE, nordihydroguaiaretic acid and BW-755 on the metabolism of arachidonic acid in human leukocytes and platelets. Prostaglandins Leukotrienes Med 13:53–60

Samelson LE, Harford J, Schwartz RH, Klausner RD (1985) A 20-KDa protein associated with the murine T-cell antigen receptor is phosphorylated in response to activation by antigen or concanavalin A. Proc Natl Acad Sci USA 82:1969–1973

Samuelsson B (1982) The leukotrienes: an introduction. Adv Prostaglandin Thromboxane Leukotriene Res 9:1–18

Samuelsson B, Goldyne M, Granstrom E, Hamberg M, Hammarstrom S, Malmsten C (1978) Prostaglandins and thromboxanes. Annu Rev Biochem 47:997–1029

Sasaki T, Hasegawa-Sasaki H (1981) Effects of anchorage-modulating doses of concanavalin A, microtubule-disrupting drugs and microfilament perturbants, cytochalasins, in the phosphatidylinositol response of rat lymphnode cells. Biochim Biophys Acta 649:449–454

Sasaki T, Hasegawa-Sasaki H (1985) Breakdown of phosphatidylinositol 4,5-bisphosphate in a T-cell leukemia line stimulated by phytohemagglutinin is not dependent on Ca^{2+} mobilization. Biochem J 227:971–979

Schellenberg RR, Gillespie E (1977) Colchicine inhibits phosphatidylinositol turnover induced in lymphocytes by concanavalin A. Nature 265:741–742

Schellenberg RR, Gillespie E (1980) Effects of colchicine, vinblastine, griseofulvin and deuterium oxide upon phospholipid metabolism in concanavalin A-stimulated lymphocytes. Biochim Biophys Acta 619:522–532

Schreiner GF, Unanue ER (1975) The modulation of spontaneous and anti-Ig-stimulated motility of lymphocytes by cyclic nucleotides and adrenergic and cholinergic agents. J Immunol 114:802–809

Schumm DE, Morris HP, Webb TE (1974) Early biochemical changes in PHA-stimulated peripheral blood lymphocytes from normal and tumor bearing rats. Eur J Cancer 10:107–113

Schwab R, Crow MK, Russo C, Weksler ME (1985) Requirements for T cell activation by OKT3 monoclonal antibody: role of modulation of T3 molecules and interleukin 1. J Immunol 135:1714–1718

Schwartz A, Nagano K, Nakao M, Lindenmayer GE, Allen JC (1971) The sodium- and potassium-activated adenosinetriphosphatase system. Methods Pharmacol 1:361–388

Segel GB, Lichtman MA (1976) Potassium transport in human blood lymphocytes treated with phytohemagglutinin. J Clin Invest 58:1358–1369

Segel GB, Lichtman MA (1981) Amino acid transport in human lymphocytes: distinctions in the enhanced uptake with PHA treatment or amino acid deprivation. J Cell Physiol 106:303–308

Segel GB, Hollander MM, Gordon BR, Klemperer MR, Lichtman MA (1975) A rapid phytohemagglutinin induced alteration in lymphocyte potassium permeability. J Cell Physiol 86:327–335

Segel GB, Lichtman MA, Hollander MM, Gordon BR, Klemperer MR (1976) Human lymphocyte potassium content during the initiation of phytohemagglutinin induced mitogenesis. J Cell Physiol 88:43–48

Segel GB, Kovach G, Lichtman MA (1979) Sodium-potassium adenosine triphosphatase activity of human lymphocyte membrane vesicles: kinetic parameters, substrate specificity, and effects of phytohemagglutinin. J Cell Physiol 100:109–118

Serhan CN, Fridovich J, Goetzl EJ, Dunham PB, Weissmann G (1982) Leukotriene B_4 and phosphatidic acid are calcium ionophores. J Biol Chem 257:4746–4752

Shackelford DA, Trowbridge IS (1984) Induction of expression and phosphorylation of the human interleukin 2 receptor by a phorbol diester. J Biol Chem 259:11706–11712

Shapiro HM, Natale PJ, Kamentsky LA (1979) Estimation of membrane potentials of individual lymphocytes by flow cytometry. Proc Natl Acad Sci USA 76:5728–5730

Shenker BJ, Gray I (1979) Cyclic nucleotide metabolism during lymphocyte transformation. Cell Immunol 43:11–21

Sherline P, Mundy GR (1977) Role of the tubulin-microtubular system in lymphocyte activation. J Cell Biol 74:371–376

Smit JW, Bloom NR, van Luyn MJA, Halie MR (1983) Lymphocytes with parallel tubular structures: morphologically a distinctive subpopulation. Blut 46:311–320

Smith JW, Steiner AL, Newberry WM, Parker CW (1971) Cyclic adenosine 3',5'-monophosphate in human lymphocytes. Alterations after phytohemagglutinin stimulation. J Clin Invest 50:432–441

Smith KA, Favata MF, Oroszlan S (1983) Production and characterization of monoclonal antibodies to human interleukin 2: strategy and tactics. J Immunol 131:1808–1815

Smith RS, Sherman NS, Coffey RG (1974) Effects of pokeweed mitogen, prostaglandin E_1, and cholera toxin on human tonsillar immunoglobulin synthesis and cyclic AMP levels. Int Arch Allergy Appl Immunol 47:586–597

Spach C, Aschkenasy A (1979) Effects of a protein-free diet on the changes in cyclic AMP and cyclic GMP levels induced by immunization in splenic T and B lymphocytes in rat. J Nutr 109:1265–1273

Stark R, Liebes LF, Nevrla D, Silber R (1982) The quantitation of actin in human lymphocytes by isoelectric focusing. Biochem Med 27:200–206

Sternholm RL, Falor WH (1970) Early biochemical changes in phytohemagglutinin-stimulated human lymphocytes of blood and lymphocytes. J Reticuloendothel Soc 7:471–483

Stoeck M, Northoff H, Resch K (1983) Inhibition of mitogen-induced lymphocyte proliferation by ouabain. J Immunol 131:1433–1437

Stolc V (1980) Stimulatory effect of ionophores on adenosine 3',5'-monophosphate content in human mononuclear leukocytes. Biochem Pharmacol 29:1991–1994

Strom TB, Lundin AP, Carpenter CB (1977) The role of cyclic nucleotides in lymphocyte activation and function. Prog Clin Immunol 3:115–153

Sugiura T, Waku K (1984) Enhanced turnover of arachidonic acid-containing species of phosphatidylinositol and phosphatidic acid of concanavalin A-stimulated lymphocytes. Biochim Biophys Acta 796:190–198

Sundquist KG, Otteskog P, Wanger L, Thorstensson R, Utter G (1980) The morphology and microfilament organization in human blood lymphocytes: effects of substratum and mitogen exposure. Exp Cell Res 130:327–337

Sunshine GH, Basch RS, Coffey RG, Cohen KW, Goldstein G, Hadden JW (1978) Thymopoietin enhances the allogeneic response and cyclic GMP levels of mouse peripheral, thymus-derived lymphocytes. J Immunol 120:1594–1599

Suzuki T, Sadasivan R, Saito-Taki T, Stechschulte DJ, Balentine L (1980) Studies of Fc gamma-receptors of human B lymphocytes: phospholipase A_2 activation of Fc gamma-receptors. Biochemistry 19:6037–6043

Svenson M, Bendtzen K (1985) Effects of cyclic GMP-agonists on cyclosporin-induced suppression of human lymphokine production. Allergy 40:529–534

Szamel M, Schneider S, Resch K (1981) Functional interrelationship between (Na$^+$ and K$^+$)-ATPase and lysolecithin acyltransferase in plasma membranes of mitogen-stimulated rabbit thymocytes. J Biol Chem 256:9198–9204

Takemoto DJ, Kaplan SA, Appleman MM (1979) Cyclic guanosine 3',5'-monophosphate and phosphodiesterase activity in mitogen-stimulated human lymphocyte. Biochem Biophys Res Commun 90:491–497

Takemoto DJ, Dunford C, Vaughn D, Kramer KJ, Smith A, Powell RG (1982) Guanylate cyclase activity in human leukemic and normal lymphocytes. Enzyme 27:179–188

Takigawa M, Waksman B (1980) Mechanisms of lymphocyte "deletion" by high concentrations of ligand. I. Cyclic AMP levels and cell death in T-lymphocytes exposed to high concentration of concanavalin A. Cell Immunol 58:29–38

Tam CF, Walford RL (1978) Cyclic nucleotide levels in resting and mitogen-stimulated spleen cell suspensions from young and old mice. Mech Ageing Dev 7:309–320

Tandon NN, Davidson LA, Titus EO (1983) Changes in (Na$^+$ and K$^+$) ATPase activity associated with stimulation of thymocytes by concanavalin A. J Biol Chem 258:9850–9855

Tatham PER, O'Flynn KO, Linch DC (1986) The relationship between mitogen-induced membrane potential changes and intracellular free calcium in human T-lymphocytes. Biochim Biophys Acta 856:202–211

Taylor MJ, Metcalfe JC, Hesketh TR, Smith GA, Moore JP (1984) Mitogens increase phosphorylation of phosphoinositides in thymocytes. Nature 312:462–465

Toh BH, Hard GC (1977) Actin co-caps with concanavalin A receptors. Nature 269:695–697

Tomar RH, Darrow TL, John PA (1981) Response to and production of prostaglandins by murine thymus, spleen, bone marrow and lymph node cells. Cell Immunol 60:335–346

Touraine JL, Hadden JW, Touraine F, Hadden EM, Estensen R, Good RA (1977) Phorbol myristate acetate: a mitogen selective for a T-lymphocyte subpopulation. J Exp Med 145:460–465

Toyoshima S, Hirata F, Axelrod J, Beppu M, Osawa T, Waxdal MJ (1982a) The relationship between phospholipid methylation and calcium influx in murine lymphocytes stimulated with native and modified Con A. Mol Immunol 19:229–234

Toyoshima S, Hirata F, Iwata M, Axelrod J, Osawa T, Waxdal MJ (1982b) Lectin-induced mitosis and phospholipid methylation. Mol Immunol 19:467–476

Trevillyan MJ, Nordstrom A, Linna TJ (1985) High tyrosine protein kinase activity in normal peripheral blood lymphocytes. Biochim Biophys Acta 845:1–9

Trotter J, Ferber E (1981) CoA-dependent cleavage of arachidonic acid from phosphatidylcholine and transfer to phosphatidylethanolamine in homogenates of murine thymocytes. FEBS Lett 128:237–241

Trotter J, Fleisch I, Schmidt B, Ferber E (1982) Acyltransferase-catalyzed cleavage of arachidonic acid from phospholipids and transfer to lysophosphatides in lymphocytes and macrophages. J Biol Chem 257:1816–1823

Tsien RY, Pozzan T, Rink TJ (1982) T-cell mitogens cause early changes in cytoplasmic free Ca^{2+} and membrane potential in lymphocytes. Nature 295:68–70

Tuil D, Vaulont S, Levin MJ, Munnich A, Moguilewsky M, Bouton MM, Brissot P, Dreyfus J-C, Kahn A (1985) Transient transcriptional inhibition of the transferrin gene by cyclic AMP. FEBS Lett 189:310–314

Udey MC, Parker CW (1982) Effects of inhibitors of arachidonic acid metabolism on alpha-aminoisobutyric acid transport in human lymphocytes. Biochem Pharmacol 31:337–345

Udey MC, Chaplin DD, Wedner HJ, Parker CW (1980) Early activation events in lectin-stimulated human lymphocytes: evidence that wheat germ agglutinin and mitogenic lectins cause similar early changes in lymphocyte metabolism. J Immunol 125:1544–1550

Ui M (1984) Islet-activating protein, pertussis toxin: a probe for functions of the inhibitory guanine nucleotide regulatory component of adenylate cyclase. Trends Pharmacol Sci 5:277–279

Valone FH, Payan DG (1985) Potentiation of mitogen-induced human T-lymphocyte activation by retinoic acid. Cancer Res 45:4128–4131

Van den Berg KJ, Betel I (1971) Early increase of amino acid transport in stimulated lymphocytes. Exp Cell Res 66:257–259

Van den Berg KJ, Betel I (1973a) Increased transport of 2-aminoisobutyric acid in rat lymphocytes stimulated with concanavalin A. Exp Cell Res 76:63–72

Van den Berg KJ, Betel I (1973b) Selective early activation of a sodium dependent amino acid transport system in stimulated rat lymphocyte. FEBS Lett 29:149–152

Van den Berg KJ, Betel I (1974a) Correlation of early changes in amino acid transport and DNA synthesis in stimulated lymphocytes. Cell Immunol 10:319–323

Van den Berg KJ, Betel I (1974b) Regulation of amino acid uptake in lymphocytes stimulated by mitogens. Exp Cell Res 84:412–418

Vanderhoek JY, Bryant RW, Bailey JM (1980) Inhibition of leukotriene biosynthesis by the leukocyte product 15-hydroxy-5,8,11,13-eicosatetraenoic acid. J Biol Chem 255:10064–10066

Verma AK (1985) Inhibition of phorbol ester-caused synthesis of mouse epidermal ornithine decarboxylase by retinoic acid. Biochim Biophys Acta 846:109–119

Wagshal A, Jegasothy B, Waksman B (1978) Regulatory substances produced by lymphocytes. VI. Cell cycle specificity of inhibitor of DNA synthesis action in L cells. J Exp Med 147:171–181

Waksman BH, Dessaint J-P, Katz SP (1980) Proteolysis, calcium and cyclic nucleotides in macrophage T-lymphocyte interaction. In: de Weck AL, Kristensen F, Landy M (eds) Biochemical characterization of lymphokines. Academic, New York, pp 435–443

Walker C, Kristensen F, Bettens F, de Weck AL (1983) Lymphokine regulation of activated (G$_1$) lymphocytes. J Immunol 130:1170–1173

Wang T, Sheppard JR, Foker JE (1978) Rise and fall of cyclic AMP required for onset of lymphocyte DNA synthesis. Science 201:155–157

Waterhouse PD, Anderson PL, Brown DL (1983) Increases in microtubule assembly and in tubulin content on mitogenically stimulated mouse splenic T lymphocytes. Exp Cell Res 144:367–376

Watson J (1975) The influence of intracellular levels of cyclic nucleotides on cell proliferation and the induction of antibody synthesis. J Exp Med 141:97–111

Watson J, Nilsen-Hamilton M, Hamilton RT (1976) The subcellular distribution of adenylate and guanylate cyclases in murine lymphoid cells. Biochemistry 15:1527–1534

Webb DR, Nowowiejski I (1981) Control of suppressor cell activation via endogenous prostaglandin synthesis: the role of T cells and macrophages. Cell Immunol 63:321–328

Webb DR, Stites DP, Perlman JD, Luong D, Fudenberg HH (1973) Lymphocyte activation: the dualistic effect of cAMP. Biochem Biophys Res Commun 53:1002–1008

Wedner HJ, Parker CW (1975) Protein phosphorylation in human peripheral lymphocytes-stimulation by phytohemagglutinin and N^6-monobutyryl cyclic AMP. Biochem Biophys Res Commun 62:808–815

Wedner HJ, Parker CW (1976) Lymphocyte activation. Prog Allergy 20:195–300

Wedner HJ, Dankner R, Parker CW (1975) Cyclic GMP and lectin-induced lymphocyte activation. J Immunol 115:1682–1687

Wedner HJ, Chan BY, Parker CS, Parker CW (1979) Cyclic nucleotide phosphodiesterase activity in human peripheral blood lymphocytes and monocytes. J Immunol 123:725–732

Weiel JE, Hamilton TA (1984) Quiscent lymphocytes express intracellular transferrin receptors. Biochem Biophys Res Commun 119:598–602

Weinstein Y, Segal S, Melmon KL (1975) Specific mitogenic activity of 8-Br-guanosine 3′,5′-monophosphate (Br-cyclic GMP) on B lymphocytes. J Immunol 115:112–117

Weiss A, Imboden J, Shoback D, Stobo J (1984) Role of T3 surface molecules in human T-cell activation: T3-dependent activation results in an increase in cytoplasmic free calcium. Proc Natl Acad Sci USA 81:4169–4173

Wess JA, Archer DL (1981) Restoration by cyclic guanosine monophosphate and extracellular calcium of butylated hydroxyanisole-suppressed primary murine thymus-dependent antibody response. Immunopharmacology 3:361–366

Whitesell RR, Johnson RA, Tarpley HL, Regen DM (1977) Mitogen-stimulated glucose transport in thymocytes. Possible role of Ca^{2+} and antagonism by adenosine 3':5'-monophosphate. J Cell Biol 72:456–469

Whitfield JF, Rixon RH, Perris AD, Youdale T (1969) Stimulation by calcium of the entry of thymic lymphocytes into the deoxyribonucleic acid-synthetic (S) phase of the cell cycle. Exp Cell Res 57:8–12

Whitfield JF, MacManus JP, Boynton AL, Gillan DJ, Isaacs RJ (1974) Concanavalin A and the initiation of thymic lymphoblast DNA synthesis and proliferation by a calcium-dependent increase in cyclic GMP level. J Cell Physiol 84:445–458

Whitfield JF, MacManus JP, Rixon AH, Boynton AL, Youdale T, Swierenga S (1976) The positive control of cell proliferation by the interplay of calcium and cyclic nucleotides: a review. In Vitro 12:1–18

Whitney RB, Sutherland RM (1972a) Enhanced uptake of calcium by transforming lymphocytes. Cell Immunol 5:137–147

Whitney RB, Sutherland RM (1972b) Requirement for calcium ions in lymphocyte transformation stimulated by phytohemagglutinin. J Cell Physiol 80:329–338

Whitney RB, Sutherland RM (1973) Characteristics of calcium accumulation by lymphocytes and alteration in the process induced by phytohemagglutinin. J Cell Physiol 82:9–20

Williams RO, Loeb LA (1973) Zinc requirement for DNA replication in stimulated human lymphocytes. J Cell Biol 58:594–601

Wolff CHJ, Akerman KEO, Andersson LC (1985) Kinetics of long term (72 hr) calcium content during mitogen activation of cultured human T lymphocytes. J Cell Physiol 123:46–50

Wright P, Quastel MR, Kaplan JG (1973) Differential sensitivity of antigen- and mitogen-stimulated human leukocytes to prolonged inhibition of potassium transport. Exp Cell Res 79:87–94

Yamamoto I, Webb DR (1975) Antigen-stimulated changes in cyclic nucleotide levels in the mouse. Proc Natl Acad Sci USA 72:2320–2324

Yamamoto Y, Fujimoto K, Ohmura T, Maeda S, Shimada K, Onoue K (1985) Interleukin 3 mRNA induction in human lymphocytes: analysis of the synergistic effect of a phorbol ester and phytohemagglutinin. J Biochem 98:49–56

Yasmeen D, Laird AJ, Hume DA, Weidemann MJ (1977) Activation of 3-O-methyl-glucose transport in rat thymus lymphocytes by concanavalin A. Biochim Biophys Acta 500:89–102

Yunis AA, Arimura GK, Kipnis DM (1963) Amino acid transport in blood cells. I. Effect of cations and amino acid transport in human leukocytes. J Lab Clin Med 62:465–476

Zimmerman TP, Schmitges CJ, Wolberg G, Deeprose RD, Duncan GS, Cuatrecasas P, Elion GB (1980) Modulation of cyclic AMP metabolism by S-adenosylhomocysteine and S-3-deazadenosylhomocysteine in mouse lymphocytes. Proc Natl Acad Sci USA 77:5639–5643

Zwiller J, Revel M-O, Malviya AN (1985) Protein kinase C catalyzes phosphorylation of guanylate cyclase in vitro. J Biol Chem 260:1350–1353

Part 2

CHAPTER 5

Generation and Measurement of Antibodies

H. F. J. SAVELKOUL, S. S. PATHAK, N. R. SABBELE, and R. BENNER

A. Introduction

The antibody (Ab) molecule has evolved to perform two distinct functions: epitope recognition and elimination of foreign antigens (Ag). Ab activity resides in immunoglobulin (Ig) molecules, each of which can interact with some of a virtually unlimited number of physicochemically different Ags. These Ags include exogenous (foreign or nonself) as well as endogenous (self) Ags, including Ig idiotopes (EICHMANN 1978; JERNE 1984; KÖHLER et al. 1984). In spite of the large variety of different Ab specificities, Ab destroy or eliminate foreign Ag by a small number of effector mechanisms. To carry out its dual function, the Ab molecule has evolved discrete globular domains: one of these domains binds Ag, whereas the others mediate effector mechanisms (EDELMAN 1973). Thus, the functional duality of the Ab molecule is reflected in its three-dimensional structure. The organization of Ab-gene clusters also reflects this duality (HONJO 1983; CALVERT et al. 1984).

A state of humoral immunity to a certain Ag is characterized by the presence of sufficient Ab in the blood to counteract the Ag and/or the ability to mediate an accelerated and increased Ab production as compared with a nonimmune state. Since the majority of the Abs produced are released into the bloodstream, it is generally assumed that the Ig levels in the serum reflect the overall activity of the humoral immune system. The total activity of all B cell clones will yield, under normal conditions, a heterogeneous spectrum of serum Ig molecules.

In disease, however, some disorders of the immune system can lead to imbalanced B cell activity, which is reflected in excessively high or low serum levels of one or more Ig classes or subclasses (RADL et al. 1972, 1978). Moreover, this imbalanced activity can lead to a restriction in serum Ig heterogeneity and the appearance of temporary or permanent homogeneous Ig components or paraproteins (RADL 1979; RADL et al. 1980). Excessive production of such components is often the result of malignant B cell transformation (McINTYRE 1979).

Insight into the regulation of the overall activity of the humoral immune system requires reliable measurement of the normal and the diseased concentration, and the heterogeneity of the various Ig classes and subclasses in the blood. Together with the determination of the numbers of Ab- and Ig-secreting cells after immunization, measurement of circulating Ab gives an insight into the regulation of Ig synthesis and Ag-specific Ab induction under normal conditions. Moreover, determination of these parameters might help in the rapid diagnosis and understanding of the underlying cause of diseases in which the B cell system is involved.

In this chapter, we will focus on the determination of Ab- and Ig-secreting cells and the measurement of circulating Ab in the mouse (all the techniques we describe here have been applied by us primarily in the species). Applications to the study of human Ab formation are mentioned in the various sections. Further information is available in the references cited.

I. B Cell Development Leading to Antibody Production

All individuals, whether mice or humans, that are not deliberately immunized, have naturally occurring Ig in their serum and at secretory sites. The Ig levels are built up and maintained by Ig-secreting cells in the various lymphoid organs. In mice, the number of these spontaneously occurring "background" Ig-secreting cells vary, as do the serum level and serum Ig heterogeneity, with the genetic background, T cell function, and exogenous antigenic load (BENNER et al. 1982a; HOOIJKAAS et al. 1984, 1985a, b).

When mice are deliberately immunized with thymus-dependent (TD) Ag, Ab-secreting cells are found, depending on the route of immunization, in the spleen, lymph nodes, gut-associated and bronchus-associated lymphoid tissues (GALT and BALT), but not in the bone marrow (BM). Upon secondary immunization of mice with TD Ag, the BM becomes the major source of Ab formation, depending on migration of reactivated memory B cells from peripheral lymphoid organs into the BM (BENNER et al. 1977). Thymus-independent (TI) Ag can also induce Ab-secreting cells in the various peripheral lymphoid organs. However, some TI antigens (e.g., lipopolysaccharides (LPS), hapten-Ficoll conjugates), induce BM Ab formation after primary immunization, while others are incapable of inducing an Ab-secreting cell response in the BM (KOCH et al. 1982a).

In vivo Ig production is usually estimated by quantitating the serum Ig concentration or the numbers of Ig-containing or Ig-secreting cells in the various lymphoid organs. It is also known that, on immunization with TD as well as TI Ag, and independent of the Ag dose, Ig with no binding capacity for the eliciting Ag are synthesized (URBAIN-VANSANTEN 1970; MOTICKA 1974; PACHMANN et al. 1974). The ratio of this so-called Ag-nonspecific response to the Ag-specific response is isotype dependent and is greater during a primary immune response than during a secondary response (BENNER et al. 1982b). Whether this is caused by Ag-nonspecific B cell growth and maturation factors, or induction of autoantibodies or anti-idiotypic antibodies, is still controversial. This nonspecific Ig production, together with Ag-specific Ab production upon immunization, is also reflected in the serum Ig fraction (CAZENAVE et al. 1974). Therefore, measurement of serum Ig levels is not a reliable measure of the capacity to produce Ag-specific Ab upon immunization. This is all the more certain since a substantial proportion of the circulating Ig is withdrawn from the circulatory system at secretory sites (VAN MUISWINKEL et al. 1979).

The improvement of in vitro culture techniques, both for murine and human B cells, allows the analysis of normal B cell development at the cellular level. Under these conditions, Ig production or secretion by B cells can also be measured by many different and reliable techniques (Sects. B and C).

Studies on B cell function in humans are mainly restricted to the functional analysis of peripheral blood mononuclear cells. In humans, study of the regulation of the Ag-induced immune response became feasible only after the development of appropriate in vitro culture techniques and Ag-specific plaque-forming cell assays.

II. Antibodies as Diagnostic Tools

It is well established that the formation of an Ag-Ab complex is the basic event for a humoral immunologic reaction. This complex formation is driven by thermodynamic principles. Together with the nature of the noncovalent bonds involved, this Ag-Ab complex formation suggests the chemical basis of the immunologic reaction. Antibodies can be studied from these immunochemical points of view as a screening system for B cell activity in fundamental immunology.

It is also obvious that Ab, because of their molecular recognition properties, can be used as detecting reagents for a variety of proteins by virtue of their high specificity and the sensitivity of Ag-Ab complex formation. A variety of soluble antigens, such as glycoproteins and lipoproteins, polysaccharides, hormones, vitamins, and haptens, whether linked to cells, bacteria, latex particles, carrier molecules, or otherwise, can thus be detected. Therefore many techniques have been designed, all based on detection of this Ag-Ab complex formation. They are applied among others in clinical chemistry, food and dairy technology, microbiology as well as in immunology, pathology, molecular biology, and endocrinology. The various techniques, some of which will be discussed in greater detail later in the chapter, have their own detection limits, sensitivity ranges, advantages, and disadvantages. It is important to note that we will discuss in this chapter only those methods that we have experience with and not review all the other methods that are available.

B. Induction of Antibody Formation

The clonal selection theory proposed by BURNET in 1959 remains one of the most important integrating concepts in immunology. When the immune system encounters an Ag, only those lymphocytes carrying the appropriate receptors will be able to bind that particular Ag. As a consequence, intracellular processes are initiated (i.e., activation) which can lead to cell division and differentiation.

An essential aspect in the discussion of activation is the cell cycle. Most of the mature $mIgM^+IgD^+$ B lymphocytes are in a resting state (G_0 phase), exhibiting a low rate of metabolic activity and no net DNA synthesis (CHAN and OSMOND 1979). Activation is a general term referring to a complex process by which the cell, after contact with the stimulating agent, progresses from the G_0 phase into the cell cycle (BLACK et al. 1980; HERZENBERG et al. 1980; Chap. 1).

I. In Vitro Antibody Formation

In studying the processes related to activation and subsequent proliferation and differentiation of B lymphocytes in vitro, specific Ag or polyclonal B cell activators (mitogens) are used. The latter stimulate a large proportion of the B cell population and thus evoke responses of sufficient magnitude to permit analysis of membrane-related and intracellular changes. Polyclonal B cell activators (PBA) can be divided roughly into two groups. One group of substances can bind to the Ag receptor (membrane-bound Ig) while mitogens of the second group bind to other (mostly unknown) membrane-associated structures. Examples of the latter category are pokeweed mitogen (PWM), LPS, purified protein derivative (PPD), dextran, and Epstein-Barr virus (EBV). PBA binding to the Ag receptor are immunoglobulin-specific antibodies (anti-Ig; anti-IgM; anti-IgD; anti-IgG; idiotype-specific antibodies) and *Staphylococcus aureus* Cowan I strain (Sta) bacteria (SIECKMANN et al. 1978; ROMAGNANI et al. 1981; PURÉ and VITETTA 1980; YOSHIZAKI et al. 1982).

PBA and Ag can be subdivided according to their requirement for T cells to facilitate the B cell response. Thymus-dependent (TD) and thymus-independent (TI) PBA and Ag can be distinguished. TD PBA and Ag can only induce a B cell response in the presence of T cell help (e.g., PWM, PPD, and most soluble proteins). In contrast, TI PBA and Ag are able to stimulate B cells in the absence of T cells (e.g., LPS, EBV, and certain polysaccharides). T cell help in the B cell response against TD PBA and Ag requires physical contact of the helper T cell and the responding B cell. The T cell recognizes the Ag, probably bound to the Ag receptor of the B cell, in context with class II molecules coded for by the major histocompatibility (MHC) complex (SCHWARTZ 1984).

The second way in which a B cell can be helped to proliferate and differentiate, is through soluble Ag-specific helper factors and/or nonspecific factors – often referred to as lymphokines – produced by activated T cells. Among these are growth factors, regulating the proliferation of activated B cells, and differentiation-inducing factors.

The initial activation of helper T cells participating in TD B cell responses is based on the dual recognition of the Ag (or polyclonal T cell activator) and class II MHC-molecules, usually present on the surface of Ag-presenting cells (APC) (VITETTA et al. 1984). The factor-dependent differentiation of B cells is thought to be a linear sequence of steps, leading from an initial activation, subsequent DNA synthesis, and cell division, to Ig production. In studying these processes two membrane Ig-binding PBA are most frequently used: anti-IgM (mice, humans) and Sta (humans) (KISHIMOTO et al. 1984; HOWARD et al. 1984; KEHRL et al. 1984).

A prerequisite for in vitro growth of normal B lymphocytes is the use of suitable culture conditions, which allow every single lymphocyte, having the capacity to be stimulated by the PBA employed, to grow and develop into a clone of cells. Growth requires, in addition to RPMI 1640 medium (for mouse lymphocyte cultures) and the presence of, for example, the mitogen LPS, growth-supporting fetal bovine serum and the use of 2-mercaptoethanol, while for maturation, mouse or rat thymus filler cells are necessary (HOOIJKAAS et al. 1982; LEFKOVITS 1972, 1979;

Chap. 12). Serum-free media have also been used (Iscove and Melchers 1978). It has been reported that macrophages are a prerequisite for the in vitro activation of B cells by LPS (Melchers and Corbel 1983). In general, every third murine splenic B cell is responsive to LPS and will grow for up to 7 days, dividing every 18 h under these in vitro culture conditions. Cultures are normally analyzed on day 5 for IgM secretion and on day 7 for the secretion of IgG, IgE or IgA in the appropriate plaque assays. For the analysis of supernatants in RIA or ELISA the cells are generally cultured up to 11 days.

We use the following culture conditions: varying numbers of mouse spleen or lymph node cells (maximally 1200 per 0.2 ml) or BM cells (maximally 6000 per 0.2 ml) are cultured in 96-well tissue culture plates (Costar 3596; Costar, Cambridge, Massachusetts) together with 7.2×10^5 irradiated (0.1 Gy) rat thymus cells to support growth and 50 µg/ml LPS B from *Escherichia coli* (026:B6; Difco Laboratories, Detroit, Michigan) in 0.2 ml RPMI 1640 medium supplemented with glutamic (4 mM), penicillin (100 IU/ml), streptomycin (50 µg/ml), 2-mercaptoethanol $(5 \times 10^{-5} M)$, and fetal bovine serum (20%) (lot B 66390302; Boehringer Mannheim GmbH, Mannheim), specifically selected for growth-supporting properties and low endogenous mitogenic acitivity. Cultures are incubated in a humidified atmosphere containing 5% CO_2 at 37 °C (Heraeus, Hanau).

II. In Vivo Antibody Formation

Several lymphoid organs are involved in Ab formation in vivo. The BM and thymus are called the "central" or "primary" lymphoid organs because they are the breeding sites for lymphocytes. The BM generates the immunocompetent virgin B lymphocytes and pre-T cells. These pre-T cells are generated independent of the presence of the thymus, the lymphoid organ to which these immature, immunoincompetent cells normally home, proliferate, and differentiate into mature immunocompetent T lymphocytes. The "peripheral" or "secondary" lymphoid organs, such as the spleen, lymph nodes, GALT, and BALT, provide the architecture and accessory cells (macrophages and dendritic cells) appropriate for Ag processing and for the presentation of Ag to the lymphocytes. In these organs, therefore, the Ag-driven differentiation of lymphocytes takes place. Within these peripheral lymphoid organs a B and T cell compartment can be recognized. Virgin B cells settle predominantly in the lymphoid follicles, whereas T cells are found within the periarteriolar lymphoid sheath (PALS) of the splenic white pulp, the paracortex of lymph nodes, and the interfollicular areas of the GALT (Van Ewijk et al. 1977; Rozing et al. 1978).

1. Primary and Secondary Responses

On primary Ag injection, small B lymphocytes can be stimulated to transform into B cell blasts in the peripheral part of the PALS. These B cell blasts proliferate and differentiate into Ab-producing plasma cells. During this differentiation, the cells migrate to the red pulp of the spleen and to the medullary cords of the lymph nodes.

Although thymic humoral factors or T cells do not influence the lymphocyte production in the BM, after Ag stimulation of B cells Ag-specific T cells can greatly enhance their response. The activated B cells give rise to clones of plasma cells which remain mainly localized in the lymphoid organs. However, their secretory products, the Ab, are carried by the blood and lymph to their sites of action.

The humoral immune response to an Ag is characterized not only by the production of plasma cells, but also by the induction of Ag-specific immunologic memory. By comparison with the primary response, the secondary response is characterized by: a shorter lag period between the encounter with Ag and Ab production; Ab production that has a higher rate and is more persistent; higher Ab titers at the peak of the response; a predominance of IgG molecules; and Ab with a higher affinity for Ag than those produced in the primary response.

Both the T and B lymphocyte population carry immunologic memory, and such cells are, in contrast to virgin cells, long-lived small cells with a life span of several weeks to several months (Sprent 1977). Furthermore, these memory cells are recirculating cells, while virgin lymphocytes are mainly nonrecirculating sessile cells (Strober and Dilley 1973). The amounts and the types (affinity, isotypes) of Ab formed vary widely with the conditions of immunization, some of which are discussed in the following sections.

2. Type of Antigen

The induction of maximal Ab production to most Ag requires the participation of Ag-specific T helper cells (hence such Ag are called thymus-dependent or TD). Upon primary immunization of mice with TD Ag, plaque-forming cells (PFC) are almost exclusively found in spleen and lymph nodes. Secondary immunization, however, induces a substantial PFC response in the BM as well. During the secondary response, the BM becomes the major source of serum Ab (Benner et al. 1974). This BM Ab formation is dependent on the immigration and the subsequent proliferation of memory B cells that are reactivated by the booster Ag in the peripheral lymphoid organs (Benner et al. 1974; Koch et al. 1982b).

Presumably, the BM lacks the appropriate microenvironment and/or the quantity or quality of cells required for the early steps in the induction of immune responses. In contrast to mouse BM, human BM has features which are characteristic of peripheral lymphoid tissues, e.g., the occurrence of follicles with germinal centers (Nieuwenhuis and Opstelten 1984). Therefore, Ab formation in human BM may not be similarly dependent on an influx of Ag-activated B cells from the periphery. Germinal centers arise as discrete sites of B cell differentiation in B cell areas of lymphoid tissues after antigenic stimulation. An important role has been suggested for germinal centers in heavy chain class switching (Kraal et al. 1982, 1985).

The characteristic kinetics of the PFC response in spleen and BM shows that the Ab-forming cell response is regulated in such a manner that the peripheral lymphoid organs respond rapidly, but only for a short period, whereas the BM response starts slowly, but accounts for a long-lasting massive production of Ab to repeated Ag challenge. Thus, the peripheral lymphoid organs provide a fast defense against the challenging Ag, while the BM provides long-lasting protection against recurrent infections (TYLER and EVERETT 1972; MENDELOW et al. 1980).

In contrast to TD Ag, certain TI antigens give rise to Ab formation in the BM during the primary response (KOCH et al. 1982a,c). The difference in capacity of the various TI Ag that we have tested to induce a PFC response in the BM does not correlate with the subdivision of TI Ag into two classes (TI-1 and TI-2) according to the response they induce in CBA/N mice. These mice are unable to raise an immune response to TI-2 Ag such as DNP-Ficoll, levan, dextran, etc. (SHER et al. 1975). It is thought that TI-2 Ag stimulate the more mature B cells that express IgD, complement receptors, Lyb-3 and Ly-5 surface Ag, and predominantly occur in the spleen (HUBER et al. 1977; AHMED et al. 1977). TI-1 Ag such as TNP-LPS and TNP-*Brucella abortus* stimulate not only the more mature B cells, but also a population of less mature B cells that are also present in the BM (MOND et al. 1977).

3. Route of Antigen Administration

Normally, lymphatic tissues are almost constantly encountering Ag from transiently invasive or indigenous microbes (normal flora of skin, intestines, etc.) and those that enter the body by inhalation (e.g., plant pollens), by ingestion (e.g., food, drugs) and by penetration of the skin.

For deliberate immunization, immunogens are usually injected into skin, (intradermally or subcutaneously, s.c), or muscle (intramuscularly, i.m.), depending on the volume injected and the irritancy of the immunogen. Intraperitoneal (i.p.) and intravenous (i.v.) injections are also used in experimental work, especially with particulate Ag. Regardless of the route, most Ag eventually become distributed throughout the body via lymphatic and vascular channels. Because most Ag are degraded in the intestines, feeding is effective only under special circumstances. Allergic responses to food are probably due to Ag that resist degradation by intestinal enzymes. Immunization can also be achieved by aerosol administration of the Ag. Ab formation is generally most prominent in the lymphoid organ draining the site of immunization. The highest bone marrow PFC responses are observed with i.v. or i.p. booster injections (BENNER et al. 1977).

Secondary immunization with a TD Ag will lead to Ab formation in the BM, independent of the route of primary immunization; i.v. and i.p. are equally effective while s.c. priming is effective only with higher doses of Ag.

Every Ag has an optimal immunogenic dose range. Much larger amounts elicit high zone tolerance. With TD Ag, but not with TI Ag, lower amounts can also cause tolerance (low dose tolerance). Also, the physical state of an Ag influences the immunogenicity: aggregated molecules of bovine γ-globulin, for instance, are immunogenic, while monomers are tolerogenic. It is thus difficult to induce tolerance to particulate Ag, which are usually highly immunogenic. The route of administration is another determinant: soluble Ag tend to be immunogenic when injected into tissues, but to be tolerogenic when given i.v.

The surface of a protein Ag consists of a complex array of overlapping, potentially antigenic determinants; in aggregates, they approach a continuum. Most determinants depend on the conformational integrity of the native protein molecule. Those to which an individual responds are determined by the structural differences between an Ag and the host's self-proteins and by host regulatory mechanisms, and this is not necessarily an inherent property of the protein molecule, reflecting restricted antigenicity or limited number of antigenic sites. As stated already, protein Ag are therefore more immunogenic when administered in aggregated than in soluble form. Thus, chemically cross-linked protein molecules (e.g., by glutaraldehyde) and Ag-Ab complexes, prepared under conditions of slight Ag excess, are usually highly immunogenic. However, when the complexes are prepared under conditions of Ab excess, their immunogenicity is greatly reduced, probably because the antigenic determinants are blocked.

The level of Ab in the serum reflects the balance between rates of synthesis and degradation. When the rates are equal, the serum Ab concentration is constant (steady state). The rate of synthesis depends on the total number of Ab-producing cells, which varies enormously with conditions of immunization. By contrast, the rate of degradation (expressed as half-life) is determined by the H chain class; e.g., IgM, IgE and IgA usually have a shorter half-life than IgG molecules.

4. Use of Adjuvants

Adjuvants are agents that, by nonspecific mechanisms, can modify the humoral or cellular immune response when injected with Ag. Adjuvants are not only able to stimulate the response to the Ag, but, depending on the conditions, they can also suppress it; furthermore, their effect can be both Ag-specific and nonspecific. A large variety of substances can act as adjuvants and their modes of action are very heterogeneous (BOREK 1977; WHITEHOUSE 1977; HILGERS et al. 1985).

Originally, most adjuvants used were of bacterial origin and were themselves good immunogens. Adjuvants such as complete Freund's adjuvant (CFA) have a strong stimulating effect on most immune responses. However, CFA also induces excessive granulopoiesis within the BM, which abolishes the ongoing Ig synthesis in this organ. Other adjuvants which do not induce excessive granulopoiesis, such as alum, do not interfere with Ab formation in the marrow. Many adjuvants probably mediate their effect by protecting the Ag for prolonged periods of time against breakdown, while they simultaneously stimulate the mononuclear phagocyte system. Adjuvant-induced immunomodulation, on the other hand, can also be mediated by macrophages.

5. Age

A variety of membrane changes can occur during aging, including the appearance of new differentiation Ag, modification of the cell membrane by continued exposure to environmental chemical haptens, quantitative differences in the expression of normal cell surface Ag (e.g., Ig idiotype by monoclonal expansion of a B cell line), changes in cholesterol: phospholipid ratio, expression of viral Ag, or by insertion into the cell membrane of altered proteins arising from somatic mutations or errors in protein synthesis (ORGEL 1973; HEIDRICK 1973; BURNET 1974; RIVNAY et al. 1979; CALLARD 1981).

The proliferation and differentiation of B cells is only moderately impaired with age, leading to a decrease in the number of effector cells generated (PRICE and MAKINODAN 1972). However, the pattern of differentiation of B cell precursors found in the BM of aged mice may be altered, since, in the in vivo transfer systems, it was suggested that BM from aged mice contained a significantly greater number of differentiated immunocomponent cells than the marrow of young mice (FARRAR et al. 1974). The age-related changes in the central lymphoid organs are to a large extent based on deficiencies in T cell function: old BM has a decreased capacity to provide the thymus with T cell progenitors because of a reduced stem cell population. Also, the number of cortisone-resistant mature thymocytes declines with age, and there is a progressive involution of the thymus after sexual maturation (TYAN 1981).

In mice, high avidity IgG Ab-forming cells preferentially decline during aging (GOIDL et al. 1976). This finding is in contrast to the notion that the secondary immune potential is less severely affected by age than the primary potential (FINGER et al. 1972). Moreover, the reponse to TD Ag is more susceptible to age-related decline than the response to the TI Ag LPS (BLANKWATER et al. 1975). Also, the responsiveness to low doses of Ag declines faster than the responsiveness to high doses (PRICE and MAKINODON 1972).

It was shown in unintentionally immunized mice that the total number of cells containing cytoplasmic immunoglobulins (c-Ig) summed over spleen, BM, mesenteric lymph nodes, and Peyer's patches, did not change appreciably during aging, in contrast to the relative contribution of the different lymphoid organs to the total (HAAIJMAN et al. 1977; HAAIJMAN and HIJMANS 1978). The majority of c-Ig cells in young mice were localized in the spleen, whereas in mice older than 6 months the predominant site was the BM. Comparative studies with athymic (nude) mice revealed that the differential role of spleen and BM during aging is not dependent on the presence of a functional thymus, but the class distribution of c-Ig is (HAAIJMAN et al. 1979). Ideally, the total number of Ig-producing cells in the various lymphoid organs should correlate with the Ig concentration in the serum. In humans, such correlations have been reported for the various Ig classes and subclasses (HIJMANS 1975; TURESSON 1976). In these studies, Ig-producing cells were enumerated by immunofluorescence. In mice, similar studies, also with immunofluorescence, did not reveal a simple linear correlation. During aging in normal mice, a slow increase of background c-Ig- positive cells was found (VAN OUDENAREN et al. 1981). However, the increase in numbers of Ig-secreting cells is more pronounced (BENNER et al. 1982a), leading to a change in the ratio between the number of Ig-producing cells found in the protein A plaque assay and by immunofluorescence. The underlying cause of these discrepancies is probably that in immunofluorescence only plasma blasts and plasma cells can be identified with certainty. However, earlier stages of the plasmacytic series are also able to produce and secrete Ig, and thus are able to cause plaques (MELCHERS and ANDERSSON 1973, 1974).

The number of Ig-producing cells per organ depends on age; during the first week of life in mice only IgM secretion is found. At 14 weeks, the number of Ig-secreting cells reaches a maximum in lymph nodes and Peyer's patches and then decreases gradually. However, the number of Ig-secreting cells in the BM increases constantly throughout life (BENNER et al. 1982a).

Qualitative aspects concerning serum Ig levels in the aging human and laboratory animal population show an increase of the average concentrations of IgG and IgA while those of IgM and IgD show a (generally nonsignificant) decrease (Buckley et al. 1974). Increased levels of IgG1 and IgG3 subclasses in volunteers over 95 years of age were found to be responsible for the elevated values of the IgG class as compared with young adult controls (Radl et al. 1975). The IgG2 and IgG4 subclasses did not seem to contribute substantially to the increased total concentration of IgG in the aged. Increased variations with age among the Ig levels of different individuals were generally found in both humans and mice. The age-related changes were, therefore, selective (Radl 1981). In old age, autoantibodies, paraproteins, and immunodeficiencies can occur at the B cell level as well as at the T cell level. This is most likely due to a selective effect, influenced by genetic factors.

6. Corticosteroid Level

The height of the primary response to an Ag, especially TD Ag, is influenced by the plasma level of corticosteroids (Van Dijk et al. 1976). This influence of corticosteroids on the immune system can be mediated by: (a) redistribution of potentially circulating lymphoid cells and mononuclear phagocytes; and (b) an effect on the function of these cells.

The distribution pattern of these cells is affected because of a shrinkage of the thymus, spleen, BM, and lymph nodes, associated with a fall in circulating lymphocytes (Fauci et al. 1976). The redistribution of these cells to the BM is apparent from the increase in the T cell number and T cell function in this compartment, and the prevention of monocyte emigration. Moreover, lymphocyte traffic within BM, spleen, and lymph nodes is almost completely arrested, and the influx of lymphocytes into lymph nodes is impaired. Another factor that contributes to the corticosteroid-dependent redistribution is lymphoid cell destruction (Fauci 1975).

The effects on the function of the lymphoid cells, exerted by corticosteroids, are different for T and B cells, the T cells being more susceptible. It has been postulated that Ag-reactive T cells are more severely depleted from the peripheral blood than mitogen-reactive T cells (Ten Berge 1983). There is a vast literature on the biochemical mode of action of steroids (see Chap. 17). Convergent data indicate the following scheme: steroids pass the cell membrane and bind to a specific cytosol receptor. The steroid-receptor complex then enters the nucleus where it interacts with DNA. This interaction may lead to alterations in transcription level and later on in translation level, the final effect resulting in modifications of enzyme synthesis – either induction of repression (Morley et al. 1984).

A study of the effects of corticosteroid treatment on continued Ig synthesis in various lymphoid organs of the same nonimmunized individual provides an example of how Ig assays such as the protein A plaque assay can be applied to determine the number and the organ distribution of the "spontaneously" occurring "background" Ig-secreting cells. Our own laboratory has performed such studies in BALB/C mice, with the synthetic corticosteroid dexamethasone sodium phosphate (DEXA). This was done for IgM-, IgG-, and IgA-secreting cells in spleen, mesenteric lymph nodes (MLN), and BM. A single injection of DEXA (16–144 mg per kilogramm body weight) markedly reduced the number of Ig-secreting cells in spleen and MLN within 1 day, but hardly affected their number in the BM (Fig. 1). The decrease was immediately followed by a recovery and, at the highest doses and especially in MLN, by an overshoot. Some 2 weeks after the initial decrease, a second decrease was found. When mice were subjected to daily treatment with DEXA for 1 week, an initial recovery pattern was found in spleen and MLN similar to that found after a single injection of a high dose. In this case, however, the effects were less dose dependent and the overshoot reaction was followed by a period of subnormal numbers of Ig-secreting cells which lasted at least 1 week. This late effect of DEXA occurred not only in spleen and MLN, but also in the BM. The most prominent effect of daily treatment with DEXA was the long-lasting decrease in the number of IgG-secreting cells, starting 1 week after withdrawal of treatment (Fig. 2). This decrease was associated with a severely decreased serum IgG level (SABBELE et al. 1983 a,b).

To study the corticosteroid-induced suppressive effect on newly formed B cells, a culture system was employed that allowed the clonal growth of every mitogen-reactive B cell up to a cell input of 1200 spleen cells or 6000 BM cells per culture (BENNER et al. 1981). *Escherichia coli* LPS were used as a mitogen which, in C57BL/6J mice, induces every third B cell to develop into a clone of Ig-secreting cells (ANDERSSON et al. 1977). A single injection of a high dose of DEXA (144 mg/kg) caused a marked decrease in the number of spleen cells and a moderate decrease in the number of BM cells. The percentage of B cells among the remaining spleen and BM cells was not affected, neither was the polyclonal response after stimulation of the remaining B cells with LPS in vitro. Thus, the population of LPS-reactive B cells seem to be neither more nor less sensitive to DEXA than the other cells of the lymphohemopoietic system. Prolonged treatment with a relatively moderate dose of DEXA (50 mg/kg) did affect the percentage of total B cells in spleen and BM as well as the subpopulation of LPS-reactive B cells.

When DEXA was added to cultures of LPS-activated B cells, the LPS-induced Ig-secreting cell response by splenic B cells and BM B cells in vitro was substantially affected (Fig. 3). It appeared that $10^{-8}M$ DEXA reduced the response of the splenic B cells by more than 80%, while a similar reduction of the response by BM B cells required a 1000-fold higher concentration (Table 1).

In "corticosteroid-resistant" species such as humans, it has been demonstrated that in vitro corticosteroids in physiologically and pharmacologically attainable concentrations cause a marked enhancement of pokeweed mitogen-(PWM)-induced PFC responses by human peripheral blood lymphocytes (FAUCI et al. 1977). The effect is exerted on the actual activation process and is probably due to a modulation of the B cell triggering signal, either directly through the B cell or via T cell regulation of B cell responses. Although there is ample evidence that corticosteroid treatment of humans decreases Ab formation, contradictory reports have also appeared showing that they can enhance the in vivo Ab formation. Thus, TUCHINDA et al. (1972) have shown that alternate-day prednisone treatment of six children with bronchial asthma enhanced the primary humoral immune response to keyhole limpet hemocyanin (KLH). The secondary response after a booster injection with the same Ag, however, was not affected.

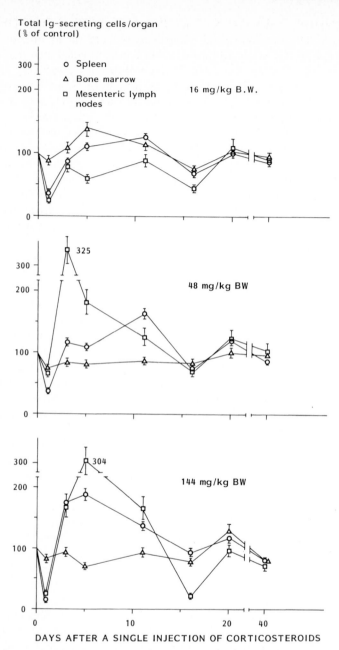

Fig. 1. Effect of a single injection of DEXA on the total number of "background" Ig-secreting cells in mouse spleen, MLN and BM. Numbers of Ig-secreting cells (IgM plus IgG plus IgA) were determined at various intervals after injection of either 16, 48, or 144 mg DEXA per kilogram body weight. At all time points, a group of BSS-treated control mice were also assayed ($N = 6$). The day 0 values (100%) were calculated as the arithmetic mean of all controls. These values are: for spleen $209\,000 \pm 10\,000$; for MLN 9000 ± 1000; and for BM $115\,000 \pm 9000$ cells

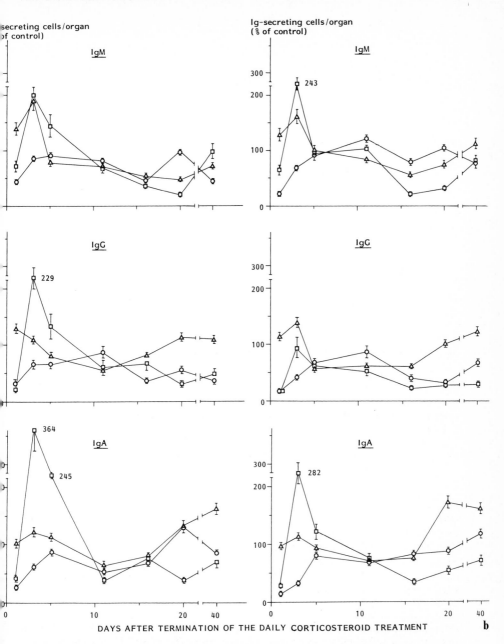

Fig. 2a,b. Effect of seven daily injections of DEXA on the number of "background" IgM-, IgG-, and IgA-secreting cells in mouse spleen (*circles*), MLN (*squares*), and BM (*triangles*). Numbers of Ig-secreting cells were determined at various intervals after the last injection of either 1 (**a**) or 16 (**b**) mg DEXA per kilogram body weight. At all time points, a group of BSS-treated control mice were also assayed ($N = 6$). The day 0 values (100%) were calculated as the arithmetic mean of all controls. The values for IgM, IgG, and IgA are: for spleen $71\,000 \pm 4000$, $58\,000 \pm 7000$, and $57\,000 \pm 4000$; for MLN 1400 ± 200, 7000 ± 1300, and 3300 ± 600; and for BM $18\,000 \pm 2000$, $31\,000 \pm 2000$, and $45\,000 \pm 3000$ cells

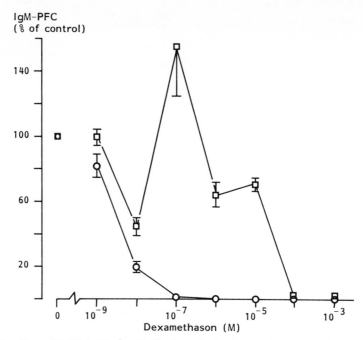

Fig. 3. The effect of DEXA (10^{-9} – 10^{-3} M) on the in vitro LPS-activated B cell response. IgM PFC (day 5) were determined after culturing 1200 spleen cells (*circles*), 6000 BM cells (*squares*) per well (0.2 ml)

Table 1. Effects of single or multiple dexamethasone injection on the in vitro polyclonal B cell response to *E. coli* lipopolysaccharide

Organ	Treatment[a]	Nucleated cells ($\times 10^{-6}$)[b]	s-Ig$^+$ cells[c] (%)	IgM PFC[d]	IgG PFC	IgA PFC
Spleen		115±8.8	45 ±2.0	18354±1135	9588± 602	713±157
Spleen	Single	25±7.0	40 ±0.9	16332± 961	7663± 785	725±109
Bone marrow		35±1.8	5.3±0.7	11334± 692	7738± 974	663±206
Bone marrow	Single	25±1.3	5.4±0.3	12786± 897	9050± 438	550±124
Spleen		102±9.8	47 ±2.2	17860± 899	6220± 490	ND
Spleen	Daily	8±1.8	21 ±3.5	10960± 766	6450± 558	ND
Bone marrow		29±4.7	5.6±0.1	14420±1043	7870±1281	ND
Bone marrow	Daily	24±1.4	2.5±0.2	6300± 603	7630± 691	ND

[a] Mice were injected intraperitoneally with either a single injection of dexamethasone (144 mg/kg) or seven daily injections of dexamethasone (50 mg/kg). Cells were harvested 1 day after the last injection.
[b] Figures represent the number of nucleated cells ($\times 10^{-6}$) per whole spleen or per two femurs.
[c] The percentage of surface Ig-positive (s-Ig$^+$) B cells was determined by immunofluorescence.
[d] The number of Ig-secreting cells (PFC) was determined in cultures of LPS-stimulated spleen cells (1200 viable nucleated cells per well) and bone marrow cells (6000 viable nucleated cells per well). IgM PFC were determined on day 5, and IgG and IgA PFC were determined on day 6 of culture.

C. Measurement of Immunoglobulin Secretion at the Cellular Level

The analysis of Ab production in different organs can be performed at the cellular level under normal in vivo or controlled in vitro conditions. Before describing the most frequently used detection techniques for Ig secretion, we shall discuss the preparation of cell suspensions from lymphoid organs of mice and humans. For quantitating the Ig-secreting cell activity, it is essential to use procedures for the preparation of cell suspensions that allow the recovery of as many viable Ig-secreting cells as possible. In the following sections, we shall discuss the procedure that, in our hands, gives the best results.

1. Cell Suspensions from Lymphoid Organs of Mice

Immediately after killing the mice, the organs to be used (spleen, lymph nodes and/or thymus), are removed and transferred to balanced salt solution (BSS). This solution is prepared according to MISHELL and DUTTON (1967). Spleen, lymph nodes, and thymus are minced with scissors and squeezed through a 100-μm mesh nylon gauze filter (Stokvis and Smits Textiel Mij., Haarlem) to give a single-cell suspension. The nylon is stretched between two aluminum rings of diameter 3 cm. The cells are gently forced through the nylon filter with a plunger, and another 4 ml BSS is used to collect the remaining cells. The pooled cells are washed by spinning down in a Heraeus-Christ centrifuge (Minifuge, Osterode AM, Harz) at 4 °C for 10 min at 500 g. Immediately thereafter, the supernatant is discarded and the packed cells resuspended in 5 ml BSS. All suspensions are kept on ice until further use. Viable and total nucleated cells are assessed simultaneously after resuspension.

For collection of the femoral BM, the killed mice are pinned ventrally to a cork tray, the forelegs and hindlegs spread apart. The skin is cut after wetting with 70% ethanol in water. The procedure for removing the femur is critical, and is as described by BENNER et al. (1981). Before isolating the BM from the femur, the residual muscle tissue is removed with a tissue paper. The marrow can most easily be isolated after cutting the head of the femur and a small piece of the greater trochanter on the upper side, and a small piece of the condyle on the lower side. By means of a 2- or 5-ml syringe equipped with a 25 G × 0.6 needle, a hole is pricked in both spongious ends of the femur and the marrow is collected by flushing the marrow cavity with 1–2 ml BSS from the syringe. Whether the marrow has been completely extracted from the femur or not can be judged from the color of the shaft. Single-cell suspensions from the BM are obtained by gently squeezing the latter through a 100-μm mesh nylon gauze filter. To calculate the number of cells in the total BM, the number of cells that occur in two femoral BM samples are multiplied by a factor of 7.94 (BENNER et al. 1981).

It should be noted that the thymus, and to a lesser extent the mesenteric lymph nodes, contain cells which are very sensitive to adverse conditions. Such conditions can lead to their lysis releasing DNA which agglutinates the rest of the cells in the suspensions.

2. Cell Suspensions of Human Origin

Most frequently, heparinized peripheral blood samples are obtained while samples of lymphoid organs such as BM or lymph nodes are occasionally available. After mincing the organs (if necessary) and aspiration of the cells through a needle, or flushing through a 100-μm mesh nylon gauze filter, mononuclear cells are collected by density centrifugation on Ficoll-Paque (density 1.077 g/cm^3; Pharmacia, Uppsala).

I. Antibody-Secreting Cell Assays

The objective of hemolytic plaque assays is to enumerate and study individual Ab-secreting cells, especially in situations where only a few such cells are present among many cells that do not release Ab. For example, with the plaque assay as few as 100 Ab-secreting PFC can be detected within a population of 10^8 spleen cells. This is very useful during the early phase of the immune response after a primary antigenic stimulus, and in attempts to induce Ab formation in vitro.

The original Jerne-type direct plaque assay detects single cells which secrete IgM Ab that bind to determinants on the target red blood cells, usually sheep erythrocytes (SRBC) (Jerne and Nordin 1963; Jerne et al. 1963). These determinants may be naturally occurring red blood cell surface Ag, or determinants artificially coupled to the red cell surface (Jerne et al. 1974). Cells secreting Ab of a class or subclass other than IgM may also be detected in this assay. Therefore rabbit Ab specific for that Ig class or subclass has to be added as developing antiserum (Dresser and Wortis 1965).

Cells secreting Ig without known Ab specificity, "background" Ig-secreting cells, can also be assayed in a hemolytic plaque assay. Two main systems have been developed to determine isotype-specific Ig-secreting cells: the reverse plaque assay (Molinaro and Dray 1974; Molinaro et al. 1978), and the protein A plaque assay (Gronowicz et al. 1976). Both are completely dependent on the presence of Ig-specific Ab on the surface of the target SRBC. In the reverse plaque assay (Sect. B.II.2), the SRBC are directly coated with the Ab molecules. In the protein A plaque assay (Sect. C.II.1), this is done indirectly by coating the target SRBC with protein A by CrCl$_3$, followed by the addition of Abs of the IgG class with high binding affinity to protein A.

As the detection of PFC depends solely on the specificity of the developing antiserum, isotype-specific assays can be performed, and it is plausible that these assays are applicable to any molecule secreted in sufficient amounts and for which a specific developing antiserum is available. For example, the secretion of albumin by hepatocytes (Primi et al. 1981).

In the original hemolytic plaque assay of Jerne and Nordin, lymphoid cells, together with a suspension of target red blood cells are immobilized in an agar gel. Cunningham (1965) and Cunningham and Szenberg (1968) proposed a modification in which the lymphoid cells and the target red blood cells are incubated in a medium, without supporting gels as monolayers, in sealed chambers. This method is simple, sensitive, and rapid for the enumeration of PFC, and is therefore used routinely throughout the different plaque assays described in this chapter.

1. Protein A Plaque Assay

Ig-secreting cells can be assayed by the hemolytic plaque assay as described by GRONOWICZ et al. (1976) and modified by VAN OUDENAREN et al. (1981). This assay is based on binding of the Fc portion of rabbit anti-Ig to *Staphylococcus aureus* protein A that has been coupled to target SRBC. Secretion of Ig by murine Ig-producing cells leads to the formation of immune complexes consisting of mouse Ig and rabbit Ab. These complexes, bound to the protein A-coated SRBC, activate complement, which leads to lysis of the target SRBC and thus to "plaque" formation. This assay detects all cells secreting Ig that are recognized by the rabbit antiserum used. So using only one type of indicator red cells and various class- or subclass-specific Ab of rabbit origin, Ig-secreting cells of various isotypes can be enumerated, regardless of the specificity of the secreted Ab.

In most strains of *S. aureus*, protein A is covalently linked to the cell wall (LÖFKVIST and SJÖQUIST 1963). This protein A binds Ig molecules with high affinity. The principal Ig class bound is IgG, although in many cases binding is restricted to certain IgG subclasses. In some species, IgM and IgA can also bind to protein A (GODING 1978). Protein A has proven to be useful for the study of Ag and receptors on the surface of intact cells, and for the detection of Ig-secreting cells. Thus, the use of protein A is now the method of choice for many preparative and analytic techniques in immunology.

For the plaque assay, *S. aureus* protein A (Pharmacia, Uppsala) is coupled to SRBC with $CrCl_3 \cdot 6H_2O$. For coupling, 1 ml protein A solution (1 mg dissolved in 1 ml 0.9% NaCl), 1 ml washed packed SRBC, 9 ml 0.9% NaCl, and 50 μl aged (over 1-year-old) solution of $CrCl_3 \cdot 6H_2O$ (0.05 M in saline) are mixed and incubated for 1.5 h at 37 °C, with shaking every 15 min. Thereafter, the cells are washed three times with 0.9% NaCl, and finally resuspended in BSS. The protein A-coated SRBC can be used in the plaque assay for at least 3 days, provided they are stored at 4 °C. Alternatively, protein A as well as other proteins can be coupled to target cells within 4 min, as described in Sect. C.II.3.b.

The protein A plaque assay is performed in BSS, using Cunningham-type chambers as described by LEFKOVITS and COSENZA (1979). These incubation chambers are prepared by placing three strips of narrow double sided adhesive tape on a microscope slide (75×25 mm), dividing it into two areas of roughly equal surface. A second slide is pressed onto the first so that the two slides are face to face and separated only by the thin strips of tape. The total volume of the two chambers is 180–200 μl.

Each sample to be tested consists of 100 μl of an appropriately diluted cell suspension, mixed with 15 μl of an optimal amount of diluted guinea pig complement purified over a Sepharose-protein A column in order to remove the IgG fraction (VAN OUDENAREN et al. 1981), 15 μl of appropriately diluted specific rabbit anti-mouse IgM, IgG, IgA, or IgE antiserum and 15 μl 17% (v/v) suspension of protein A-coated SRBC. The rabbit antiserum used is purified over a Sepharose-protein A column as described by GODING (1978) in order to isolate the protein A-binding fraction of Ig.

Each sample is mixed and distributed over both chambers of a set of slides. The chambers are sealed by carefully dipping the slide edges into a melted mixture of equal portions of paraffin (Paramat, Gurr Ltd., High Wycombe) and wax

(ACF Chemifarma NV, Maarssen). Subsequently, the chambers are placed on a tray and incubated at 37 °C for 4–5 h. the Ig-secreting PFC are counted under a dissecting microscope with dark-field illumination. Careful handling of the chambers avoids distortion of the plaque morphology. Since its introduction, the protein A plaque assay has been succesfully employed for the detection of Ig-secreting cells of a variety of species, including humans (HAMMERSTRÖM et al. 1979; SMITH et al. 1979; HAMMERSTRÖM et al. 1980).

2. Reverse Plaque Assay

The presence of contaminating Ig molecules in the guinea pig complement used for protein A, as well as reverse plaque assays, reduces the number of plaques and their size by competitive inhibition of the binding of the specific rabbit anti-Ig molecules via the protein A to the target SRBC. For the protein A plaque assay, this problem can be overcome by affinity chromatography of the guinea pig complement on a protein A-Sepharose column (VAN OUDENAREN et al. 1981).

In the reverse plaque assay, developed by MOLINARO and DRAY (1974), SRBC are directly coated with Ab by the chromium chloride coupling method (see Sect. C.II.4.a). This assay is based on diffusion of the Ig (e.g., mouse Ig) from the Ig-secreting cells into an agar gel containing SRBC coated with rabbit anti-mouse Ig. Localized hemolysis occurs around the cells on addition of a rabbit anti-mouse Ig developing antiserum and complement. The method, essentially a modification of Mancini's single radial immunodiffussion assay, has the same incubation time of 48 h, but a greater sensitivity (0.1 µg/ml compared with 100 µg/ml). Ig-secreting cells form hemolytic plaques independent of the Ab specificity of the secreted Ig. This assay can therefore be applied to enumerate subpopulations of Ig-secreting cells on the basis of the isotype, allotype, or idiotype they secrete (MOLINARO et al. 1978).

The protein A plaque assay, however, is more economical since it requires a smaller amount of rabbit Ig-specific Abs. Moreover, affinity purification of the developing Ig-specific Ab, required in the reverse plaque assay, is not necessary in the protein A assay. Furthermore, the same batch of protein A-coated SRBC can be used to enumerate Ig-secreting cells in cell suspensions obtained from different species.

3. Antigen-Specific Plaque Assays

The PFC assay can be adapted to the detection of cells forming Abs to Ag, such as proteins, polypeptides, polysaccharides, and a variety of haptens. The only requirement is that the red cells be coated to exhibit an adequate density of Ag determinants without causing excessive fragility of the red cells or altering their susceptibility to lysis by complement.

Two general approaches to coupling determinants to red cells are used: the chemical approach, where the Ag or haptens are directly coupled to the red cells, or the immunologic approach, where proteins or haptens are conjugated to erythrocyte-specific Abs which then attach to red cells by virtue of their Ab activity. This is most effectively accomplished by using monovalent Fab fragments of erythrocyte-specific Abs. Such conjugates, which should not by themselves lyse in the presence of complement, have been described (STRAUSBAUCH et al. 1970; MILLER and WARNER 1971).

In the direct plaque assay, the only Abs detected are of the IgM class, since IgG, IgA, and IgE Abs are not efficient enough in complement binding to mediate cell lysis under these experimental conditions. To detect antibodies of the non-IgM isotype, the so-called indirect plaque assay has to be applied. In the latter assay, an IgG-, IgA- or IgE-specific rabbit antiserum is added, which will bind to Ab of the relevant Ig class produced by the cell suspension and bound to the indicator erythrocyte. The class-specific Abs cross-link the coating Abs and generate conditions for efficient complement binding and hence for cell lysis. Since direct plaques will also develop, it is essential to note that the number of such "facilitated" or "indirect" plaques can, in principle, be determined by subtracting from the number of plaques developed with the antiserum the number of plaques obtained in its absence. In the following section, an example of a protein-Ag-specific as well as a number of hapten-specific plaque assays will be given.

a) Coupling of Haptens to Target Cells for Use in Plaque Assays

Haptenic groups may be linked directly to the erythrocyte surface, or be attached as a hapten-protein conjugate which is especially useful to space out the haptenic group or when the coupling conditions are damaging to the red cell membrane.

The widely used nitrophenyl derivatives 2,4-dinitrophenyl (DNP) and 2,4,6-trinitrophenyl (TNP) are completely cross-reactive. Preferably, TNP is coupled to SRBC by using water-soluble trinitrobenzenesulfonic acid (TNBS) as the active form, essentially as described by RITTENBERG and PRATT (1969). Briefly, 30 mg TNBS (Eastman Kodak Co., Rochester) is dissolved in 4 ml sodium cacodylate buffer (0.28 M, pH 6.9) (BDH Chemicals Ltd., Poole). Together with 1 ml washed, packed SRBC, the mixture is wrapped in foil and incubated for 10 min at room temperature on a rotor. Subsequently, the cells are washed twice in glycylglycine (0.05 M in BSS) and then twice in BSS. Cells are resuspended to 17% (v/v) in BSS. When 3 mg TNBS is used for coupling to 1 ml SRBC, cells are referred to as TNP_3-SRBC instead of TNP_{30}-SRBC in the protocol described.

Other nitrophenyl derivatives such as 4-hydroxy-5-iodo-3- nitrophenyl (NIP) or 4-hydroxy-3,5-dinitrophenyl (NNP) are coupled to SRBC by adding, e.g., 0.4 or 4 mg and 0.2 or 2 mg of the hapten succinimide active esters (Biosearch, San Rafael) per milliliter washed, packed SRBC. The coated cells are referred to as $NIP_{0.4}$-SRBC, NIP_4-SRBC, $NNP_{0.2}$-SRBC, and NNP_2-SRBC, respectively. This mild coupling procedure is essentially as described by POHLIT et al. (1979): SRBC (1 ml) are resuspended in 10 ml carbonate-bicarbonate buffer (0.12 M, pH 9.2). Addition of the esters is as follows: for NNP_2-SRBC, 50 µl 40 mg/ml solution is used, for $NNP_{0.2}$-SRBC 50 µl 4 mg/ml solution, while for NIP_4 100 µl 40 mg/ml, and for $NIP_{0.4}$ 100 µl 4 mg/ml solution is used. These ester solutions are added dropwise to the mixture.

The coupling mixture is wrapped in foil and incubated for 40 min at room temperature on a rotor. Cells are then washed in saline and BSS (twice), and finally resuspended in BSS and adjusted to a 17% solution (HOOIJKAAS et al. 1983; HOOIJKAAS et al. 1985).

b) Coupling of Proteins to Target Cells for Use in Plaque Assays

For the coupling of large protein Ags to target cells for use in complement-dependent lysis, it is essential that indicator cells of optimal sensitivity are produced. The simplest procedure for coating red cells with proteins such as ovalbumin and chicken γ-globulin (KOCH and BENNER 1982), is the one that makes use of $CrCl_3$ as coupling agent, according to the method described by GOLD and FUDENBERG (1967). We recently described a rapid procedure in which different proteins such as protein A or ovalbumin can be coupled to SRBC within 4 min (SAVELKOUL et al. 1988). This procedure is also based on $CrCl_3$ as the coupling agent, but it can essentially be prepared fresh in order to give more reproducible coupling ratios compared with the aged solutions that are routinely used (PERUCCA et al. 1969; SWEET and WELBORN 1971; KOFLER and WICK 1977; LING et al. 1977; TRUFFA-BACHI and BORDENAVE 1980). SRBC are washed four times (5 min, 1500 g) in 10 volumes freshly prepared $CrCl_3$ in saline (12.5 µg/ml). For coupling, 1 ml washed, packed SRBC, 1 ml protein A or ovalbumin in saline (1 mg/ml), and 1 ml $CrCl_3$ in saline (1 mg/ml) are mixed and incubated for 4 min at room temperature. Subsequently, 20 volumes 1% fetal calf serum (FCS) in saline is added, and the cells are washed in this solution three times for 5 min at 600 g. Finally, the cells are resuspended in BSS and used within 3 days of preparation.

4. Practical Aspects of Plaque-Forming Cell Assays

a) $CrCl_3$ Technique

The simplest procedure for coating red cells with proteins such as protein A (Sect. C.II.1 and C.II.3.b) and ovalbumin (Sect. C.II.3.b), and the one requiring the least protein, is the use of chromium chloride ($CrCl_3$), according to the method described by GOLD and FUDENBERG (1967). The coupling conditions that produce indicator cells of optimal sensitivity must be found empirically (BURNS and PIKE 1981). Relevant points to consider are: an optimal protein concentration should be between 0.25 and 2.5 mg/ml, and phosphate ions, which terminate the reaction, should be excluded from the mixture until coupling has been completed. For a given number of SRBC, the volume of $CrCl_3$ solution may vary, but the final concentration of $CrCl_3$ per cell must be kept constant. The same holds true for the desired protein to be coupled.

   For unknown reasons, aged solutions of $CrCl_3$ usually have to be used for the coupling reaction. In our alternative method we use a freshly prepared $CrCl_3$ solution for reproducible coupling. Moreover, by prewashing the cells in a low concentration of $CrCl_3$, the coupling time can be decreased to 4 min. Stopping the reaction by washing with a 1% FCS solution prevents clumping of the cells, which is a well-known problem with the $CrCl_3$ coupling method.

   Most important, optimal conditions for sensitization of red cells, i.e., optimal for hemagglutination and reverse plaque assays, are inadequate for plaque assays. Such cells have a low density of determinants so that the rate of attachment of the secreted Ab to red cells is too low to cause a plaque. Dependence on a high degree of coupling varies with the stage of the immune response (the affinity of the Ab), and the Ig class of the PFC. Other protein coupling procedures, e.g., with carbodiimide, benzidine, and benzoquinone will not be discussed here (for details see TERNYNCK and AVRAMEAS 1976; DRESSER 1978).

b) Inhibition Techniques

Inhibition of plaque formation by free Ag or hapten confirms the specificity of the plaques. The avidity of the Ab produced by the PFC can be analyzed by measuring this inhibition: high avidity Ab plaque formation is inhibited by lower concentrations of free Ag or hapten than are necessary for inhibition of plaque formation by low avidity Ab (JERNE et al. 1974; FAZEKAS DE ST GROTH 1979).

c) Optimization of Plaque Formation

Optimal hemolytic plaque formation requires carefully controlled reagents and conditions. A batch of SRBC should be selected on the basis of a low autohemolytic activity. Most batches of guinea pig complement are most effective at a $1:20$ final dilution of fresh serum or a $1:10$ dilution after passage of the guinea pig complement through a protein A-Sepharose column.

SRBC in Alsever's solution should be aged for 1–3 weeks, since fresh cells are less susceptible to lysis while older cells are excessively fragile. The optimal final red cell concentration is 2%, thus 17 μl 17% (v/v) suspension of Ag or protein A-coated SRBC per 147 μl incubation mixture.

Prolonged incubation times (up to 4–5 h) do not affect plaque morphology and numbers, provided the guinea pig complement and developing rabbit antiserum have been carefully absorbed with the target red blood cells in order to remove Abs that can lyse the whole monolayer of target red blood cells. After incubation at 37 °C and 40 °C, approximately the same number of plaques are found, while lower temperatures cause a reduction in plaque numbers.

d) Assessment of Plaques

True plaques must fulfill the following criteria:

1. Microscopic examination must reveal the Ab-releasing cell in the center of a plaque and not tissue fragments that cause false plaques.
2. Toward the periphery of a plaque, a diluting effect of lysed SRBC should be visible, since the concentration of Ab becomes too low to cause lysis.
3. Plaques should be round and not sharp-edged like air bubbles.
4. Plaques are never totally clear, that is, lysis of the red cell monolayer is never complete. Fully transparent, clean plaques in the monolayer are almost always the result of bacterial activity, since the plaque assays described are essentially performed under nonsterile conditions.

e) Counting of the PFC

It is essential, when the Cunningham liquid layer plaque assay is used, that the number of PFC are counted immediately after the incubation. The convenient range of PFC counted per slide is 30–150 PFC. Outside this range the counts are less reliable. Plaques can be counted under low magnification ($\times$ 20–40) under dark-field illumination with a dissecting microscope.

The frequency distribution of the number of plaques in each of a large number of slides containing PFC from a single population is not normal, but follows a Poisson distribution. This means that the estimate of variance is equal to the total number of plaques counted. The variance of the square root of the plaque count or its 2 SD range is ± 1. Thus, the 95% Poisson confidence range associated with a plaque count of 100 is from 9^2 (81) to 11^2 (121). In these circumstances, it is necessary to calculate the geometric means of the data. However, with a group of animals (involving some nonresponders), the arithmetic mean calculated for the whole group will give a closer approximation to the mean response of responders than the geometric mean (JERNE et al. 1974).

The plaque counts are expressed either as PFC per whole organ or as PFC per 10^6 viable nucleated cells. This can easily be done for spleen and lymph nodes, with a sample from a cell suspension made from the whole organ. But for the total BM, this is not feasible. Since the BM from femurs can easily be isolated, a conversion factor has been determined: the PFC response of the total BM can be calculated to be 7.94 times the response by the BM from two femurs (BENNER et al. 1981). If the samples are taken from cultures, then the number of PFC may be expressed per culture, per 10^6 input cells, or per 10^6 recovered viable cells.

f) Plaque Size

The size of the plaques depends on both the quality and quantity of Abs released: cells secreting high-affinity Ab will produce smaller plaques than low affinity Ab, given the same number of Ab molecules secreted per unit time. The smallest recognizable plaque is about 0.1 mm, corresponding to the angular resolution of the human eye.

Another important factor is the epitope density of the Ag determinants on the indicator red cells: higher epitope density leads to smaller plaques for a given number of Ab molecules. Also, the production rate of the Ab-secreting cell (the number of Ab molecules secreted per cell per unit time) determines the size of the plaque. This might be related to the isotype of the secreted Ab, since large plaques are usually found when tested for IgM-secreting cells, medium sized plaques for IgG-secreting cells, and small plaques for IgE-secreting cells.

5. Solid Phase Enzyme-Linked Immunospot Assay

Hemolytic plaque assays have been used extensively for evaluating the kinetics of the humoral immune response and the regulatory mechanisms underlying proliferation and maturation of B lymphocytes to Ab-secreting cells. These assays have, as outlined in Sect. II.4, several inherent limitations when the assay is applied to soluble protein Ags.

Inconsistent results have generally been associated with difficulties in coupling enough Ag onto the target red cells, the instability of the Ag-coated target red cells, variable "lysability" of different batches of target red cells, uncertainty about the isotype involved in the formation of direct plaques, and the inability to quantitate the Ab molecules secreted. Methods have been described in which the Ag is adsorbed onto polystyrene or nitrocellulose surfaces (SEDGWICK and HOLT 1983; CZERKINSKY et al. 1983; MOORE and CALKINS 1983; HOLT et al. 1984; MÖLLER and BORREBAECK 1985; HOLT and PLOZZA 1986). Application of Ab-secreting cells results in an immobilized Ag specific focus of the Ig produced. These foci are subsequently developed in an enzyme-linked immunosorbent assay (ELISA) by the addition of the appropriate enzyme-anti-Ig conjugate and an enzyme substrate in agarose which yields an insoluble product after incubation, resulting in clearly visible spots of different size and intensity. Apart from Ag-specific Ig, isotype-specific Ig can also be determined in this ELISPOT assay by means of protein A-coated surfaces.

The procedure we use is essentially according to SEDGWICK and HOLT (1983) with some modifications. Proteins (e.g., ovalbumin) are coated at a concentration of 2 µg/ml in 10 mM phosphate-buffered saline (PBS) pH 7.2, in 100 µl per well of polyvinylchloride microtiter plates (Titertek, Flow, Irvine) for 1 h at 37 °C. Plates are then washed three times with PBS and subsequently the remaining active binding sites are blocked with PBS containing 1% bovine serum albumin (BSA) (Boseral, Organon Teknika, Oss). The wells are washed once with PBS-BSA containing 0.05% Tween-20 (Merck-Schuchard, Munich). After drying, the wells are slowly filled with the cell suspensions, washed twice with PBS, and diluted in PBS-BSA or BSS-BSA. The most suitable cell densities must be determined critically, by testing many different inputs, e.g., 10^6–10^3 cells/ml. These cell suspensions are incubated on a stable surface for 2 h at 37 °C. Incubation times can be prolonged up to 16 h at 4 °C by working under sterile conditions. Cells are then resuspended in culture medium containing BSA, and plates are incubated in a 5% CO_2 atmosphere. Cells are discarded by flicking the plate and washing once with 0.05% Tween-20 in distilled water to lyse the remaining cells. Subsequently, the plates are washed thoroughly with PBS-BSA-Tween for 2 h at 37 °C before applying a suitable conjugate. Conjugates can be prepared according to KEARNEY et al. (1979), by coupling the enzyme alkaline phosphatase to specific affinity purified Abs.

The plates are washed three times in PBS-BSA-Tween and dried before the substrate is added. The substrate buffer is prepared as follows: 150 mg $MgCl_2 \cdot 6H_2O$, 0.1 ml Triton X-405 (Sigma, St. Louis), and 1.0 g sodium azide are dissolved in a small volume of distilled water and 95.8 ml 0.1 M 2-amino- 2-methyl-1-propanol buffer is added with stirring. Distilled water is added to about 90% of the final volume, and the pH adjusted to 10.25 with concentrated HCl. The solution is left overnight at 20 °C and the pH readjusted. Distilled water is then added to bring the volume to 1.0 l and the buffer stored at 4 °C. A 2.3 mM solution of the substrate 5-bromo-4-chloro-3-indolyl phosphate (5-BCIP, Sigma, St. Louis) is prepared in stirred 0.1 M 2-amino-2- methyl-1-propanol buffer in a light-protected bottle, and the substrate is filtered through a 0.45-µm filter about 1 h after preparation to sterilize the solution and to remove any insoluble material. The solution should then be stored at 4 °C in the dark.

For use in the assay, the substrate is mixed with agarose. A 3% (w/v) solution of agarose (type I, Sigma, St. Louis) is prepared in distilled water, divided into 3-ml aliquots, and stored at 4 °C. On the day of assay, one aliquot is heated and, when the agarose is liquefied, it is cooled to 40 °C. Subsequently, a mixture of 12 ml substrate (prewarmed to 40 °C) and 3 ml agarose is prepared, and 100 µl of this is immediately added to each well of the plate, and placed on a level surface. After 5 min, when the mixture has solidified, the plates are covered and incubated at 37 °C until blue dots, each representing an Ig-secreting cell, are clearly visible (30–60 min). Spots can be easily counted with a light microscope equipped with a × 17.5 magnifier (Bellco Glass Inc., Vineland).

Critical points to note in this procedure are:

1. Filtration of the substrate solution to avoid the occurrence of false spots above the agarose/solid phase interface;
2. Addition of a protein (such as BSA) in all washing and incubation steps to prevent a high number of small false spots;
3. Avoidance of cell movement during the incubation of the cell suspensions and movement of the agarose during spot development, which could result in diffuse spots;
4. The likelihood of a lack of sufficient isotype specificity of the conjugated antiserum, especially with many of the commercially available conjugates.

6. Immunofluorescence Assays

Cells producing Ig are morphologically characterized by an increased amount of basophilic cytoplasm. Their morphology can range from lymphoblast to plasma cell. Many of these cells can be enumerated by means of immunofluorescence with heterologous Abs specific for the Ig produced (HIJMANS et al. 1969; HIJMANS and SCHUIT 1972). The availability of fluorescent reagents of high activity and specificity is a crucial requirement for reliable results. In practice, the choice is mainly between fluorescein isothiocyanate (FITC) and tetramethylrhodamine isothiocyanate (TRITC). Although many conjugates are commercially available, they can be prepared easily as described by BERGGUIST and NILSSON (1974) and GODING (1976). It has been found in cell suspensions of murine lymphoid organs that enumerations of the Ig-producing cells by immunofluorescence and by the protein A plaque assay do not always give similar results (VAN OUDENAREN et al. 1984). The protein A plaque assay was found to detect as many or several times more Ig-producing cells than the immunofluorescence assay, depending on the age and antigenic load of the mice, and on the Ig class and organ studied. To detect intracytoplasmic Ig-containing (c-Ig) cells, the cells have to be fixed with reagents that allow the fluorescent antibody to enter them.

Therefore, cell suspensions of peripheral blood nucleated cells, or of lymphoid organs, are prepared, washed, resuspended, and diluted to $0.5–2 \times 10^6$/ml in PBS containing 1% BSA (Organon Teknika, Oss) at pH 7.8. Subsequently, cytocentrifuged (Nordic, Tilburg) preparations are made by spinning down (5 min, 1000 rpm) 50 μl of the cell suspensions to be tested on slides precoated with 100 μl PBS-BSA. After air-drying for 15 min, the location of the cells is marked by encircling them with a glass pencil. The slides are then fixed in ethanol containing 5% acetic acid for 15 min at $-20\ °C$, washed for 30 min in PBS while stirring, and dried by wiping with a fine paper tissue, avoiding the cell spot. Because the cells are spun in a monolayer of diameter about 5–7 mm, they can be easily stained with a small volume (15–20 μl) FITC- or TRITC-conjugated antiserum. This is done for 30 min at room temperature in a humidified chamber. The conjugates are diluted in PBS-BSA containing 10–20 mM sodium azide to prevent bacterial growth. Excess conjugate is removed by flicking the slides and washing for 15 min in PBS. The slides are then dried and mounted in glycerol/PBS (9 : 1) containing phenylenediamine 1 mg/ml (stored at $-20\ °C$) to prevent fading of the fluorochrome. A coverslip is sealed to the slide with paraffin wax. For evaluation of immunofluorescence staining, fluorescence microscopes have to be used, preferably equipped with phase contrast and an epi-illumination system (HIJMANS et al. 1981). The Ig class distribution of the c-Ig cells can be determined by means of combinations of TRITC- and FITC-labeled antisera specific for the heavy chains of IgM, IgG, IgA, IgD, and IgE. It is also possible to perform indirect staining in that the cells are first exposed to the relevant antiserum at the appropriate dilution and then, after washing, to a fluorescent antiserum to detect the first Ab as an Ag.

Fluorescent labeled Abs are widely used for the detection of membrane-bound glycoproteins. However, such membrane labeling can well be combined with detection of c-Ig. For the detection of membrane-bound Ig or other membrane glycoproteins, cell suspensions need not be fixed. They are carefully washed (5 min at 100 g at 4 °C) three times with PBS-BSA to remove serum proteins or proteins secreted by the cells themselves. The pellet is resuspended and adjusted to a cell density of $1–2 \times 10^7$ cells/ml. From this suspension, 50 µl is mixed with an equal volume of the appropriate conjugated antiserum and incubated for 30 min in melting ice. Then 2 ml ice- cold PBS-BSA is added and cells are washed twice with cold PBS-BSA. Then, the cells are cytocentrifuged (direct staining) or stained once more with one or two other Abs conjugated to other fluorochromes, before preparing slides (double or triple staining). To block remaining active sites of the heterologous antiserum, cells are incubated with normal serum of the species in which the antiserum was induced.

By such techniques much has been learned about the differentiation and maturation pathway (or pathways) of B cells both in mice and humans, depending on their membrane-bound as well as intracytoplasmic markers. Since many, if not all, differentiation stages of normal human B cell development seem to be paralleled by leukemic disorders, these techniques are extremely valuable in the detection of malignant cells (VAN DONGEN et al. 1984, 1985).

D. Measurement of Circulating Immunoglobulins

As outlined in the Sect. A.II, Ab can be used as detecting reagents for a variety of molecules (e.g., Ig) by virtue of their molecular recognition properties. A vast literature exists on different techniques developed to detect Ig in a qualitative, semiquantitative, or quantitative way. Such assays are based on different molecular properties of Ab, Ag or Ab-Ag complexes. As will be discussed later, in this respect it is important to note that different Ig isotypes, because of differences in protein (antigenic) structure, can behave differently in the various assays, resulting in false conclusions. In all of these assays, detection and, if possible, quantitation is based on detecting (anti-isotypic) Abs and the specificity, affinity, and titer of these Abs determines the reliability of the assay. The formation of Ag-Ab complexes on which all known assays are based, determines the conditions under which the assays should be performed. Most Ab-Ag complex formation occurs optimally at a pH of 6.5–7.0, although the reaction is not greatly affected between pH 5.5 and 5.8. Monoclonal Ab, however, can show drastic changes in specificity with altering pH. The rate of association can be increased by lowering the ionic strength of the buffer, especially when dealing with Ab of relatively low affinity ($K_a < 10^5 \ M^{-1}$). In many reactions, the affinity of Ab specific for a certain Ag is increased by incubation at lower temperature (4 °C instead of room temperature or 37 °C). Changes in reaction temperature do influence the reaction speed, but only minor changes occur in the affinity constant. The stability of the Ag-Ab complex under both in vivo and in vitro conditions depends largely on noncovalent interactions, mainly hydrophobic forces and hydrogen bonds and, to a lesser extent, on electrostatic interactions. These hydrophobic forces contribute to the overall shape of a protein molecule in an aqueous system when the hydrocarbon-like parts of the protein chain are close together and the polar parts of the chain are in contact with the solvent.

The specificity of an Ab is dependent on the degree of cross-reactivity with closely related antigenic determinants. Such interactions mostly occur with a lower affinity. The following sections describe a number of assays that are routinely performed in our laboratory.

I. Precipitation-Based Assays

When an optimal concentration of Ag with multiple antigenic determinants is present in a solution together with Ab, a large three-dimensional network is formed that precipitates out of solution. Protein Ag with molecular weights of 40–60 kdalton only precipitate under narrow optimal concentrations (equivalence zone of the so-called Heidelberger-Kendall curve). Polysaccharides, viruses, and denatured or very large proteins result in very broad curves. This reaction is especially sensitive to changes in pH, ionic strength, or temperature. The affinity of the Ab used determines the rate at which the precipitate is formed. It can be envisaged that Abs of the IgM class have a greater ability to form complexes than Abs of the IgG or IgA classes.

Detection of the developed precipitate is based on the visibility of the sediment. The sensitivity of detection can be increased by allowing the Ag and the Ab to diffuse into an agar gel. At the point where Ag and Ab meet in an equivalent concentration ratio, they will form an insoluble precipitate. Since the excess of Ag or Ab will remain soluble outside the equivalence zone and can be washed out of the gel, the remaining precipitate can be stained by a regular protein staining method (e.g., Coomassie Brilliant Blue, silver staining, etc.). In the original double-immunodiffusion technique (according to Ouchterlony) it is very difficult to asses the concentration of an Ag because of the need to keep both the reagent concentrations within the equivalence zone. The same holds true for two quantitative modifications: single radial immunodiffusion (SRID; MANCINI et al. 1965) and the rocket electroimmunoassay (LAURELL 1966). In SRID a known amount of Ab is mixed in the gel, restricting the amount of the unknown Ag that can be determined after concentric diffusion has resulted in circular precipitate formation. The diameter of such a precipitation circle is proportional to the Ag concentration. In the rocket electrophoresis technique, an Ag is moved (by a unidirectional electric field) into an Ab-containing agarose gel. When precipitation occurs, a stationary precipitate is formed which has the appearance of a rocket. Its length is related to the Ag concentration.

The accuracy of quantitation of Ig levels is highly dependent on the quality of the reference standard that is tested in parallel, and from which the absolute values are derived. For quantitation of murine Ig, we employed SRID as well as rocket electrophoresis while the quantitation is based on a secondary standard consisting of normal mouse serum, which is generally more reliable than a primary standard of a myeloma protein (MINK and BENNER 1979; MINK et al. 1980). To determine the absolute Ig concentration in human sera SRID is also commonly used (DE BRUYN et al. 1982; KORNMAN-VAN DEN BOSCH et al. 1984).

Another branch of precipitation-based techniques consists of immunoelectrophoresis (IEP) and immunofixation. In IEP, mixtures of Ag are separated in a unidirectional electric field in an agar gel. Subsequently, slots are cut out of the agar next to the sample wells and filled with an isotype-specific antiserum. Diffusion of the Ab is allowed and at the optimal Ag:Ab ratio a precipitation bow is formed. Any serum proteins can be identified in this way, provided the specific Ab is available. The technique is primarily qualitative, but is extremely valuable in the detection of monoclonal gammopathies, both in mice and humans (RADL et al. 1980; RADL 1981). Immunofixation is a more sensitive modification of IEP, employing the same Ag separation in a electric field, but the separated Ag are detected by overlaying the gel with an Ab-impregnated strip of cellulose acetate or filter paper. This technique is used for sera of experimental animals as well as for sera and cerebrospinal fluid samples from patients suffering from gammopathies or multiple sclerosis (CEJKA and KITHIER 1976; RADL 1981).

II. Agglutination-Based Assays

Agglutination occurs when Abs react with Ag determinants, either on native antigens or artificially attached to molecules, cells, or particles. Apart from these direct agglutination reactions by Ab directed against Ag determinants on the surface of red blood cells (so-called hemagglutination reactions), bacteria, and molds, indirect agglutination reactions also occur when Ab is directed against soluble Ag passively adsorbed or chemically coupled to the surface of red blood cells or inert particles such as latex, carbon, bentonite, collodion, or Sepharose beads to which a second (detecting) Ab is added as a developing reagent. It is obvious that in these assays IgM Ab are also more effective than IgG or IgA Ab. Sometimes, the agglutinating capacity of Ab can be improved by adding heterologous Ab specific for the light chain or Fc part of the heavy chain of the agglutinating Ab.

Another kind of agglutination-like assay for detecting Ig secretion is the rosette-forming cell assay. In this assay, isotype-specific Ab are coupled to erythrocytes, so that they form rosettes when incubated with Ab-secreting cells (HAEGERT 1981).

All the techniques described so far are semiquantitative in that the detection of formation of an Ag-Ab precipitate in solution or gel, or an Ag-Ab agglutinate, are limited to the smallest visible complexes. Therefore, much effort has been directed toward improving the detection of such complexes in solution, based on Rayleigh light scattering. For the absolute quantitative determination of Ab in human sera, techniques such as nephelometry and turbidimetry have thus been used (DE BRUYN et al. 1982).

III. Ligand-Binding Assays

Since the introduction of radioimmunoassay (RIA), a variety of immunoassays have been developed in which the detection of Ig is based on a labeled isotype-specific Ab ligand. Many different labels are available for this purpose: radioisotopes, enzymes, fluorescent dyes, stable free radicals, electron-dense components, etc. Here, we will deal with enzyme immunoassays (EIA). Moreover, we will focus on heterogeneous assays in which the bound and the free fraction of the ligand are physically separated by a washing procedure, and in which the Ag (Ig) to be determined is, either directly or indirectly, physically attached to a solid phase (e.g., the well of a microtiter plate or Terasaki tray). Therefore, such assays are called enzyme-linked immunosorbent assays (ELISA).

For the detection of the antigen-specific fraction or the total amount of a particular Ig isotype in serum we apply a two-site system. In both cases, the Ig to be determined is sandwiched between the known Ag or an anti-isotypic catching Ab adsorbed to a solid phase and an enzyme-labeled second Ab, respectively. Both the catching and the detecting Ab are heterologous compared with the Ig to be determined. After adsorbing the Ag or catching Ab to the solid phase, all subsequent incubations are done until equilibrium has been reached and competition can no longer occur between the labeled and unlabeled ligand involved. Moreover, all other reagents, except the sample, are in slight excess, so that the amount of Ig present in the sample, is the only limiting factor. In this way, the signal is directly related to the amount of Ig bound. Other EIAs, whether competitive, homologous, one-site, homogeneous, or nonequilibrium, will not be discussed here. The reader is refered to the available review articles (SCHUURS and VAN WEEMEN 1977; WISDOM 1976) and books (VOLLER et al. 1981; AVRAMEAS 1983; BIZOLLON 1984). Especially for use in sandwich ELISA the quality of the antisera is extremely important in determining the specificity and the sensitivity of the assay (SHIELDS and TURNER 1986). Some relevant points to consider before performing ELISA will be described, after which essential parameters such as sensitivity, detection limit, and accuracy will be discussed.

1. Assay Setup

The majority of ELISA techniques are performed in microtiter plates because a lot of equipment facilitating easy and automatic handling is commercially available. In a moderately sensitive ELISA system, a serum sample of 100 µl is enough to determine the concentration of IgM or IgG Ab (STOKES et al. 1982; OHLSON and ZETTERSTREND 1985; SCOTT et al. 1985; JENUM 1985). This holds for mice as well as humans. Simultaneous detection of a number of Ig classes, especially rare ones such as IgD, IgE, autoantibodies, or idiotype-specific Abs, however, does require a fair amount of serum. In a number of instances, e.g., during longitudinal studies of sera from mice or children, it is often difficult to acquire enough serum to perform the various assays. Moreover, during the production of monoclonal Ab, investigators want to test for Ig production by the hybrid cells as soon as possible following fusion, thus only very small amounts of medium are available for assay. The amount of reagents required for such micro-ELISAs is also fairly large. These problems led to our decision to perform ELISA in 60-well Terasaki trays with 5-µl samples per well.

2. Coating of Solid Phases

In microtiter systems, different solid phases can be used to ensure protein adsorption in sufficiently high amounts, including polystyrene, polyvinyl chloride, polypropylene, polycarbonate, nitrocellulose, silicones, etc. For the Terasaki system only, clear polystyrene plates are available and these can be coated easily and reproducibly. Most proteins are adsorbed on plastic surfaces, probably owing to hydrophobic interactions between the nonpolar plastic matrix and protein molecules which have a net charge of zero. The rate and the extent of coating depends on the diffusion coefficient of the adsorbing molecule, the ratio of the surface area to be coated to the volume of the coating solution, the concentration of the adsorbing substances, as well as the temperature and the duration of the adsorption process. With regard to the last two items 3 h at 37 °C or overnight at 4 °C is generally found to be suitable. Moreover, to ensure sufficient saturation of the solid phase, the sample for coating is dissolved, preferably in a high ionic strength buffer (0.1 M sodium carbonate buffer) at a high pH (9.6) (ENGVALL and PERL-MANN 1972). coating is also improved by preincubation of the desired protein at elevated temperature (10 min, 70 °C) to aggregate the protein (PARISH and HIGGINS 1982). During coating, microtiter plates show a distinct "edge effect." Wells at the edges of a plate adsorb more protein than those in the interior (KRICKA et al. 1980).

There is evidence that, during the setup and performance of the assay, 30%–40% of the adsorbed protein is released from the solid phase, depending on the total amount adsorbed (METZGER et al. 1981). This is a prozone phenomenon known as the "hook effect" (PESCE et al. 1983; KLASEN and RIGUTTI 1983). Such an effect can greatly influence the sensitivity and precision of a one-site ELISA, but does not affect sandwich ELISA systems (SCHUURS and VAN WEEMEN 1977).

We have also tried to coat plates by allowing them to dry completely (1 h at 37 °C, or 15 min with a fan) so as to ensure a 100% coating of protein. We anticipate that, under these conditions, a higher degree of protein denaturation will also occur so that the overall sensitivity of the assay is not improved (H. F. SAVEL-KOUL and S. S. PATHAK 1986, unpublished work). Since the reproducibility of the assay depends heavily on the quality of the coating reaction, we use a two-site system with, preferably, a standard coat of a heterologous monoclonal catching Ab specific for the isotype of the Ig molecule to be assayed.

To detect polyclonal Ab (serum) or monoclonal Ab (hybridoma supernatant) against cell surface antigenic determinants, monolayers of cells are coated to the solid phase with a very low concentration of glutaraldehyde (0.02% for 15 min at room temperature; STOCKER and HEUSSER 1979; LANSDORP et al. 1980; VAN SOEST et al. 1984). Such a low concentration of glutaraldehyde does not alter the conformation of antigenic determinants at the cell surface (VAN EWIJK et al. 1984).

When testing the occurrence of Ab directed against small Ag, it is advisable to precoat the plates with a polylysine spacer, while in the case of haptens hapten-carrier conjugates are preferably used for coating. The conformation of Ag determinants, however, can be altered more by such procedures than by the coating process itself.

Coated plates can be stored either wet in PBS with 1–2 mM sodium azide at 4 °C or dry in a dessicator for periods of up to 4 weeks. After the coating has been completed, trays have to be washed and all the remaining binding sites saturated with an unrelated protein (1% w/v BSA or 0.02% w/v gelatin in 1 M Na$_2$CO$_3$ buffer or PBS) and incubated for 0.5–1 h at 37 °C. Husby et al. (1983) have suggested the use of 0.1% v/v human serum albumin preincubated at 56°C for 30 min to reduce nonspecific binding. In all the subsequent washing and incubation steps, this protein is present along with a small amount (0.05% v/v) of Tween-20, a nonionic detergent, to prevent nonspecific adsorption (Schønheyder and Anderson 1984).

3. Choice and Preparation of Ligand

The sensitivity of ELISA systems depends heavily on the quality and the specificity of the detecting Ab. For use in ELISA, the heterologous Ab that are generally employed are purified out of hyperimmune sera. After immunization of the animal with the purified Ag or Ig, there is an increase in Ab quality and affinity. We shall discuss this in greater detail in Sect. D.III.5.

In addition, the specific activity and the turnover number (or molecular activity) of the enzyme to be applied for conjugating the detecting Ab play a major role. We have decided to use the enzyme β-galactosidase from *Escherichia coli* (EC 3.2.1.23) for a number of reasons. First, the enzyme is available with high specific activity (400 units/mg), it has a high turnover number (12 500 substrate molecules transformed per molecule of enzyme per minute) and it is sufficiently large (540 kdalton) to be linked to Ab by a number of chemical methods with a good degree of retention of enzymatic and immunologic activity. Second, the conjugate is soluble and stable under the assay conditions, and can be stored for prolonged times. Finally, the enzyme itself is absent from the sample and so are alternative substrates, inhibitors, and other disturbing factors.

Several methods have been successfully used to link enzymes to Abs (for reviews see Kennedy et al. 1976; Schuurs and Van Weemen 1977; Avrameas et al. 1978; O'Sullivan and Marks 1981). The most popular cross-linking methods employ either succinimidyl-3-2-pyridyldithiopropionate (SPDP) and the one-step and two-step glutaraldehyde method, in which the homobifunctional aldehyde reacts with the amino residues in the protein to form a Schiff's base, or the periodate oxidation method, in which carbohydrate residues of the enzyme are oxidized to form aldehyde groups, or m-maleimidobenzoyl-N-hydroxysuccinimide ester (MBS), a heterobifunctional reagent coupling to sulfhydryl residues on the enzyme molecule.

We have employed the one-step glutaraldehyde method of Avrameas and Ternynck (1969). The Ab to be coupled is extensively dialyzed against 0.1 M potassium phosphate buffer, pH 7.8. Routinely, we couple 1 ml Ab solution containing 5–10 mg protein per milliliter. Of the enzyme β-galactosidase (specific activity 600 units/mg; Boehringer Mannheim GmbH, Mannheim) 2 mg is dissolved in 1 ml of the same buffer. The reaction mixture is prepared by mixing 1 ml enzyme (2 mg/ml) with 1 ml Ab (4 mg/ml) and 10 µl v/v glutaraldehyde solution (TAAB, Reading), stored in the dark at 4 °C. The reaction is allowed to occur for

30 min at room temperature on an end-over-end mixer. The reaction is then blocked by the addition 1 ml 1 M lysine (Sigma, St. Louis) in the same buffer and left overnight at 4 °C. Extensive dialysis against PBS is performed and, after addition of either 1% BSA or 0.02% gelatin or glycerol to a final concentration of 50% v/v, the conjugate is stored at 4 °C. With these additions, the conjugate is stable for a few months, while in the absence of these additives activity is lost within a few weeks.

Another way of performing an Ag-specific ELISA is by employing a conjugate of a biotinylated Ag and an avidin-labeled enzyme. The extremely high affinity constant of avidin-biotin binding ($K_a = 10^{15} M^{-1}$) ensures a high degree of enzyme bound specifically to the Ig in the sample (YOLKEN et al. 1983; BOORSMA 1983; ALEVY and BLYNN 1986).

In sandwich ELISA, enzyme-labeled protein A can also be used (ENGVALL 1978; SUROLIA and PAIN 1981; LANGONE 1982). This method can be useful when assaying Ig with no binding affinity for protein A, e.g., rat monoclonal Ab directed against mouse cell surface determinants (VAN SOEST et al. 1984) or Ag-specific and total mouse IgE (SAVELKOUL et al. 1985). Another advantage is the use of unlabeled isotype-specific detecting Ab having very high affinity for protein A (e.g., rabbit IgG class hyperimmune fractions). In this way various unlabeled isotype-specific antisera can be used as detecting Ab. Coupling of protein A β-galactosidase is performed with MBS according to the method described by DEELDER and DE WATER (1981).

4. Substrate Reaction and Product Detection

We use the substrate 4-methylumbelliferylgalactoside (Sigma, St. Louis) which generates a highly fluorescent ketone (umbelliferone) on cleavage by β-galactosidase. The setup of our assay system enables an automatic fluorescent measurement of the reaction end point. The performance characteristics of these ELISAs compares favorably with those of equivalent assay systems using colorigenic substrates such as o-nitrophenyl-β-galactopyranoside, in that the minimal detection limits are 10^{-9} and $10^{-5} M$, respectively.

The microfluorometric analysis of the individual wells of the Terasaki trays is performed as described by DE JOSSELIN DE JONG et al. (1980) and VAN SOEST et al. (1984). The readings are expressed in arbitrary fluorescence units (AFU). The substrate is dissolved at 0.25 mg/ml in 0.05 M potassium phosphate buffer, pH 7.8, with 10 mM MgCl$_2$ by heating to 60 °C. After dissolving the substrate the solution is cooled, aliquoted, and can then be stored at -20 °C for a few months. The solution is heated again to 60 °C to dissolve the substrate before use. It should be realized that all incubation steps are performed as binding reactions, so they are continued until equilibrium is reached. The substrate incubation time should always be kept constant (e.g., 60 min).

5. Quantitation in Immunoassays

Quantitation based on ELISA results is generally employed in three essential different ways. One procedure is based on interpolation on a standard calibration curve (VAN WEEMEN et al. 1978; MASSEYEFF 1978; HILL and LIU 1981; BORZINI et al. 1981; GIALLONGO et al. 1982; TSANG et al. 1983; BLECKA et al. 1983; HAMADA et al. 1983; SAVELKOUL et al. 1985). This procedure is often hampered by the lack of reproducibility of the standard curve, the limited number of standard points, and the uncertainty of the geometry of the curve at low concentration. We routinely prepare calibration graphs by assaying six replicates of eight standard dilutions. The second procedure is based on the Langmuir adsorption isotherm. This can be extended, for example, by Scatchard analysis of myeloma monoclonal Ab reactive against haptens (PORSTMANN et al. 1984; PESCE et al. 1978; JACOBSEN and STEENSGAARD 1984). When an oligoclonal antiserum is involved with a few Ab with different affinities for an Ag (MOYLE et al. 1983), an index of heterogeneity can be introduced leading to a Sips analysis (STEWARD and PETTY 1972; LEW 1984). Both these analyses of the binding curves allow the determination of affinity constants and estimation of the unknown Ig (Ag) concentration. This does not hold for real polyclonal Ab against multideterminant Ag (ROHOLT et al. 1972). In such situations, a third method of empirically derived equations is used. Starting from theories developed for RIA, a basic equation is used from which a number of empirical equations are derived (FERNANDEZ et al. 1983). Moreover, a number of equations have been formulated to describe the shape of the dilution curve in such an assay. Apart from a spline function, $Y = A + B/x + C/x^2$, an empirial polynomial equation has been used (GORDON et al. 1985).

Especially noteworthy is the four-parameter log-logit plot which is very useful for microprocessor-based data analysis (UKRAINCIK and PIKNOSH 1981; DUGGLEBY 1981; RITCHIE et al. 1983; CAULFIELD and SCHAFFER 1984). The general form of this equation may be expressed as

$$Y = (a–d)/[1 + (X/c)^b] + d$$

and

$$\text{logit } Y = \ln [Y/(100\text{-}Y)] = b \ln (X) + k$$

where: a = the response when $X = 0$; b = the slope of the curve; c = the concentration resulting from a response at 50% of $(a–d)$; k = const; and d = value of control (infinite X dilution).

Commonly, a calibration curve of fluorescence (AFU) versus the logarithm of the dilution of the standard is plotted, and used to determine the concentration of the Ig in the samples. In our experience, however, probably because of differing affinities of the Ig for the coat, the standard and the sample curves often have different slopes complicating interpretation of the data obtained. BUTLER et al. (1978, 1985) considered the logarithmic transformation of the mass law and concluded that the system can become independent of affinity when log-log plots are used.

While it is assumed that the ratio of solid phase Ag to added Ab in the so-called linear region of the log-log ELISA titration curve is such that all Ab becomes bound to solid phase Ag, this has not been empirically demonstrated. If ELISAs are influenced by affinity (BUTLER et al. 1978; BUTLER 1981), the amount of Ab bound in this linear region may be less than 100%. The nature of such binding curves may also be influenced by avidity and heterogeneity.

The binding of detection reagents (Ab-enzyme conjugates) at high concentrations of primary Ab appears to be sterically inhibited in direct proportion to the size of the conjugate system used for detection, leading to a marked deviation from linearity in this region of the binding curve. Discrepancies between the slope of the binding curve for the primary Ab and the binding of the detection system in the linear region of the titration plot result from changing ratios of bound enzyme to bound primary Ab, rather than altered activity of the former. Alternatively, the standard curve can be transformed into a four-parameter log-logit fit from which the sample Ig concentration can be determined.

Controversy has arisen over whether the ELISA measures Ab concentration or Ab affinity (BUTLER et al. 1978). As a discontinuous solid phase assay usually comprises two cycles of three washes and a second Ab step, during which time the first Ab may be dissociating, it would not be surprising if low affinity Abs are not detected. Because low affinity Abs may predominate early in an immune response (and hence are important in the early diagnosis of infections) and may be important immunopathologically (STEWARD and STEENSGAARD 1983), it was considered worthwhile to investigate the influence of Ab affinity in ELISA.

The study of the effect of affinity on in vitro assays has until recently depended on immune sera raised in vivo. These sera contain a heterogeneous population of Abs of varying class and affinity, so that interpretation of results is based on overall affinity estimation. Although often called average affinity, the affinity value estimated empirically for a particular antiserum may not represent the mean, mode, or median. This is due to the fact that, so far, there is no satisfactory experimental or mathematical way of describing the distribution of affinites of the Abs in an antiserum in terms of its shape (which may be a skewed gaussian or bimodal distribution) or its range (STEWARD and STEENSGAARD 1983). Monoclonal Ab techniques now provide the opportunity of studying individual homogeneous Abs of known affinity, class, and concentration.

6. Features of Enzyme Immunoassays

Some common characteristics of ligand-binding immunoassays determine the quality and the final applicability of such an assay. These are the specificity, sensitivity, precision and reproducibility, and practicability.

The *specificity* of the assay depends to a large extent on the quality of the detecting Ab employed. As mentioned earlier, these Ab are purified out of hyperimmune sera and need to be of a high affinity to be of use as a detecting reagent. However, it was not until studies by EISEN and SISKIND (1964), using the DNP-hapten system, that thermodynamically precise measurements of Ab affinity were made. These studies clearly showed that the affinity of rabbit Ab for DNP produced following immunization with DNP-bovine γ-globulin in complete Freund's adjuvant (CFA) increase progressively. These authors demonstrated the effect of Ag dose on affinity maturation. With lower doses of Ag, the rate of affinity maturation is greater than with higher doses. Lower doses resulted in some affinity maturation, but low levels of Ab (SISKIND et al. 1968). Early in an immune response, when Ag is not limited, cells bearing receptors of a wide range of affinities (including low affinity) will capture Ag and be stimulated. However, as Ag becomes limited, cells bearing receptors of higher affinity will preferentially bind Ag and produce Ab. Thus, decreasing Ag exerts a selective pressure for the production of progressively higher affinity Ab.

Since the specificity of such Ab is most commonly tested in immunodiffusion or immunoelectrophoresis, retesting of the Ab in a new and more sensitive system is necessary (SHIELDS and TURNER 1986). Often, additional affinity purification of the Ab is necessary when employing commercially available conjugates. When using the conjugate, two factors have to be taken into consideration: first, the maximum enzymatic activity must be retained, and second, the affinity of the Ab part of the molecule must remain unaltered. Thus, the formulation (pH, molarity, presence of activators, etc.) of the conjugate buffer plays a major role in the specificity and the sensitivity of the assay. Also, direct binding of the conjugate to the solid phase, which is only slightly reduced by the use of detergents, should be checked and the conjugate should therefore be employed at the highest possible dilution. In a sandwich or two-site assay, as described in this section, a much better sensitivity is reached by the double recognition of the Ig carrying at least two Ag determinants, by the catching Ab or the Ag immobilized on the solid phase and the detecting Ab. Moreover, in such an assay (after calibration) there is no need to use pure Ag for coating.

The *sensitivity* of an assay is usually defined as the lowest amount or concentration giving a response which differs significantly from the zero concentration response (detection limit). Apart from the factors which largely determine the specificity, other assay conditions play a role in the sensitivity, such as washing buffers and the method of washing, optimal reagent dilutions (determined by checkerboard titrations), nature and molecular weight of the Ag (for Ag-specific assays), sample dilution to avoid interference, diluent ionic strength and pH, incubation period and temperature, and the molar ratio of enzyme label per detecting Ab. Also, the detection efficiency of the high energy product affects the sensitivity of the assay. Most of the sensitive and quantitative assays described achieve detection limits for Ab variety from 2 to 20 fmol/ml (for example, IgG with a molecular weight of 150 kdalton implies a detection range of 0.3–3 ng/ml (KATO et al. 1975 a,b,c, 1976).

The *precision and reproducibility* of the assay are reflected by the slope of the log dose-response curve and the standard deviation of the individual readings at a certain dose of Ag. The steeper the log dose-response curve and the smaller the standard deviation, the higher will be the precision of the assay.

The *practicability* of the assay refers not only to the speed and ease of performance of the assay, but also to the possibility of automation of steps such as washing, addition of coating, conjugates, substrate, etc. and especially data collection and calculation of results.

7. Recommended Procedure for a Sandwich ELISA for Murine Circulating Antibodies

a) Clear polystyrene 60-well Terasaki trays are coated with 5 µl per well of 1–10 µg rat monoclonal isotype-specific mouse Ab or purified Ag per milliliter coating buffer (0.1 M Na_2CO_3 buffer, pH 9.6) in all wells. After the addition of distilled water, the lid on each tray is closed and the trays are incubated overnight at 4 °C.

b) Trays are washed three times with PBS, three times with PBS containing 0.05% v/v Tween-20 (PBS-Tw), and three times with PBS containing 0.02% gelatin with low Bloom number (PBS-Gel). Wells are filled with PBS-Gel, the lids are closed, and the trays are incubated for 30 min at 37 °C.

c) Serum samples are diluted four to eight times with a dilution factor of 2, 3.3, or 10, after which 5 µl per well is applied very carefully with a standardized calibrated pipette (Hamilton, Bonaduz). Two rows of each plate are filled with PBS-Gel: one as a blank and the other as a serum control. Trays are closed in a humidified atmosphere (for this and all subsequent steps) and incubated for 1 h at room temperature.

d) Samples are removed from the wells by sucking out the liquid with a replicator (Biotec, Basel). Plates are washed extensively with PBS-Tw-Gel three times, with intermittent drying.

e) The detecting antibody-β-galactosidase conjugate is applied to all eight rows plus the serum control row. The conjugate is diluted in PBS with 10 mM $MgCl_2$, 0.05% Tween, and 0.02% gelatin (PBS-Tw-Gel), and plates are incubated for 30 min at 37 °C, or 60 min at room temperature.

f) After extensive washing (five times with PBS-Tw-Gel), 5 µl per well 3.7 M substrate solution (4-methylumbelliferyl-β-D-galactopyranoside) is applied and plates are incubated for exactly 60 min at 37 °C.

g) Finally, to each well 5 µl stopping buffer (0.1 M Na_2CO_3 buffer, pH 10.4) is added and the resulting fluorescence is determined in an automatic inverted microfluorimeter.

Acknowledgments. We gratefully acknowledge Mr. A. van Oudenaren for stimulating discussions, Ms. G. de Korte for assistance in the preparation of the manuscript. These studies are supported by the Netherlands Asthma Foundation.

References

Ahmed A, Sher I, Sharrow SO, Smith AH, Paul WE, Sachs DH, Sell KW (1977) B-lymphocyte heterogeneity: development and characterization of an alloantiserum which distinguishes B-lymphocyte differentiation alloantigens. J Exp Med 145:61

Alevy YG, Blynn JCM (1986) An avidin-biotin ELISA assay for the measurement of de novo IgE synthesis in culture supernatants. J Immunol Methods 87:273

Andersson J, Coutinho A, Lernhardt W, Melchers F (1977) Clonal growth and maturation to immunoglobulin secretion in vitro of every growth-inducible B lymphocyte. Cell 10:27

Avrameas S, Ternynck T (1969) The cross-linking of proteins with glutaraldehyde and its use for the preparation of immunoadsorbants. Immunochemistry 6:53

Avrameas S, Ternynck T, Guesdon TL (1978) Coupling of enzymes to antibodies and antigens. Scand J Immunol 8 [Suppl 7]:7

Avrameas SA, Druet P, Masseyeff R, Feldman G (eds) (1983) Immunoenzymatic techniques. Elsevier, Amsterdam, p 159

Benner R, Meima F, Van der Meulen GM, Van Ewijk W (1974) Antibody formation in mouse bone marrow. III. Effects of route of priming and antigen dose. Immunology 27:747

Benner R, Van Oudenaren A, De Ruiter H (1977) Antibody formation in mouse bone marrow. IX. Peripheral lymphoid organs are involved in the initiation of bone marrow antibody formation. Cell Immunol 34:125

Benner R, Van Dongen JJM, Van Oudenaren A (1978) Corticosteroids and the humoral immune response of mice. I. Differential effect of corticosteroids upon antibody formation to sheep red blood cells in spleen and bone marrow. Cell Immunol 41:52

Benner R, Rijnbeek A-M, Bernabé RR, Martinez-Alonso C, Coutinho A (1981 a) Frequencies of background immunoglobulin-secreting cells in mice as a function of organ, age, and immune status. Immunobiology 158:225

Benner R, Van Oudenaren A, Koch G (1981 b) Induction of antibody formation in mouse bone marrow. In: Lefkovits I, Pernis B (eds) Immunological methods, vol 2. Academic, New York, p 247

Benner R, Van Oudenaren A, Björklund M, Ivars F, Holmberg D (1982a) "Background" immunoglobulin production: measurement, biological significance and regulation. Immunol Today 3:243

Benner R, Rijnbeek AM, Van Oudenaren A, Coutinho A (ed) (1982 b) Quantitative aspects of the non-specific humoral immune response to sheep erythrocytes. In: Nieuwenhuis P, Van den Broek H, Hanna MG (eds) In vivo immunology. Plenum, New York, p 703

Bergquist NR, Nilsson P (1974) The conjugation of immunoglobulins with tetramethylrhodamine isothiocyanate by utilization of dimethylsulfoxide (DMSO) as a solvent. J Immunol Methods 5:189

Bizollon CA (1984) Monoclonal antibodies and new trends in immunoassay. Elsevier, Amsterdam

Black SJ, Tokuhisa T, Herzenberg LA, Herzenberg LA (1980) Memory B cells at successive stages of differentiation: expression of surface IgD and capacity for a self renewal. Eur J Immunol 10:846

Blankwater MJ, Levert LL, Hijmans W (1975) Age-related decline in the antibody response to E. coli lipopolysaccharide in New Zealand mice. Immunology 28:847

Blecka LJ, Shaffar M, Dworschack R (1983) Inhibitor enzyme immunoassays for the quantitation of various haptens: a review. Avrameas SA, Druet P, Masseyeff R, Feldman G (eds) Immunoenzymatic techniques. Elsevier, Amsterdam

Boorsma DM (1983) Conjugation methods and biotin-avidin systems. In: Bullock GR, Petrusz P (eds) Techniques in immunochemistry. Academic, London, p 154

Borek F (1977) Adjuvants. In: Sela M (ed) The antigens. Academic, New York, p 369

Borzini P, Tedesco F, Greppi N, Rebulla P, Parravicini A, Sirchia G (1981) An immunoenzymatic assay for the detection and quantitation of platelet antibodies: the platelet β-galactosidase test (PGT). J Immunol Methods 44:323

Buckley CE, Buckley EG, Dorsey FC (1974) Longitudinal changes in serum immunoglobulin levels in older human. Fed Proc Fed Am Soc Exp Biol 33:2036

Burnet FM (1959) The clonal selection theory of acquired immunity. Cambridge University Press, Cambridge

Burnet FM (1974) Intrinsic mutagenesis: a genetic approach to ageing. Medical and Technical Publishers, St Leonardgate, Lancaster

Burns GF, Pike BL (1981) Spontaneous reverse hemolytic plaque formation. I. Technical aspects of the protein A assay. J Immunol Methods 41:269

Butler JE (1981) The amplified ELISA: principles and applications for the comparative quantitation of class and subclass antibodies and the distribution of antibodies and antigens in biochemical separates. Methods Enzymol 738:482

Butler JE, Peterman JH, Koertge TF (1985) The amplified enzyme-linked immunosorbent assay (a-ELISA). In: Ngo TT, Lenhoff HM (eds) Enzyme-mediated immunoassay. Plenum, New York, p 241

Callard RE (1981) Aging of the immune system. In: Kay MMB, Makinodan T (eds) CRC Handbook of immunology in aging. CRC Press, Boca Raton, Fl, p 103

Calvert JE, Maruyama S, Tedder TF, Webb CF, Cooper MD (1984) Cellular events in the differentiation of antibody-secreting cells. Semin Hematol 21:226

Caulfield MJ, Shaffer D (1984) A computer program for the evaluation of ELISA data obtained using an automated microtiter plate absorbance reader. J Immunol Methods 74:205

Cazenave PA, Ternynck T, Avrameas S (1974) Similar idiotypes in antibody-forming cells and in cells synthesizing immunoglobulins without the detectable antibody function. Proc Natl Acad Sci USA 71:4500

Cejka J, Kithier C (1976) A simple method for the classification and typing of monoclonal immunoglobulins. Immunochemistry 13:629

Chan FPH, Osmond DG (1979) Maturation of bone marrow lymphocytes. III. Genesis of Fc receptor-bearing "null" cells and B lymphocyte subtypes defined by concomitant expression of surface IgM, Fc, and complement receptors. Cell Immunol 47:366

Cunningham AJ (1965) A method of increased sensitivity for detecting single antibody-forming cells. Nature 207:1106

Cunningham AJ, Szenberg A (1968) Further improvements in the plaque technique for detecting single antibody-forming cells. Immunology 14:599

Czerkinsky CC, Nilsson LA, Nygren H, Ouchterlony Ö, Tarkowski A (1983) A solid-phase enzyme-linked immunospot (ELISPOT) assay for enumeration of specific antibody secreting cells. J Immunol Methods 65:109

De Bruyn AM, Klein F, Neumann H, Sandkuyl LA, Vermeeren R, Le Blansch G (1982) The absolute quantification of human IgM and IgG: standardization and normal values. J Immunol Methods 48:339

De Josselin de Jong JE, Jongkind JF, Ywema HR (1980) A scanning inverted microfluorometer with electronic shutter control for automatic measurements in micro-test plates. Anal Biochem 102:120

Deelder AM, De Water R (1981) A comparative study on the preparation of immunoglobulin-galactosidase conjugates. J Histochem Cytochem 29:1273

Delespesse G, Ishizaka K, Kishimoto T (1975) Rabbit lymphocyte populations responding to haptenic and carrier determinants for DNA synthesis. J Immunol 114:1065

Dresser DW (1978) Assays for immunoglobulin-secreting cells. In: Weir DM (ed) Handbook of Experimental Immunology. Blackwell, Oxford, vol 2, chap 28.1

Dresser DW, Wortis HH (1965) Use of an antiglobulin serum to detect cells producing antibody with low haemolytic efficiency. Nature 208:859

Duggelby RG (1981) A nonlinear regression program for small computers. Anal Biochem 110:9

Edelman GM (1973) Antibody structure and molecular immunology. Science 180:830

Eichmann K (1978) Expression and function of idiotypes on lymphocytes. Adv Immunol 26:195

Eisen HN, Siskind GW (1964) Variations in the affinities of antibodies during the immune response. Biochemistry 3:996

Engvall E (1978) Preparation of enzyme-labelled staphylococcal protein A and its use for detection of antibodies. Scand J Immunol 8 [Suppl 7]:25

Engvall E, Perlmann P (1972) Enzyme-linked immunosorbent assay, ELISA. III. Quantitation of specific antibodies by enzyme-labelled anti-immunoglobulin in antigen-coated tubes. J Immunol 109:129

Farrar JJ, Longhman BE, Nordin AA (1974) Lymphopoietic potential of bone marrow cells from aged mice: comparison of the cellular constituents of bone marrow from young and aged mice. J Immunol 112:1244

Fauci AS (1975) Mechanisms of corticosteroid action on lymphocyte subpopulations. I. Redistribution of circulating T and B lymphocytes in the bone marrow. Immunology 25:669

Fauci AS, Dale DC, Balow JE (1976) Glucocorticosteroid therapy: mechanisms of action and clinical considerations. Ann Intern Med 84:304

Fauci AS, Pratt KR, Whalen G (1977) Activation of human lymphocytes. IV. Regulatory effects of corticosteroids on the triggering signal in the plaque-forming cell response of human peripheral blood B lymphocytes to polyclonal activation. J Immunol 199:598

Fazekas De St Groth (1979) The quality of antibodies and cellular receptors. In: Lefkovits I, Pernis B (eds) Immunological methods, vol 1. Academic, New York, p 1

Fernandez AA, Stevenson GW, Abraham GE, Chiamori NJ (1983) Interrelation of the various mathematical approaches to radioimmunoassay. Clin Chem 29:184

Finger H, Beneke G, Emmerling P, Bertz R, Plager L (1972) Secondary antibody-forming potential of aged mice, with special reference to the influence of adjuvant on priming. Gerontologia 18:77

Giallongo A, Kochoumian L, King TP (1982) Enzyme and radioimmunoassays for specific murine IgE and IgG with different solid-phase immunosorbents. J Immunol Methods 52:279

Goding J (1976) The chromium chloride method of coupling antigens to erythrocytes: definition of some important parameters. J Immunol Methods 10:61

Goding J (1978) Use of staphylococcal protein A as an immunological reagent. J Immunol Methods 20:241

Goding JW (1976) Conjugation of antibodies with fluorochromes: modifications to the standard methods. J Immunol Methods 13:215

Goidl EA, Innes JB, Weksler ME (1976) Loss of IgG and high avidity plaque-forming cells and increased suppressor cell activity in aging mice. J Exp Med 144:1037

Gold ER, Fudenberg HH (1967) Chromic chloride: a coupling reagent for passive hemagglutination reactions. J Immunol 99:858

Gordon J, Rordorf DM, Rosenthal M, Sun YZ (1985) Immunoblotting and dot immunobinding. In: Habermehl RO (ed) Rapid methods and automation in microbiology and immunology. Springer, Berlin Heidelberg New York Tokyo, p 103

Gronowicz E, Coutinho A, Melchers F (1976) A plaque assay for all cells secreting Ig of a given type or class. Eur J Immunol 6:588

Haaijman JJ, Hijmans W (1978) The influence of age on the immunological activity and capacity of the CBA mouse. Mech Ageing Dev 7:375

Haaijman JJ, Schuit HRE, Hijmans W (1977) Immunoglobulin containing cells in different lymphoid organs of the CBA mouse during its lifespan. Immunology 32:427

Haaijman JJ, Slingerland-Teunissen J, Benner R, Van Oudenaren A (1979) The distribution of cytoplasmic immunoglobulin containing cells over various lymphoid organs of congenitally athymic (nude) mice as a function of age. Immunology 36:271

Haegert DG (1981) Rosette tests for T and B lymphocyte immunoglobulin. Immunol Today 2:200

Hamada S, Michadek SM, Torii M, Morisaki J, McGhee JR (1983) An enzyme-linked immunosorbent assay (ELISA) for quantifications of antibodies to *Streptococcus mutans* surface antigens. Mol Immunol 20:453

Hammarström L, Bird AG, Britton S (1979) Pokeweed mitogen induced differentiation of human B cells: evaluation by a protein A haemolytic plaque assay. Immunology 38:181

Hammarström L, Bird AG, Smith CIE (1980) Mitogenic activation of human lymphocytes: a protein A plaque assay evaluation of polyclonal B-cell activators. Scand J Immunol 11:1

Heidrick ML (1973) Imbalanced cyclic-AMP and cyclic-GMP levels in concanavalin-A stimulated spleen cells from aged mice. J Cell Biol 57:139a

Herzenberg LA, Black SJ, Tokuhisa T, Herzenberg LA (1980) Memory B cells at successive stages of differentiation. Affinity maturation and the role of IgD receptors. J Exp Med 151:1071

Hijmans W (1975) In: Silvestri LG (ed) The immunological basis of connective tissue disorders. North-Holland, Amsterdam, p 293

Hijmans W, Schuit HRE (1972) Immunofluorescence studies on immunoglobulins in the lymphoid cells of human peripheral blood. Clin Exp Immunol 11:483

Hijmans W, Schuit HRE, Klein F (1969) An immunofluorescence procedure for the detection of intracellular immunoglobulins. Clin Exp Immunol 4:457

Hijmans W, Haaijman JJ, Schuit HRE (1981) In: Adler WH, Nordin AA (eds) Immunological techniques applied to aging research. CRC Press, Boca Raton, FL, p 141

Hilgers LAT, Snippe H, Jange M, Willers JMN (1985) Combinations of two synthetic adjuvants: synergistic effects of a surfactant and a polyanion on the humoral immune response. Cell Immunol 92:203

Hill PN, Liu FT (1981) A sensitive enzyme-linked immunosorbent assay for the quantitation of antigen-specific murine IgE. J Immunol Methods 45:51

Holt PG, Plozza TM (1986) Enumeration of antibody-secreting cells by immunoprinting: sequential readout of different antibody isotypes on individual cell monolayers employing the ELISA plaque assay. J Immunol Methods 93:167

Holt PG, Cameron KJ, Stewart GA, Sedgwick JD, Turner KJ (1984) Enumeration of human immunoglobulin-secreting cells by the ELISA-plaque methods: IgE and IgG isotypes. Clin Immunol Immunopathol 30:159

Honjo T (1983) Immunoglobulin genes. Ann Rev Immunol 1:499

Hooijkaas H, Preesman AA, Benner R (1982) Low dose x-irradiation of thymus filler cells in limiting dilution cultures of lipopolysaccharide-reactive B cells reduces the background immunoglobulin-secreting cells without affecting growth-supporting capacity. J Immunol Methods 51:323

Hooijkaas H, Preesman AA, Van Oudenaren A, Benner R, Haaijman JJ (1983) Frequency analysis of functional immunoglobulin C and V gene expression in murine B cell at various ages. J Immunol 131:1629

Hooijkaas H, Benner R, Pleasants JR, Wostmann BS (1984) Isotypes and specificities of immunoglobulins produced by germfree mice fed chemically defined ultrafiltered "antigen-free" diet. Eur J Immunol 14:1127

Hooijkaas H, Van der Linde-Preesman AA, Benne S, Benner R (1985a) Frequency analysis of the antibody specificity repertoire in mitogen-reactive B cells and "spontaneous" occuring "background" plaque-forming cells in nude mice. Cell Immunol 92:154

Hooijkaas H, Van der Linde-Preesman AA, Bitter WM, Benner R, Pleasants JR, Wostmann BS (1985b) Frequency analysis of functional immunoglobulin C and V gene expression by mitogen-reactive B cells in germfree mice fed chemically defined ultrafiltered "antigen-free" diet. J Immunol 134:2223

Howard M, Nakanishi K, Paul WE (1984) B cell growth and differentiation factors. Immunol Rev 78:185

Huber B, Gershon RK, Cantor H (1977) Identification of a B-cell surface structure involved in antigen-dependent triggering: absence of this structure on B cells from CBA/N mutant mice. J Exp Med 145:10

Husby S, Nielson U, Jensenius JC, Erb K (1983) Increased non-specific protein binding in ELISA with serum samples pre-incubated at elevated temperatures. In: Avrameas SA, Druet P, Masseyeff R, Feldman G (eds) Immunoenzymatic techniques. Elsevier, Amsterdam, p 155

Iscove NN, Melchers F (1978) Complete replacement of serum by albumin, transferrin, and soybean lipid in cultures of lipopolysaccharide-reactive B cells. J Exp Med 147:923

Jacobsen C, Steensgaard J (1984) Binding properties of monoclonal anti-IgG antibodies: analysis of binding curves in monoclonal antibody systems. Immunology 51:423

Jenum PA (1985) Antibodies against chlamydia measured by an ELISA method. Acta Pathol Microbiol Immunol Scand [C] 93:175

Jerne NK (1984) Idiotypic networks and other preconceived ideas. Immunol Rev 79:5

Jerne NK, Nordin AA (1963) Plaque formation in agar by single antibody-producing cells. Science 140:405

Jerne NK, Nordin AA, Henry C (1963) The agar plaque technique for recognizing antibody-producing cells. In: Amos B, Koprowski H (eds) Cell-bound antibodies. Wistar Institute Press, Philadelphia, p 109

Jerne NK, Henry C, Nordin AA, Fuji H, Koros AMC, Lefkovits I (1974) Plaque forming cells: methodology and theory. Transplant Rev 18:130

Kato K, Hamaguchi Y, Fukui H, Ishikawa E (1975a) Enzyme-linked immunoassay: novel method for synthesis of the insulin-β-D-galactosidase conjugate and its applicability for insulin assay. J Biochem 78:235

Kato K, Hamaguchi Y, Fukui H, Ishikawa E (1975b) Enzyme-linked immunoassay: a simple method for synthesis of the rabbit antibody-β-D-galactosidase complex and its general applicability. J Biochem 78:423

Kato K, Fukui H, Hamaguchi Y, Ishikawa E (1976) Enzyme-linked immunoassay: conjugation of the FAB fragment of rabbit IgG with β-D-galactosidase from E. coli and its use for immunoassay. J Immunol 116:1554

Kato K, Hamaguchi Y, Fukui H, Ishikawa E (1976) Enzyme-linked immunoassay: conjugation of rabbit anti-(human immunoglobulin G) Antibody with β-D-galactosidase from *Escherichia coli* and its use for human immunoglobulin G assay. Eur J Biochem 62:285

Kearney JF, Radbruch A, Liesegang B, Rajewsky K (1979) A new mouse myeloma cell line that has lost immunoglobulin expression but permits the construction of antibody secreting hybrid cell lines. J Immunol 123: 1548

Kehrl JH, Muraguchi A, Butler JL, Kalkoff RJM, Fauci AS (1984) Human B cell activation, proliferation and differentiation. Immunol Rev 78:75

Kennedy JH, Kricka LJ, Wilding P (1976) Protein-protein coupling reactions and the applications of protein conjugates. Clin Chim Acta 70:1

Kishimoto T, Yoshizaki K, Komoto M, Okada M, Kuritani T, Kikutani H, Shimizu K, Nakagawa T, Nakagawa N, Miki Y, Kishi H, Fukunaga K, Yoshikubo T, Taga T (1984) B cell growth and differentiation factors and mechanism of B cell activation. Immunol Rev 78:97

Klasen E, Rigutti A (1983) A solid phase EIA which allows coating of peptides and water-insoluble protein showing no "hook effect" immunoreactivity of hemoglobin. In: Avrameas SA, Druet P, Masseyeff R, Feldman G (eds) Immunoenzymatic techniques. Elsevier, Amsterdam, p 159

Koch G, Benner R (1982) Differential requirement for B memory and T memory cells in adoptive antibody formation in mouse bone marrow. Immunology 45:697

Koch G, Lok BD, Van Oudenaren A, Benner R (1982a) The capacity and mechanism of bone marrow antibody formation by thymus-independent antigen. J Immunol 128:1479

Koch G, Lok BD, Benner R (1982b) The proliferative activity of antibody forming cells in the mouse bone marrow. Adv Exp Biol Med 149:75

Koch G, Lok BD, Benner R (1982c) Antibody formation in mouse bone marrow during secondary type response to thymus-independent antigens. Immunology 163:484

Kofler R, Wick G (1977) Some methodologic aspects of the chromium chloride method for coupling antigen to erythrocytes. J Immunol Methods 16:201

Köhler H, Urbain J, Cazenave PA (1984) Idiotypy in biology and medicine. Academic, Orlando

Kornman-van den Bosch HJ, De Bruijn AM, Klein F (1984) The effect of the diffusion medium on quantification of human IgM by radial immunodiffusion. J Immunol Methods 73:437

Kraal G, Weisman IL, Butcher EC (1982) Germinal centre B cells: antigen specificity and changes in heavy chain class expression. Nature 298:377

Kraal G, Weisman IL, Butcher EC (1985) Germinal center cells: antigen specificity, heavy chain class expression and evidence of memory. Adv Exp Med Biol 186:145

Kricka LJ, Carter TJN, Burt SM, Kennedy JH, Holder RL, Halliday MI, Telford ME, Wisdom GB (1980) Variability in the adsorption properties of microtitre plates used as solid supports in enzyme immunoassay. Clin Chem 26:741

Langone JJ (1982) Use of labeled protein A in quantitative immunochemical analysis of antigens and antibodies. J Immunol Methods 51:3

Lansdorp PM, Astaldi GCB, Oosterhof F, Janssen MC, Zeijlemaker WP (1980) Immunoperoxidase procedures to detect monoclonal antibodies against cell surface antigens. Quantitation of binding and staining of individual cells. J Immunol Methods 39:393

Laurell CB (1966) Quantitative estimation of proteins by electrophoresis in agarose gel containing antibodies. Anal Biochem 15:45

Lefkovits I (1972) Induction of antibody-forming cell clones in microcultures. Eur J Immunol 2:360

Lefkovits I (1979) Limiting dilution analysis. In: Lefkovits I, Pernis B (eds) Immunological methods, vol 1. Academic, New York, p 355

Lefkovits I, Cosenza H (1979) Assay for plaque-forming cells. In: Lefkovits I, Pernis B (eds) Immunological methods, vol 1. Academic, New York, p 277

Lew AM (1984) The effect of epitope density and antibody affinity on the ELISA as analysed by monoclonal antibodies. J Immunol Methods 72:171

Ling NR, Bishop S, Jefferis R (1977) Use of antibody-coated red cells for the sensitive detection of antigen and in rosette tests for cells bearing surface immunoglobulins. J Immunol Methods 15:279

Löfkvist T, Sjöguist J (1963) Purification of staphylococcal antigens with special reference to antigen A (Jensen). Int Arch Allergy 23:289

Mancini G, Vaerman JP, Carbonara AO, Heremans JF (1965) Immunochemical quantitation of antigens by single radial immunodiffusion. Immunochemistry 2:235

Masseyeff R (1978) Assay of tumour-associated antigens. Scand J Immunol 8 [Suppl 7]:83

McIntyre OR (1979) Multiple myeloma. N Engl J Med 30:193

Melchers F, Andersson J (1973) Synthesis, surface deposition and secretion of immunoglobulin M in bone marrow-derived lymphocytes before and after mitogenic stimulation. Transplant Rev 14:76

Melchers F, Andersson J (1974) B cell activation: three steps and their variations. Cell 37:715

Melchers F, Corbel C (1983) Studies on B-cell activation in vitro. Ann Inst Pasteur/Ann Immunol (Paris) 134D:63

Mendelow B, Grobicki D, Katz J, Metz J (1980) Separation of normal nature bone marrow plasma cells. Br J Haematol 45:251

Metzger WJ, Butler JE, Swanson P, Reinders E, Richerson HB (1981) Amplification of the enzyme-linked immunosorbent assay for measuring allergen-specific IgE and IgG antibody. Clin Chem 11:523

Miller JFAP, Warner NL (1971) The immune response of normal, irradiated and thymectomized mice to fowl immunoglobulin G as detected by a hemolytic plaque technique. Int Arch Allergy 40:59

Mink JG, Benner R (1979) Serum and secretory immunoglobulin levels in preleukaemic AKR mice and three other mouse strains. Adv Exp Med Biol 114:605

Mink JG, Radl J, Van den Berg P, Haaijman JJ, Van Zwieten MJ, Benner R (1980) Serum immunoglobulins in nude mice and their heterozygous littermates during ageing. Immunology 40:539

Mishell RI, Dutton RW (1967) Immunization of dissociated spleen cell cultures from normal mice. J Exp Med 126:423

Molinaro CA, Drays S (1974) Antibody coated erythrocytes as a manifold probe for antigens. Nature 248:515

Molinaro CA, Carey Hanly W, Dray S, Molinaro GA (1978) Identifying immunoglobulin isotypes, allotypes and idiotypes by a hemolytic assay in gel. J Immunol Methods 21:89

Möller SA, Borrebaeck CAK (1985) A microfilter assay for the detection of antibody-producing cells in vitro. In: Habermehl KO (ed) Rapid methods and automation in microbiology and immunology. Springer, Berlin Heidelberg New York Tokyo, p 123

Mond JJ, Lieberman R, Inman JK, Mosier DE, Paul WE (1977) Inability of mice with a defect in B-lymphocyte maturation to respond to phosphorylcholine on immunogenic carriers. J Exp Med 146:1138

Moore J, Calkins C (1983) Formation of antigen specific foci as a complement independent assay for individual antibody-secreting cells. J Immunol Methods 63:377

Morley J, Hanson JM, Youlten LJF (1984) Mediators of allergy. In: Lessof MH (ed) Allergy, immunological and clinical aspects. Wiley, Chichester, p 45

Moticka EJ (1974) The non-specific stimulation of immunoglobulin secretion following specific stimulation of the immune system. Immunology 27:401

Moyle WR, Lin C, Corson RL, Ehrlich PH (1983) Quantitative explanation for increased affinity shown by mixtures of monoclonal antibodies: importance of circular complex. Mol Immunol 20:439

Nieuwenhuis O, Opstelten D (1984) Functional anatomy of germinal centres. Am J Anat 170:421

Ohlson S, Zetterstrand K (1985) Detecting circulating immune complexes by PEG precipitation combined with ELISA. J Immunol Methods 77:87

Orgel LE (1973) Ageing of clones of mammalian cells. Nature 243:441

O'Sullivan MJ, Marks V (1981) Methods for the preparation of enzyme-antibody conjugates for use in enzyme immunoassay. Methods Enzymol 73:147

Pachmann K, Killander D, Wigzell H (1974) Increase in intracellular immunoglobulins in the majority of splenic lymphoid cells after primary immunization. Eur J Immunol 4:138

Paige CJ, Schreier MH, Sidman CL (1982) Mediators from cloned T helper cell lines affect immunoglobulin expression by B cells. Proc Natl Acad Sci USA 79:4756

Parish Cr, Higgins TJ (1982) Latex bead rosetting method for cell-surface antigens. J Immunol Methods 53:367

Perucca PJ, Faulk WP, Fudenberg HH (1969) Passive immune lysis with chromic chloride-treated erythrocyte. J Immunol 102:812

Pesce AJ, Ford DI, Gaizates MA (1978) Qualitative and quantitative aspects of immunoassays. Scand J Immunol 8 [Suppl 7]:1

Pesce AJ, Krieger NJ, Michael GJ (1983) Theories of immunoassay employing labelled reagents with emphasis on heterogeneous enzyme immunoassays. In: Avreamas SA, Druet P, Masseyeff R, Feldman G (eds) Immunoenzymatic techniques. Elsevier, Amsterdam, p 127

Pohlit HM, Haas W, von Boehmer H (1979) Haptenation of viable biological carriers. In: Lefkovits I, Pernis B (eds) Immunological methods, vol 1. Academic, New York, p 181

Porstmann T, Porstmann B, Micheel B, Schmidt EH, Herzmann H (1984) Characterization by Scatchard plots of monoclonal antibody enzyme conjugates directed against alpha-1-foetoprotein. J Immunol Methods 66:277

Price GB, Makinodan T (1972) Immunologic deficiencies in senescence. I. characterization of intrinsic deficiencies. J Immunol 108:403

Primi D, Triglia RP, Chen P, Lewis GK, Goodman JW (1981) A hemolytic plaque assay for the estimation of lymphokine-secreting cells. In: Pick E, Landy M (eds) Lymphokines, a forum for regulatory cell products, vol 2. Academic, New York, p 273

Puré E, Vitetta ES (1980) Induction of murine B cell proliferation by insolubilized anti-immunoglobulin. J Immunol 125:1240

Radl J (1979) The influence of the T immune system on the appearance of homogeneous immunoglobulins in man and experimental animals (a mini review). In: Lowenthal A (ed) The proceedings of the advanced study institute on humoral immunity in neurological diseases. Plenum, New York, p 517

Radl J (1981) Immunoglobulin levels and abnormalities in aging humans and mice. In: Adler WH, Nordin AA, Adelman RC (eds) CRC Handbook of immunology in aging. CRC Press, Boca Raton, FL, p 121

Radl J, Dooren LJ, Eijsvoogel VP, Van Went JJ, Hijmans W (1972) An immunological study during post-transplantation follow-up of a case of severe combined immunodeficiency. Clin Exp Immunol 10:367

Radl J, Sepers JM, Skvaril F, Morell A, Hijmans W (1975) Immunoglobulin pattern in humans over 95 years of age. Clin Exp Immunol 22:84

Radl J, Hollander CF, Van den Berg P, De Glopper E (1978) Idiopathic paraproteinaemia. I. Studies on an animal model – the ageing C57Bl/KaLwRij mouse. Clin Exp Immunol 33:395

Radl J, Mink JG, Van den Berg P, Van Zwieten MJ, Benner R (1980) Increased frequency of homogeneous immunoglobulins in the sera of nude athymic mice with age. Clin Immunol Immunopathol 17:469

Ritchie DG, Nickerson JM, Fuller GM (1983) Two simple programs for the analysis of data from enzyme-linked immunosorbent assay (ELISA) on a programmable desk-top calculator. Methods Enzymol 92:577

Ritterberg MB, Pratt KL (1969) Anti-trinitrophenyl (TNP) plaque assay. Primary response of BALB/c mice to soluble and particulate immunogen. Proc Soc Exp Biol Med 132:575

Rivnay B, Globerson A, Shinitzky M (1979) Viscosity of lymphocyte plasma-membrane in ageing mice and its possible relation to serum cholesterol. Mech Ageing Dev 10:71

Roholt DA, Grossberg AL, Yagi Y, Pressman D (1972) Limited heterogeneity of antibodies. Resolution of hapten binding curves into linear components. Immunochemistry 9:961

Romagnani S, Giudizi MG, Biagiotti T, Almerigogna T, Maggi E, Del Prete G, Ricci M (1981) Surface immunoglobulins are involved in the interaction of protein A with human B cells and in the triggering of B cell proliferation induced by protein A-containing *Staphylococcus aureus*. J Immunol 127:1307

Rozing J, Brons NHC, Van Ewijk W, Benner R (1978) B lymphocyte differentiation in lethally irradiated and reconstituted mice. A histological study using immunofluorescent detection of B lymphocytes. Cell Tissue Res 189:19

Sabbele NR, Van Oudenaren A, Benner R (1983a) The effect of corticosteroids upon the number and organ distribution of "background" immunoglobulin-secreting cells in mice. Cell Immunol 77:308

Sabbele NR, Van Oudenaren A, Hooijkaas H, Benner R (1983b) Effects of corticosteroids and cyclophosphamide upon the murine B cell system. In: Weimar W, Marquet RL, Bijnen AB, Ploeg RJ (eds) Proceedings of the modern trends in clinical immunosuppression. Erasmus University Press, Rotterdam, p 167

Savelkoul HFJ, Soeting PWC, Benner R, Radl J (1985) Quantitation of murine IgE in an automatic ELISA system. In: Klaus GGB (ed) Microenvironments in the lymphoid system. Plenum, New York, p 757

Savelkoul HFJ, Greeve AAM, Rijkers GT, Marwitz PA, Benner R (1988) Rapid procedure for coupling of protein antigens to red cells to be used in plaque assays by prewashing in chromium chloride. J Immunol Methods (in press)

Schønheyder H, Andersen P (1984) Effects of bovine serum albumin on antibody determination by the enzyme-linked immunosorbent assay. J Immunol Methods 72:251

Schuurs AHWM, Van Weemen BK (1977) Enzyme-immunoassay. Clin Chim Acta 81:1

Schwartz RH (1984) The role of products of the major histocompatibility complex in T cell activation and cellular interactions. In: Paul WE (ed) Fundamental immunology. Raven, New York, p 379

Scott H, De Rognum J, Brandtzaeg P (1985) Performance testing of antigen-coated polystyrene microplates for ELISA measurements of serum antibodies to bacterial and dietary antigens. Acta Pathol Microbiol Immunol Scand [C] 93:117

Sedgwick JD, Holt PG (1983) A solid-phase immunoenzymatic technique for the enumeration of specific antibody secreting cells. J Immunol Methods 57:301

Sher I, Ahmed A, Strong DM, Steinberg AD, Paul WE (1975) X-linked B-lymphocyte immune defect in CBA/HN mice. I. Studies of the function and composition of spleen cells. J Exp Med 141:788

Shields JG, Turner MW (1986) The importance of antibody quality in sandwich ELISA systems; evaluation of selected commercial reagents. J Immunol Methods 87:29

Sieckmann DG, Asofsky R, Mosier D, Zitron I, Paul WE (1978) Activation of mouse lymphocytes by anti-immunoglobulin. I. Parameters of the proliferative response. J Exp Med 147:814

Siskind GW, Dunn P, Walker JC (1968) Studies on the control of antibody synthesis. II. Effect of antigen dose and of suppression by passive antibody on the affinity of antibody synthesized. J Exp Med 127:55

Smith CIE, Hammarström L, Bird AG (1979) Lipopolysaccharide and lipid A-induced human blood lymphocyte activation as detected by a protein A plaque assay. Eur J Immunol 9:619

Sprent J (1977) Recirculating lymphocytes. In: Marchalonis JJ (ed) The lymphocyte structure and function. Marcel Dekker, New York, p 43

Steward MW, Petty RE (1972) The antigen binding characteristics of antibody pools of different relative affinity. Immunology 23:881

Steward MW, Steensgaard J (1983) Antibody affinity: thermodynamic aspects and biological significance. CRC Press, Boca Raton, FL

Stocker JW, Heusser CH (1979) Methods for binding cells to plastic: application to a solid-phase radioimmunoassay for cell-surface antigens. J Immunol Methods 26:87

Stokes RP, Cordwell A, Thompson RA (1982) A simple, rapid ELISA method for the detection of DNA antibodies. J Clin Pathol 35:566

Strausbauch P, Sulica A, Givol D (1970) General method for the detection of cells producing antibodies against haptens and proteins. Nature 227:68

Strober S, Dilley J (1973) Maturation of B lymphocytes in the rat. I. Migration pattern, tissue distribution and turnover rate of unprimed and primed B lymphocytes involved in the adoptive antidinitrophenyl response. J Exp Med 138:1331

Surolia A, Pain D (1981) Preparation of protein A-enzyme monoconjugate and its use as a reagent in enzyme immunoassays. Methods Enzymol 73:176

Sweet GH, Welborn FL (1971) Use of chromium chloride as the coupling agent in a modified plaque assay of cells producing anti-protein antibody. J Immunol 106:1407

Ten Berge (1983) The influence of immunosuppressive drugs on human immunocompetence. Thesis, University Amsterdam

Ternynck T, Avrameas S (1976) A new method using p-benzoquinone for coupling antigens and antibodies to marker substances. Ann Inst Pasteur/Ann Immunol (Paris) 127C:197

Truffa-Bachi P, Bordenave GR (1980) A reverse hemolytic plaque assay for the detection and the enumeration of immunoglobulin allotype-secreting cells. Cell Immunol 50:261

Tsang VC, Wilson BC, Peralta JM (1983) Quantitative, single tube, kinetic dependent enzyme-linked immunosorbent assay (K-ELISA). Methods Enzymol 92:391

Tuchinda M, Newcomb RW, De Vald BL (1972) Effect of prednisone treatment on the human immune response to keyhole limpet hemocyanin. Int Arch Allergy 42:533–544

Turesson I (1976) Distribution of immunoglobulin-containing cells in human bone-marrow and lymphoid tissues. Acta Med Scand 199:293

Tyan ML (1981) Marrow stem cells during development and aging. In: Kay MMB, Makinodan T (eds) CRC Handbook of immunology in aging. CRC Press, Boca Raton, FL, p 87

Tyler RW, Everett NB (1972) Radioautographic study of cellular migration using parabiotic rats. Blood 39:249

Ukraincik K, Piknosh W (1981) Microprocessor-based radioimmunoassay data analyses. Methods Enzymol 74:497

Urbain-Vansanten G (1970) Concomitant synthesis, in separate cells on nonreactive immunoglobulins and specific antibodies after immunization with tobacco mosaic virus. Immunology 19:783

Van Dijk H, Testerink J, Noordegraaf E (1976) Stimulation of the immune response against SRBC by reduction of corticosteroids plasma levels. Cell Immunol 25:8

Van Dongen JJM, Hooijkaas H, Hählen K, Benne K, Bitter WM, Van der Linde-Preesman AA, Tettero ILM, Van de Rijn R, Hilgers J, Van Zanen GE, Hagemeijer A (1984) Detection of minimal residual disease in TdT positive T cell malignancies by double immunofluorescence staining. In: Löwenberg B, Hagenbeek A (eds) Minimal residual disease in acute leukemia. Martinus Nijhoff, The Hague, p 67

Van Dongen JJM, Hooijkaas H, Comans-Bitter WM, Hählen K, De Klein A, Van Zanen GE, Van 't Veer MB, Abels J, Benner R (1985) Human bone marrow cells positive for terminal deoxynucleotidyl transferase (TdT), HLA-DR, and a T cell marker may represent prothymocytes. J Immunol 135:3144

Van Ewijk W, Rozing J, Brons NHC, Klepper D (1977) Cellular events during primary immune response in the spleen. A fluorescence-, light-, and electromicroscopic study in germfree mice. Cell Tiss Res 183:471

Van Ewijk W, Van Soest PL, Verkerk A, Jongkind JF (1984) Loss of antibody binding to prefixed cells: fixation parameters for immunocytochemistry. Histochem J 16:179

Van Muiswinkel WB, De Laat AMM, Mink JG, Van Oudenaren A, Benner R (1979) Serum immunoglobulin levels in mice, determination of the low IgA level in AKR mice by an irradiation-resistant factor. Int Arch Allergy Appl Immunol 60:240

Van Oudenaren A, Hooijkaas H, Benner R (1981) Improvement of the protein A plaque assay for immunoglobulin-secreting cells by using immunoglobulin-depleted guinea pig serum as a source of complement. J Immunol Methods 43:219

Van Oudenaren A, Haaijman JJ, Benner R (1984) Frequencies of background cytoplasmic Ig-containing cells in various lymphoid organs of athymic asplenic (lasat) athymic, asplenic and normal BALB/c mice. Immunology 42:437

Van Soest PL, De Josselin de Jong J, Lansdorp PM, Van Ewijk W (1984) An automatic fluorescence micro-ELISA system for quantitative screening of hybridoma supernatants using a protein-A-β-galactosidase conjugate. Histochemic J 16:21

Van Weemen BK, Bosch AMG, Dawson EC, Van Hell H, Schuurs AHWM (1978) Enzyme immunoassay of hormones. Scand J Immunol 8 [Suppl 7]:73

Vitetta ES, Brooks K, Chen YW, Isakson P, Jones S, Layton J, Mishra GC, Puré E, Weiss E, Word C, Yuan D, Tucker P, Uhr JW, Krammer PH (1984) T cell derived lymphokines that induce IgM and IgG secretion in activated murine B cells. Immunol Rev 78:137

Voller A, Bartlelett A, Bidwell D (ed) (1981) Immunoassay for 80's. University Park Press, Baltimore

Whitehouse MW (1977) The chemical nature of adjuvants. In: Glynn LE, Steward M (eds) Immunochemistry. An advanced textbook. Wiley, Chichester, p 571

Wisdom BG (1976) Enzyme-immunoassay. Clin Chem 22:1243

Yang WC, Miller SC, Osmond DG (1978) Maturation of bone-marrow lymphocytes. II. Development of Fc and complement receptors and surface immunoglobulins studied by rosetting and radioautography. J Exp Med 148:1251

Yolken RH, Leister FJ, Whitcomb LS, Santosham M (1983) Enzyme immunoassays for the detection of bacterial antigen utilizing biotin-labeled antibody and peroxidase-biotin-avidin complex. J Immunol Methods 56:319

Yoshizaki K, Nakagawa T, Kaieda T, Muraguchi A, Yamamura Y, Kishimoto T (1982) Induction of proliferation and Igs-production in human B leukemic cells by anti-immunoglobulins and T cell factors. J Immunol 128:1296

Monoclonal Antibodies to Lymphocyte Surface Molecules as Probes for Lymphocyte Functions

M. A. TALLE and G. GOLDSTEIN

A. Introduction

Since the introduction of hybridoma technology by KOHLER and MILSTEIN in 1975, countless monoclonal antibodies (mAb) to lymphocyte surface molecules have been created. The resultant detection and characterization of important lymphocyte surface molecules has facilitated the definition of regulatory and effector functions of human lymphocytes at the molecular level. Restricted expression on an interesting subset of cells has usually been the criterion of selection, but the mAb thus selected has often been utilized to determine the function of the cells bearing the antigen, to characterize the function of the molecule itself, and, in some instances, to provide an essential reagent in determining the structure of the molecule, either by conventional protein techniques or by gene cloning.

This chapter focuses on lymphocyte surface markers which participate in human immune function and which have been identified or largely characterized by mAbs. The first group includes those involved in T lymphocyte activation. This group also includes those molecules which function as receptors for defined growth factors or components of complement as well as molecules associated with leukocyte adhesion. The second group consists of molecules whose chief function is thought to be recognition of structures such as class I and class II major histocompatibility complex (Mhc) molecules or antigens presented on the surfaces of interacting cells. Assignment of a lymphocyte surface marker to a particular group is somewhat arbitrary since several of the molecules, particularly T4, T8, LFA-1, and LFA-3, are involved with both cell recognition and other functions.

The review of specific lymphocyte molecules is preceded by a general discussion on the production of mAbs, with emphasis on approaches to immunization and screening, and pitfalls to avoid for successful hybridoma isolation.

B. Methods for Monoclonal Antibody Generation

The theory of mAbs and hybridoma technology is lucidly presented in a book by GODING (1983), including details of mAb production, purification, and modification as well as antigen characterization.

I. Immunization Strategies

The method of immunization one chooses frequently depends on how much is known about the antigen. Many of the mAbs that recognize lymphocyte surface molecules were produced without any knowledge of their target antigen. mAbs with restricted patterns of reactivity with various human lymphocyte types were generated by KUNG et al. 1980, and these opened a new era in defining human T cell differentiation antigens. Enriched populations of intact human T lymphocytes were used as the immunogens in this instance, and mAbs reactive with the immunizing cell type, but unreactive with other leukocytes, were isolated and used to characterize the molecule or molecules they defined. A similar strategy has been used to identify functionally important structures of B lymphocytes and many other cell types.

mAb technology is built on three fundamental points: (a) a given B lymphocyte produces immunoglobulin of a single antigen-binding specificity; (b) the B lymphocyte can be immortalized by fusing it with a myeloma cell; and (c) the hybrid can be cloned. Thus, even if the immunogen consists of the myriad of antigens contained within a population of intact cells, isolation of a hybrid cell producing mAb reactive with a single antigen is feasible. The number of stable hybrids resulting from the fusion of a myeloma line with spleen cells from an immunized animal is proportional to the number of antigen-activated B cells present in the spleen. Therefore, a fusion performed with spleen cells from an animal immunized with a complex immunogen such as whole cells will lead to a greater number of stable hybrids than one in which the immunogen was an isolated protein. Detection and isolation of the stable hybrid cells producing mAb of desired specificity becomes more difficult with increased fusion frequency if the cells are not adequately diluted during plating; the greater the number of antibodies with differing specificity within a given culture supernatant in one well, the more likely it is that there will be antibodies masking the presence of the specificity being sought. If a simple and rapid screen is not available, it is often advantageous to immunize with cells enriched for the antigen. Alternatively, one can produce asynchronous clonal expansions by immunizing with cells displaying some of the antigens of the immunizing cell type (but not the desired ones) 5–7 days prior to the final prefusion boost with the immunizing cells. For example, if mAbs specific for T lymphocytes are sought, a preboost immunization with granulocytes followed by a final immunizing boost with T cells will lower the overall fusion frequency, but will enrich for stable hybrids producing T cell-specific antibodies (M. A. TALLE 1985, unpublished work). The success of this in vivo enrichment method is presumably a consequence of inducing B cells reactive with antigens shared by T cells and granulocytes to reach an inappropriate stage of differentiation for formation of stable hybridomas. Optimal fusion frequency occurs 3–5 days after immunization, and B cells that respond to the preimmunogen will therefore be less likely to be at a fusible differentiation stage 9–11 days later.

mAbs to serologically or biochemically defined antigens can be generated with splenocytes from animals immunized with enriched preparations of the immunogen. Antigens to which polyclonal or monoclonal sera exist can be purified by immunoaffinity. Since elution of a protein antigen from an antibody frequently results in denaturation of the antigens, it may be desirable to immunize with the intact antigen–antibody complex.

This can be achieved by immunoprecipitating the antigen from detergent-solubilized membranes and using an anti-antiserum or staphylococcal protein A to cross-link the antigen–antibody complexes. These aggregates are washed several times, and the detergent is removed by acetone precipitation of the protein (HAGER and BURGESS 1980). Removal of the detergent, which is critical for the survival of the animal being immunized, may in some instances partially denature the antigen. Whereas antigen–antibody complexes are immunogenic aggregates, soluble protein antigens are tolerogenic and must be presented mixed in an adjuvant. The first immunization is given in Freund's complete adjuvant, and subsequent injections in Freund's incomplete adjuvant, either intraperitoneally or subcutaneously. It is wise to test the immunized sera for antigen-binding activity prior to the final boost. Fusion is performed 3–5 days after the final boost, which should be administered in soluble form without adjuvant, either intravenously or intraperitoneally. The frequency of hybridomas producing antibodies to a given antigen will naturally be higher if purified antigen rather than whole cells is the immunogen.

II. Fusion

Spleens are removed from animals 3–5 days after the final antigen challenge. If there is uncertainty regarding the ability of the animal to respond to a given antigen, the serum should be tested for antibody titer. Under most circumstances, either the BALB/c strain or an F_1 hybrid of BALB/c is used for mAb generation. This stems from the fact that the mutant myeloma lines that were selected for the absence of hypoxanthine-guanine phosphoribosyl transferase (HGPRT) activity were derived from BALB/c myeloma lines. If an immune response to a given antigen cannot be mounted by a BALB/c, then other strains can be used; however, the resulting hybridomas may be less stable, and ascites production becomes more difficult if the appropriate F_1 strain is not available.

The HGPRT$^-$ myeloma cell lines most frequently used for fusion are P3-NS1-Ag4-1 (NS1) (KOHLER et al. 1976), SP2/O-Ag-14 (SP2) (SHULMAN et al. 1978), and X63-Ag8.653 (KEARNEY et al. 1979). Both the SP2 and X63-Ag8.653 lines have lost the ability to synthesize endogenous heavy and light immunoglobulin chains, whereas the NS1 line produces, but does not secrete κ chains. Hybridomas resulting from fusion with NS1 produce immunoglobulin molecules containing light chains derived from either NS1 or the fused B cell.

The methods employed for fusion vary nearly as much as the number of individuals performing the technique. In the method described by GALFRE and MILSTEIN (1981), cells are treated with polyethylene glycol (PEG) for 1 min and the PEG is gradually diluted over the next several minutes. Alternatively, the cells can be mixed with PEG and briefly centrifuged (200 g). After 5–7 min, the PEG is rapidly diluted (GEFTER et al. 1977). Many variables have been studied within these methods, and ranges for good fusion frequency have been determined. PEG (average molecular weight of either 1000 or 1500) gives satisfactory results at concentrations of 30%–50%, pH values between 7.0 and 8.5, and temperatures of 25–

40 °C. The toxicity of the PEG increases with concentration and time. The ratio of splenocytes to myeloma cells is generally in the range of 10:1 to 6:1. Once an appropriate combination of variables resulting in high fusion frequency has been determined by an investigator, these can be expected to yield consistently efficient fusions, provided one possesses good tissue culture skills (FRESHNEY 1983).

Cells are placed in hypoxanthine aminopterin thymidine (HAT) selective medium immediately following fusion or they may be "rested" in normal medium for 24 h. Although the HGPRT reversion rate is low, it is wise to test the myeloma line for aminopterin sensitivity with each fusion. The products of a fusion are usually plated into 100–1000 tissue culture wells, depending chiefly on the ease of the antibody screen and the expected fusion frequency. If a good fusion frequency can be expected, there are several reasons to plate cells at a low density (feeder cells can be added if the density is very low). Multiple hybridomas in a single well, which produce distinct antibodies to a given antigen, may mask the presence of a desirable antibody. For example, a culture supernatant containing both anti-leukocyte-reactive as well as anti-T cell-restricted antibodies would be excluded in a screen intended to select for reactivity restricted to T cells. We have performed fusions from which >90% of the resulting stable hybridomas have produced antibodies reactive with the immunogen. Analysis of the mAbs produced could be performed only if the cells were plated at a density of one cell per well. Generally, however, the percentage of hybridomas producing antibodies to the immunogen is lower, and up to ten hybridomas per well can provide interpretable data. This number can be even higher if a highly specific screen is available, but then one is faced with increasing difficulty in cloning the hybridoma of interest.

III. Screening

A screen for mAbs should be fast, sensitive, economical, accurate, and reproducible; it should be developed prior to fusion. Screens for detecting antibodies to cell surface antigens are usually indirect, utilizing antisera to mouse immunoglobulin labeled with either an isotope, a fluorochrome, or an enzyme to detect binding of antibody to the cell surface. However, assays which measure immune functions have also been used successfully.

Sheep or goat anti-mouse immunoglobulin can be gently labeled to high specific activity with ^{125}I ($t_{1/2} = 60$ days) using either chloramine-T or Iodogen. Antibody prepared in this way can be stored at 4 °C for at least 2 weeks without appreciable loss of antigen-binding activity. A panel of cells can be rapidly assessed for the presence of antigen reactive with a given culture supernatant, however, the level of ^{125}I bound does not reveal what percentage of the cell population expresses antigen.

An enzyme-linked immunosorbent assay (ELISA) is a particularly useful screening method if the antigen is available in a partially purified form or remains intact in the membrane fraction of cells extracted with detergent. If the antigen preparation can be freed of detergent, ELISA plates can be directly coated; membranes containing detergent must be anchored to the plate indirectly via polyclonal or monoclonal antisera. The ELISA is therefore most often used to detect additional antibodies to known surface molecules and soluble proteins. Intact cells capable of adhering to plastic can be used as the antigen source for an ELISA, provided the level of endogenous enzyme activity is low. Use of cell suspensions in an ELISA suffers from poor reproducibility, owing to accidental loss of cells during the many washes and centrifugations required. A variety of enzymes coupled to anti-mouse immunoglobulin are available from many suppliers. No special equipment is required, but automated scanners which measure the optical densities of 96 wells in less than 2 min facilitate screening.

Fluorochromes, particularly fluorescein, covalently coupled to anti-mouse immunoglobulin are the most widely used reagents for detection of monoclonal antibodies to cell surface antigens. Analysis of the stained cells, either by microscopy or by flow cytometry, is more time consuming than the other methods, but this technique is worthwhile because of the additional information gained. One learns not only what percentage of a given population of cells bears antigen, but also the relative density and heterogeneity of antigen expression by cells within that population. Analysis by flow cytometry has the added advantage that a mixed population of cells differing in light scattering properties can be measured independently of fluorescence. For example, a single portion of whole blood can be stained with fluorescent antibody and lymphocytes, monocytes, and granulocytes can each be analyzed independently for expression of antigen. In addition, it is now possible to analyze cells for the presence of more than one antigen by staining with multiple (usually two) fluorochromes.

Testing the effect of culture supernatants in immunologic assays is the most direct means of obtaining mAbs to molecules involved in immune function. The nature of the assay determines to a certain extent the range of molecules that can be identified. If T cell proliferation is the readout, then T cells stimulated with allogeneic non-T cells can be blocked at many points, and antibodies to a wide range of target proteins may be detected. Replication of interleukin 2- (IL-2)-dependent cloned T cells, stimulated only with IL-2, will be blocked by a more limited number of antibodies. Glycoproteins required for cytotoxic T cell function have been identified by screening for mAbs able to block ^{51}Cr release in a T cell-mediated lympholysis assay (SANCHEZ-MADRID et al. 1982). Similarly, testing culture supernatants in assays designed to measure immunoglobulin (Ig) production by B cells or assays for B cell growth and differentiation factors should lead to the identification of additional important functional surface proteins.

IV. Cloning

Initial screening is usually performed on culture supernatants from mixed populations of hybridoma cells. Several methods are available to isolate the desired hybridoma. Cloning by limiting dilution in the presence of feeder cells (usually murine thymocytes) is generally successful, and hybridomas should be diluted such that the frequency of growth in the microtiter plate will be one in three wells (see Chap. 12). Cloning frequency among hybridomas is highly variable so that it is necessary to plate cells at several densities to be assured of the proper growth frequency. Cells cloned twice at the proper growth frequency have a high probability of clonality. Cloning can also be performed in soft agar, but clones derived in this manner will subsequently need to be expanded in tissue culture (see Chap. 12). If a scheme exists for identifying the desired hybridoma directly, such as a fluorochrome-tagged antigen, then cloning can be accomplished most easily by sorting on a flow cytometer. If very large quantities of a particular antibody will be required over a period of years, then a seed lot of the hybridoma should be prepared, or it may become necessary to reclone to ensure maintenance of cells producing the desired antibody.

C. Functional Molecules

A large number of antigens having relatively restricted patterns of expression on leukocytes have been defined by mAbs (Table 1). Some of these antigens are restricted to cells of a particular lineage whereas others are more widely expressed. In a few instances, a function can be ascribed to the recognized antigen, leading to a further characterization. The molecules included in this section are those whose function has been elucidated largely through the availability of mAbs.

Table 1. Lymphocyte surface molecules defined by monoclonal antibodies

Molecule (cluster designation)	Molecular weight (Kdalton)		Function	Distribution
	Reduced	Non-reduced		
T1 (CD5)	gp67	gp67	Positive sigmal mediation	Pan-T/some B-CLL
T3 (CD3)	gp20 p20 gp25	gp20 (δ) p20 (ε) gp25 (γ)	Signal transduction	Mature T; associated with T cell Ag receptor
T11 (CD2)	gp50	gp50	E rosette receptor; signal mediation	Pan-T
T9	gp90	gp180	Binds transferrin	Proliferating cells
TAC (CD25)	gp55	gp55	Binds interleukin 2	Normal activated lymphocytes
CR2 (CD21)	gp160	gp140	Binds C3d	B cells
CR3 (CD11b)	gp165 gp95	gp165 (α) gp95 (β)	Binds C3bi	Monocytes; granulocytes; large granular lymphocytes
LFA-1 (CD18)	gp177 gp95	gp177 (α) gp95 (β)	Adhesion	Hematopoietic lineage
LFA-3	gp60	gp60	Adhesion (?)	Wide distribution
T4 (CD4)	gp55	gp51	Class II HLA recognition (?)	Mature T cell subset
T8 (CD8)	gp32	gp70	Class I HLA recognition (?)	Mature T cell subset
Ti	gp90	gp37–45 (β) gp45–55 (α)	Antigen recognition	Mature T cells; associated with T3

B-CLL, chronic lymphocytic leukemia of B cell origin; gp, glycoprotein; p, protein.

I. T Cell Lineage Restricted

1. T3-CD3

A key T lymphocyte differentiation antigen which remained undefined until the introduction of hybridoma technology is identified by the monoclonal antibody OKT3 (KUNG et al. 1979). It was subsequently designated CD3 (IUIS-WHO 1985). CD3 is expressed by all mature peripheral T cells, but by only a fraction of cells within the thymus. Medullary thymocytes express CD3 at a high density, whereas cortical thymocytes bear less CD3. Phenotypic (REINHERZ et al. 1980 b) and functional studies (UMIEL et al. 1982) indicate that the high density CD3 medullary cells are the mature cells capable of executing T cell-specific functions.

OKT3 immunoprecipitates a 20 kdalton (δ) glycoprotein (VAN AGTHOVEN et al. 1981); however, under less stringent washing conditions, glycoproteins of 25 (γ), 37 (α), and 44 (β) kdalton are detected (BORST et al. 1982). A fifth member of the complex has been described as a nonglycosylated 20 kdalton protein (ε) and details of the biosynthesis of the γ, δ, and ε components have been published (BORST et al. 1983; KANELLOPOULOS et al. 1983; PESSANO et al. 1985). mAbs to surface structures unique to individual antigen-responsive T cell clones (clonotype-specific antibodies) immunoprecipitate glycoproteins similar in size to the α and β chains of the CD3 complex. Modulation of these antigens from the cell surface by the clonotype-specific antibodies results in the concurrent loss of OKT3 reactivity (MEUER et al. 1983 a). This suggests that the clonotypic structures are the α and β components of the CD3 complex. Direct evidence for this is provided by immunoprecipitation of chemically cross-linked cell membranes. Under these conditions, clonotype-specific antibodies precipitate an additional protein which, after cleavage of the cross-linker, migrates in a polyacrylamide gel to a position indistinguishable from the CD3 δ chain. Similarly, immunoprecipitation of cross-linked membranes by a CD3-specific antibody, which otherwise precipitates only the γ and δ proteins, results in detection of two additional proteins indistinguishable in size from the α and β chains detected by clonotype-specific antisera (BRENNER et al. 1985).

Although mAbs to the CD3 γ, δ, and ε components of murine T cells have not yet been obtained, clonotype-specific antibodies to the α and β chains do exist. Immunoprecipitation with these reagents reveals an additional 32 kdalton disulfide-linked homodimer (ζ) as part of the CD3 complex. The existence of this component in the human T cell has not been reported (SAMELSON et al. 1985).

The CD3 antigen is involved in numerous T cell-specific functions. Addition of OKT3 mAb to cultures of T cells blocks the proliferative response to both soluble antigens and allogeneic cells, and inhibits the generation of cytotoxic T cells in mixed lymphocyte cultures; it also abrogates the ability of T cells to provide help to B cells in antibody production (REINHERZ et al. 1980 a). Lysis of allogeneic target cells by uncloned allospecific cytotoxic T lymphocytes (CTL) is blocked by OKT 3 (CHANG et al. 1981) as are cytotoxic T cell clones directed toward either class I or class II Mhc antigens (SPITS et al. 1982). Of the mAbs to lymphocyte surface structures able to interfere with CTL, CD3-specific antibodies are unique in that they inhibit CTL-mediated lympholysis by interfering with a step subsequent to killer target recognition and adhesion (TSOUKAS et al. 1982; LANDE-

GREN et al. 1982). CD3-specific antibodies have been shown to activate T cell clones as well as alloantigen-primed uncloned T cells to lyse targets nonspecifically (LEEUWENBERG et al. 1985; MENTZER et al. 1985a; SPITS et al. 1985a). The mechanism of anti-CD3-mediated nonspecific cytolysis is Fc dependent, and may be a consequence of bridging the target cell via its Fc receptors to the cytolytic cell bearing CD3. Binding of anti-CD3 to the killer T cell would result in activation of its lytic components and their localized release in the vicinity of the target cell (MENTZER et al. 1985a).

Normal resting T cells can be activated to proliferate by anti-CD3. As little as 10^{-12} M OKT3 mimics this antigen-like effect (VAN WAUWE et al. 1980). Aggregated human IgG and its Fc fragments inhibit the mitogenicity of OKT3, presumably by binding to monocyte Fc receptors (VAN WAUWE and GOOSSENS 1981; LOONEY and ABRAHAM 1984). Mitogenesis by OKT3 requires accessory monocytes. The precise mechanism by which monocytes promote anti-CD3-induced mitogenesis has not yet been elucidated, but variability among individual proliferative responses induced by CD3-specific antibodies of IgG1 isotype suggests a polymorphism of human monocyte Fc receptors for murine IgG1 antibodies (TAX et al. 1983; KANEOKA et al. 1983). The requirement for monocytes in an IgG2a anti-CD3-driven proliferative response can be circumvented by anchoring the anti-CD3 to an anti-mouse immunoglobulin-coated plastic tissue culture dish. This suggests that at least one function of the monocyte is to cross-link or conformationally alter CD3 molecules (CEUPPENS et al. 1985).

Activation of T cells by anti-CD3 is mediated by increases in concentrations of intracellular inositoltrisphosphates which release Ca^{2+} from intracellular stores (see Chaps. 3 and 4). The elevation of the intracellular Ca^{2+} concentration provides a signal leading to IL-2 production and presumably other activation events (WEISS et al. 1984; IMBODEN and STOBO 1985).

Isolation of cDNA clones encoding the CD3 δ-glycoprotein permitted the elucidation of its amino acid sequence (VAN DEN ELSEN et al. 1984). The molecule consists of two functional domains: an NH terminal extracellular domain of 79 residues, with two N-linked oligosaccharides, and a cytoplasmic domain of 44 amino acids. There is no sequence homology with members of the T cell receptor/immunoglobulin/Mhc multigene family, or with the murine Thy-1 antigen. Northern blot analysis shows CD3 δ-chain mRNA to be restricted to cells of T lineage, and southern blots indicate that the CD3 δ-chain is represented as a single-copy gene (VAN DEN ELSEN et al. 1984).

In summary, the molecule of the T cell surface with which OKT3 reacts is noncovalently associated with the T cell antigen recognition molecule and appears to be an essential component, mediating signal transduction. Reaction of OKT3 with this molecule alone, or clearing of the CD3–antigen recognition complex by modulation after exposure to OKT3 in vitro (REINHERZ et al. 1982) or in vivo (CHATENOUD et al. 1982) effectively blocks T cell function.

2. T1-CD5

Another functional T cell surface molecule originally identified by the mAb OKT1 (KUNG et al. 1979; REINHERZ et al. 1979a) and subsequently by many others is designated CD5 (IUIS-WHO 1985). The 64 kdalton glycoprotein (Fox et al. 1982; VAN AGTHOVEN et al. 1981) is expressed by all peripheral blood T cells and several transformed T cell lines, but not by normal peripheral blood B cells, null cells, monocytes, granulocytes, or transformed B cell lines. It is absent from stem cell precursors in the bone marrow, but is expressed by approximately 90% of thymocytes (Fox et al. 1982) and therefore appears on the T cell surface earlier than the T3 antigen. Surprisingly, this otherwise T cell-restricted antigen is present on most chronic lymphocytic leukemias of B cell origin and is a diagnostic indicator for that malignancy (BOUMSELL et al. 1980; ROYSTON et al. 1980).

The precise function of CD5 has not yet been determined, but two interesting phenomena have been observed. CD5 appears to be involved in induction of helper function by $CD4^+$ T cells which function in the differentiation of B cells to immunoglobulin-producing cells. Cultures of $CD4^+$ cells with OKT1 or OKT1-F(ab')2 for 3 h in the presence of non-sheep red blood cell (SRBC) rosetting peripheral blood leukocytes [E-rosette($-$)] results in the production of a factor or factors, which drive the differentiation of B cells to immunoglobulin-producing cells (THOMAS et al. 1984a). Supernatants of $CD4^+$ cells cultured with OKT1 in the absence of E^- cells do not provide the same activity, suggesting that interaction of CD5 with OKT1 effects B cell differentiation indirectly via an E-rosette($-$) cell subpopulation. More recently, CD5-specific antibodies have been shown to enhance the anti-CD3-induced proliferation of T cells under conditions of suboptimal monocyte participation, suggesting a regulatory role for CD5 in T cell proliferation (LEDBETTER et al. 1985). Further study is required to define the function of this T cell differentiation molecule more completely.

3. T11-CD2

Lymphocytes of T lineage had been defined operationally as that subset of lymphocytes [E-rosette($+$)] able to form nonimmune rosettes with SRBC (JONDAL et al. 1972; FORLAND 1972). The T cell differentiation antigen which imparts that ability has been identified by a variety of mAbs as a 50 kdalton glycoprotein (KUNG et al. 1980; KAMOUN et al. 1981; HOWARD et al. 1981; VERBI et al. 1982) designated CD2 (IUIS-WHO 1985). CD2 is expressed by all thymocytes and peripheral blood E-rosette($+$) T cells, surface immunoglobulin-negative (sIg^-) tonsil cells, and 10% of bone marrow cells. The CD2 antigen density is greater on thymocytes than it is on peripheral T cells, and its presence on all thymocytes indicates that its appearance precedes that of CD5 and CD3. CD2 is expressed only on uncultured leukemias and transformed leukemic cell lines determined to be T cell in origin by other markers. Evidence that CD2 represents the receptor for SRBC is threefold: (a) a high positive correlation exists between cells able to form rosettes with SRBC and cells bearing CD2; (b) many mAbs directed toward CD2 block the ability of cells to form rosettes with SRBC; and (c) modulation of CD2 from the cell surface by interaction with an anti-CD2 mAb under appropriate conditions results in the loss of the ability to form rosettes.

CD2 was first shown to be a functionally significant T cell differentiation antigen by VAN WAUWE et al. (1981). They observed that the addition of an anti-CD2 mAb (OKT11A) to lymphocytes cultured with alloantigen, lectins, or soluble antigen blocked the proliferative response triggered by these stimuli. Binding of radiolabeled OKT11A was not reduced in the presence of the lectins, and they concluded that the inhibition of lectin-induced proliferation was not due to direct binding competition by OKT11A. Furthermore, proliferation was not blocked at the antigen recognition level since anti-CD2 mAbs added to cultures as late as 48 h – 72 h after soluble antigen or alloantigen were able to prevent lymphocyte proliferation (Tadmori et al. 1985).

Like CD3-specific antibodies, certain anti-CD2-specific antibodies are able to block specific T cell-mediated lympholysis (CTL); however, unlike anti-CD3s, which block at a post-effector–target cell conjugate stage, anti-CD2s block conjugate formation (Krensky et al. 1984). The inhibitory effect is greatest if the antibody is bound to the effector and not the target cell (Krensky et al. 1983). In addition to preventing specific T cell-mediated lympholysis, antibodies to certain CD2 epitopes are able to block NK cell-mediated lysis (Martin et al. 1983). The mechanism of inhibition and its relationship to T cell-mediated lysis has not yet been determined.

At least four distinct epitopes have been identified on CD2 by mAbs (Bernard et al. 1982; Meuer et al. 1984). Normal resting peripheral T cells bear only two of the epitopes, one of which defines the receptor for SRBC. Two additional epitopes are fully displayed only after activation or membrane perturbation of resting T cells. Identification of these hidden epitopes led to the discovery that interaction of certain combinations of anti-CD2 with CD2 can produce T cell activation.

The epitope defined by D-66 is partially masked on resting T cells by sialic acid residues, but is readily detected on immature and activated T cells. Incubation of T cells with D-66 and an anti-CD2 directed to the epitope which defines the SRBC receptor results in a strong, monocyte-dependent proliferative response (Brottier et al. 1985). The monocyte requirement is bypassed by exogenous IL-2, and expression of IL-2 receptors is induced in the absence of monocytes.

The epitope defined by anti-T11$_3$ appears on activated T cells, but is not detected on immature T cells. Unlike D-66, anti-T11$_3$ is mitogenic for T cells in cooperation with an mAb directed to the resting CD2 epitope not associated with SRBC binding. Induction of proliferation by this anti-CD2 combination is not monocyte dependent (Meuer et al. 1984). Interestingly, CD3$^-$ thymocytes can be induced to proliferate by the anti-CD2/anti-T11$_3$ pair only in the presence of exogenous IL-2, but IL-2 receptor expression by these cells occurs in the absence of exogenous IL-2 (Fox et al. 1985). It has not been reported whether monocytes can replace exogenous IL-2 in this system. Discovery of the natural ligand for CD2 will be important for understanding the regulation of T cells via CD2.

II. Growth Factor Receptors

Functional surface proteins not restricted to T lineage lymphocytes include receptors for molecules necessary for cell proliferation. The characterization of two such receptors, namely the receptors for IL-2 and transferrin, has been greatly accelerated by the availability of mAbs to these structures.

1. Tac: Receptor for IL-2

IL-2, formerly known as T cell growth factor, is a 14.5 kdalton peptide produced by T cells in response to lectin- or antigen-induced stimulation (see Chap. 8). It permits the establishment of long-term lines and clones of untransformed T cells that have distinct biologic function and antigen specificity (SMITH 1980). The observation that [³H] IL-2 binds to cells that respond to IL-2 and not to other cells suggested the existence of a specific receptor for this polypeptide (ROBB et al. 1981).

UCHIYAMA et al. (1981) prepared an mAb, termed anti-Tac (T cell activation antigen), which reacted with the IL-2-dependent T cell line derived from a patient with mycosis fungoides, but did not react with a transformed B cell line established from the same patient. The antigen recognized by this antibody was found on activated T cells, but not on freshly separated, resting T cells, B cells, or monocytes, or on IL-2-independent transformed T cell lines or B cell lines. IL-2-dependent cultured T cells were, however, reactive with anti-Tac.

The fact that anti-Tac prevented the proliferation of cloned T cell lines induced by IL-2 and that anti-Tac blocked the binding of IL-2 to Tac-bearing cells suggested that anti-Tac and IL-2 might bind to the same molecule (MIYAWAKI et al. 1982; LEONARD et al. 1982). This was confirmed by sequential immunoprecipitation of extracts of radiolabeled Tac-positive T-cell blasts with IL-2 covalently bound to Affigel (Biorad, Richmond) and anti-Tac coupled to Sepharose. All material capable of binding to IL-2 on its support was removed by preincubation with anti-Tac on its support (ROBB and GREENE 1983).

The T cell receptor for IL-2, as defined by anti-Tac, is a glycoprotein of 55–65 kdalton. N- and O-linked oligosaccharides contribute 20–25 kdaltons to the total size, and the molecule is both sulfated and phosphorylated (WANO et al. 1984; LEONARD et al. 1985a). The primary translation product does not bind IL-2. Post-translational processing results in precursor forms of 33, 35, and 37 kdaltons which, although not fully glycosylated, can bind IL-2 (LEONARD et al. 1985a).

Receptors of both high and low affinity are present on activated T cells. The latter bind with a several thousandfold lower affinity and are at least tenfold more abundant (ROBB et al. 1984). The functional significance of this finding is unknown at present, as is the mechanism by which IL-2 regulates the expression of its own receptors (WELTE et al. 1984).

The expression of Tac on malignancies of B cell lineage (KORSMEYER et al. 1983) prompted careful investigation of normal activated B cells. TSUDO et al. (1984) demonstrated by two-color immunofluorescence the expression of Tac antigen on sIg⁺ B cells activated with Staphylococcus aureus Cowan I (SAC). Furthermore, activated B cells could be induced to proliferate by IL-2, and IL-2-induced proliferation could be inhibited by anti-Tac (WALDMANN et al. 1984). Anti-Tac was also shown to block SAC-induced secretion of Ig by B cells. The Tac antigens immunoprecipitated from T and B cells were found to be indistinguishable on the basis of chymotryptic peptide analysis (MITTLER et al. 1985; BOYD et al. 1985).

Molecular cloning of cDNA encoding the human IL-2 receptor revealed the presence of two species of mRNA (1.5 and 3.5 kilobases) in several cell types bearing IL-2 receptors (LEONARD et al. 1984; NIKAIDO et al. 1984). The deduced protein sequence suggested a short intracytoplasmic positively charged domain with two potential phosphorylation sites at the carboxy terminus, a 19 amino acid hydrophobic transmembrane region, and a 219 residue extracellular domain with two potential N-linked glycosylation sites. Cloning of the gene itself (Leonard et al. 1985 b) led to the identification of two transcription initiation sites in normal activated T cells and the existence of an additional site in HTLV-I-infected adult T leukemia cells. The significance of the third initiation site as well as the many alternative mRNA splicing possibilities in both types of cells remains to be determined.

2. T9: Receptor for Transferrin

A surface glycoprotein important for lymphocyte as well as nonlymphoid cell proliferation is the receptor for transferrin, an iron transport protein found in serum. mAbs to the receptor were isolated and partially characterized prior to their identification as anti-transferrin receptor antibodies. OKT9 was derived from a mouse immunized both with lymphocytes isolated from a patient with acute T lymphoblastic leukemia and with thymocytes (Kung et al. 1980). This antibody binds to a subset of thymocytes (Reinherz et al. 1980 b) as well as a wide variety of leukemia and tumor cell lines, immature hematopoietic cells, fetal thymus and liver, and normal, activated, but not resting lymphocytes (Sutherland et al. 1981). Similarly, B3/25, an antibody derived by immunization with a hematopoietic cell line, K562, was shown to bind to all cultured human hematopoietic cell lines tested, and expression of B3/25 was shown to be related to cell proliferation (Omary et al. 1980).

Analysis of B3/25 immunoprecipitates from detergent-lysed, radiolabeled cells by SDS–polyacrylamide gel electrophoresis under reducing and nonreducing conditions revealed a disulfide-bonded dimer consisting of two subunits, each 110 kdaltons (Omary et al. 1980). The antigen recognized by B3/25 was shown to be a glycoprotein containing an asparagine-linked complex, high mannose oligosaccharides and covalently bound fatty acid (Omary and Trowbridge 1981). Structural studies with OKT9 revealed an antigen of similar size. The T9 antigen is a phosphorylated transmembrane molecule, the major part of which is extracellular (Schneider et al. 1982; Terhorst et al. 1981).

The size of the antigen identified by OKt9 and B3/25, and its association with cell proliferation led to its identification as the receptor for transferrin. Goding and Burns (1981) showed by peptide mapping that both OKT9 and transferrin, if coupled to agarose, precipitated identical proteins; Sutherland et al. (1981) and Trowbridge and Omary (1981) precipitated radiolabeled transferrin bound to its receptor with OKT9 and B3/25, respectively. The availability of mAbs to the transferrin receptor has facilitated the generation of another mAb (42/6) to the same receptor, capable of specifically inhibiting transferrin-mediated iron uptake (Trowbridge and Lopez 1982). Antibody 42/6 inhibits the growth of CEM cells in tissue culture and establishes the functional importance of the cell surface transferrin receptor. mAbs have also been used to monitor the transfer of the human transferrin receptor gene into mouse fibroblasts (Newman et al. 1983), the cell type from which the gene was subsequently cloned (Kuhn et al. 1984). The primary amino acid sequence of the transferrin receptor has been deduced from cDNA clones (SCHNEIDER et al. 1984; MCCLELLAND et al. 1984). Unlike many surface glycoproteins, there is no NH_2 terminal signal peptide, and the NH_2 terminus remains cytoplasmic. It consists of 62 residues, among which are four serines which could function as phosphate acceptors. A 26 residue, hydrophobic, transmembrane segment is followed by the large 648 residue extracellular COOH terminus. This model is consistent with earlier trypsin cleavage data (SCHNEIDER et al. 1982). The protein has no homology to any other known protein.

III. Receptors for Components of Complement

Fragments of the third component of the complement system have been reported to have a variety of immunoregulatory activities (WEILER et al. 1982; FEARON and WONG 1983). mAbs which identify the cellular receptors for some of these fragments can help define the consequences of receptor–ligand interaction.

1. CR2: Receptor for C3d

The first CR2-binding mAb was isolated on the basis of its identification of a B cell-specific antigen, B2 (NADLER et al. 1981). The B2 antigen is restricted to the sIg^+ cells of the blood, certain tumors of B cell origin, and Epstein–Barr virus (EBV)-transformed B cell lines. Tissue distribution studies with anti-B2 and other mAbs to this antigen, namely HB-5 (TEDDER et al. 1984) and OKB7 (MITTLER et al. 1983; KNOWLES et al. 1984), demonstrate the predominance of B2-bearing cells in the primary and secondary follicles and mantle zones of lymphoid tissues, and the complete absence of the antigen from a number of nonlymphoid tissues. The antigen is found neither in fetal liver nor on plasma cells; it is expressed by pre-B cells containing cytoplasmic IgM, and by mature circulating B cells, but is lost with further differentiation. Thus, B2 is a highly restricted B cell differentiation antigen.

The cellular distribution of B2 prompted IIDA et al. (1983) to examine its relationship to CR2, a B lymphocyte surface molecule with high affinity for the C3d fragment of the third component of complement. They prepared radiolabeled B cell membranes which were allowed to adsorb to either anti-B2-coated Sepharose beads or C3-Sepharose beads. The eluted material in both instances was 140 kdalton and had a common pI. In addition, the material eluted from the C3-Sepharose was shown to bind specifically to anti-B2 Sepharose and C3d-Sepharose. Anti-B2 was unable, however, to inhibit completely the binding of C3d-coated erythrocytes to B cells. Complete inhibition of binding was observed only in the presence of cross-linking goat anti-mouse immunoglobulin. This suggests that the epitopes on CR2 recognized by C3d and anti-B2 are distinct. Similarly, *S. aureus* cells containing bound HB-5 and HB-5 antigen specifically adhere to C3d-coated erythrocytes (WEIS et al. 1984). Inhibition of binding of C3d-coated erythrocytes to B cells by HB-5 occurs only if HB-5 is cross-linked with anti-mouse immunoglobulin. OKB7, however, directly blocks C3d rosetting, indicating a close association of the B7 epitope with the C3d-binding site on CR2 (RAO et al. 1985).

Evidence that EBV and fragments of the third component of complement bind to a closely related or identical receptor on B cells has existed for several years. The HB-5 mAb was used to demonstrate that a single molecule performs both of these receptor functions. SB cell lysates containing HB-5 antigen, when bound by immunoaffinity to HB-5-coated protein A particles, specifically bind ^{125}I-labeled EBV (FINGEROTH et al. 1984).

EBV is a well-known T cell-independent polyclonal B cell stimulator. Antibodies to CR2 (EBV receptor) have recently been shown to induce proliferation and Ig secretion in peripheral blood B cells; however, soluble or bound C3 fragments have not had a similar effect (WILSON et al. 1985; NEMEROW et al. 1985). Unlike EBV stimulation, anti-CR2-induced proliferation is T cell dependent. Interestingly, not all anti-CR2-specific antibodies are mitogenic; the restriction is not isotype related, but rather epitope dependent. At least four functionally distinct epitopes on CR2 have now been defined by mAbs. These are distinguished by the ability of the mAb to inhibit binding of EBV and/or C3d, or to induce B cell proliferation and/or differentiation. These reagents may provide the means to elucidate the mechanism by which EBV activates B cells and the role of C3d in its interaction with CR2.

2. CR3: Receptor for C3bi

The leukocyte surface molecule defined by the mAbs Mac-1, OKM1, OKM9, OKM10, and Mo1 is expressed: (a) by the majority of large, adherent, Ia$^+$ peripheral blood monocytes required for soluble antigen-induced T cell proliferation; (b) by smaller nonadherent Ia$^-$T3$^-$ peripheral blood mononuclear cells that include null cells and large granular lymphocytes; (c) by a subset of T cells bearing low levels of T3 antigen; and (d) by granulocytes (BREARD et al. 1980; AULT and SPRINGER 1981; TODD et al. 1981; TALLE et al. 1983). Immunoprecipitation of detergent lysates of monocytes or granulocytes with these antibodies reveals a noncovalently linked heterodimer consisting of a 165 kdalton α chain polypeptide and a 95 kdalton β chain polypeptide. The β subunit is associated with two other distinct α subunits, each with unique cellular distribution, which comprise a family of leukocyte adhesion glycoproteins (SANCHEZ-MADRID et al. 1983). The aforementioned mAbs bind to epitopes confined to the 165 kdalton α chain. A cellular distribution pattern similar to that of Mac-1 has been described for CR3, a complement receptor which mediates adhesion of monocytes and granulocytes to C3bi-sensitized particles (ROSS and LAMBRIS 1982).

Evidence that Mac-1 has C3bi-binding activity was first presented by BELLER et al. (1982). Binding of C3bi-coated erythrocytes, but not C3b-coated erythrocytes, which bind to CR1, was diminished by preincubation of human granulocytes with anti-Mac-1. Additional evidence was provided by WRIGHT et al. (1983). Down regulation of monocyte surface molecules by interaction with mAbs OKM1, OKM9, OKM10, or IB4 anchored to a solid support resulted in the specific loss of C3bi, but not C3b-binding capacity. Among those antibodies, each of which recognizes a distinct epitope on the Mac-1 antigen, only OKM10 directly inhibited attachment of C3bi-coated particles. Furthermore, protein A-Sepharose beads containing either IB4 or OKM1, but not OKM10 and specific antigen derived from cell lysates were able to bind C3bi. mAbs to other monocyte surface proteins were unable to mediate binding of C3bi. The recognition site for C3bi is most precisely defined by OKM10 on the α subunit, but IB4 and other antibodies which bind the β subunit (HILDRETH and AUGUST 1985) are able to partially block C3bi attachment. This effect is most likely indirect since cells that are devoid of the Mac-1 α subunit, but express large amounts of the β subunit in conjunction with other α subunits, do not possess CR3 activity.

IV. Leukocyte Adhesion Molecules LFA-1 and LFA-3

The mAbs which define LFA-1 and LFA-3 were discovered through implementation of a functional screen designed to identify surface molecules associated with human T lymphocyte-mediated cytolysis. Each of these antibodies was isolated for its ability to inhibit anti-HLA-DR-specific cytotoxic T cell activity. The LFA-1 antigen is a heterodimeric glycoprotein consisting of noncovalently associated 177 kdalton (α) and 95 kdalton (β) subunits. Its expression is widely distributed within cells of hematopoietic lineage. It is found on peripheral blood lymphocytes, monocytes, granulocytes, and large granular lymphocytes as well as most thymocytes and approximately 40% of cells in the bone marrow. LFA-3 is a 60 kdalton monomeric glycoprotein and is not restricted to the hematopoietic lineage (SANCHEZ-MADRID et al. 1982; KRENSKY et al. 1983).

Preincubation of effector or target cells with anti-LFA-1 or anti-LFA-3 demonstrated that anti-LFA-1 inhibits T cell-mediated lympholysis at the level of the effector cell, whereas anti-LFA-3 blocks the target cell (KRENSKY et al. 1983). Unlike CD3-specific antibodies which allow effector:target conjugate formation, both anti-LFA-1 and anti-LFA-3 prevent the binding of effectors to targets (KRENSKY et al. 1984). The possibility exists, therefore, that LFA-1 and LFA-3 function as mutual ligands. Arguments against this hypothesis are as follows: 1. Anti-LFA-1, but not anti-LFA-3, blocks NK-mediated cytolysis, even though LFA-3 is expressed by the NK target K562 (KRENSKY et al. 1984). 2. Treatment of target cells with trypsin results in the loss of anti-LFA-3 inhibition of T cell-mediated lympholysis as well as loss of the LFA-3 epitope defined by anti-LFA-3, whereas inhibition of T cell-mediated lympholysis by anti-LFA-1 is markedly enhanced if trypsinized target cells are used. The possibility remains, however, that an LFA-3 trypsin-insensitive epitope functions as the LFA-1 ligand (GROMKOWSKI et al. 1985). 3. mAbs to LFA-1, but not LFA-3, prevent spontaneous intercellular aggregation of the B lymphoblastoid line JY (MENTZER et al. 1985 b).

Additional evidence for the intercellular adhesive function of LFA-1 is provided from experiments in which the antiproliferative effects of antibodies to LFA-1 were measured. Most of the stimuli which induce proliferation of T lymphocytes require cellular interaction. For example, in the mixed lymphocyte reaction, responder T cells interact with allogeneic HLA-DR-bearing stimulator cells; stimulation of T cells by soluble antigens or anti-CD3 mAbs occurs only in the presence of adherent monocytes. Anti-LFA-1 mAbs inhibit T cell proliferation in all these circumstances where cellular interaction is required (KRENSKY et al. 1983; DONGWORTH et al. 1985). Conversely, direct stimulation of T cells by pairs of CD2-specific antibodies or by anti-CD3 coupled to Sepharose is not impaired by LFA-1-specific antibodies.

LFA-1, like Mac-1 (CR3), (see Sect. C.III.2) belongs to glycoprotein family comprised of distinct α subunits and common β subunits. The α or β subunit specificity for a number of mAbs has been determined by dissociation of the subunits at alkaline pH prior to immunoprecipitation. An mAb with β chain specificity (T51/18) was shown to immunoprecipitate three distinct α chains from radiolabeled granulocytes corresponding to LFA-1 (177 kdalton), Mac-1 (165 kdalton), and a novel p150 (150 kdalton). Clearing granulocyte lysates with the anti-β subunit mAb prior to adding various anti-α chain-specific mAbs resulted in substantial reduction in the amount of α chain precipitated. Cross-linking of radiolabeled cell lysates with a cleavable bifunctional reagent and subsequent immunoprecipitation with α subunit-specific mAbs and analysis by sodium dodecylsulfate–polyacrylamide gel electrophoresis (SDS–PAGE) revealed an $\alpha_1\beta_1$ stoichiometry. Isoelectric focusing and SDS–PAGE on the cleaved immunoprecipitates demonstrated identical β subunits and distinct α subunits (SANCHEZ-MADRID et al. 1983). NH_2 terminal sequence analysis of murine LFA-1 and Mac-1 α chains showed 33% homology. The α subunits are therefore structurally related. In addition, the murine LFA-1 α subunit NH_2 terminus shares homology with human interferons α and β, 35% and 26%, respectively (SPRINGER et al. 1985). The functional relationship of the α subunits is as yet unknown; however, a newly developed mAb to the p150 (α) subunit, anti-Leu-M5, does not inhibit many of the functions affected by antibodies to LFA-1 or Mac-1 (LANIER et al. 1985).

Deficiency of the Mac-1, LFA-1, p150,95 family of glycoproteins results in a heritable disease characterized clinically by recurrent bacterial infections, progressive periodontitis, delayed wound healing, and persistent granulocytosis. Granulocytes from these patients have depressed phagocytic function and are deficient in adherence, chemotaxis, and antibody-dependent cell-mediated cytotoxicity (ADCC). The ADCC defect is manifested by lack of effector : target cell adhesion. Granulocyte Fc receptor function is normal in these patients. Since all members of the Mac-1, LFA-1, p150,95 antigen family are deficient in this disease and because normal α subunit precursors are synthesized, but not assembled with the β subunit, it is believed that the primary genetic defect is in the β subunit (SPRINGER et al. 1984; SPRINGER and ANDERSON 1985; KOHL et al. 1984). Further studies of functional defects of cells from these patients should extend the understanding of this interesting group of surface glycoproteins.

D. Recognition Molecules

There are a limited number of T lymphocyte-restricted antigens which appear to be involved in the recognition of cell surface components associated with immune function.

I. T4 and T8: Class II and Class I Recognition Molecules

The T cell differentiation antigens CD4 (defined by mAb OKT4/Leu-3) and CD8 (defined by mAb OKT8/Leu-2) are expressed by mutually exclusive, mature T cell subsets. The $CD8^+$ (T8) subset is generally associated with cytotoxic and suppressor function and corresponds to the T cell subset originally identified by the anti-TH$_2$ heteroserum (REINHERZ et al. 1980c). Lyt-2 is the murine homolog of CD8 (ZAMOYSKA et al. 1985). The CD4$^+$ (T4) subset, first identified by the mAb OKT4 (KUNG et al. 1979), is historically associated with helper or inducer function in many assays (REINHERZ et al. 1979b,c). L3T4 is the murine homologue (DIALYNAS et al. 1983). Assignment of CD4-bearing and CD8-bearing cells to distinct functional subsets has been contradicted, however, by the observation that CD4$^+$ cells can exhibit both suppressor (THOMAS et al. 1981) and cytotoxic (MORETTA et al. 1981) behavior. Similarly, irradiated, activated OKT8$^+$ cells can amplify the plaque-forming cell response under conditions of suboptimal help by fresh OKT4$^+$ cells (THOMAS et al. 1984b).

The highly restricted expression of CD4 and CD8 prompted numerous investigators to explore the functions of the molecules with mAbs to various epitopes. Evidence that CD4 and CD8 participate in cellular recognition events derives from experiments in which CD4-specific antibodies blocked cytotoxicity by CD4$^+$ cells (REINHERZ et al. 1982), blocked proliferation of CD4$^+$ cells to alloantigen and soluble antigen (ENGLEMAN et al. 1981a, 1983; BIDDISON et al. 1982, 1983), and prevented CD4$^+$-induced B cell differentiation (ROGOZINSKI et al. 1984). Similar observations were made with CD8$^+$ cells and CD8-specific antibodies. Inhibition of cytotoxicity was shown to result from prevention of effector–target adhesion and not at a postconjugate event, as occurs with CD3-specific antibodies (PLATSOUCAS 1984; LANDEGREN et al. 1982; BIDDISON et al. 1984b). Not all anti-CD4 or anti-CD8 mAbs are equally effective at inhibiting cytotoxicity (BIDDISON et al. 1984a), and it is likely, therefore, that specific epitopes on the CD4 and CD8 molecules are involved in cellular interactions. Some cytotoxic T cell clones are not susceptible to intervention by mAbs (MORETTA et al. 1984), but this may be dependent on the overall affinity of the effector for the target (BIDDISON et al. 1984a).

The target structures recognized by CD4 and CD8 appear to be monomorphic regions of Mhc class II and Mhc class I molecules, respectively. Bulk cultures of CD4$^+$ cells or long-term lines or clones of CD4$^+$ cells kill targets or proliferate in response to cells that share Mhc class II antigens with the original stimulator. mAbs to monomorphic determinants of class II molecules inhibit the cytotoxicity. Conversely, CD8$^+$ cells respond to class I structures and are blocked by mAbs to monomorphic regions of class I molecules (ENGLEMAN et al. 1981b; MEUER et al. 1982; KRENSKY et al. 1982a, b; BALL and STASTNY 1982; BIDDISON et al. 1982, 1983). Direct demonstration of CD4 association with Mhc class II or CD8 with Mhc class I molecules has not, however, been achieved.

In addition to the Mhc recognition function attributed to CD4 and CD8, a role for transduction of a negative signal has been postulated. An anti-CD4 mAb has been shown to block anti-CD3-induced proliferation of CD4$^+$, but not CD8$^+$ cells in a system independent of class II-bearing cells (BANK and CHESS 1985). Moreover, when CD4$^+$ or CD8$^+$ cytotoxic T cell clones are triggered nonspecifically (by lectins or CD3-specific antibodies) to kill targets negative for Mhc class II or Mhc class I molecules, respectively, lysis is inhibited by the appropriate anti-CD4 or anti-CD8 mAbs (FLEISCHER et al. 1986). The consequences of an Mhc molecule–CD4/CD8 interaction may therefore be more than intercellular adhesion.

The CD8 glycoprotein is a covalent dimer of two 32 kdalton subunits on mature peripheral T cells, although it can exist in the thymus as covalent heteromultimers consisting of associations of the 32 kdalton subunits with 46 kdalton subunits. The 46 kdalton subunit is identical to the cortical thymocyte restricted marker CD1 (T6) which is also found associated noncovalently with β_2 microglobulin and is therefore Mhc class I in character (TERHORST et al. 1981; SNOW and TERHORST 1983; SNOW et al. 1985). CD4 is a 60 kdalton monomeric glycoprotein (TERHORST et al. 1980). Genes encoding CD4 and CD8 have been cloned and the protein structures deduced are strikingly similar. Both molecules are integral membrane glycoproteins which share amino acid sequence homology with the immunoglobulin supergene family. Each has an extracellular NH_2 terminal domain, part of which is homologous to an immunoglobulin light chain V region, a transmembrane stretch homologous to that of Mhc class II β chains, and a charged cytoplasmic domain. Overall, however, CD4 and CD8 share a low sequence homology (LITTMAN et al. 1985; SUKHATME et al. 1985; MADDON et al. 1985).

The foregoing illustrates the contribution hybridoma technology has made toward identifying and understanding the role of CD4 in the immune response. Additional interest in mAbs to CD4 stems from the fact that they have recently become important in defining the means by which the human retrovirus HTLV-III/LAV infects T cells. Treatment of $CD4^+$ T cells with anti-CD4 mAbs blocks HTLV-III/LAV binding, syncytia formation, and infectivity (DALGLEISH et al. 1984; KLATZMANN et al. 1984; McDOUGAL et al. 1985). Moreover, CD4 has been coprecipitated with the viral envelope glycoprotein gp110, which indicates that CD4 may function as part of the virus receptor (McDOUGAL et al. 1986). Anti-CD4 mAbs may figure prominently in the development of vaccines and therapies for acquired immunodeficiency syndrome (AIDS).

II. T Cell Receptor for Antigen

Prior to the mAb era, the receptor for antigen on T cells remained elusive. An mAb to a murine T cell lymphoma was developed which identified a tumor-specific molecule composed of disulfide-linked protein subunits of 39 and 41 kdalton. Analysis of the surface proteins of T and B cells from various sources by two dimensional SDS–PAGE revealed structures of similar size only on T cells. A heteroserum to the affinity-purified, tumor-specific molecule was used to immunoprecipitate similar structures from different T cell populations and two-dimensional tryptic peptide maps revealed constant and variable peptides within each protein subunit (ALLISON et al. 1982; McINTYRE and ALLISON 1983). The tumor-specific molecule could not be identified as the T cell receptor for antigen, however, since its antigenic specificity was unknown and it could not therefore be assigned an antigen-specific function.

The availability of functional T cell clones permitted the development of mAbs to "clonotypic" structures. Cloned T cell lines with defined antigenic specificity and function were used as immunogens, and antibodies reactive with the immunizing T cell clones, but not other T cell clones were identified. The anti-clonotypic mAbs blocked or stimulated antigen-specific responses of only the appropriate T cell clone and specifically immunoprecipitated similar, but not identical structures from the appropriate clone in parallel experiments. These structures each contained variable and constant peptide regions (HASKINS et al. 1983; KAYE et al. 1983; MEUER et al. 1983a; SAMELSON et al. 1983; STAERZ et al. 1984).

Production of mAbs to a clonotypic structure on a class I-directed cytotoxic human T cell clone permitted MEUER et al. (1983a) to study the relationship of the clonotypic structure to other known human T cell surface molecules. Antibody-induced modulation experiments and competitive binding studies showed CD3 to be closely associated with the clonotypic structure (MEUER et al. 1983a, b). Biochemical evidence for the CD3 association was provided by OETTGEN et al. (1984). The human clonotypic heterodimer consists of a 45–55 kdalton (α) subunit and a 37–45 kdalton (β) subunit. Both deglycosylated peptide backbones are 33–34 kdalton. Clonotype-specific antibodies to tumor cell lines have permitted the isolation of sufficient quantities of α and β chain for partial amino acid sequence determination. Sequence data has been used to confirm the cloning of genes encoding these proteins. The genes for the T cell receptor resemble Ig genes in both overall structure and the requirement for DNA rearrangement before expression. Most information regarding the fine structure of the T cell receptor has been deduced from cDNA sequences and is the subject of several review articles (MAK and YANAGI 1984; DAVIS 1985; HOOD et al. 1985; KAYE et al. 1984). The recent observation that the mAb WT-31 (TAX et al. 1983) recognizes a constant region of the T cell receptor (SPITS et al. 1985b) will permit direct analysis of its structure and biosynthesis from T cells for which no anti-clonotypic mAbs exist.

E. Summary

The ability to utilize hybridization to immortalize and clone antibody-producing B cells at a high frequency has provided a powerful tool for the identification and understanding of many molecules involved in immune function. Only a small percentage of antigens expressed in a restricted fashion within the immune system have as yet been clearly associated with a given function; undoubtedly, steady progress in this area will continue. Identification of novel epitopes on known molecules may also help elucidate their function, as was demonstrated with CD2. Monoclonal antibodies are now indispensable not only in categorizing the cell surface effector and regulatory molecules of the immune system, but also as probes for their function.

Note in proof: The literature review for this article was completed in late 1985. Significant advances, too numerous to mention here, have added extensively to our knowledge of lymphocyte surface proteins.

References

Allison JP, McIntyre BW, Bloch D (1982) Tumor-specific antigen of murine T-lymphoma defined with monoclonal antibody. J Immunol 129:2293–2300

Ault KA, Springer TA (1981) Cross reaction of a rat anti-mouse phagocyte specific monoclonal antibody (anti-Mac-1) with human monocytes and natural killer cells. J Immunol 126:359–364

206   M. A. Talle and G. Goldstein

Ball EJ, Stastny P (1982) Cell-mediated cytotoxicity against HLA-D-region products expressed in monocytes and B lymphocytes. IV: Characterization of effector cells using monoclonal antibodies against human T-cell subsets. Immunogenetics 16:157–169

Bank I, Chess L (1985) Perturbation of the T4 molecule transmits a negative signal to T cells. J Exp Med 162:1294–1303

Beller DI, Springer TA, Schreiber RD (1982) Anti-Mac-1 selectively inhibits the mouse and human type three complement receptor. J Exp Med 156:1000–1009

Bernard A, Gelin C, Raynal B, Pham D, Gosse C, Boumsell L (1982) Phenomenon of human T cells rosetting with sheep erythrocytes analyzed with monoclonal antibodies. "Modulation" of a partially hidden epitope determining the conditions of interactions between T cell and erythrocytes. J Exp Med 155:1317–1333

Biddison WE, Rao PE, Talle MA, Goldstein G, Shaw S (1982) Possible involvement of the OKT4 molecule in T cell recognition of class II HLA antigens. Evidence from studies of cytotoxic T lymphocytes specific for SB antigens. J Exp Med 156:1065–1076

Biddison WE, Rao PE, Talle MA, Goldstein G, Shaw S (1983) Possible involvement of the T4 molecule in T cell recognition of class II HLA antigens: evidence from studies of proliferative responses to SB antigens. J Immunol 131:152–157

Biddison WE, Rao PE, Talle MA, Goldstein G, Shaw S (1984a) Possible involvement of the T4 molecule in T cell recognition of class II HLA antigens. Evidence from studies of CTL-target cell binding. J Exp Med 159:783–797

Biddison WE, Rao PE, Talle MA, Boselli CM, Goldstein G (1984b) Distinct epitopes on the T8 molecule are differentially involved in cytotoxic T cell function. Hum Immunol 9:117–130

Borst J, Prendiville MA, Terhorst C (1982) Complexity of the human T lymphocyte-specific cell surface antigen T3. J Immunol 128:1560–1565

Borst J, Alexander S, Elder J, Terhorst C (1983) The T3 complex on human T lymphocytes involves four structurally distinct glycoproteins. J Biol Chem 258:5135–5141

Boumsell L, Coppin H, Pham D, Raynal R, Lemerle J, Dausset J, Bernard A (1980) An antigen shared by a human T cell subset and B cell chronic lymphocytic leukemia cells. J Exp Med 152:229–234

Boyd AW, Fisher DC, Fox DA, Schlossman SF, Nadler LM (1985) Structural and functional characterization of IL 2 receptors on activated human B cells. J Immunol 134:2387–2392

Breard J, Reinherz EL, Kung PC, Goldstein G, Schlossman SF (1980) A monoclonal antibody reactive with human peripheral blood monocytes. J Immunol 124:1943–1953

Brenner MB, Trowbridge IS, Strominger JL (1985) Cross-linking of human T cell receptor proteins: association between the T cell idiotype β subunit and the T3 glycoprotein heavy subunit. Cell 40:183–190

Brottier P, Boumsell L, Gelin C, Bernard A (1985) T cell activation via CD2[T,gp50] molecules: accessory cells are required to trigger T cell activation via CD2-D66 plus CD2-9.6/T11$_1$ epitopes. J Immunol 135:1624–1631

Ceuppens JL, Bloemmen FJ, van Wauwe JP (1985) T cell unresponsiveness to the mitogenic activity of OKT 3 antibody results from a deficiency of monocyte Fc receptors for murine IgG2a and inability to cross-link the T3-Ti complex. J Immunol 135:3882–3886

Chang TW, Kung PC, Gingras SP, Goldstein G (1981) Does OKT3 monoclonal antibody react with an antigen-recognition structure on human T cells? Proc Natl Acad Sci USA 78:1805–1808

Chatenoud L, Baudrihaye MF, Kreis H, Goldstein G, Schindler J, Bach J-F (1982) Human in vivo antigenic modulation induced by the anti-T cell OKT3 monoclonal antibody. Eur J Immunol 12:979–982

Dalgleish AG, Beverly PCL, Clapham PR, Crawford DH, Greaves MF, Weiss RA (1984) The CD4 (T4) antigen is an essential component of the receptor for the AIDS retrovirus. Nature 312:763–767

Davis MM (1985) Molecular genetics of the T cell-receptor beta chain. Annu Rev Immunol 3:537–560

Dialynas DP, Quan ZS, Wall KA, Pierres A, Quintans J, Loken MR, Pierres M, Fitch F (1983) Characterization of the murine T cell surface molecule, designated L3T4, identified by monoclonal antibody GK1.5: similarity of L3T4 to the human Leu-3/T4 molecule. J Immunol 131:2445–2451

Dongworth DW, Gotch FM, Hildreth JEK, Morris A, McMichael AJ (1985) Effects of monoclonal antibodies to the α and β chains of the human lymphocyte function-associated (H-LFA-1) antigen on T lymphocyte functions. Eur J Immunol 15:888–892

Engleman EG, Benike CJ, Glickman E, Evans RL (1981 a) Antibodies to membrane structures that distinguish suppressor/cytotoxic and helper T lymphocyte subpopulations block the mixed leukocyte reaction in man. J Exp Med 153:193–198

Engleman EG, Benike CJ, Grumet FC, Evans RL (1981 b) Activation of human T lymphocyte subsets: helper and suppressor/cytotoxic T cells recognize and respond to distinct histocompatibility antigens. J Immunol 127:2124–2129

Engleman EG, Benike CJ, Metzler C, Gatenby PA, Evans RL (1983) Blocking of human T lymphocyte functions by anti-Leu-2 and anti-Leu-3 antibodies: differential inhibition of proliferation and suppression. J Immunol 130:2623–2628

Fearon DT, Wong WW (1983) Complement ligand-receptor interactions that mediate biological responses. Annu Rev Immunol 1:243–271

Fingeroth JD, Weis JJ, Tedder TF, Strominger JL, Biro PA, Fearon DT (1984) Epstein-Barr virus receptor of human B lymphocytes is the C3d receptor CR2. Proc Natl Acad Sci USA 81:4510–4514

Fleischer B, Schrezenmeier H, Wagner H (1986) Function of the CD4 and CD8 molecules on human cytotoxic T lymphocytes: regulation of T cell triggering. J Immunol 136:1625–1628

Forland SS (1972) Binding of sheep erythrocytes to human lymphocytes. A probable market of T lymphocytes. Scand J Immunol 1:269–277

Fox DA, Hussey RE, Fitzgerald KA, Bensussan A, Daley JF, Schlossman SF, Reinherz EL (1985) Activation of human thymocytes via the 50KD T11 sheep erythrocyte binding protein induces the expression of interleukin 2 receptors on both T3$^+$ and T3$^-$ populations. J Immunol 134:330–335

Fox RI, Harlow D, Royston I, Elder J (1982) Structural characterization of the human T cell surface antigen (p67) isolated from normal and neoplastic lymphocytes. J Immunol 129:401–405

Freshney RI (1983) Culture of animal cells. A manual of basic technique. Liss, New York

Galfre G, Milstein C (1981) Preparation of monoclonal antibodies: strategies and procedures. Methods Enzymol 73:1–46

Gefter ML, Margulies DH, Scharff MD (1977) A simple method for polyethylene glycol-promoted hybridization of mouse myeloma cells. Somat Cell Genet 3:231–236

Goding JW (1983) Monoclonal antibodies: principles and practice. Academic, London

Goding JW, Burns GF (1981) Monoclonal antibody OKT-9 recognizes the receptor for transferrin on human acute lymphocytic leukemia cells. J Immunol 127:1256–1258

Gromkowski SH, Krensky AM, Martz E, Burakoff SJ (1985) Functional distinctions between the LFA-1, LFA-2, and LFA-3 membrane proteins on human CTL are revealed with trypsin-pretreated target cells. J Immunol 134:244–249

Hager DA, Burgess RR (1980) Elution of proteins from sodium dodecyl sulfate-polyacrylamide gels, removal of sodium dodecyl sulfate, and renaturation of enzymatic activity: results with sigma subunit of *Escherichia coli* RNA polymerase, wheat germ DNA topoisomerase, and other enzymes. Anal Biochem 109:76–86

Haskins K, Kubo R, White J, Pigeon M, Kappler J, Marrack P (1983) The major histocompatibility complex-restricted antigen receptor on T cells. I. Isolation with a monoclonal antibody. J Exp Med 157:1149–1169

Hildreth JEK, August JT (1985) The human lymphocyte function-associated (HLFA) antigen and a related macrophage differentiation antigen (HMac-1): functional effects of subunit-specific monoclonal antibodies. J Immunol 134:3272–3280

Hood L, Kronenberg M, Hunkapiller T (1985) T cell antigen receptors and the immunoglobulin supergene family. Cell 40:225–229

Howard FD, Ledbetter JA, Wong J, Bieber CP, Stinson EB, Herzenberg LA (1981) A human T lymphocyte differentiation marker defined by monoclonal antibodies that block E-rosette formation. J Immunol 126:2117–2122

Iidia K, Nadler L, Nussenzweig V (1983) Identification of the membrane receptor for the complement fragment C3d by means of a monoclonal antibody. J Exp Med 158:1021–1033

Imboden JG, Stobo JD (1985) Transmembrane signalling by the T cell antigen receptor. Perturbation of the T3-antigen receptor complex generates inositol phosphates and releases calcium ions from intracellular stores. J Exp Med 161:446–456

Iuis-Who (1985) Nomenclature subcommittee. J Immunol 134:659–660

Jondal M, Holm G, Wigzell H (1972) Surface markers on human T and B lymphocytes. I. A large population of lymphocytes forming nonimmune rosettes with sheep red blood cells. J Exp Med 136:207–215

Kamoun M, Martin JP, Hansen JA, Brown MA, Siadak AW, Nowinski RC (1981) Identification of a human T lymphocyte surface protein associated with the E-rosette receptor. J Exp Med 153:207–212

Kanellopoulos JM, Wigglesworth NM, Owen MJ, Crumpton MJ (1983) Biosynthesis and molecular nature of the T3 antigen of human T lymphocytes. EMBO J 2:1807–1814

Kaneoka H, Perez-Rojas G, Sasasuki T, Benike CJ, Engleman EG (1983) Human T lymphocyte proliferation induced by a PAN-T monoclonal antibody (Anti-Leu 4): heterogeneity of response is a function of monocytes. J Immunol 131:158–164

Kaye J, Porcelli S, Tite J, Jones B, Janeway CA Jr (1983) Both a monoclonal antibody and antisera specific for determinants unique to individual cloned helper T cell lines can substitute for antigen and antigen-presenting cells in the activation of T cells. J Exp Med 158:836–856

Kaye J, Jones B, Janeway CA Jr (1984) The structure and function of T cell receptor complexes. Immunol Rev 81:39–64

Kearney JF, Radbruch A, Liesegang B, Rajewsky K (1979) A new mouse myeloma cell line which has lost immunoglobulin expression but permits the construction of antibody in secreting hybrid cell lines. J Immunol 123:1548–1550

Klatzmann D, Champagne E, Chamaret S, Gruest J, Guetard D, Hercend T, Gluckman J-C, Montagnier L (1984) T-lymphocyte T4 molecule behaves as the receptor for human retrovirus LAV. Nature 312:767–768

Knowles DM II, Tolidjan B, Marboe CC, Mittler RS, Talle MA, Goldstein G (1984) Distribution of antigens defined by OKB monoclonal antibodies on benign and malignant lymphoid cells and on nonlymphoid tissues. Blood 63:886–896

Kohl S, Springer TA, Schmalstieg FC, Loo LS, Anderson DC (1984) Defective natural killer cytotoxicity and polymorphonuclear leukocyte antibody-dependent cellular cytotoxicity in patients with LFA-1/OKM-1 deficiency. J Immunol 133:2972–2978

Kohler G, Milstein C (1975) Continuous cultures of fused cells secreting antibody of predefined specificity. Nature 256:495–497

Kohler G, Howe SC, Milstein C (1976) Fusion between immunoglobulin-secreting and non-secreting myeloma cell lines. Eur J Immunol 6:292–295

Korsmeyer SJ, Greene WC, Cossman J, Hsu SM, Jensen JP, Neckers LM, Marshall SL et al. (1983) Rearrangement and expression of immunoglobulin genes and expression of Tac antigen in hairy cell leukemia. Proc Natl Acad Sci USA 80:4522–4526

Krensky AM, Reiss CS, Mier JW, Strominger JL, Burakoff JJ (1982a) Long-term human cytolytic T-cell lines allospecific for HLA-DR6 antigen are OKT4$^+$. Proc Natl Acad Sci USA 79:2365–2369

Krensky AM, Clayberger C, Reiss CS, Strominger JL, Burakoff SJ (1982b) Specificity of OKT4$^+$ cytotoxic T lymphocyte clones. J Immunol 129:2001–2003

Krensky AM, Sanchez-Madrid F, Robbins E, Nagy JA, Springer TA, Burakoff SJ (1983) The functional significance, distribution, and structure of LFA-1, LFA-2, and LFA-3: cell surface antigens associated with CTL-target interactions. J Immunol 131:611–616

Krensky AM, Robbins E, Springer T, Burakoff SJ (1984) LFA-1, LFA-2, and LFA-3 antigens are involved in CTL-target conjugation. J Immunol 132:2180–2182

Kuhn LC, McClelland A, Ruddle FH (1984) Gene transfer, expression and molecular cloning of the human transferrin receptor gene. Cell 37:95–103

Kung PC, Goldstein G, Reinherz EL, Schlossman SF (1979) Monoclonal antibodies defining distinctive human T cell surface antigens. Science 206:347–349

Kung PC, Talle MA, DeMaria M, Butler M, Lifter J, Goldstein G (1980) Strategies for generating monoclonal antibodies defining human T lymphocyte differentiation antigens. Transplant Proc [Suppl 1] 12:141–146

Landegren U, Ramstedt U, Axberg I, Ullberg M, Jondal M, Wigzell H (1982) Selective inhibition of human T cell cytotoxicity at levels of target recognition or initiation of lysis by monoclonal OKT3 and Leu-2a antibodies. J Exp Med 155:1579–1584

Lanier LL, Arnaout MA, Schwarting R, Warner NL, Ross G (1985) p150/95, Third member of the LFA-1/CR3 polypeptide family identified by anti-Leu M5 monoclonal antibody. Eur J Immunol 15:713–718

Ledbetter JA, Martin PJ, Spooner CE, Wofsy D, Tsu TT, Beatty PG, Gladstone P (1985) Antibodies to Tp67 and Tp44 augment and sustain proliferative responses of activated T cells. J Immunol 134:2331–2336

Leeuwenberg JFM, Spits H, Tax WJM, Capel PJA (1985) Induction of nonspecific cytotoxicity by monoclonal anti-T3 antibodies. J Immunol 134:3770–3775

Leonard WJ, Depper JM, Uchiyama T, Smith KA, Waldmann TA, Greene WC (1982) A monoclonal antibody that appears to recognize the receptor for human T-cell growth factor; partial characterization of the receptor. Nature 300:267–269

Leonard WJ, Depper JM, Crabtree GR, Rudikoff S, Pumphrey J, Robb RJ, Kronke M et al. (1984) Molecular cloning and expression of cDNAs for the human interleukin-2 receptor. Nature 311:626–631

Leonard WJ, Depper JM, Kronke M, Robb RJ, Waldmann TA, Greene WC (1985a) The human receptor for T-cell growth factor. Evidence for variable post-translation processing, phosphorylation, sulfation, and the ability of precursor forms of the receptor to bind T-cell growth factor. J Biol Chem 260:1872–1880

Leonard WJ, Depper JM, Kanehisa M, Kronke M, Peffer NJ, Svetlik PB, Sullivan M, Greene WC (1985b) Structure of the human interleukin-2 receptor gene. Science 230:633–639

Littman DR, Thomas Y, Maddon PJ, Chess L, Axel R (1985) The isolation and sequence of the gene encoding T8: a molecule defining functional classes of T lymphocytes. Cell 40:237–246

Looney RJ, Abraham GN (1984) The Fc portion of intact IgG blocks stimulation of human PBMC by anti-T3. J Immunol 133:154–156

Mac TW, Yanagi Y (1984) Genes encoding the T cell antigen receptor. Immunol Rev 81:221–233

Maddon PJ, Littman DR, Godfrey M, Maddon DE, Chess L, Axel R (1985) The isolation and nucleotide sequence of a cDNA encoding the T cell surface protein T4: a new member of the immunoglobulin gene family. Cell 42:93–104

Martin PJ, Longton G, Ledbetter JA, Newman W, Braun MP, Beatty PG, Hansen JA (1983) Identification and functional characterization of two distinct epitopes on the human T cell surface protein Tp50. J Immunol 131:180–185

McClelland A, Kuhn LC, Ruddle FH (1984) The human transferrin receptor gene: genomic organization, and the complete primary structure of the receptor deduced from a cDNA sequence. Cell 39:267–274

McDougal JS, Mawle A, Cort SP, Nicholson JKA, Cross GD, Scheppler-Campbell JA, Hicks D, Sligh J (1985) Cellular tropism of the human retrovirus HTLV-III/LAV. I. Role of T cell activation and expression of the T4 antigen. J Immunol 135:3151–3162

McDougal JS, Kennedy MS, Sligh JM, Cort SP, Mawle A, Nicholson JKA (1986) Binding of HTLV-III/LAV to T4$^+$ T cells by a complex of the 110K viral protein and the T4 molecule. Science 231:382–395

McIntyre BW, Allison JP (1983) The mouse T cell receptor: structural heterogeneity of molecules of normal T cells defined by xenoantiserum. Cell 34:739–746

Mentzer SJ, Barbosa JA, Burakoff SJ (1985a) T3 monoclonal antibody activation of nonspecific cytolysis: a mechanism of CTL inhibition. J Immunol 135:34–38

Mentzer SJ, Gromkowski SH, Krensky AM, Burakoff SJ, Martz E (1985b) LFA-1 membrane molecule in the regulation of homotypic adhesions of human B lymphocytes. J Immunol 135:9–11

Meuer SC, Schlossman SF, Reinherz EL (1982) Clonal analysis of human cytotoxic T lymphocytes: T4$^+$ and T8$^+$ effector T cells recognize products of different major histocompatibility complex regions. Proc Natl Acad Sci USA 79:4395–4399

Meuer SC, Fitzgerald KA, Hussey RE, Hodgdon JC, Schlossman SF, Reinherz EL (1983a) Clonotypic structures involved in antigen-specific human T cell function. Relationship to the T3 molecular complex. J Exp Med 157:705–719

Meuer SC, Acuto O, Hussey RE, Hodgdon JC, Fitzgerald KA, Schlossman SF, Reinherz EL (1983b) Evidence for the T3-associated 90K heterodimer as the T-cell antigen receptor. Nature 303:808–810

Meuer SC, Hussey RE, Fabbi M, Fox D, Acuto O, Fitzgerald KA, Hodgdon JC, et al. (1984) An alternative pathway of T cell activation: a functional role for the 50 Kd T11 sheep erythrocyte receptor protein. Cell 36:897–906

Mittler RS, Talle MA, Carpenter K, Rao PE, Goldstein G (1983) Generation and characterization of monoclonal antibodies reactive with human B lymphocytes. J Immunol 131:1754–1761

Mittler R, Rao P, Olini G, Westberg E, Newman W, Hoffmann M, Goldstein G (1985) Activated human B cells display a functional IL 2 receptor. J Immunol 134:2393–2399

Miyawaki T, Yachie A, Uwadana N, Ohzeki S, Nagaoki T, Taniguchi N (1982) Functional significance of Tac antigen expressed on activated human T lymphocytes: Tac antigen interacts with T cell growth factor in cellular proliferation. J Immunol 129:2474–2478

Moretta L, Mingari MC, Sekaly PR, Moretta A, Chapuis B, Cerottini J-C (1981) Surface markers of cloned human T cells with various cytolytic activities. J Exp Med 154:569–574

Moretta A, Pantaleo G, Mingari MC, Moretta L, Cerottini J-C (1984) Clonal heterogeneity in the requirement for T3, T4 and T8 molecules in human cytolytic T lymphocyte function. J Exp Med 159:921–934

Nadler LM, Stashenko P, Hardy R, van Agthoven A, Terhorst C, Schlossman SF (1981) Characterization of a human B cell-specific antigen (B2) distinct from B1. J Immunol 126:1941–1947

Nemerow GR, McNaughton ME, Cooper NR (1985) Binding of monoclonal antibody to the Epstein Barr virus (EBV)/CR2 receptor induces activation and differentiation of human B lymphocytes. J Immunol 135:3068–3073

Newman R, Domingo D, Trotter J, Trowbridge I (1983) Selection and properties of a mouse L-cell transformant expressing human transferrin receptor. Nature 304:643–645

Nikaido T, Shimizu A, Ishida N, Sabe H, Teshigawara K, Maeda M, Uchiyama T, Yodoi J, Honjo T (1984) Molecular cloning of cDNA encoding human interleukin-2 receptor. Nature 311:631–635

Oettgen HC, Kappler J, Tax WJM, Terhorst C (1984) Characterization of the two heavy chains of the T3 complex on the surface of human T lymphocytes. J Biol Chem 259:12039–12048

Omary MB, Trowbridge IS (1981) Biosynthesis of the human transferrin receptor in cultured cells. J Biol Chem 256:12888–12892

Omary MB, Trowbridge IS, Minowada J (1980) Human cell-surface glycoprotein with unusual properties. Nature 286:888–891

Pessano S, Oettgen H, Bhan AK, Terhorst C (1985) The T3/T cell receptor complex: antigenic distinction between the two 20-kd T3 (T3-δ and T3-E) subunits. EMBO J 4:337–344

Platsoucas CD (1984) Human T cell antigens involved in cytotoxicity against allogeneic or autologous chemically modified targets. Association of the Leu2a/T8 antigen with effector-target binding and of the T3/Leu 4 antigen with triggering. Eur J Immunol 14:566–577

Rao PE, Wright SD, Westberg EF, Goldstein G (1985) OKB7, a monoclonal antibody that reacts at or near the C3d binding site of human CR2. Cell Immunol 93:549–555

Reinherz EL, Kung P, Goldstein G, Schlossman S (1979a) A monoclonal antibody with selective reactivity with mature human thymocytes and all peripheral human T cells. J Immunol 123:1312–1317

Reinherz EL, Kung PC, Goldstein G, Schlossman SF (1979b) Separation of functional subsets of human T cells by a monoclonal antibody. Proc Natl Acad Sci USA 76:4061–4065

Reinherz EL, Kung PC, Goldstein G, Schlossman SF (1979c) Further characterization of the human inducer T cell subset defined by monoclonal antibody. J Immunol 123:2894–2896

Reinherz EL, Hussey RE, Schlossman SF (1980a) A monoclonal antibody blocking human T cell function. Eur J Immunol 10:758–762

Reinherz EL, Kung PC, Goldstein G, Levey RH, Schlossman SF (1980b) Discrete stages of human intrathymic differentiation: analysis of normal thymocytes and leukemic lymphoblasts of T-cell lineage. Proc Natl Acad Sci USA 77:1588–1592

Reinherz EL, Kung PC, Goldstein G, Schlossman SF (1980c) A monoclonal antibody reactive with the human cytotoxic/suppressor T cell subset previously defined by a heteroserum termed TH_2. J Immunol 124:1301–1307

Reinherz EL, Meuer S, Fitzgerald KA, Hussey RE, Levine H, Schlossman SF (1982) Antigen recognition by human T lymphocytes is linked to surface expression of the T3 molecular complex. Cell 30:735–743

Robb RJ, Greene WC (1983) Direct demonstration of the identity of T cell growth factor binding protein and the TAC antigen. J Exp Med 158:1332–1337

Robb RJ, Munck A, Smith KA (1981) T cell growth factor receptors. Quantitation, specificity, and biological relevance. J Exp Med 154:1455–1474

Robb RJ, Greene WC, Rusk CM (1984) Low and high affinity cellular receptors for interleukin 2. Implications for the level of Tac antigen. J Exp Med 160:1126–1146

Rogozinski L, Bass A, Glickman E, Talle MA, Goldstein G, Wang J, Chess L, Thomas Y (1984) The T4 surface antigen is involved in the induction of helper function. J Immunol 132:735–739

Ross GD, Lambris JD (1982) Identification of a C3bi-specific membrane complement receptor that is expressed on lymphocytes, monocytes, neutrophils, and erythrocytes. J Exp Med 155:96–110

Royston I, Majda J, Baird S, Yanamoto G, Meserve B, Griffiths J (1980) Human T cell antigen defined by monoclonal antibody: the 65000 dalton antigen is found on CLL cells bearing surface immunoglobulin. J Immunol 125: 725–731

Samelson LE, Germain RN, Schwartz RH (1983) Monoclonal antibodies against the antigen receptor on a cloned T-cell hybrid. Proc Natl Acad Sci USA 80:6972–6976

Samelson LE, Harford JB, Klausner RD (1985) Identification of the components of the murine T cell antigen receptor complex. Cell 43:223–231

Sanchez-Madrid F, Krensky AM, Ware CF, Robbins E, Strominger JL, Burakoff SJ, Springer TA (1982) Three distinct antigens associated with human T-lymphocyte-mediated cytolysis: LFA-1, LFA-2, and LFA-3. Proc Natl Acad Sci USA 79:7489–7493

Sanchez-Madrid F, Nagy JA, Robbins E, Simon P, Springer TA (1983) A human leukocyte differentiation family with distinct α-subunits and a common β subunit: the lymphocyte function-associated antigen (LFA-1), the C3bi complement receptor (OKM1/MAC-1), and the p150,95 molecule. J Exp Med 158:1785–1803

Schneider C, Sutherland R, Newman R, Greaves M (1982) Structural features of the cell surface receptor for transferrin that is recognized by the monoclonal antibody OKT9. J Biol Chem 257:8516–8522

Schneider C, Owen MJ, Banville D, Williams JG (1984) Primary structure of human transferrin receptor deduced from the mRNA sequence. Nature 311:675–678

Shulman M, Wilde CD, Kohler G (1978) A better cell line for making hybridomas secreting specific antibodies. Nature 276:269–270

Smith KA (1980) T cell growth factor. Immunol Rev 51:337–357

Snow PM, Terhorst C (1983) The T8 antigen is a multimeric complex of two distinct subunits on human thymocytes but consists of homomultimeric forms on peripheral blood T lymphocytes. J Biol Chem 258:14675–14681

Snow PM, van de Rijn M, Terhorst C (1985) Association between the human thymic differentiation antigens T6 and T8. Eur J Immunol 15:529–532

Spits H, Borst J, Terhorst C, de Vries JE (1982) The role of T cell differentiation markers in antigen-specific and lectin-dependent cellular cytotoxicity mediated by $T8^+$ and $T4^+$ human cytotoxic T cell clones directed at class I and Class II MHC antigens. J Immunol 129:1563–1569

Spits H, Yssel H, Leeuwenberg J, de Vries JE (1985 a) Antigen-specific cytotoxic T cell and antigen-specific proliferating T cell clones can be induced to cytolytic activity by monoclonal antibodies against T3. Eur J Immunol 15:88–91

Spits H, Borst J, Tax W, Capel PJA, Terhorst C, de Vries JE (1985 b) Characteristics of a monoclonal antibody (WT-31) that recognizes a common epitope on the human T cell receptor for antigen. J Immunol 135:1922–1928

Springer TA, Anderson DC (1985) Functional and structural interrelationships among the Mac-1, LFA-1 family of leukocyte adhesion glycoproteins, and their deficiency in a novel heritable disease. In: Springer AA (ed) Hybridoma technology in the biosciences and medicine. Plenum, New York, pp 191–206

Springer TA, Thompson WS, Miller LJ, Schmalstieg FC, Anderson DC (1984) Inherited deficiency of the Mac-1, LFA-1, p150,95 glycoprotein family and its molecular basis. J Exp Med 160:1901–1918

Springer TA, Teplow DB, Dreyer WT (1985) Sequence homology of the LFA-1 and Mac-1 leukocyte adhesion glycoproteins and unexpected relation to leukocyte interferon. Nature 314:540–542

Staerz UD, Pasternack MS, Klein JR, Benedetto JD, Bevan MJ (1984) Monoclonal antibodies specific for a murine cytotoxic T-lymphocyte clone. Proc Natl Acad Sci USA 81:1799–1803

Sukhatme VP, Sizer KC, Vollmer AC, Hunkapiller T, Parnes JR (1985) The T cell differentiation antigen Leu-2/T8 is homologous to immunoglobulin and T cell receptor variable regions. Cell 40:591–597

Sutherland R, Delia D, Schneider C, Newman R, Kemshead J, Greaves M (1981) Ubiquitous cell-surface glycoprotein on tumor cells is proliferation-associated receptor for transferrin. Proc Natl Acad Sci USA 78:4515–4519

Tadmori W, Reed JC, Nowell PC, Kamoun M (1985) Functional properties of the 50 Kd protein associated with the E-receptor on human T lymphocytes: suppression of IL-2 production by anti-p50 monoclonal antibodies. J Immunol 134:1709–1716

Talle MA, Rao PE, Westberg E, Allegar N, Makowski M, Mittler RS, Goldstein G (1983) Patterns of antigenic expression on human monocytes as defined by monoclonal antibodies. Cell Immunol 78:83–99

Tax WJM, Willems HW, Reekers PPM, Capel PJA, Koene RAP (1983) Polymorphism in mitogenic effect of IgG1 monoclonal antibodies against T3 antigen on human T cells. Nature 304:445–447

Tedder TF, Clement LT, Cooper MD (1984) Expression of C3d receptors during human B cell differentiation: immunofluorescence analysis with the HB-5 monoclonal antibody. J Immunol 133:678–683

Terhorst C, van Agthoven A, Reinherz E, Schlossman S (1980) Biochemical analysis of human T lymphocyte differentiation antigens T4 and T5. Science 209:520–521

Terhorst C, van Agthoven A, LeClair K, Snow P, Reinherz E (1981) Biochemical studies of the human thymocyte cell-surface antigens T6, T9 and T10. Cell 23:771–780

Thomas Y, Rogozinski L, Irigoyen OH, Friedman S, Kung PC, Goldstein G, Chess L (1981) Functional analysis of human T cell subsets defined by monoclonal antibodies. IV. Induction of suppressor cells within the OKT4[+] population. J Exp Med 154:459–467

Thomas Y, Glickman E, DeMartino J, Wang J, Goldstein G, Chess L (1984 a) Biologic functions of the OKT1 T cell surface antigen. I. The T1 molecule is involved in helper function. J Immunol 133:724–728

Thomas Y, Rogozinski L, Rabbani L, Chess A, Goldstein G, Chess L (1984 b) Functional analysis of T cell subsets defined by monoclonal antibodies. VI. Distinct and opposing immunoregulatory functions within the OKT8[+] population. J Mol Cell Immunol 1:103–110

Todd RF III, Nadler LM, Schlossman SF (1981) Antigens on human monocytes identified by monoclonal antibodies. J Immunol 126:1435–1442

Trowbridge IS, Lopez F (1982) Monoclonal antibody to transferrin receptor blocks transferrin binding and inhibits human tumor cell growth in vitro. Proc Natl Acad Sci USA 79:1175–1179

Trowbridge IS, Omary MB (1981) Human cell surface glycoprotein related to cell proliferation is the receptor for transferrin. Proc Natl Acad Sci USA 78:3039–3043

Tsoukas CD, Carson DA, Fong S, Vaughan JH (1982) Molecular interactions in human T cell-mediated cytotoxicity to EBV. II. Monoclonal antibody OKT3 inhibits a postkiller-target recognition/adhesion step. J Immunol 129:1421–1425

Tsudo M, Uchiyama T, Uchino H (1984) Expression of Tac antigen on activated normal human B cells. J Exp Med 160:612–617

Uchiyama T, Broder S, Waldmann TA (1981) A monoclonal antibody (anti-Tac) reactive with activated and functionally mature human T cells. I. Production of anti-Tac monoclonal antibody and distribution of Tac (+) cells. J Immunol 126:1393–1397

Umiel T, Daley JF, Bhan AK, Levey RH, Schlossman SF, Reinherz EL (1982) Acquisition of immune competence by a subset of human cortical thymocytes expressing mature T cell antigens. J Immunol 129:1054–1060

Van Agthoven A, Terhorst C, Reinherz E, Schlossman S (1981) Characterization of T cell surface glycoproteins T1 and T3 on all human peripheral T lymphocytes and functionally mature thymocytes. Eur J Immunol 11:18–21

Van den Elsen P, Shepley BA, Borst J, Coligan JE, Markham AF, Orkin S, Terhorst C (1984) Isolation of cDNA clones encoding the 20K T3 glycoprotein of human T-cell receptor complex. Nature 312:413–418

Van Wauwe J, Goossens J (1981) Mitogenic actions of Orthoclone OKT3 on human peripheral blood lymphocytes: effects of monocytes and serum components. Int J Immunopharmacol 3:203–208

Van Wauwe JP, de Mey JR, Goossens JG (1980) OKT3: a monoclonal anti-human T lymphocyte antibody with potent mitogenic properties. J Immunol 124:2708–2713

Van Wauwe J, Goossens J, Decock W, Kung P, Goldstein G (1981) Suppression of human T-cell mitogenesis and E-rosette formation by the monoclonal antibody OKT11A. Immunology 44:865–871

Verbi W, Greaves MF, Schneider C, Koubek K, Janossy G, Stein H, Kung P, Goldstein G (1982) Monoclonal antibodies OKT11 and OKT11A have pan-T reactivity and block sheep erythrocyte receptors. Eur J Immunol 12:81–86

Waldmann TA, Goldman CK, Robb RJ, Depper JM, Leonard WJ, Sharrow SO, Bongiovanni KF, Korsmeyer SJ, Greene WC (1984) Expression of interleukin 2 receptors on activated human B cells. J Exp Med 160:1450–1466

Wano Y, Uchiyama T, Fukui K, Maeda M, Uchino H, Yodoi J (1984) Characterization of human interleukin 2 receptor (Tac antigen) in normal and leukemic T cells: co-expression of normal and aberrant receptors on HUT-102 cells. J Immunol 132:3005–3010

Weiler JM, Ballas ZK, Needham BW, Hobbs MV, Feldbush EJ (1982) Complement fragments suppress lymphocyte immune responses. Immunol Today 3:238–243

Weis JJ, Tedder TF, Fearon DT (1984) Identification of 145,00 M_r membrane protein as the C3d receptor (CR2) of human B lymphocytes. Proc Natl Acad Sci USA 81:881–885

Weiss A, Imboden J, Shoback D, Stobo J (1984) Role of T3 surface molecules in human T-cell activation: T3-dependent activation results in an increase in cytoplasmic free calcium. Proc Natl Acad Sci USA 81:4169–4173

Welte K, Andreeff M, Platzer E, Holloway K, Rubin BY, Moore MAS, Mertelsmann R (1984) Interleukin 2 regulates the expression of TAC antigen on peripheral blood T lymphocytes. J Exp Med 159:1390–1403

Wilson BS, Platt JL, Kay NE (1985) Monoclonal antibodies to the 140,000 mol wt glycoprotein of B lymphocyte membranes (CR2 receptor) initiate proliferation of B cells in vitro. Blood 66:824–829

Wright SD, Rao PE, van Voorhis WC, Craigmyle LS, Iida K, Talle MA, Westberg EF, Goldstein G, Silverstein SC (1983) Identification of the C3bi receptor of human monocytes and macrophages by using monoclonal antibodies. Proc Natl Acad Sci USA 80:5699–5703

Zamoyska R, Vollmer AC, Sizer KC, Liaw CW, Parnes JR (1985) Two Lyt-2 polypeptides arise from a single gene by alternative splicing patterns of mRNA. Cell 43:153–163

Interleukin 1 Production from Various Cells and Measurement of its Multiple Biologic Activities

C. A. DINARELLO

A. Introduction

Interleukin 1 (IL-1) now refers to a family of polypeptides which are produced by the host in response to injury, infection, and various immunologic reactions. To date, two forms have been cloned. Recombinant IL-1s confirm the multiple and diverse biologic properties that had been described previously for natural IL-1s. IL-1 is unique among the lymphokines. Unlike IL-2, colony-stimulating factors, or the interferons, IL-1 has been known by many names, each one reflecting a different biologic property (reviewed in DINARELLO 1984). For example, it had been described for its ability to produce fever (endogenous pyrogen activity), to induce acute phase changes (leukocytic endogenous mediator), to stimulate synovial cell prostaglandin E_2 and collagenase release (mononuclear cell factor), to augment mitogen and antigen responses in B cells (B cell-activating factor), to activate T cells and induce IL-2 and IL-2 receptors (lymphocyte-activating factor), to induce cartilage breakdown (catabolin), to initiate muscle proteolysis (muscle proteolysis-inducing factor), and to stimulate bone resorption (osteoclast-activating factor).

At the beginning of 1985, the issue of whether a single molecule was capable of eliciting so many diverse changes in a variety of cells remained unresolved. In late 1984, two forms of IL-1 had been cloned and the complete amino acid sequences (derived from the cDNAs) were described. A human blood monocyte IL-1 cDNA was first reported in October at the Fourth International Lymphokine Conference (AURON et al. 1984) and the report of a mouse cDNA cloned from the macrophage cell line P388D was published in November (LOMEDICO et al. 1984). From these two different amino acid sequences, it was clear that there was more than a single IL-1 gene coding for IL-1.

The two sequences correlated with two of the isoelectric focusing points of IL-1; the human cDNA coded for the pI 7 form and the mouse cDNA coded for the pI 5 form. These two forms can also be called β and α, respectively. Although the human homolog of the mouse IL-1-α form has been reported (MARCH et al. 1985; GUBLER et al. 1986), the human IL-1-β is the dominant form at both the mRNA and protein level. In human cells, particularly human blood monocytes, the amount of mRNA coding for the IL-1-β form approaches 5% of the total polyadenylated RNA which exceeds the IL-1-α form by a factor of 100 or more. Analysis of the protein sequences revealed that they shared a common region near the carboxy terminus which, being conserved, probably represented, or was associated with, a putative active site (AURON et al. 1985). During 1985, these two forms were expressed in bacterial and mammalian cells and recombinant forms of IL-1 were made available. For the general area of IL-1 research, the recombinant IL-1s have been very important because they were needed to confirm the multiple biologic activities attributed to this substance. For the most part, recombinant IL-1 of either form induces the same broad spectrum of biologic responses which had been reported for IL-1s purified from cell cultures (reviewed in DINARELLO 1986). Even the most optimistic of the early investigators working with the IL-1 molecules could hardly have predicted the biologic significance of its various and diverse effects. It is increasingly clear that IL-1 is involved in nearly every organ system or homeostatic mechanism which changes during the host's defense against infection, injury, malignancy, inflammation, or antigenic challenge. What remains unclear is whether IL-1 participates in normal physiology or cellular function in the absence of infection or injury. IL-1 seems to be a biologically fundamental molecule; this concept is supported by the fact that IL-1 is old (estimated at 400 million years) and evolved before lymphocytes and immunoglobulins.

B. Production of IL-1 In Vitro

I. IL-1 Induction from Peripheral Blood Monocytes

1. Unstimulated/Stimulated Cells

The peripheral blood monocyte is probably the most potent source of IL-1. Mononuclear cells are usually separated from whole heparinized blood with Ficoll–Hypaque or commercially available lymphocyte-separating media. The latter may be contaminated with endotoxins, which will result in stimulation of IL-1 production from apparently "unstimulated" cells. As little as 100 pg/ml endotoxin is sufficient to induce IL-1 production from blood monocytes, particularly human blood monocytes. Some investigators have reported that 50 pg/ml endotoxin induces IL-1 from these cells (DUFF and ATKINS 1982; DINARELLO and KRUEGER 1986). The mononuclear cells do not need to be separated into populations of lymphocytes and monocytes for routine IL-1 production unless the experimental design includes this consideration.

Cells are usually suspended in low endotoxin content Eagle's minimal essential medium containing 10 mM HEPES buffer, penicillin, and streptomycin. Monocytes do not require L-glutamine for IL-1 synthesis. As noted already, the endotoxin concentration should be less than 100 pg/ml. The choice of serum depends on the stimulus employed. In general, 1%–5% v/v autologous serum, and for human cells pooled AB serum, can be used. Regardless of the serum source, all sera should be heat inactivated at 56 °C for 30 min, and then centrifuged (10 000 g) to remove aggregates. These procedures reduce the likelihood of nonspecific stimulation of IL-1 production from resting mononuclear cells. Fetal calf serum is often contaminated with endotoxin or growth factors, which can result in IL-1 production; use of fetal calf serum in IL-1 production is not indicated under normal conditions.

In addition to low endotoxin culture media, the concentration of cells and the ratio of vessel surface size to cell number are important considerations in obtaining minimal IL-1 production from unstimulated cells. Mononuclear cells crowded in a pellet at the bottom of an upright tube can become "autostimulated" and produce IL-1 by close cell contact

(DINARELLO 1981). The optimal concentration range seems to be $1-5 \times 10^6$ mononuclear cells/ml in flat-bottom wells so that there are between 1 and 5×10^6 cells/cm². Under these conditions, the supernatant medium does not contain significant IL-1 (DINARELLO et al. 1984c). The level of "significant" IL-1 is, of course, relative to the assay employed; however, as discussed later, IL-1 mRNA synthesis and translation occurs as a result of contact with culture vessel surfaces. Therefore, there is never an "unstimulated" monocyte in culture in terms of IL-1 production. Circulating cells in blood, when carefully harvested so as not to perturb them, do not have detectable IL-1 mRNA nor IL-1 protein (AURON et al. 1984). During the first hour of culture, there is evidence of IL-1 RNA transcription and translation of protein despite no apparent source of stimulant, i.e., endotoxin or other known monocyte activators. Nevertheless, under these conditions, the amount of IL-1 found in the supernatant medium after 24–48 h is low or undetectable by several assay methods.

2. Intracellular/Extracellular IL-1

Until recently, most investigations concerning the production of IL-1 were based on the presence of IL-1 activity in the supernatant medium. There is now sufficient evidence that IL-1 is initially synthesized as a 31 kdalton precursor polypeptide which is then "processed" or "cleaved" to a 17 kdalton peptide which is the size found in cell culture supernatants. IL-1 (23 kdalton) can also be found in the supernatants of stimulated monocytes (DINARELLO et al. 1985). The evidence is derived from the molecular cloning of IL-1 (AURON et al. 1984; LOMEDICO et al. 1984), metabolically labeled IL-1 (GIRI et al. 1985), and biologic activity following gel filtration in physiologic media (DINARELLO et al. 1974; LEPE-ZUNIGA et al. 1985; SAHASRABUDDHE et al. 1985). The IL-1 31 kdalton precursor lacks a clear signal peptide. This lack of a signal peptide has been demonstrated in both forms of IL-1 (AURON et al. 1984; LOMEDICO et al. 1984). Hence, the mechanism for cleavage and transport remains unclear. Furthermore, IL-1 has been found on the surface of macrophages (KURT-JONES et al. 1985a) and this "membrane-bound" IL-1 may represent IL-1 which is trapped in the cell membrane as it is being processed or transported.

The early studies by the late Dr. Phyllis BODEL (1970) had established that, 4 h following stimulation by *Staphylococcus albus*, human blood monocytes contained detectable levels of intracellular IL-1. In her studies on protein synthesis inhibitors and IL-1 production, the endogenous pyrogen fever assay was used. Extracellular IL-1 was found after 9 h, and the kinetics of production and release demonstrated that intracellular levels of IL-1 were elevated and then slowly depleted as extracellular IL-1 increased in the supernatant. The method used for extracting the intracellular IL-1 was multiple cycles of freeze-thawing in physiologic media. More recently, LEPE-ZUNIGA et al. (1985) have reported that sonication and the use of nonionic detergents facilitated the extraction of intracellular IL-1. Intracellular IL-1 appears as several high molecular weight species on gel filtration (70, 45, and 26 kdalton) (LEPE-ZUNIGA et al. 1985), but with 8 mM CHAPS detergent, the multiple molecular weights of the extracellular IL-1 were observed around 15 kdalton. This was also shown with a hypotonic buffer (SAHASRABUDDHE et al. 1985). These results suggest that some of the intracellular IL-1 is likely to be aggregated or bound to high molecular weight proteins.

At present, it seems that an assessment of IL-1 production must include a separate analysis of both the intracellular and extracellular compartment (GERY et al. 1981; Lepe-Zuniga and Gery 1984). For example, some cells (astrocytes) do not release much IL-1, but have considerable levels of intracellular IL-1 following stimulation (Fontana et al. 1982b, 1984). B cell IL-1 production may also have a similar pattern (Kurt-Jones et al. 1985b).

3. Activators of IL-1 Production and Release

Activators of IL-1 production seem to have two roles: (a) they increase mRNA levels; and (b) they contribute to the processing and transport of IL-1 into the extracellular compartment. This latter mechanism has received considerable attention. Depending on the type of stimulus or activator, IL-1 release may be considerable; however some activators induce large amounts of IL-1 mRNA and intracellular protein synthesis without appreciable release. For example, stimulation of human blood monocytes by *Staphylococcus aureus* exotoxins, particularly the exotoxin associated with toxic shock syndrome, yields large amounts of extracellular IL-1 (Ikejima et al. 1984), while endotoxin (lipopolysaccharide from gram-negative bacteria) stimulation of human blood monocytes results in increased mRNA and large amounts of IL-1 with two-thirds of the IL-1 activity remaining intracellular (Lepe-Zuniga and Gery 1984). On the other hand, stimuli such as silica or zymosan particles result in very high levels of extracellular as well as intracellular IL-1. Part of the mechanism by which silica, zymosan, or other particulate activators increase extracellular IL-1 is through cell damage. Increased levels of lactate dehydrogenase are observed in macrophage cultures stimulated with silica (Gery et al. 1981).

The differences in IL-1 production compared with release are difficult to evaluate using biologic activity as an indicator of IL-1 protein. Biologic assays are vulnerable to the effects of IL-1-inhibiting substances. There is increasing evidence that IL-1 activity on T cells such as thymocytes is inhibited by macrophage products released with IL-1 (Arend et al. 1985). In addition to inhibitors, the activity of IL-1 precursor protein is thought to be less than that of the mature form (March et al. 1985; Dinarello et al. 1986a). The latter is particularly troublesome since intracellular IL-1 is mostly precursor IL-1. The ideal assessment of intracellular or extracellular IL-1 should make use of an assay system which is not vulnerable to such inhibitory effects. Using immunoprecipitation of methionine or tritiated leucine metabolically radiolabeled IL-1 affords a method for both molecular characterization (size on SDS–PAGE) and semiquantitation (determination of radioactivity). Radioimmunoassays using antibodies which recognize epitopes common to both precursor and processed IL-1 are also useful (Lisi et al. 1987).

It is still unclear how activation of cells leads to IL-1 mRNA transcription, translation, and release. Activators of IL-1 production also induce PGE_2 production and the magnitude of the PGE_2 response correlates with the amount of IL-1 produced. However, inhibition of PGE_2 synthesis by cyclooxygenase-blocking drugs, such as aspirin or indomethacin, do not reduce, but rather increases IL-1 production (Dinarello et al. 1984a; Chap. 15). On the other hand, inhibitors of phospholipase, or lipoxygenation of arachidonic acid results in decreased IL-1 production (Dinarello et al. 1984b), and recent evidence suggests that this inhibition takes place at the transcriptional level.

Table 1. Inducers of IL-1 production

Viruses (influenza, Newcastle disease, Epstein-Barr, cytomegalovirus)
Gram-negative bacteria (lipopolysaccharide endotoxins, synthetic lipid A derivatives)
Gram-positive bacteria (exotoxins, i.e., toxic shock syndrome toxin-1, enterotoxins A–F;
     erythrogenic toxins)
Yeasts (polysaccharide capsules)
Spirochetes
Antigen-antibody complexes
C5a; phorbol myristate acetate; bile salts; etiocholanolone; thrombin
Silica; glucocerebroside
Muramyl peptides; peptidogylcans
Tumor necrosis factor (cachectin); lymphotoxin
Colony-stimulating factors

Corticosteroids, BW755C (DINARELLO et al. 1984a), and the 5-lipoxygenase inhibitor U60,257 reduce IL-1 production by a variety of activators. Adding these drugs 1–2 h after activation does not affect IL-1 production as much as when these agents are present prior to stimulation, These data are consistent with the concept that cell membrane perturbation by IL-1-inducing substances releases arachidonic acid, and the lipoxygenase metabolites formed from this fatty acid are linked to gene expression and processing. This concept is also consistent with the observation that leukotriene B_4 (LTB_4) is a direct activator of IL-1 production (KUNKEL et al. 1985). On the other hand, cyclooxygenase products such as PGE_2, which increase cAMP concentration, reduce IL-1 production (KNUDSEN and STROM 1985). Table 1 lists several substances which induce IL-1 production.

Several lymphocyte products stimulate IL-1 production, but it is presently unclear whether these substances are directly inducing IL-1 transcription or are involved primarily with IL-1 precursor processing and transport. Considerable attention has been focused on the ability of IFN-γ to induce IL-1 (PALLADINO et al. 1984); however, on close examination, IFN-γ apparently does not directly induce IL-1, but rather augments IL-1 production by agents such as muramyl dipeptides or endotoxin (DAMAIS et al. 1985; DINARELLO and KENT 1985). IFN-α has a similar action (ARENZANA-SEISDEDOS and VIRELIZIER 1983). Since most commercial culture media contain 1–5 ng/ml endotoxin, the addition of IFN-γ or IFN-α results in a dose-dependent increase in IL-1 production. However, in endotoxin-free media or in the presence of polymyxin B, the addition of IFN-γ or IFN-α does not result in extracellular IL-1 generation. On the other hand, tumor necrosis factor (TNF, also called cachectin; see Chap. 11), lymphotoxin, and colony-stimulating factors induce IL-1 in the absence of endotoxin or other IL-1 inducers (DINARELLO et al. 1986b).

II. Cell Sources of IL-1

1. Fixed Macrophagic Cells

The previous section has dealt with blood monocytes as a source of IL-1; fixed macrophages are considered as a separate population. These cells are often located in strategic blood-filtering organs and are involved in primary phagocytic defense mechanisms against invading microorganisms. For example, there are fixed macrophages lining the alveolar space, in the lamina propria, and in the dermis. Fixed macrophagic cells also make up the lining of blood-filtering organs, for example, the Kupfer cells of the liver, the splenic sinusoidal cells, and lymph node macrophages. Peritoneal macrophages are also part of the primary phagocytic defense mechanism since these cells would be involved with microorganisms derived from intestinal perforations. Several studies have shown that peritoneal, splenic, and alveolar cells produce IL-1 when stimulated in vitro. The different methods used to remove and purify these cells from other tissue cells may affect IL-1 production. Most studies involving IL-1 production from peritoneal cells employ agents such as oil or thioglycolate, and these agents may not only raise the total number of peritoneal macrophages in the peritoneal cavity, but may also "prime" the macrophage for subsequent stimulation in vitro. Several biologically active molecules such as tuftsin, while not IL-1 inducers, lower the threshold of peritoneal macrophages to exogenous stimuli such as endotoxin. Such "priming" may also be part of the mechanism by which pretreatment of blood monocytes with interferons increases endotoxin-induced IL-1 production. Another example is that human alveolar cells from cigarette smokers produce IL-1 when stimulated in vitro, but alveolar macrophages from nonsmokers do not (WEWERS et al. 1984).

Langerhans' cells isolated from the skin can be separated from keratinocytes by adherence techniques and, when stimulated, these cells produce IL-1 (SAUDER et al. 1984a). Using a similar method, dendritic cells from human synovium can also be separated from other synovial cells and produce IL-1 on stimulation (DUFF et al. 1985).

2. Keratinocytes

Freshly isolated keratinocytes, which produce large amounts of keratin, also produce IL-1. Several keratinocyte lines of human or mouse origin produce IL-1 without any apparent stimulant, but increase production when incubated with endotoxin or toxic shock syndrome toxin-1 (reviewed in SAUDER 1984). Keratinocyte-derived IL-1 exists in multiple molecular weight species (15–50 kdalton) and has three different isoelectric points of 7.4, 6.1, and 5.1, forms characteristic of human blood monocyte IL-1 (SAUDER et al. 1984b). Keratinocyte IL-1 also shares with monocyte-derived IL-1 such multiple biologic activities as fever induction (SAUDER 1984), chemotaxis of neutrophils and monocytes (SAUDER et al. 1984b; LUGER et al. 1983a), and a 4 kdalton fragment also stimulates muscle proteolysis (SAUDER 1984). Keratinocyte-derived IL-1 is the source of IL-1 found in the cornified epidermis (GAHRING and DAYNES 1985). Rabbits irradiated with ultraviolet light have circulating levels of IL-1, and it seems probable that this may be keratinocyte derived (ANSEL et al. 1983; GAHRING et al. 1984). It has also been speculated that keratinocyte IL-1 production may be involved in a variety of skin lesions, including acute sunburn, or as a result of treatment with ultraviolet B phototherapy for certain skin diseases (KONNIKOV et al. 1986).

3. B Cell IL-1

SCALA et al. (1984a) were the first to demonstrate that Epstein–Barr virus-infected human B cell lines produce IL-1. These cells also release an IL-1-inhibiting substance which may be the same inhibitor substance described by others and isolated from human blood, urine, and joint fluid (DINARELLO et al. 1982; KIMBALL et al. 1984; WOOD et al. 1983; FONTANA et al. 1982a). Circulating B cells isolated from the blood of apparently healthy humans can be stimulated by a variety of agents to produce IL-1 (MATSUSHIMA et al. 1985a). Many of these agents, such as *Staphylococcus aureus* Cowan strain, anti-μ, and endotoxin are used as stimulators of B cell activity, and part of their stimulation may be mediated via IL-1 induction. Recently, IL-1 from a human Epstein–Barr virus-infected line has been purified to homogeneity and the NH_2 terminus amino acid sequence is different from that of either form of human monocyte IL-1 (RIMSKY et al. 1986). Other evidence suggests that B cell IL-1 is antigenically distinct from human monocyte IL-1 (VALENTINE et al. 1986). A considerable amount of the B cell-derived IL-1 may be membrane-bound (KURT-JONES et al. 1985b), and this finding is consistent with several studies implicating B cells as antigen-presenting cells in which IL-1 could not be detected. An explanation for this may be that the IL-1 is bound and stimulates T cell activation in its bound form.

4. Large Granular Lymphocytes (Natural Killer Cells)

These cells are also known as natural killer (NK) cells, and have been purified from human blood and shown to release IL-1 upon stimulation with endotoxin or tumor cell targets (SCALA et al. 1984b; HERMAN and RABSON 1984; HERMAN et al. 1984, 1985). Patients with large tumor burdens have circulating NK cells which produce little IL-1 and have a markedly reduced ability to bind and lyse tumor targets. IL-1 production and killing capacity increase when these cells are pretreated with IFN-α. IL-1 itself has only a slightly enhancing effect on NK cell killing capacity, but potentiates NK activity by interferons and IL-2 (DEMPSEY et al. 1982). However, IL-1 production from NK cells may be vital to the binding of killer cells to their targets (HERMAN et al. 1984).

5. Mesangial Cells

Rat mesangial cell lines produce IL-1 (LOVETT et al. 1983a), and this IL-1 is active in both the thymocyte and fever assay (LOVETT et al. 1985). The rat IL-1 derived from mesangial cells has been subjected to several purification procedures, and this mesangial cell IL-1 has multiple molecular weights and changed forms (LOVETT et al. 1985). In addition to stimulating thymocytes and the thermoregulatory center, mesangial cell IL-1 has also been shown to act as a growth factor for these cells (LOVETT et al. 1983b).

6. Astroglia, Microglia, and Glioma Cell IL-1 Production

Brain astrocytes present antigen and express major histocompatibility complex class II antigens on their cell surface. In addition, these neural cells produce IL-1

(FONTANA et al. 1982b). Human glioma cell lines produce an IL-1 which is anti-genically related to human monocyte IL-1. Mice injected with endotoxin intra-peritoneally develop fever for several hours, and astrocytes separated from other neural tissue contain large amounts of intracellular IL-1 (FONTANA et al. 1984). In fact, astrocyte IL-1 may play an important role in fever induction. Astrocyte-derived IL-1 induces PGE_2 production from glioma cell lines (FONTANA et al. 1982b). IL-1 also stimulates glial cell proliferation, and locally produced IL-1 may be involved with central nervous system tissue scarring, also known as gliosis (GIULIAN and LACHMAN 1985). Recent studies have also focused on other central nervous system cells, the microglia, as a potent source of IL-1 (GIULIAN et al. 1985). The relative production of IL-1 from microglia seems to be 10- to 50-fold greater than that from astrocytes. This is not surprising since microglia are con-sidered as brain tissue macrophages.

7. IL-1 Production from Blood Vessel Cells

The two major blood vessel cells, endothelium and smooth muscle, both produce IL-1. Endothelial cells have been reported by several groups to produce IL-1 (WINDT and ROSENWASSER 1984; SHANAHAN and KORN 1984; STERN et al. 1985; LIBBY et al. 1986a; MIOSSEC et al. 1986). In general, IL-1 production from endo-thelial cells is an inducible event, and endotoxin is a particularly effective stimulus compared with other well-known inducers of monocyte IL-1 (MIOSSEC et al. 1986). Freshly isolated adult human saphenous vein endothelium or newborn umbilical artery endothelium, and cell lines derived from these cells have been used. The endothelial cell IL-1 is neutralized by anti-monocyte IL-1 (LIBBY et al. 1986a; STERN et al. 1985) and, by means of a cDNA probe to the human mono-cyte IL-1 β sequence, endothelial cell IL-1 mRNA has been shown to increase within 1 h. In contrast, with the IL-1-α cDNA, little or no IL-1 mRNA corre-sponding to this IL-1 was observed.

Smooth muscle cell lines of human origin produce IL-1 which is similar to monocyte IL-1 by immunoprecipitation and mRNA hybridization (LIBBY et al. 1986b). The findings that both blood vessel-derived cells produce IL-1 may be im-portant to the understanding of the pathologic processes in vasculitis since endo-thelial cells are activated by IL-1 to increase their adhesiveness for leukocytes and procoagulant activity (reviewed in DINARELLO 1986). Therefore, in disease pro-cesses such as antigen–antibody complex-mediated diseases, or tissue injury and vessel disruption, endothelial and/or smooth muscle IL-1 likely acts as an autocoid and may contribute to the progression of the lesion.

8. Epithelial Cells

Epithelial cell IL-1 production has been reported in two studies: (a) IL-1 from the gingival epithelial cell (CHARON et al. 1982), and (b) IL-1 from the corneal epithe-lium (LUGER et al. 1983a). In the gingiva, local IL-1 production clearly plays an important role since IL-1 stimulates bone resorption (GOWEN et al. 1984; RI-CHARDSON et al. 1985), and osteoclast-activating factor has been shown to have the same polypeptide sequence as IL-1-β (DEWHIRST et al. 1985). IL-1 production by corneal epithelium is also of considerable potential clinical significance since IL-1 is chemotactic for neutrophils, monocytes, and lymphocytes (SAUDER et al. 1984 b; LUGER et al. 1983 a; MIOSSEC et al. 1983).

C. Production of IL-1 In Vivo

I. Detection of IL-1 in the Circulation

IL-1-like substances have been identified in the circulation of rabbits during fever (reviewed in ATKINS and BODEL 1974), of mice following injection of various IL-1 inducers including muramyl dipeptides (STARUCH and WOOD 1985; IKEJIMA and DINARELLO 1985), and of humans during normal physiologic changes as well as in diseased subjects (CANNON and KLUGER 1983; CANNON and DINARELLO 1985 a, b; CLOWES et al. 1983; DINARELLO et al. 1984 b). The detection of IL-1 in human plasma or serum has been difficult, owing to circulating inhibitors of IL-1, particularly inhibitors of T cell proliferation assays. In order to remove such inhibitors, most investigators have employed gel filtration, using either standard methods or high performance liquid chromatography (KOCK and LUGER 1985). Fractions eluting from columns are then individually assayed. Although this is a tedious method, it effectively separates IL-1 from its inhibitors as well as separating IL-1 into its different molecular weight fragments. The IL-1 inhibitors are in the range 30–90 kdalton, whereas the IL-1 species are 17, 4, and 2 kdalton (CANNON and DINARELLO 1985 a, b). T cell assays for IL-1 detected all three species, but other assays, such as fever in rabbits, do not detect the 4 kdalton IL-1 fragment (DINARELLO et al. 1984 b). Fragmentation of IL-1 into low molecular weight subunits seems particularly characteristic of human IL-1. The fragmentation seems to be part of post-translation events, and sequence homology between the two peptide sequences of IL-1-α and IL-1-β has indicated a 4–6 kdalton peptide location which may represent the fragment possessing the so-called active site (AURON et al. 1985).

Detection of IL-1 in mouse serum has been less problematic. Mouse serum apparently does not contain sufficient amounts of the T cell inhibitors, and therefore the serum is diluted and assayed directly on T cells (STARUCH and WOOD 1985). In both humans and mice, anti-IL-1 have been used to demonstrate the IL-1 specificity (CANNON and DINARELLO 1985 b; IKEJIMA and DINARELLO 1985) since the action of circulating IL-2 can be misinterpreted as an IL-1 effect in T cell assays.

II. Detection of IL-1 in Synovial Fluid

Many of the multiple biologic activities of IL-1 have been implicated in the progression and inflammatory process of either rheumatoid or osteoarthritis. Biologic properties, such as T cell IL-2 production and Il-2 receptor expression (KAYE and JANEWAY 1985; KAYE et al. 1984; WILLIAMS et al. 1985), and B cell activation (PETERS et al. 1985; FALKOFF et al. 1984; LIPSKY 1985) contribute to the immunologic alterations seen in these patients. In addition, the induction of collagenase and PGE$_2$ synthesis from synovial fibroblasts by IL-1 plays an important role in the destructive component of the disease (KRANE et al. 1982, 1985; DAYER et al. 1986). IL-1 has also been shown to have properties identical to those of osteoclast-activating factor (RICHARDSON et al. 1985; GOWEN et al. 1984; Chap. 11). Thus, the detection of IL-1 in human joint fluid has, unquestionably, helped to clarify the role of IL-1 in joint disease. However, as with human serum or plasma, inhibitors of IL-1 have made detection difficult. By means of anti-human monocyte-IL-1 immobilized on Sepharose 4B, IL-1 has been detected in synovial effusions from patients with a variety of arthropathies (WOOD et al. 1983). Using other methods, investigators have also reported IL-1 in human joint fluids (FONTANA et al. 1982a).

III. Detection of IL-1 in Urine

Similar to the studies on human blood levels of IL-1, human urine analysis requires gelfiltration to separate IL-1 from its inhibitors (KIMBALL et al. 1984). In fact, considerable information concerning the IL-1 T cell inhibitor (or inhibitors) has been derived from urine obtained from febrile patients (LIAO et al. 1984, 1985; BALAVOINE et al. 1985). The IL-1 present in human urine chromatographs at 17, 4, and 2 kdalton, and these IL-1 fragments possess both T cell and fibroblast proliferative properties. The inhibitor is approximately 30–50 kdalton, and blocks the ability of purified IL-1 to induce T cell proliferative responses (LIAO et al. 1984, 1985) and, in some studies, to induce PGE_2 and collagenase from human synovial cells (BALAVOINE et al. 1985). SCHWYZER and FONTANA (1985) have also described an IL-1 inhibitor purified from human glioma cells. It is important, however, to note that these IL-1 inhibitors are specific for the IL-1–T cell interaction since they have no effect on IL-2-driven lymphocyte proliferation. These IL-1 inhibitors may play a role in some aspects of immunosuppression in humans (LOTZ et al. 1986).

IV. Detection of IL-1 in Peritoneal Fluid

Patients undergoing chronic peritoneal dialysis for renal failure are susceptible to sclerosing peritonitis and its severe life-threatening complications (SHALDON et al. 1985). Since IL-1 induces fibroblast proliferation (SCHMIDT et al. 1984) and is a direct inducer of collagen mRNA (CANALIS 1985; KRANE et al. 1985), detecting IL-1 in the peritoneal fluid of these patients would implicate IL-1 in the pathologic process. By methods similar to those for human plasma or urine, IL-1 has been detected in the peritoneal fluid of nearly all patients undergoing such therapy (DINARELLO and WYLER 1984). Since these patients receive 2–3 l fluid per day, concentrations of endotoxin below those detectable by the standard *Limulus* assay may be inducing the IL-1. For example, levels of endotoxin of 10 pg/ml represent a dose of 30 ng per patient per day. Since 100 ng endotoxin (3 mg/kg) injected intravenously in humans induces fever, IL-1, and several components of the acute phase response (ELIN et al. 1981), such amounts of endotoxin are likely contributing to IL-1 production in the peritoneal cavity. The IL-1 detected in human peritoneal fluid possesses T lymphocyte and fibroblast proliferating properties.

D. Assays for IL-1

I. Lymphocyte Activation Assays

Table 2 lists the multiple biologic properties of recombinant IL-1. However, the most sensitive and least ambiguous of the many assays for IL-1 is that of augmentation of lymphocyte proliferative responses to mitogens and antigens. This test also seems to be the most sensitive and specific assay for IL-1. Many of the acute-phase inducing assays for IL-1 (i.e., fever, neutrophilia, hypozincemia, hypoferremia, and induction of hepatic acute phase protein synthesis) are also sensitive to TNF (cachectin) (reviewed in DINARELLO 1986; DINARELLO et al. 1986b). T cell assays for IL-1 are based on the ability of IL-1 to induce IL-2 or IL-2 receptors in the presence of antigen or mitogen (WILLIAMS et al. 1985; KAYE and JANEWAY 1984). As such, IL-1 does not induce IL-2 by itself; therefore, the IL-1 T Cell assay is an augmentation of T cell responses to mitogens or antigens. In the ideal assay,

Table 2. Multiple biologic properties of recombinant IL-1

In vivo
Fever in rabbits, mice, rats, guinea pigs
Hypozincemia, hypoferremia
Decreased cytochrome P-450 enzyme activity
Neutrophilia
Slow wave sleep induction
Hepatic acute phase protein synthesis
Increased survival rate in immunosuppressed mice
Increased bacterial clearance in immunosuppressed mice
Increased cortisone levels in mice and rats
Increased ACTH levels in mice and rats
Increased accumulation of neutrophils in skin
Loss of body mass (weight loss)
Chemotaxis of lymphocytes and monocytes
Increased IL-2 receptors (human)
Increased IL-2 production (human)
Synergism with IL-2 in natural killer cell assay (human)
Proliferation of dermal fibroblasts
Induction of fibroblast and endothelial granulocyte-macrophage colony-stimulating factor activity
Induction of endothelial cell procoagulant activity
Induction of human endothelial cell leukocyte adhesion molecules
Induction of human endothelial cell neutrophil adhesion
Production of PGE: in: (a) human dermal fibroblasts; (b) human synovial fibroblasts; and (c) rabbit hypothalamic cells
Production of PGI_2 in human endothelial cells
Decreased hepatocyte albumin synthesis
Increased neutrophil and monocyte thromboxane synthesis
Degranulation of human basophils (histamine release)
Cytotoxic for human melanoma cells
Cytotoxic for human β islet cells (insulin-producing)
Increased collagenase production by (a) human synovial fibroblasts; and (b) rabbit chondrocytes
Increased bone resorption

the amount of mitogen is suboptimal and, in the presence of IL-1, there is a severalfold increase in IL-2 and/or IL-2 receptor production. With murine thymocytes, both the T cell responding to the IL-1 and the T cell responding to the IL-2 are present and the assay is self-contained. However, one can also employ a two-step assay in which IL-1 in the presence of mitogen or antigen induces IL-2 which is removed after 48 h and then incubated with an IL-2-dependent cell line, such as a cloned cytotoxic T lymphocyte (CTL) line. CTL cells are highly sensitive to IL-2, and hence the two-step assay has the potential for greater sensitivity. A murine T cell line, cloned by KAYE et al. (1984) and called D10.G4.1, is highly sensitive to IL-1, and the mechanism of IL-1 action on these cells is apparently related to the induction of IL-2 receptors rather than IL-2 generation (KAYE and JANEWAY 1984). Other cell lines have been described and utilized in the same two-step method (CONLON 1983).

Despite their sensitivity, T cell assays for IL-1 are sensitive to several inhibitors found in plasma, urine, synovial fluid, and peritoneal cavities (as discussed already). In addition, T cell proliferation is severely reduced by lipoproteins. It has also been shown that infection of human peripheral blood mononuclear cells by cytomegalovirus results in production of high levels of inhibiting substance (RODGERS et al. 1985). These inhibitors (95 kdalton) are clearly produced by the monocytes and when they are separated by gel filtration, one can measure the IL-1 induced as a result of the viral injections. It is presently unclear whether these inhibitors are related to those present in plasma and other body fluids. With human synovial monocytes from patients with rheumatoid arthritis, a similar monocyte inhibitor was detected which severely reduced T cell responses to mitogen (LOTZ et al. 1986). Although PGE_2 present in cell supernatants inhibits T cell responses to IL-1, it can be removed by dialysis. In view of this, T cell assays for IL-1 should be carried out with dialyzed samples.

II. Induction of Acute Phase Responses

Recombinant IL-1 induces gene expression for several hepatic acute phase proteins (RAMADORI et al. 1985; PERLMUTTER et al. 1986). However, in vitro assays, although sensitive, are vulnerable to the effects of inhibiting substances. On the other hand, the in vivo induction of fever, neutrophilia, and other acute phase responses can be induced with crude monocyte supernatants, apparently without seeing the effect of inhibitors. This may, in part, be explained by the fact that inhibitors of IL-1 injected into the circulation are rapidly inactivated or diluted to levels where they are no longer effective. Until recently, in vivo assays for IL-1 have been very useful, particularly in the use of recombinant IL-1, which has yielded a large body of evidence confirming previous claims that IL-1 induced a generalized acute phase response. However, these assays can no longer be considered specific for IL-1 since recombinant tumor necrosis factor (TNF) (also called cachectin) possesses the same biologic properties as IL-1, with the exception of T cell activation (reviewed in DINARELLO 1986; Chap. 11). In addition, although TNF induces a large spectrum of acute phase changes, it also induces IL-1 production from human blood monocytes (DINARELLO et al. 1986b) and endothelial cells (LIBBY et al. 1986a). Table 3 compares the biologic poperties of IL-1 and

Table 3. Comparison of biologic activities of IL-1[a] and TNF (cachectin)[b]

Property	Recombinant IL-1	Recombinant TNF
Fever	+	+
Hypothalamic PGE	+	+
Inhibition of lipoprotein lipase activity	+	+
Induction of synovial collagenase and PGE_2	+	+
Decreased hepatic albumin synthesis	+	+
Increased hepatic acute phase protein synthesis	+	+
Neutrophil activation	+	+
T cell activation	+	−
Induction of IL-1	+	+
Leukocyte adherence to endothelial cells	+	+
Endothelial procoagulant activity	+	+
Cytotoxicity	+	+

[a] Human recombinant IL-1 (β and α).
[b] Human recombinant TNF (α).

TNF. It should be noted that IL-1 and TNF do not share amino acid homologies and seem to have separate receptors.

The production of fever remains one of the most important assays for IL-1. In such assays, one makes use of the fact that IL-1 is an endogenous pyrogen. Endogenous pyrogens are polypeptides which, when injected intravenously or intraperitoneally, act on the brain and initiate fever within minutes. In the first descriptions in 1943 and 1948, and then later in the 1950s, an endogenous pyrogen was characterized as a heat-labile protein derived from activated leukocytes which induced monophasic fever in rabbits. The fever pattern was, and still remains, critical to the definition of an endogenous pyrogen. Following intravenous injection, the rectal temperature begins to increase within 10–12 min, followed by a rapid rise in body temperature, usually 0.15 °C–0.25 °C every 10 min, and reaching peak elevation approximately 50–60 min following the injection. Thereafter, a rapid fall in rectal temperature begins and temperature returns to preinjection values approximately 2–3 h after the initial injection.

The fever pattern of endogenous pyrogens is characteristic. Nevertheless, it must be distinguished from fever due to endotoxin (bacterial lipopolysaccharide from gram-negative organisms) or muramyl dipeptides (DINARELLO et al. 1978). Endotoxin fever can also appear to be rapid in onset and monophasic; however, in general, endotoxin fever is usually slower in onset than endogenous pyrogen fever, and endotoxin fever reaches maximal elevation 70–90 min following intravenous injection in rabbits. Nevertheless, the fever due to endotoxin can be easily confused with endogenous pyrogen fever, particularly when endotoxins are present in serum or albumins. The distinction between endogenous pyrogen and endotoxin can be clarified by using inhibition of endotoxin with polymyxin B which blocks the biologic properties of all endotoxins by interference with the active Lipid A moiety. Endogenous pyrogens are not affected by polymyxin B. They are also heat labile (70 °C, 30 min) whereas temperatures as high as 90 °C have no effect on endotoxins. Finally, endogenous pyrogens are negative in the *Limulus* lysate test for endotoxins.

At the time of the introduction of the interleukin nomenclature, it had already been reported that purified human monocyte endogenous pyrogen exhibited potent lymphocyte-activating factor properties (ROSENWASSER et al. 1979). In fact, it was shown that an endogenous pyrogen with an isoelectric point of 7 which had been purified to homogeneity from human blood monocytes was the same molecule the immunologists had described as IL-1 (DINARELLO et al. 1977). MURPHY et al. (1980) came to the same conclusion with purified rabbit endogenous pyrogens. Recent reports have confirmed the initial observations that endogenous pyrogen purified from macrophagic cells to a single band on SDS–PAGE is, in fact, indistinguishable from IL-1 activity (DINARELLO et al. 1985; HANSON and MURPHY 1984; MATSUSHIMA et al. 1985b).

The most extensive study on the pyrogenicity of recombinant IL-1 species has been made with the human pI 7 (β) form (DINARELLO et al. 1986a, b). When the IL-1 is expressed in *Escherichia coli*, considerable care must be taken to rule out an effect of contaminating endotoxins. Endotoxins produce fever in rabbits at concentrations as low as 1 ng/kg. Recombinant human IL-1-β intravenously injected into rabbits results in typical endogenous pyrogen fever at 100 ng/kg. The endotoxin concentration of these recombinant IL-1 species was below the minimal pyrogenic dose in rabbits. In addition, the endogenous pyrogen fever was unaffected by polymyxin B and was also observed when IL-1 was injected into the endotoxin-resistant mouse C3H/HeJ. Thus, these experiments confirm the original reports which used materials purified from leukocytes.

III. Assays for IL-1 Employing its Catabolic and Inflammatory Properties

These assays are based on the ability of IL-1 to induce several proteases from synovial fibroblasts, bone cells, chondrocytes, and muscle tissue (KRANE et al. 1982, 1985; DAYER et al. 1986; WOOD et al. 1985; SAKLATVALA et al. 1985; SAKLATVALA and SARSFIELD 1985; GOWEN et al. 1984; RICHARDSON et al. 1985). In addition, PGE_2 production can also be measured. The difficulty with these assays is that many interfering substances can yield false negative results. For example, IFN-γ blocks the IL-1-induced changes in these assays (RICHARDSON et al. 1985). Another problem is that TNF is also active in these assays (DAYER et al. 1985). This is further complicated by the fact that crude or semipurified preparations containing TNF will induce IL-1 in some of these assays because they contain contaminating tissue macrophages. However, in testing for effects with either purified IL-1 or recombinant IL-1 species, these assays are highly specific and unlike the T or B cell assays, the IL-1 acts directly on cells. IL-1 also directly induces IFN-β from human fibroblasts (VAN DAMME et al. 1985).

Properties of IL-1 used for assay are its ability to stimulate endothelial cell leukocyte adherence (DUNN and FLEMING 1985), procoagulant activity (BEVILACQUA et al. 1985), and PGI_2 synthesis (ROSSI et al. 1985). However, some of these effects are also induced by TNF. Once again, since endothelial cells produce IL-1 in response to TNF (LIBBY et al. 1986a), one must be aware of the possibility that the effects of TNF on endothelial cells are via the induction of IL-1.

Acknowledgments. The author thanks Angela Vanstory for her help in preparing the manuscript. These studies were supported, in part, by NIH Grant AI 15614 and from funds from Cistron Biotechnology, Inc., Pine Brook, NJ.

References

Ansel JC, Luger TA, Green I (1983) The effect of in vitro and in vivo UV irradiation on the production of ETAF activity by human and murine keratinocytes. J Invest Dermatol 81:519–523

Arend WP, Joslin FG, Massoni RJ (1985) Effects of immune complexes on production by human monocytes of interleukin-1 or an interleukin-1 inhibitor. J Immunol 134:3868–3875

Arenzana-Seisdedos F, Virelizier J-L (1983) Interferons as macrophage activating-factors. II. Enhanced secretion of interleukin-1 by lipopolysaccharide stimulated human monocytes. Eur J Immunol 13:437–440

Atkins E, Bodel P (1974) Fever. In: Zweibach BW, Grant L, McCluskey RT (eds) The inflammatory process, vol 2. Academic, New York, pp 467–514

Auron PE, Webb AC, Rosenwasser LJ, Mucci SF, Rich A, Wolff SM, Dinarello CA (1984) Nucleotide sequence of human monocyte interleukin-1 precursor cDNA. Proc Natl Acad Sci USA 81:7907–7911

Auron PE, Rosenwasser LJ, Matsushima K, Copeland T, Dinarello CA, Oppenheim JJ, WEbb AC (1985) Human and murine interleukin-1 possess sequence and structural similarities. J Mol Immunol 2:169–177

Balavoine J-F, Rochemonteix B, Cruchaud A, Dayer J-M (1985) Collagenase- and PGE_2-stimulating activity (interleukin-1-like) and inhibitor in urine from a patient with monocytic leukaemia. In: Kluger MJ, Oppenheim JJ, Powanda MC (eds) The physiologic, metabolic, and immunologic actions of interleukin-1. Liss, New York, pp 429–436

Bevilacqua MP, Pober JS, Wheeler ME, Mendrick D, Cotran RS, Gimbrone MA Jr (1985) Interleukin-1 (IL-1) acts on vascular endothelial cells to increase their adhesivity for blood leukocytes. Fed Proc 44:1494

Bodel P (1970) Studies on the mechanism of endogenous pyrogen production. I. Investigation of new protein synthesis by stimulated human blood leukocytes. Yale J Biol Med 43:145–163

Canalis E (1984) Effect of cortisol on periosteal and nonperiosteal collagen and DNA synthesis in cultured rat calvariae. Calcif Tissue Int 36:158–166

Cannon JG, Dinarello CA (1985a) Increased plasma interleukin-1 activity in women after ovulation. Science 227:1247–1249

Cannon JG, Dinarello CA (1985b) Multiple interleukin-1 activities in luteal phase human plasma. Br J Rheumatol 24:226–229

Cannon JG, Kluger MJ (1983) Endogenous pyrogen activity in human plasma after exercise. Science 220:617–619

Charon JA, Luger TA, Mergenhagen SE, Oppenheim JJ (1982) Increased thymocyte-activating factor in human gingival fluid during gingival inflammation. Infect Immun 38:1190–1195

Clowes GHA Jr, George BC, Villee CA Jr, Saravis CA (1983) Muscle proteolysis induced by a circulating peptide in patients with sepsis or trauma. N Engl J Med 308:545–552

Conlon PJ (1983) Rapid biologic assay for the detection of interleukin-1. J Immunol 131:1280–1282

Damais C, Parant M, Chedid L (1985) Synergistic enhancement of interleukin-1 (IL-1) production by human monocytes stimulated with gamma-interferon and MDP. J Leuk Biol 37:692

Dayer J-M, Beutler B, Cerami A (1985) Cachectin/tumor necrosis factor stimulates synovial cells and fibroblasts to produce collagenase and prostaglandin E_2. J Exp Med 162:2163–2166

Dayer J-M, de Rochemonteix, Burrus B, Demczuk S, Dinarello CA (1986) Human recombinant interleukin-1 stimulates collagenase and prostaglandin E-2 production by human synovial cells. J Clin Invest 77:645–648

Dempsey RA, Dinarello CA, Mier JW, Rosenwasser LJ, Allegretta M, Brown TE, Parkinson DR (1982) The differential effects of human leukocytic pyrogen/lymphocyte activating factor, T-cell growth factor and interferon on human natural killer activity. J Immunol 129:2504–2510

Dewhirst FE, Stashenko PP, Mole JE, Tsuramachi T (1985) Purification and partial sequence of human osteoclast-activating factor: identity with interleukin-1 beta. J Immunol 135:2562–2568

Dinarello CA (1981) Demonstration of a human pyrogen-inducing factor during mixed leukocyte reactions. J Exp Med 153:1215–1224

Dinarello CA (1984) Interleukin-1. Rev Infect Dis 5:51–95

Dinarello CA (1986) Interleukin-1: amino acid sequences, multiple biological activities and comparison with tumor necrosis factor (cachectin). Year in Immunol 2:68–89

Dinarello CA, Kent EF Jr (1985) Chemical characterization of an interleukin-1-inducing substance derived from human mixed leukocyte reactions: interleukin-1-inducing substance is not γ-interferon. Yale J Biol Med 58:101–113

Dinarello CA, Krueger JM (1986) Induction of interleukin-1 by synthetic and naturally-occurring muramyl peptides. Fed Proc 45:2545–2548

Dinarello CA, Wyler DJ (1984) Isolation of interleukin-1 from CAPD lavage fluid: lymphocyte and fibroblast-activating factor properties of interleukin-1. Blood Purif 2:48

Dinarello CA, Goldin NP, Wolff SM (1974) Demonstration and characterization of two distinct human leukocytic pyrogens. J Exp Med 139:1269–1381

Dinarello CA, Renfer L, Wolff SM (1977) Human leukocytic pyrogen: purification and development of a radioimmunoassay. Proc Natl Acad Sci USA 74:4624–4627

Dinarello CA, Elin R, Chedid L, Wolff SM (1978) The pyrogenicity of the synthetic adjuvant muramyl dipeptide and two structural analogues. J Infect Dis 138:760–767

Dinarello CA, Rosenwasser LJ, Wolff SM (1982) Demonstration of a circulating thymocyte suppressor factor during endotoxin fever in humans. J Immunol 127:2517–2519

Dinarello CA, Bishai I, Rosenwasser LJ, Coceani F (1984a) The influence of lipoxygenase inhibitors in the in vitro production of human leukocytic pyrogen and lymphocyte activating factor (interleukin-1). Int J Immunopharmacol 6:43–50

Dinarello CA, Clowes GHA Jr, Gordon AH, Saravis CA, Wolff SM (1984b) Cleavage of human interleukin-1: isolation of a peptide fragment from plasma of febrile humans and activated monocytes. J Immunol 133:1332–1338

Dinarello CA, O'Connor JV, LoPreste G, Swift RL (1984c) Human leukocytic pyrogen test to detect pyrogenic material in growth hormone from recombinant E. coli. J Clin Microbiol 20:323–329

Dinarello CA, Bernheim HA, Cannon JG, LoPreste G, Warner SJC, Webb AC, Auron PE (1985) Purified, ^{35}S-met, ^{3}H-leu-labeled human monocyte interleukin-1 with endogenous pyrogen activity. Br J Rheumatol [Supl] 24:59–64

Dinarello CA, Cannon JG, Mier JW, Bernheim JA, LoPreste G, Lynn DL, Love RN, et al. (1986a) Multiple biological activities of human recombinant interleukin-1. J Clin Invest 77:1734–1739

Dinarello CA, Cannon JG, Wolff SM, Bernheim HA, Beutler B, Cerami A, Figari IS, Palladino MA Jr, O'Connor JV (1986b) Tumor necrosis factor (cachectin) is an endogenous pyrogen and induces production of interleukin-1. J Exp Med 163:1433–1450

Duff GW, Atkins E (1982) The detection of endotoxin by in vitro production of endogenous pyrogen: comparison with limulus amebocyte lysate gelation. J Immunol Methods 52:323–331

Duff GW, Forre O, Waalen K, Dickens E, Nuki G (1985) Rheumatoid arthritis synovial dendritic cells produce interleukin-1. Br J Rheumatol 24:94–97

Dunn CJ, Fleming WE (1985) The role of interleukin-1 in the inflammatory response with particular reference to endothelial cell-leukocyte adhesion. In: Kluger MJ, Oppenheim JJ, Powanda MC (eds) The physiologic, metabolic, and immunologic actions of interleukin-1. Liss, New York, pp 45–54

Elin RJ, Wolff SM, McAdam KP, Chedid L, Audibert F, Bernard C, Oberling F (1981) Properties of reference *Escherichia coli* endotoxin and its phthalylated derivative in humans. J Infect Dis 144:329–336

Falkoff RJM, Butler JL, Dinarello CA, Fauci AS (1984) Direct effects of a monoclonal B cell differentiation factor and of purified interleukin-1 on B cell differentiation. J Immunol 133:692–696

Fontana A, Hengartner H, Weber E, Fehr K, Grob PJ, Cohen G (1982a) Interleukin-1 activity in the synovial fluid of patients with rheumatoid arthritis. Rheumatol Int 2:49–53

Fontana A, Kristensen F, Dubs R, Gemsa D, Weber E (1982b) Production of prostaglandin E and an interleukin-1-like factor by cultured astrocytes and C6 glioma cells. J Immunol 129:2413–2419

Fontana A, Weber E, Dayer JM (1984) Synthesis of interleukin-1/endogenous pyrogen in the brain of endotoxin-treated mice: a step in fever induction? J Immunol 133:1696–1698

Gahring LC, Daynes RA (1985) The presence of functionally active ETAF/IL-1 in normal human stratum corneum. In: Kluger MJ, Oppenheim JJ, Powanda MC (eds) The physiologic, metabolic, and immunologic actions of interleukin-1. Liss, New York, pp 375–384

Gahring LC, Baltz M, Pepys MB, Daynes R (1984) Effect of ultraviolet radiation on production of epidermal cell thymocyte-activating factor/interleukin-1 in vivo and in vitro. Proc Natl Acad Sci USA 81:1198–1202

Gery I, Davies P, Derr J, Krett N, Barranger JA (1981) Relationship between production and release of lymphocyte-activating factor (interleukin-1) by murine macrophages. Cell Immunol 64:293–303

Giri JG, Lomedico PT, Mizel SB (1985) Studies on the synthesis and secretion of interleukin-1. I. A 33,000 molecular weight precursor for interleukin-1. J Immunol 134:343–349

Giulian D, Lachman LB (1985) Interleukin-1 stimulation of astroglial proliferation after brain injury. Science 228:497–499

Giulian D, Baker TJ, Young DG, Shih L-CN, Brown DC, Lachman LB (1985) Interleukin-1 as a mediator of brain cell growth. In: Kluger MJ, Oppenheim JJ, Powanda MC (eds) The physiologic, metabolic, and immunologic actions of interleukin-1. Liss, New York, pp 133–142

Gowen M, Wood DD, Ihrie EJ, Meats JE, Russell RGG (1984) Stimulation by human interleukin-1 of cartilage breakdown and production of collagenase and proteoglycanase by human chrondrocytes but not human osteoblasts in vitro. Biochim Biophys Acta 797:186–193

Gubler U, Chua AO, Stern AS, Hellmann CP, Vitek MP, DeChiara TM, Benjamin WR, et al. (1986) Recombinant human interleukin-1-α: purification and biological characterization. J Immunol 136:2492–2497

Hanson DF, Murphy PA (1984) Demonstration of interleukin-1 activity in apparently homogeneous specimens of the pI 5 form of rabbit endogenous pyrogen. Infect Immun 45:483–490

Herman J, Rabson AR (1984) Prostaglandin E_2 depresses natural cytotoxicity by inhibiting interleukin-1 production by large granular lymphocytes. Clin Exp Immunol 57:380–384

Herman J, Kew MC, Rabson AR (1984) Defective interleukin-1 production by monocytes from patients with malignant disease. Interferon increases IL-1 production. Cancer Immunol Immunother 16:182–185

Herman J, Dinarello CA, Kew MC, Rabson AR (1985) The role of interleukin-1 in tumor-NK cell interactions: correction of defective NK cell activity in cancer patients by treating target cells with IL-1. J Immunol 135:2882–2886

Ikejima T, Dinarello CA (1985) Studies on the pathogenesis of interleukin-1-mediated toxic shock syndrome: toxin-induced IL-1 production. J Leuk Biol 37:714

Ikejima T, Dinarello CA, Gill DM, Wolff SM (1984) Induction of human interleukin-1 by a product of *Staphylococcus aureus* associated with toxic shock syndrome. J Clin Invest 73:1312–1320

Kaye J, Janeway CA Jr (1984) Induction of receptors for interleukin-2 requires T-cell Ag: Ia receptor crosslinking and interleukin-1. Lymphokine Res 3:175–182

Kaye J, Gillis S, Mizel SB, Shevach EM, Malik TR, Dinarello CA, Lachman LB, Janeway CA Jr (1984) Growth of a cloned helper T-cell line induced by a monoclonal antibody specific for the antigen receptor: interleukin-1 is required for the expression of receptors for interleukin-2. J Immunol 133:1339–1345

Kimball ES, Pikeral SF, Oppenheim JJ, Rossio JL (1984) Interleukin-1 activity in normal human urine. J Immunol 133:256–261

Knudsen PJ, Strom TB (1985) Elevated intracellular cAMP levels inhibit interleukin-1 production by the tumour cell line U937. Br J Rheumatol 24:65–67

Kock A, Luger TA (1985) High-performance liquid chromatographic separation of distinct epidermal cell-derived cytokines. J Chromatogr 326:129–136

Konnikov N, Pincus SH, Dinarello CA (1986) Ultraviolet B therapy enhances plasma interleukin-1 activity. J Invest Dermatol (in press)

Krane SM, Goldring SR, Dayer J-M (1982) Interactions among lymphocytes, monocytes and other synovial cells in the rheumatoid synovium. In: Pick E, Landy M (eds) Lymphokines, vol 7. Academic, New York, pp 75–95

Krane SM, Dayer J-M, Simon LS, Byrne MS (1985) Mononuclear cell-conditioned medium containing mononuclear cell factor (MCF), homologous with interleukin-1, stimulates collagen and fibronectin synthesis by adherent rheumatoid synovial cells: effects of prostaglandin E_2 and indomethacin. Coll Relat Res 5:99–117

Kunkel SL, Chensue SW, Spengler M, Geer J (1985) Effects of arachidonic acid metabolites and their metabolic inhibitors on interleukin-1 production. In: Kluger MJ, Oppenheim JJ, Powanda MC (eds) The physiologic, metabolic, and immunologic actions of interleukin-1. Liss, New York, pp 297–307

Kurt-Jones EA, Beller DI, Mizel SB, Unanue ER (1985a) Identification of a membrane-associated interleukin-1 in macrophages. Proc Natl Acad Sci USA 82:1204–1208

Kurt-Jones EA, Kiely JM, Unanue ER (1985b) Conditions required for expression of membrane IL-1 on B-cells. J Immunol 135:1548–1550

Lepe-Zuniga JL, Gery I (1984) Production of intra- and extracellular interleukin-1 (IL-1) by human monocytes. Clin Immunol Immunopathol 31:222–230

Lepe-Zuniga JL, Zigler JS Jr, Zimmermann ML, Gery I (1985) Differences between intra- and extracellular interleukin-1. Mol Immunol 22:1387–1392

Liao Z, Grimshaw RS, Rosenstreich DL (1984) Identification of a specific interleukin-1 inhibitor in the urine of febrile patients. J Exp Med 159:126–135

Liao Z, Haimovitz A, Chen Y, Chan J, Rosenstreich DL (1985) Characterization of a human interleukin-1 inhibitor. J Immunol 134:3882–3886

Libby P, Ordovas JM, Auger KR, Robbins AH, Birinyi LK, Dinarello CA (1986a) Inducible interleukin-1 gene expression in adult human vascular endothelial cells. Am J Pathol 124:179–186

Libby P, Ordovas JM, Dinarello CA (1986b) Regulated expression by human vascular smooth muscle cells of a gene for the inflammatory mediator interleukin-1 (IL-1). J Clin Invest 78:1432–1438

Lipsky PE (1985) Role of interleukin-1 in human B-cell activation. Contemp Top Mol Immunol 10:195–217

Lisi PJ, Chu CW, Koch GA, Endnes S, Lonnemann G, Dinarello CA (1987) Development and use of a radioimmunoassay for human interleukin-1 β. Lymphokine Res 6:229–244

Lomedico PT, Gubler U, Hellman CP, Dukovich M, Giri PG, Pan YE, Collier K, Semionow R, Chua AO, Mizel SB (1984) Cloning and expression of murine interleukin-1 in Escherichia coli. Nature 312:458–462

Lotz M, Tsoukas CD, Fong S, Dinarello CA, Carson DA, Vaughan JD (1986) Release of lymphokines following Epstein Barr virus infection in vitro. II. A monocyte dependent inhibitor of interleukin-2 and gamma interferon in rheumatoid arthritis. J Immunol 136:3643–3648

Lovett DH, Ryan JL, Sterzel RB (1983a) A thymocyte-activating factor derived from glomerular mesangial cells. J Immunol 130:1796–1801

Lovett DH, Ryan JL, Sterzel RB (1983 b) Stimulation of rat mesangial cell proliferation by macrophage interleukin-1. J Immunol 131:2830–2836

Lovett DH, Sterzel RB, Ryan JL, Atkins E (1985) Production of an endogenous pyrogen by glomerular mesangial cells. J Immunol 134:670–672

Luger TA, Charon JA, Colot M, Micksche M, Oppenheim JJ (1983 a) Chemotactic properties of partially purified human epidermal cell-derived thymocyte activating factor (ETAF) for polymorphonuclear and mononuclear cells. J Immunol 131:816–820

Luger TA, Grabner G, Sztein MB, Smolin G (1983 b) A corneal cytokine triggers the in vivo synthesis of serum amyloid A by hepatocytes. Opthalmic Res 15:121–125

March CJ, Mosley B, Larsen A, Cerretti DP, Braedt G, Price V, Gillis S, et al. (1985) Cloning, sequence and expression of two distinct human interleukin-1 complementary DNAs. Nature 315:641–646

Matsushima K, Procopio A, Abe H, Scala G, Ortaldo JR, Oppenheim JJ (1985 a) Production of interleukin-1 activity by normal human peripheral blood B lymphocytes. J Immunol 135:1132–1136

Matsushima K, Durum SK, Kimball ES, Oppenheim JJ (1985 b) Purification of human interleukin-1 and identity of thymocyte co-mitogenic factor, fibroblast proliferation factor, actue phase protein inducing factor, and endogenous pyrogen. Cell Immunol 29:290–301

Miossec P, Yu C, Ziff M (1983) Lymphocyte chemotactic activity of human interleukin-1. J Immunol 133:2007–2011

Miossec P, Cavender D, Ziff M (1986) Production of interleukin-1 by human endothelial cells. J Immunol 136:2486–2491

Murphy PA, Simon PL, Willoughby WF (1980) Endogenous pyrogens made by rabbit peritoneal exudate cells are identical with lymphocyte-activating factors made by rabbit alveolar macrophages. J Immunol 124:2498–2501

Palladino MA, Svedersky LP, Shepard HM, et al. (1984) Interleukin regulation of the immune system "IRIS." In: Zoon KG, et al. (eds) Interferon research, clinical application, and regulatory considerations. Elsevier, New York, pp 139–148

Perlmutter DH, Dinarello CA, Punsal P, Colten HR (1986) Cachectin/tumor necrosis factor regulates hepatic acute phase gene expression. J Clin Invest 78:1349–1354

Peters M, Butler JL, Margolick JB, Gerrard TL, Dinarello CA, Fauci AS (1985) Synergy of helper factors in the differentiation of in vivo preactivated antigen-specific human B cells. Cell Immunol 91:33–42

Ramadori G, Sipe JD, Dinarello CA, Mizel SB, Colten HR (1985) Pretranslational modulation of acute phase hepatic protein synthesis by murine recombinant interleukin-1 and purified human IL-1. J Exp Med 162:930–942

Richardson HJ, Skjodt H, Bunning BAD, Gowen J, Dinarello CA, Russell RGG (1985) Interactions between IF-gamma and IL-1 on the proliferation of and proteinase production by human chondrocytes bone cells. Calcif Tissue Int [Suppl] 38:S27

Rimsky L, Wakasugi H, Ferrara P, Robin P, Capdevielle J, Tursz T, Fradelizi D, Bertoglio J (1986) Purification to homogeneity and NH_2-terminal amino acid sequence of a novel interleukin-1 species derived from a human B-cell line. J Immunol 136:3304–3310

Rodgers BC, Scott DM, Mundin J, Sissons JG (1985) Monocyte-derived inhibitor of interleukin-1 induced by human cytomegalovirus. J Virol 55:527–532

Rosenwasser LJ, Dinarello CA, Rosenthal AS (1979) Adherent cell function in murine T-lymphocyte antigen recognition. IV. Enhancement of murine T-cell antigen recognition by human leukocytic pyrogen. J Exp Med 150:709–714

Rossi V, Breviario F, Ghezzi P, Dejava E, Mantovani A (1985) Interleukin-1 induces prostacylclin in vascular cells. Science 229:174–176

Sahasrabuddhe CG, Dinarello CA, Martin B, Maizel AL (1985) Intracellular human IL-1: a precursor for the secreted monokine. Lymphokine Res 4:205–213

Saklatvala J, Sarsfield SJ (1985) Purification to homogeneity of two IL-1-like proteins from pig leukocytes. In: Kluger MJ, Oppenheim JJ, Powanda MC (eds) The physiologic, metabolic and immunologic actions of interleukin-1. Liss, New York

Saklatvala J, Sarsfield SJ, Townsend Y (1985) Pig interleukin-1. Purification of two immunologically different leukocyte proteins that cause cartilage resorption, lymphocyte activation, and fever. J Exp Med 162:1208–1222

Sauder DN (1984) Epidermal cytokines: properties of epidermal cell thymocyte-activating factor (ETAF). Lymphokine Res 3:145–151

Sauder DN, Dinarello CA, Morhenn BV (1984a) Langerhans cell production of interleukin-1. J Invest Dermatol 82:605–607

Sauder DN, Mounessa NL, Watz SI, Dinarello CA, Gallin JI (1984b) Chemotactic cytokines: the role of leukocytic pyrogen and epidermal cell thymocyte-activating factor in neutrophil chemotaxis. J Immunol 132:828–832

Scala G, Kuang YD, Hall RE, Mohmore AV, Oppenheim JJ (1984a) Accessory cell function of human B cells. I. Production of both interleukin-1-like activity and an interleukin-1 inhibitory factor by an EBV-transformed human B cell line. J Exp Med 159:1637–1652

Scala G, Allavena P, Djeu JY, Kasahara T, Ortaldo JR, Herberman RB, Oppenheim JJ (1984b) Human large granular lymphocytes are potent producers of interleukin-1. Nature 309:56–59

Schmidt JA, Oliver CN, Lepe-Zuniga JL, Green I, Gery I (1984) Silica-stimulated monocytes release fibroblast proliferation factors identical to interleukin-1. A potential role for interleukin-1 in the pathogenesis of silicosis. J Clin Invest 73:1462–1472

Schwyzer M, Fontana A (1985) Partial purification and biochemical characterization of a T-cell suppressor factor produced by human glioblastoma cells. J Immunol 134:1003–1009

Shaldon S, Koch KM, Quellhorst E, Lonnemann G, Dinarello CA (1985) CAPD is a second class treatment. Contrib Nephrol 44:163–172

Shanahan W, Korn J (1984) Endothelial cells express IL-1-like activity as assessed by enhancement of fibroblast PGE synthesis. Clin Res 32:666A

Staruch MJ, Wood DD (1985) Reduction of serum interleukin-1-like activity after treatment with dexamethasone. J Leuk Biol 37:193–207

Stern DM, Bank I, Nawroth PP, Cassimeris J, Kisiel W, Fenton JW, Dinarello CA, Chess L, Jaffee EA (1985) Self-regulation of procoagulant events on the endothelial cell surface. J Exp Med 162:122–1235

Valentine M, Lotz M, Dinarello CA, Carson DA, Vaughan JH (1986) Lymphoblastoid B cell lines produce an interleukin-1-like activity that can be serologically distinct from macrophage interleukin-1. Lymphokine Res 5:173–183

Van Damme J, de Ley J, Opdenakker G, Billiau A, de Somer P (1985) Homogeneous interferon-inducing 22K factor is related to endogenous pyrogen and interleukin-1. Nature 314:266–268

Wewers MD, Rennard SI, Hance AJ, Bitterman PB, Crystal RG (1984) Normal human alveolar macrophages obtained by bronchoalveolar lavage have a limited capacity to release interleukin-1. J Clin Invest 74:2208–2218

Williams JM, DeLoria D, Hansen JA, Dinarello CA, Loertscher R, Shapiro HM, Strom TB (1985) The events of primary T-cell activation can be staged by use of sepharose-bound anti-T3 (64.1) monoclonal antibody and purified interleukin-1. J Immunol 135:2249–2255

Windt MR, Rosenwasser LJ (1984) Human vascular endothelial cells produce interleukin-1. Lymphokine Res 3:175A

Wood DD, Ihrie EJ, Dinarello CA, Cohen PL (1983) Isolation of an interleukin-1-like factor from human joint effusions. Arthritis Rheum 26:975–983

Wood DD, Bayne EK, Goldring MB, Gowen M, Hamerman D, Humes JL, Ihrie EJ, Lipsky PE, Staruch MJ (1985) The four biochemically distinct species of human interleukin-1 all exhibit similar biologic activities. J Immunol 134:892–895

CHAPTER 8

Production and Measurement of Interleukin 2 and Interleukin 3

B. M. STADLER, K. HIRAI, and J.-F. GAUCHAT

A. Introduction

In 1979, at the Second International Lymphokine Workshop, it was decided to revise the nomenclature for antigen-nonspecific T cell proliferation and helper factors (AARDEN et al. 1979). The term "interleukin" was created as a common denominator for lymphokines acting among different leukocytes. Since then, the field of lymphokine research has made great progress. This is in part due to the many new technical developments which have been applied to lymphokine research, such as improved tissue culture techniques (Chap. 12), the availability of monoclonal antibodies (Chap. 6), and better biochemical separation techniques followed by the possibility of microsequencing. The greatest impact on lymphokine research was the use of recombinant DNA technology which allowed a molecular understanding of many lymphokines.

B. Interleukin 2 (IL-2)

I. The T Cell Growth Factor, IL-2

Antigen-nonspecific T cell proliferation and helper factors were termed interleukin 2 (IL-2) because it was felt that these mitogenic factors might be a family of different helper factors, and that T cell growth factor might be one of the factors of the IL-2 family (SMITH and RUSCETTI 1981). Now that the biologic and molecular characteristics of IL-2 are well understood, it has become obvious that the T cell growth factor is indeed IL-2.

1. Biologic Characteristics

MORGAN et al. (1976) observed that the addition of tissue culture medium, conditioned by T cell mitogen-stimulated human peripheral blood lymphocytes (PBL), to human leukemic blood or bone marrow, resulted in the in vitro proliferation of a homogeneous population of nonleukemic lymphoblasts. Based on surface phenotyping as well as functional data, it was concluded that the cells replicating in the presence of such conditioned media were normal human T lymphocytes (for review see RUSCETTI and GALLO 1981). Initially, IL-2-containing conditioned medium was used for the in vitro proliferation of antigen-specific murine cytolytic T lymphocytes (GILLIS and SMITH 1977a, b) and helper T lymphocytes (WATSON 1979). The growth of these T cells was strictly dependent on the presence of IL-2. Subsequently, culture conditions were improved and it became possible to establish cytolytic human T cell lines (GILLIS et al. 1978a). By means of IL-2 it then became possible to clone *human* helper T cell lines. Also, continued growth of these cloned T cell lines remained dependent on the presence of IL-2. Based on such data, it was concluded that IL-2 is a T cell-specific growth factor.

Later, it was also found that natural killer cells can proliferate in the presence of IL-2 (TIMONEN et al. 1982; KURIBAYASHI et al. 1981). More recently, it has been found that other cells, including macrophages and B cells, also respond to IL-2. Furthermore, some murine IL-2-dependent cell lines also respond to recombinant human IL-2 (STADLER et al. 1985b; WARREN et al. 1985).

Further understanding of the biologic role of IL-2 originated from experiments showing that activated T cells are able to absorb IL-2 activity from conditioned medium (BONNARD et al. 1979). Such data suggested that activated T cells might have a specific receptor for IL-2. A monoclonal antibody against the IL-2 receptor, obtained by immunizing mice with lymphoblasts (Chap. 6), helped to characterize activated T cells. The anti-IL-2 receptor monoclonal antibody (anti-Tac) also allowed final characterization of the IL-2 receptor and its cloning by molecular biology techniques (LEONARD et al. 1984; NIKAIDO et al. 1984).

2. Molecular Characteristics

Several groups initially characterized human IL-2 as a glycoprotein with molecular weight 15–19 kdalton (GILLIS et al. 1980; MIER and GALLO 1980) and it was found that IL-2 produced by normal T cells was charge heterogeneous (ROBB and SMITH 1981; STADLER et al. 1982). Since then, several groups have cloned the gene for human IL-2 (TANIGUCHI et al. 1983; DEVOS et al. 1983; DEGRAVE et al. 1983; CLARK et al. 1984; HOLBROOK et al. 1984). The IL-2 gene encodes for 153 amino acids, the first 20 of which appear to constitute a signal polypeptide, and do not appear in the secreted protein. The gene is expressed as a single mRNA species from a single-copy gene.

II. Production

Resting T cells are triggered by antigens or alloantigens to enter the cell cycle (STADLER et al. 1980; Chap. 1). For in vitro production of IL-2, this first signal can be mimicked by the addition of T cell lectins, such as phytohemagglutinin or concanavalin A. As illustrated in Fig. 1, in the early phase G_1 of the cell cycle, T cells display receptors for IL-2, and also start producing IL-2, in either an autocrine or a paracrine fashion. The interaction of IL-2 with its receptor results in a shift of the cells through the G_1 phase of the cell cycle, which is then followed by the S phase (KRISTENSEN et al. 1982). Thus, for in vitro production of IL-2, it is not necessary that the cells proliferate. On the contrary, if proliferation is inhibited, e.g., by supraoptimal lectin concentrations, increased IL-2 levels can be retrieved from supernatants of cell cultures. It has also been reported that IL-2 is diminished in culture supernatants with increasing time. This utilization of IL-2 can be prevented by the addition of blockers for the G_1/S phase of the cell cycle which results in increased IL-2 supernatant levels (STADLER et al. 1981). By the

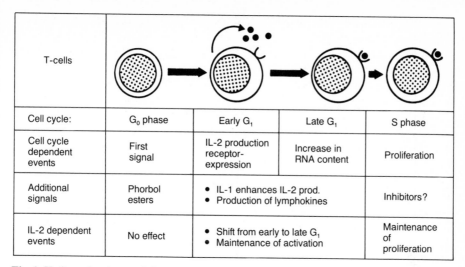

T-cells				
Cell cycle:	G_0 phase	Early G_1	Late G_1	S phase
Cell cycle dependent events	First signal	IL-2 production receptor-expression	Increase in RNA content	Proliferation
Additional signals	Phorbol esters	• IL-1 enhances IL-2 prod. • Production of lymphokines		Inhibitors?
IL-2 dependent events	No effect	• Shift from early to late G_1 • Maintenance of activation		Maintenance of proliferation

Fig. 1. IL-2 production and the early phase of the T cell cycle

addition of phorbol esters, T cells are temporarily blocked within the G_1 phase of the cell cycle, resulting in prolonged IL-2 production (STADLER et al. 1981). IL-1 has also been shown to enhance IL-2 production when added to activated T cells (GILLIS and MIZEL 1981; Chap. 7). In summary, optimal IL-2 production can be achieved in vitro by optimal stimulation of T cells, resulting in an accumulation of most of the cells in the G_1 phase of the cell cycle and, at the same time, inhibiting cell proliferation.

III. Measurement

The most important in vitro property of IL-2 is the long-term maintenance of T cell lines (GILLIS and SMITH 1977 a, b). The strict IL-2 dependence of T cell lines can be used for bioassay, and GILLIS et al. (1978 b) have developed a microassay using such IL-2-dependent T cell lines. Figure 2 shows results of a microassay as it is used routinely in our laboratory. The IL-2-dependent cell line CTLL (BAKER et al. 1979) is cultured at low cell concentrations (5×10^3 cells per 96-well plate) in the presence of serial dilutions of a standard amount of IL-2 (arbitrarily defined as 100 units/ml). Cells are cultured for 40 h and then proliferation is estimated by a 6-h pulse with [^{3}H] thymidine. Assessment of incorporated [^{3}H] thymidine yields a standard curve with plateau cpm values which are decreased in the presence of decreasing IL-2 concentrations. This standard curve is plotted in log-log fashion, and linear regression analysis is used to define the standard titer of our standard IL-2 preparation (Fig. 2). Experimental IL-2 samples to be determined are analyzed in the same way and then compared with the standard titer by the following formula

$$\frac{\text{Reciprocal experimental titer}}{\text{Reciprocal standard titer}} \times 100 = \text{Units of experimental sample.}$$

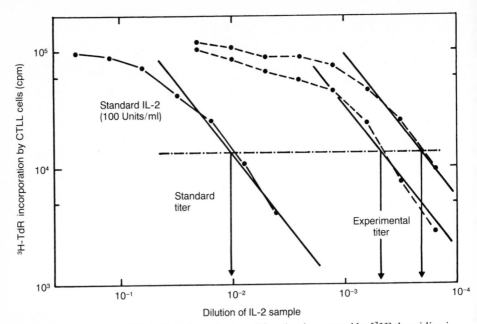

Fig. 2. Measurement of IL-2. IL-2-dependent proliferation is assessed by [³H] thymidine incorporation by 5×10^3 IL-2-dependent CTLL cells in 96-well plates after 40 h by a 6-h pulse (*full line*). Cells are cultured in the presence of twofold dilutions of a standard IL-2 preparation arbitrarily defined as 100 units/ml. In the same assay, samples to be determined for IL-2 content are also serially diluted and plotted (*broken lines*). Data points below maximal thymidine incorporation are used for linear regression analysis. The resulting parallel linear regression curves are compared in the middle of the regression lines (usually 10%–30% of maximal thymidine uptake). The reciprocals of the experimental titers are divided by the standard titer and multiplied by 100 to yield to units of IL-2 in the unknown IL-2-containing samples

    As long as parallel curves are obtained from sample data, even crude conditioned media can be quantified by such a procedure. This microassay allowed the quantification of IL-2 long before it was available in pure form for standardization purposes.

    The biologic assay for IL-2 is extremely sensitive but can lead to false results due to the presence of other biologically active mediators. For many years, different research groups have tried to generate monoclonal antibodies against IL-2 in order to construct immunologic assays for the specific measurement of IL-2. We have generated monoclonal antibodies against IL-2 (STADLER and OPPENHEIM 1982; STADLER et al. 1982) which have been helpful in the study of the in vitro role of IL-2. However, only since 1986 have radioimmunoassays or enzyme-linked immunoassays been commercially available for the detection of IL-2. Some of these assays detect 50 pg/ml IL-2. The biologic assay is still at least ten times more sensitive. Nevertheless, it can safely be predicted that many bioassays for lymphokines will be replaced by immunologic methods in the near future.

IV. Standardization

In 1983, attempts were made to standardize IL-2 (DUMONDE and PAPERMASTER 1984) using both the mouse assay as described already and human target cells to determine IL-2 potency. Such microassays, based on [³H] thymidine incorporation, were also compared with actual cell growth assays where the number of proliferating cells is determined after long-term growth. At that time, all methods used resulted in good agreement in the determination of IL-2. Now, standardization is much easier in that recombinant IL-2 is available. Figure 3 shows that the addition of human recombinant IL-2 material or homogeneously purified IL-2 results in identical curves in the microassay based on mouse target cells. Thus, purified recombinant IL-2 can now serve as a standard preparation for determining IL-2 levels. For example, from experiments as shown in Fig. 3, we now know that our arbitrary standard of 100 units actually contains 0.5 ng/ml IL-2. It is hoped that immunologic methods will also help in standardizing IL-2 preparations.

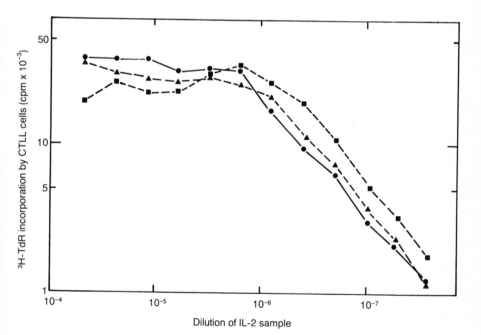

Fig. 3. Standardization of IL-2. Proliferation of IL-2-dependent CTLL cells in the presence of normal and recombinant IL-2. Thymidine incorporation by CTLL cells in the presence of a homogeneously purified IL-2 sample (200 µg/ml) derived from lectin-stimulated PBL (Biotest AG, Frankfurt, Federal Republic of Germany) (*circles*) or in the presence of recombinant IL-2 obtained from Biogen SA, Geneva, Switzerland (*triangles*), or Cetus Corp., Emeryville, CA, United States (*squares*). Both preparations of rIL-2 are 99% pure and at a concentration of 1 mg/ml

V. Measurement of IL-2 mRNA by Northern Blot Analysis

A human IL-2 complementary DNA (cDNA) clone was first isolated from cells of the Jurkat T cell line (Taniguchi et al. 1983). IL-2 cDNAs were then also cloned from normal T lymphocytes (Devos et al. 1983; Clark et al.1984; Rosenberg et al. 1984). The deduced IL-2 amino acid sequence was found to be identical and comprised 153 amino acids with a 20 amino acid signal peptide. The isolation of a cDNA (cognate to the IL-2 mRNA) was followed by the cloning and characterization of the unique IL-2 chromosomal gene (Degrave et al. 1983; Fujita et al. 1983; Holbrook et al.1984). The IL-2 gene consists of four exons separated by 91, 2292, and 1364 base pair introns. Functional properties of sequences preceding the IL-2 gene have been studied, and a region of about 200 base pairs has been mapped which might be responsible for the cell type and induction-specific expression of the IL-2 gene (Fujita et al. 1986).

The availability of IL-2 cDNA as a probe has allowed one to analyze cellular RNA for IL-2-specific mRNA. A mRNA of about 900 nucleotides has been detected by Northern blot analysis in poly A$^+$ RNA isolated from activated T lymphocytes, as well as from T cell lines such as Jurkat (Taniguchi et al. 1983; Clark et al. 1984). For Northern blot analysis, aliquots of total, cytoplasmic, or poly A$^+$ RNA are denatured, fractionated according to their size by electrophoresis, transferred, and fixed to a membrane. The band of IL-2 mRNA is revealed by hybridization with a radiolabeled cDNA probe, followed by autoradiography. We are presently using the following procedure: total RNA is isolated by the guanidium thiocyanate–CsCl method (Chirgwin et al. 1979). Briefly, cultures are lysed in a mixture of a powerful denaturing agent (guanidium thiocyanate) and a strong reducing agent (2-mercaptoethanol) which rapidly inactivates ribonucleases (Chirgwin et al. 1979; McCandliss et al. 1981). The higher density of RNA in CsCl (i.e., 1.9; protein 1.3; DNA 1.7) allows one to isolate RNA by centrifugation through a CsCl cushion of density 1.7 (Glisin et al. 1974; Chirgwin et al. 1979).

Aliquots of purified RNA are then denatured with formaldehyde and subjected to agarose electrophoresis (Ledrach et al. 1977). The resolved RNA is electrotransferred on nylon membrane (GeneScreen Instruction Manual 1983; Stellweg and Dahlberg 1980; Khandjian 1986) and covalently fixed by UV irradiation (Khandjian 1986). IL-2 mRNA is revealed by hybridization with purified cDNA inserts (Dretzen et al. 1981) labeled to high specific activity with ^{32}P by random priming (Feinberg and Vogelstein 1983) followed by stringent washes (Khandjian 1986) and autoradiography with intensifying screens (Laskey 1980). Prehybridization and hybridization are performed with 50% formamide (Thomas 1980, 1983) in the presence of volume excluders (either dextran sulfate or polyethylene glycol; Wahl et al. 1979; Amasino 1986). This type of procedure provides a high degree of sensitivity (1–10 pg RNA) (Collins and Hunsaker 1985; Berent et al. 1985).

Figure 4 illustrates the use of this technique: the IL-2 mRNA level was measured in RNA isolated from PBL (obtained from three donors) and stimulated either with phytohemagglutinin (PHA)±phorbol myristate acetate (PMA), CD3-specific antibody±PMA, or PMA alone. Figure 4 illustrates the advantage

IL-2 m RNA

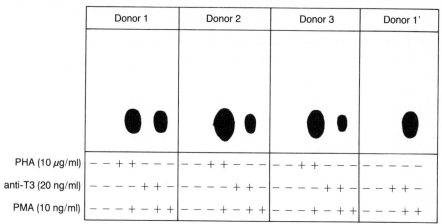

	Donor 1	Donor 2	Donor 3	Donor 1'
PHA (10 µg/ml)	− − + + − − −	− − + + − − −	− − + + − − −	− − − − − −
anti-T3 (20 ng/ml)	− − − − + + −	− − − − + + −	− − − − + + −	− − + + −
PMA (10 ng/ml)	− − − + − + +	− − − + − + +	− − − + − + +	− − − + +

Fig. 4. IL-2 mRNA revealed by Northern blot analysis. Human mononuclear cells were stimulated with phytohemagglutinin CD3-specific antibody (anti-T3 = BMA 030) or phorbol myristate acetate (PMA) as indicated by the *plus* and *minus* signs. 2 µg RNA was subjected to gel electrophoresis prior to blotting. Autoradiographic exposure was performed for 4 h

of the Northern blot analysis: background (e.g., artifacts of either the membrane or ribosomal RNA) can easily be distinguished from the signal of the IL-2 mRNA. On the other hand, a single autoradiographic exposure allows measurement of the IL-2 mRNA in only a limited range. These methods could also detect the weak signal for IL-2 mRNA in cells stimulated by PHA alone (data not shown), but in this case the film is strongly overexposed for IL-2 mRNA in cultures stimulated by PHA+PMA or anti-CD3+PMA, while such an overexposure reveals weaker signals, it will not allow one discriminate among the overexposed stronger signals. Another limitation of this technique is the number of lymphocytes necessary for RNA isolation. The minimal amount of cells per determination is limited by the RNA isolation procedure. With the original method (CHIRGWIN et al. 1979) at least 30–40 × 10^6 lymphocytes are required. Below this number the yield of RNA is decreased and is subject to variation (J.-F. GAUCHAT 1987, unpublished work). With smaller volumes and smaller centrifugation tubes (0.8 ml), 10–15 × 10^6 mononuclear cells are sufficient. At present, this may still be too large a number of cells for the study of cell subpopulations. However, some of these limitations can be eliminated by working with dot hybridization procedures.

IV. Measurement of IL-2 mRNA by Microdot Hybridization

An alternative method to Northern blot analysis is dot hybridization (KAFATOS et al. 1979; THOMAS 1980) or "dot blot." For this procedure, RNA is not subjected to electrophoresis, but directly dotted on the hybridization membrane. The technique is less time consuming than Northern blot analysis and allows one to use serial dilutions of RNA, which permit more quantitative comparisons between samples. On the other hand, in this assay, it is more difficult to exclude false-positive results due to background signals (e.g., with rRNA). We use RNA purified by the guanidium thiocyanate–CsCl procedure (CHIRGWIN et al. 1979) or isolated by selective ethanol precipitation from guanidium–HCl cell lysates (COX 1968; CHELEY and ANDERSON 1984). Aliquots of RNA are denatured with formaldehyde (LEDRACH et al. 1977), adsorbed on nylon$^+$ membrane (Compas, Genofit) with a slot-blotter apparatus (CHELEY and ANDERSON 1984), and fixed by UV irradiation (KHANDJIAN 1986).

Hybridization with a radiolabeled IL-2 cDNA insert is performed as described for Northern blot analysis in the presence of 10% polyethylene glycol as a volume excluder. With the micromethod described by CHELEY and ANDERSON (1984) based on a single step of guanidium–HCl ethanol precipitation, it is possible to use as few as 10^6 lymphocytes for each RNA isolation. Figure 5 shows that the coefficients of variation between individual dots (<12) and selective RNA precipitations (<11) are very good. We have also compared our results obtained with RNA isolated by the guanidium–CsCl or the micromethod of CHELEY

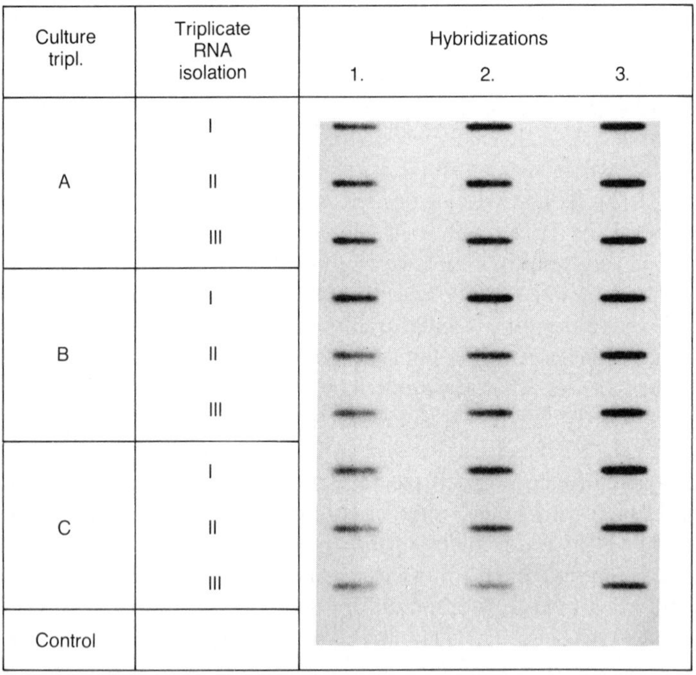

Fig. 5. Measurement of IL-2 mRNA by microdot hybridization assay. PBL were isolated from one individual donor, and triplicate cultures (3×10^6 cells) were incubated ± 20 ng BMA 030 (CD3-specific antibody) plus 10 ng PMA for 20 h. Total RNA was isolated three times from a third of the cultures (1×10^6 cells). Three aliquots (each 10% of the total volume) of the RNA were denatured, dotted on an nylon$^+$ membrane, fixed by UV irradiation, and hybridized with a ^{32}P-labeled probe specific for IL-2 mRNA. The membrane was subjected to autoradiography for 8 h

and ANDERSON. For the measurement of IL-2 mRNA, the sensitivity was equivalent and the background with RNA derived from unstimulated cells was very low (no signal could be detected, even after prolonged exposure times). However, owing to the low cell number and the RNA extraction procedure, the signal measured by the micromethod is related to the number of cells used and not based on a defined RNA concentration as in Northern blot analysis. In order to improve interexperimental comparisons, we are using as a reference standard different dilutions of a large stock of RNA isolated from Jurkat cells stimulated for 6 h with PHA and PMA.

In comparison with biologic assays which determine biologic activities, hybridization techniques have both advantages and disadvantages. The techniques described here measure RNA steady state levels, reflecting the accumulation of specific mRNA in the cells. However, it seems that different stimulations of T cells which lead to identical supernatant IL-2 levels may still lead to different levels of specific mRNA (GAUCHAT et al. 1986). This suggests that, under certain conditions, relatively more mRNA is produced than is actually translated into protein. The hybridization procedure enables one to reveal individual blots successively with different cDNA probes (e.g., specific for other lymphokines, or surface receptors for lymphokines). Presently, in situ hybridizations also allow one to study lymphokine production in mixed cell populations by microscopic identification of individual cells containing the specific mRNAs. Such techniques will finally demonstrate how many cells within a mixed cell population or tissue section are actively producing a given lymphokine.

C. Interleukin 3 (IL-3)

The hematopoietic system is organized into three compartments: the stem cell, the committed progenitor cell, and mature cell populations. Stem cells can either self-renew or give rise to a series of committed progenitor cells of several distinct lineages. These progenitor cells can then undergo a number of cell divisions which are accompanied by differentiation to mature hematopoietic cells (METCALF 1985). Growth and differentiation of committed progenitor cells are influenced by a family of factors called colony-stimulating factors (CSFs) because they induce the formation of colonies of maturing progeny cells in solid or semisolid cultures. All the CSFs are glycoproteins and are active in stimulating cell proliferation at 10^{-11}–10^{-13} M concentrations. For example, there are three major glycoprotein CSFs controlling granulocyte and macrophage populations in the mouse (GM-CSF, G-CSF, M-CSF; METCALF 1985). Furthermore, these lineages are influenced by a multi-CSF activity, also called interleukin 3 (IL-3) (IHLE et al. 1981 a). In contrast to most of the CSF molecules, IL-3 has no cell lineage restriction (RENNICK et al. 1985).

Four murine and four human CSFs have been purified to homogeneity and complementary DNA has been cloned for murine GM-CSF (GOUGH et al. 1984) and IL-3, as well as for human GM-CSF (WONG et al. 1985; LEE et al. 1985; CANTRELL et al. 1985; FUNG et al. 1984; YOKOTA et al. 1984), human urinary CSF (KAWASAKI et al. 1985), and human G-CSF (NAGATA et al. 1985; SOUZA et al. 1986).

There is now evidence that the fourth human CSF, namely IL-3, has also been cloned (YANG et al. 1986).

I. The Multilineage-Specific Hematopoietic Growth Factor, IL-3

1. Biologic Characteristics

IL-3 was initially believed to be a growth factor for immature T cells (IHLE et al. 1981 a; 1981 b). Later, it was found that the same molecular entity (IL-3) was identical to other factors such as: burst-promoting activity (ISCOVE et al. 1982), P cell-stimulating factor (SCHRADER et al. 1981; SCHRADER 1981), mast cell growth factor (TERTIAN et al. 1981; YUNG et al. 1981), and multi-CSF activity (IHLE et al. 1983). It is now generally accepted that IL-3 promotes self-renewal of stem cells, induces proliferation and development of megakaryocytes, granulocytes, macrophages, erythroid, and mast cell precursor cells, as well as the formation of mixed colonies from multipotential progenitor cells.

2. Molecular Characteristics

Murine IL-3 is a glycoprotein of molecular weight 23–28 000 (IHLE et al. 1983; CLARK-LEWIS et al. 1984). After removal of carbohydrate groups by endoglycosidase F, the peptide has a molecular weight of 15 000, but still retains all its biologic activities. Murine IL-3 has been molecularly cloned and its amino acid sequence has been determined (FUNG et al. 1984; YOKOTA et al. 1984). The molecule has no sequence homology to other cloned CSF molecules, erythropoietin, or IL-2. IL-3 and GM-CSF are single-copy genes and are both located on chromosome 11. Human IL-3 has significant sequence homology with murine IL-3 and a similar gene structure organization to murine IL-3 (YANG et al. 1986).

II. Production

The CSFs are not exclusively of lymphocyte or even hematopoietic origin. There is clear evidence that other cells such as fibroblasts and epithelial cells produce one or more of the CSFs (METCALF 1985). IL-3 is produced by T lymphocytes (NABEL et al. 1981; IHLE et al. 1981 b), but the commonest source for in vitro use is the WEHI-3B cell line which is of myelomonocytic origin (WARNER et al. 1969). Furthermore, it has been shown that epithelial cells (LUGER et al. 1985) and astrocytes produce IL-3 activity (FREI et al. 1985). Murine spleen cell cultures stimulated with lectins (as described for the production of IL-2; see Sect. B.II) produce measurable IL-3 activities (HASTHORPE 1980; RAZIN et al. 1981). The most commonly used source of murine IL-3 is still the WEHI-3B cell line which constitutively produces large amounts of IL-3 (LEE et al. 1982), owing to retroviral insertion near the IL-3 gene (YMER et al. 1985).

III. Measurement

In view of the multifaceted activities of murine IL-3, many different assays are presently used for its determination. These include: the induction of the enzyme

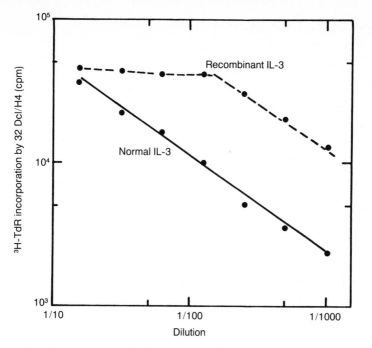

Fig. 6. Measurement of IL-3 activity. Proliferation of IL-3-dependent mast cell-like cells in the presence of normal or recombinant IL-3. 32 Dcl/H4 cells were cultured at a density of 10^4 cells per well and pulsed with thymidine after 18 h culture. Normal IL-3 was derived from culture supernatant of the WEHI-3B cell line, while recombinant IL-3 was derived from supernatants of the COS 7 cell line transfected with the IL-3 gene (DNAX)

20-α-hydroxysteroid dehydroxygenase (WEINSTEIN 1977) in nu/nu splenic lymphocytes (IHLE et al. 1981 a); the assessment of erythroid colonies in the presence of erythropoietin (burst-promoting activity assay, ISCOVE et al. 1982); the production of mast cell-like cells from bone marrow or spleen cells (SCHRADER et al. 1981; SCHRADER 1981). However, the most important additions to these methods available for the measurement of IL-3 are clonal populations of IL-3-dependent cells which can be maintained in liquid culture (DEXTER et al. 1980; SAKAKEENY and GREENBERGER 1982; GREENBERGER et al. 1983). Such IL-3-dependent cell lines can be used in a very similar fashion to that described for the determination of IL-2. The cell lines quickly die in culture in the absence of IL-3. Figure 6 shows an experiment where a subclone of the 32 Dcl line (SAKAKEENY and GREENBERGER 1982) is used for bioassay (STADLER et al. 1985a, b). Dilution curves of IL-3-containing samples can be quantified according to an experimental standard or, even better, by the addition of recombinant murine IL-3. IL-3 can be quantified with the identical experimental procedures described for the determination of IL-2 (Sect. B.III). However, it is important to note that the use of such an assay as the sole measuring principle for IL-3 is dangerous as it is known that some IL-3-dependent lines also respond to other lymphokines or growth factors (HAPEL et al. 1984).

D. Human IL-3 Like Factors

Many of the immunologically reactive mediators are not species restricted. There-fore, we have used murine IL-3-dependent cell lines to search for the putative hu-man IL-3 activity. Based on the 32 Dcl/H4 subclone, we have found a factor in human supernatants that maintained the growth of murine IL-3-dependent cells (STADLER et al. 1985 a, b). Figure 7 shows titration curves of supernatants from the WEHI-3B cell (containing murine IL-3) or from human PBL stimulated with lectins. We have purified this human activity and found that it also induced pro-liferation of human mast cell-like cells from normal bone marrow (STADLER et al. 1987). Because of this functional analogy to murine IL-3 which induces in vitro mast cell growth and maintains growth of IL-3-dependent cell lines, we have termed this factor "human IL-3-like activity." It has been noted that some IL-3-dependent cell lines also respond to other types of growth factors. WARREN et

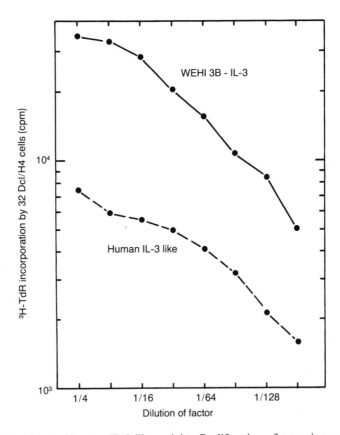

Fig. 7. Measurement of human IL-3-like activity. Proliferation of a murine mast cell-like cell in response to murine IL-3 or human IL-3-like factor (*broken line*). Murine IL-3 was derived from the WEHI-3B cell line, while human IL-3-like activity was semipurified from lectin-stimulated human PBL

al. (1985) and ourselves have been able to show that the 32 Dcl line also responds to IL-2 (Fig. 8). Other cell lines have been described that respond to GM-CSF. While it can be shown that recombinant IL-2 and recombinant GM-CSF have a clear effect on the IL-3-dependent cells line 32 Dcl/H4, it must be noted that these growth factors have been used in high concentrations in order to yield a significant proliferative response. Figure 8 shows also that other factors such as basophil-promoting activity, recombinant IL-1-α and IL-1-β, normal alpha interferon, or recombinant gamma interferon have absolutely no effect on the proliferation of 32 Dcl cells. Human IL-3-like activity is biochemically easily separable from other lymphokines such as IL-2 or urinary CSF. Most interestingly, IL-3 activity was also shown to be different from a factor that induced the growth of human basophil-like cells (TADOKORO et al. 1983; OGAWA et al. 1983; STADLER et al. 1985a, b; ISHIZAKA et al. 1985). The Il-3-dependent murine cell line 32 Dcl/H4 can also discriminate between GM-CSF and the human IL-3-like activity. Rabbit

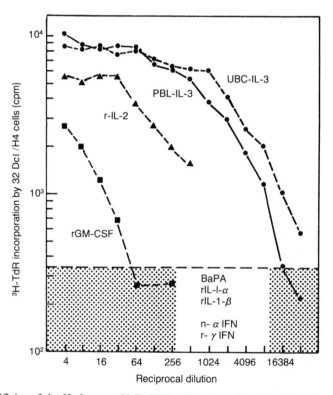

Fig. 8. Specificity of the IL-3 assay. 32 Dcl/H4 cells were cultured in the presence of serial dilutions of IL-3 derived from: human PBL (*circles, full line,* 1500 units/ml); UBC 5637-derived IL-3 (*circles, broken-line,* 1800 units/ml); recombinant IL-2 (*triangles, broken line* Cetus Corp., Emeryville, CA, United States, 1ug/ml); recombinant GM-CSF (*squares, broken line,* Biogen AG, 10000 units/ml). Background proliferation (*stippled area*) was obtained with recombinant IL-1-α and IL-1-β (100 ng/ml), recombinant gamma interferon (4×10^4 units/ml), purified normal alpha interferon (2×10^5 units/ml), and semipurified basophil-promoting activity (BaPA, 20-fold concentration of usual supernatant content)

anti-recombinant GM-CSF does not neutralize human IL-3-like activity (B. M. STADLER 1986, unpublished work; antiserum and GM-CSF obtained from Biogen SA, Geneva, Switzerland).

Thus, clearly some biologic evidence has been accumulated indicating that this IL-3-like factor might be analogous to human IL-3. However, final purification and amino acid sequencing of the human IL-3-like activity isolated from the urinary bladder carcinoma line 5637 has revealed that this activity is homologous to human G-CSF (A. WALZ et al., manuscript in preparation). WELTE et al. (1985) have purified a pluripotent hematopoietic CSF from the same line, which was also homologous to G-SCF. WATSON et al. (1986) also used the 32 Dcl cell line for the purification of a human hematopoietic growth factor which was finally identified as human G-CSF.

Thus, the use of IL-3-dependent mouse cell lines has not led to the discovery of human IL-3, but has shown that the biologic role of the human hematopoietic factors termed G-CSF has yet to be clarified (WATSON et al. 1986). The findings described also clearly demonstrate the limitations of bioassays for the detection of new biologic activities.

E. Conclusions

IL-2 and IL-3 are exquisite examples of the importance of technological developments in the field of lymphokine research. Both factors have been purified and characterized because of the development of relatively specific and sensitive biologic microassays. The microassays were reproducible and allowed quantification of the respective lymphokines. It can be foreseen that such assays might be replaced by immunologic methods for the determination of supernatant and serum lymphokine levels. However, cell lines that are specifically dependent on a given lymphokine may still play a role in the assessment of biologic activity in the future. The availability of cDNA probes for lymphokines and their surface receptors makes it possible to replace some of the biologic assays and to measure the specific mRNAs for as many lymphokines as there are cDNA probes available.

Acknowledgments. We thank Professor W. Fiers, University of Ghent, Belgium, for providing the IL-2 cDNA probe. We thank Cetus Corp., Emeryville CA, United States, and Biogen SA, Geneva, Switzerland, for providing recombinant IL-2, and Biotest AG, Frankfurt, Federal Republic of Germany, for the natural IL-2. We are grateful to Ms. M. Bader for assistance in the preparation of the manuscript. This work was in part supported by grants from the Swiss National Science Foundation (grant numbers 3.249-085 and 3.998-0.84).

References

Aarden LA, Brunner TK, Cerottini JC, Dayer JM, de Weck AL, Dinarello CA, Di Sabato G, Farrar JJ, Gery I, Gillis S, Handschumachher RE, Henney CS, Hoffmann MK, Koopman WJ, Karane SM, Lachman LB, Lefkowits I, Mishell RI, Mizel SB, Oppenheim JJ, Paetkau V, Plate J, Röllinghoff M, Rosenstreich D, Rosenthal AS, Rosenwasser LJ, Schimpl A, Shin HS, Simon PL, Smith KA, Wagner H, Watson JD, Wecker E, Wood DD (1979) Letter to the editor. Revised nomenclature for antigen non-specific T cell proliferation and helper factors. J Immunol 123:2928–2929

Amasino RM (1986) Acceleration of nucleic acid hybridization rate by polyethylene glycol. Anal Biochem 152:304–307

Baker PE, Gillis S, Smith KA (1979) Monoclonal cytolytic T-Cell lines. J Exp Med 149:273–278

Berent SL, Mahmoudi M, Torczynski RM, Bragg PW, Bollon AP (1985) Comparison of oligonucleotide and long DNA fragments as probes in DNA and RNA dot, southern, northern, colony and plaque hybridizations. Biotechniques 3:208–220

Bonnard GD, Yasaka K, Jacobson D (1979) Ligand-activated T cell growth factor-induced proliferation: absorption of T cell growth factor by activated T cell. J Immunol 123:2794–2708

Cantrell MA, Anderson D, Cerretti DP, Price V, McKereghan K, Tushinski RJ, Mochizuki DY, Larsen A, Grabstein K, Gillis S, Cosman D (1985) Cloning, sequence, and expression of a human granulocyte/macrophage colony-stimulating factor. Proc Natl Acad Sci USA 82:6250–6254

Cheley S, Anderson R (1984) A reproducible microanalytical method for the detection of specific RNA sequences by dot-blot hybridization. Anal Biochem 137:15–19

Chirgwin JM, Przybyla AE, MacDonald RJ, Rutter WJ (1979) Isolation of biologically active ribonucleic acid from sources enriched in ribonuclease. Biochemistry 18:5294–5299

Clark SC, Arya SK, Wong-Staal F, Matsumoto-Kobayashi M, Kay RM, Kaufman RJ, Brown EL, Shoemaker C, Copeland T, Oroszlan S, Smith K, Sarngadhapan MG, Lindner SG, Gallo RC (1984) Human T-cell growth factor: partial amino acid sequence, cDNA cloning, and organization and expression in normal and leukemic cells. Proc Natl Acad Sci USA 81:2543–2547

Clark-Lewis I, Kent SBH, Schrader JW (1984) Purification to apparent homogeneity of a factor stimulating the growth of multiple lineages of hemopoietic cells. J Biol Chem 259:7488–7494

Collins ML, Hunsaker WR (1985) Improved hybridization assays employing tailed oligonucleotide probes: a direct comparison with 5'-end-labeled oligonucleotide probes and nick-translated plasmid probes. Anal Biochem 151:211–224

Cox RA (1968) The use of guanidium chloride in the isolation of nucleic acids. Methods Enzymol 12:120–129

Degrave W, Tavernier J, Duerinck F, Plaetinck G, Devos R, Fiers W (1983) Cloning and structure of the human interleukin 2 chromosomal gene. EMBO J 2:2349–2353

Devos R, Plaetinck G, Cheroutre H, Simons G, Degrawe W, Tavernier J, Remaut E, Fiers W (1983) Molecular cloning of human interleukin 2 cDNA and its expression in E. coli. Nucl Acids Res 11:4307–4323

Dexter TM, Garland J, Scott D, Scolnick E, Metcalf D (1980) Growth of factor-dependent hemopoietic precursor cell lines. J Exp Med 152:1036–1047

Dretzen G, Bellard M, Sassone-Corsi P, Chambon P (1981) A reliable method for the recovery of DNA fragments from agarose and acrylamide gels. Anal Biochem 112:295–298

Dumonde DC, Papermaster BW (1984) Towards the standardization of lymphokines: First Report of the Lymphokine Standardization Subcommittee of the International Union of Immunological Societies, PAHO, Washington, DC, November 1983. Lymphokine Res 3:193–226

Feinberg AP, Vogelstein B (1983) A technique for radiolabeling DNA restriction endonuclease fragments to high specific activity. Anal Biochem 132:6–13

Frei K, Bodmer S, Schwerdel C, Fontana A (1985) Astrocytes of the brain synthesize interleukin 3-like factors. J Immunol 135:1044–1047

Fujita T, Takaoka C, Matsui H, Taniguchi T (1983) Structure of the human interleukin-2 gene. Proc Natl Acad Sci USA 80:7437–7441

Fujita T, Shibuya H, Ohashi T, Yamanishi K, Taniguchi T (1986) Regulation of human interleukin-2 gene: functional DNA sequences in the 5' flanking region for the gene expression in activated T lymphocytes. Cell 46:401–407

Fung MC, Hapel AJ, Ymer S, Cohen DR, Johnson RM, Campell HD, Young IG (1984) Molecular cloning of cDNA for murine interleukin 3. Nature 307:233–237

Gauchat JF, Walker C, De Weck AL, Stadler BM (1986) Relation of supernatant IL-2 to steady state levels of IL-2 mRNA. Lymphokine Res 5:s43–s47

GeneScreen Instruction Manual (1983), Catalog No. NEF-972, New England Nuclear, Boston

Gillis S, Mizel SB (1981) T cell lymphoma model for the analysis of interleukin 1 mediated T-cell activation. Proc Natl Acad Sci USA 78:1133–1137

Gillis S, Smith KA (1977a) Long term culture of tumor-specific cytotoxic T cells. Nature 268:154–156

Gillis S, Smith KA (1977b) In vitro generation of tumor-specific cytotoxic lymphocytes. Secondary allogeneic mixed tumor-lymphocyte of normal murine spleen cells. J Exp Med 146:468–482

Gillis S, Baker PE, Ruscetti FW, Smith KA (1978a) Long-term culture of human antigen-specific cytotoxic T cell lines. J Exp Med 148:1093–1098

Gillis S, Ferm MM, Ou W, Smith KA (1978b) T cell growth factor: parameters of production and a quantitative microassay for activity. J Immunol 120:2027–2032

Gillis S, Smith KA, Watson JD (1980) Biochemical and biological characterization of lymphocyte regulatory molecules. II. Purification of a class of rat and human lymphokines. J Immunol 124:1954–1962

Glisin V, Crkvenjakov R, Byus C (1974) Ribonucleic acid isolated by cesium chloride centrifugation. Biochemistry 13:2633–2637

Gough NM, Gough J, Metcalf D, Kelso A, Grail D, Nicola NA, Burgess AW, Dunn AR (1984) Molecular cloning of cDNA encoding a murine haematopoietic growth regulator, granulocyte-macrophage colony stimulating factor. Nature 309:763–767

Greenberger JS, Eckner RJ, Sakakeeny M, Marks P, Reid D, Nabel G, Hapel A, Ihle JN, Humphries KC (1983) Interleukin 3-dependent hematopoietic progenitor cell lines. Fed Proc 42:2762–2771

Hapel AJ, Warren HS, Hume DA (1984) Different colony-stimulating factors are detected by the "interleukin-3"-dependent cell lines FDC-P1 and 32 Dcl-23. Blood 64:786–790

Hasthorpe S (1980) A hemopoietic cell line dependent upon a factor in pokeweed mitogen-stimulated spleen cell conditioning medium. J Cell Physiol 105:379–384

Holbrook NJ, Smith KA, Fornace AJ Jr, Comeau CM, Wiskocil RL, Crabtree GR (1984) T-cell growth factor: complete nucleotide sequence and organization of the gene in normal and malignant cells. Proc Natl Acad Sci USA 81:1634–1638

Ihle JN, Pepersack L, Rebar L (1981a) Regulation of T cell differentiation: in vitro induction of 20-a-hydroxysteroid dehydrogenase in splenic lymphocytes from athymic mice by a unique lymphokine. J Immunol 126:2184–2189

Ihle JN, Lee JC, Rebar L (1981b) T cell recognition of Moloney leukemia virus proteins. III. T cell proliferative responses against gp70 are associated with the production of a lymphokine inducing 20-α-hydroxysteroid dehydrogenase in splenic lymphocytes. J Immunol 127:2565–2570

Ihle JN, Keller J, Oroszlan S, Henderson LE, Copeland TD, Fitch F, Prystowsky MB, Goldwasser E, Schrader JW, Palaszynski E, Dy M, Lebel B (1983) Biologic properties of homogeneous interleukin 3. I. Demonstration of WEHI-3 growth factor activity, mast cell growth factor activity, P cell-stimulating factor activity, colony-stimulating factor activity, and histamine-producing cell-stimulating factor activity. J Immunol 131:282–287

Iscove NN, Roitsch CA, Williams N, Guilbert LJ (1982) Molecules stimulating early red cell, granulocyte, macrophage, and megakaryocyte precursors in culture. Similarity in size, hydrophobicity and charge. J Cell Physiol [Suppl] 1:65–71

Ishizaka T, Dvorak AM, Conrad DH, Niebyl JR, Marguette JP, Ishizaka K (1985) Morphologic and immunologic characterization of human basophils developed in cultures of cord blood mononuclear cells. J Immunol 134:532–540

Kafatos FC, Jones CW, Efstratiadis A (1979) Determination of nucleic acid sequence homologies and relative concentrations by a dot hybridization procedure. Nucl Acids Res 7:1540–1552

Kawasaki ES, Ladner MB, Wang AM, Arsdell JV, Kim Warren M, Coyne MY, Schweickart VL, Lee MT, Wilson KJ, Boosman A, Stanley ER, Ralph R, Mark DF (1985) Molecular cloning of a complementary DNA encoding human macrophage-specific colony-stimulating factor (CSF-1). Science 230:291–296

Khandjian EW (1986) UV crosslinking of RNA to Nylon membrane enhances hybridization signals. Mol Biol Rep 11:107–115

Kristensen F, Walker C, Bettens F, Joncourt F, de Weck AL (1982) Assessment of IL-1 and IL-2 effects on cycling and non cycling murine thymocytes. Cell Immunol 74:140–149

Kuribayashi K, Gillis S, Kern DE, Henney CS (1981) Murine NK cell cultures: effects of interleukin 2 and interferon on cell growth and cytotoxic reactivity. J Immunol 126:2321–2327

Laskey RA (1980) The use of intensifying screens or organic scintillators for visualizing radioactive molecules resolved by gel electrophoresis. Methods Enzymol 65:363–371

Ledrach H, Diamond D, Wozney JM, Boedtker H (1977) RNA molecular weight determination by gel electrophoresis under denaturing conditions, a critical reexamination. Biochemistry 16:4743–4751

Lee F, Yokota T, Otsuka T, Gemmell L, Larson N, Luh J, Arai KI, Rennick D (1985) Isolation of cDNA for a human granulocyte-macrophage colony-stimulating factor by functional expression in mammalian cells. Proc Natl Acad Sci USA 82:4360–4364

Lee JC, Hapel AJ, Ihle JN (1982) Constitutive production of a unique lymphokine (IL-3) by the WEHI-3 cell line. J Immunol 128:2393–2398

Leonard WJ, Depper JM, Crabtree GR, Rudikoff S, Pumphrey J, Robb RJ, Krönke M, Svetlik PB, Peffer NJ, Waldmann TA, Greene WC (1984) Molecular cloning and expression of cDNAs for the human interleukin-2 receptor. Nature 311:626–631

Luger TA, Wirth U, Köck A (1985) Epidermal cells synthesize a cytokine with interleukin 3-like properties. J Immunol 134:915–919

McCandliss R, Sloma A, Pestka S (1981) Isolation and cell-free translation of human interferon mRNA from fibroblasts and leukocytes. Methods Enzymology 79:51–59

Metcalf D (1985) The granulocyte-macrophage colony stimulating factors. Science 229:16–22

Mier JW, Gallo RC (1980) Purification and some characteristics of human T cell growth factor from PHA stimulated lymphocyte conditioned medium. Proc Natl Acad Sci USA 77:6134–6138

Morgan DA, Ruscetti FW, Gallo RC (1976) Selective in vitro growth of T lymphocytes from normal human bone marrow. Science 193:1007–1008

Nabel G, Galli SJ, Dvorak AM, Dvorak HF, Cantor H (1981) Inducer T lymphocytes synthesize a factor that stimulated proliferation of cloned mast cells. Nature 291:332–334

Nagata S, Tsuchiya M, Asano S, Kaziro Y, Yamazaki T, Yamamoto O, Hirata Y, Kubota N, Oheda M, Nomura H, Ono M (1985) Molecular cloning and expression of cDNA for human granulocyte colony-stimulating factor. Nature 319:415

Nikaido T, Shimizu A, Ishida N, Sabe H, Teshigawara K, Maeda M, Uchiyama T, Yodoi J, Honjo T (1984) Molecular cloning of cDNA encoding human interleukin-2 receptor. Nature 311:631–635

Ogawa M, Nakahata T, Leary AR, Stark OK, Ishizaka K, Ishizaka T (1983) Suspension culture of human mast cell/basophils from umbilical cord blood mononuclear cells. Proc Natl Acad Sci USA 80:4494–4498

Razin E, Corden-Cardoj C, Good RA (1981) Growth of a pure population of mouse mast cells in vitro with conditioned medium derived from concanavalin A-stimulated splenocytes. Proc Natl Acad Sci USA 78:2559–2561

Rennick DM, Lee FD, Yokota T, Arai KI, Cantor H, Nabel GJ (1985) A cloned MCGF cDNA encodes a multilineage hematopoietic growth factor: multiple activities of interleukin 3. J Immunol 134:910–914

Robb RJ, Smith KA (1981) Heterogeneity of human T-cell growth factor(s) due to variable glycosylation. Mol Immunol 18:1087–1094

Rosenberg SA, Grimm EA, McGrogan M, Doyle M, Kawasaki E, Koths K, Mark DF (1984) Biological activity of recombinant human interleukin 2 produced in *Escherichia coli*. Science 223:1413–1414

Ruscetti RW, Gallo RC (1981) Human T lymphocytes growth factor: regulation of growth and function of lymphocytes. Blood 57:379–394

Sakakeeny MA, Greenberger JS (1982) Granulopoiesis longevity in continuous bone marrow cultures and factor-dependent cell line generation: significant variation among 28 inbred mouse strains and outbred stocks. J Natl Cancer Inst 68:305–317

Schrader JW (1981) The in vitro production and cloning of the P cell, a bone marrow-derived null cell that expresses H-2 and Ia-antigens, has mast cell-like granules, and is regulated by a factor released by activated T cells. J Immunol 126:452–458

Schrader JW, Lewis SJ, Clark-Lewis I, Culvenor JG (1981) The persisting (P) cell: histamine content, regulation by a T cell-derived factor, origin from a bone marrow precursor, and relationship to mast cells. Proc Natl Acad Sci USA 78:323–327

Smith KA, Ruscetti FW (1981) T cell growth factor and the culture of cloned functional T cells. Adv Immunol 31:137–175

Souza LM, Boone TC, Gabrilove J, Lai PH, Zsobo KM, Murdock DC, Chazin VR, Bruszewski J, Lu H, Chen K, Barentdt J, Platzer E, Moore M, Mertelsmann R, Welte K (1986) Recombinant human granulocyte colony-stimulating factor: effects on normal and leukemic myeloid cells. Science 232:61

Stadler BM, Oppenheim JJ (1982) Human interleukin-2. Biological studies using purified IL-2 and monoclonal anti IL-2 antibodies. In: Mizel SB (ed) Lymphokines 6. Lymphokines in antibody and cytotoxic responses. Academic, New York, pp 117–135

Stadler BM, Kristensen F, de Weck AL (1980) Thymocyte activation by cytokines: direct assessment of G_0-G_1 transition by flow cytometry. Cell Immunol 55:436–444

Stadler BM, Dougherty SF, Farrar JJ, Oppenheim JJ (1981) Relationship of cell cycle to recovery of IL-2 activity from human mononuclear cells, human and mouse T cell lines. J Immunol 127:1936

Stadler BM, Berenstein EH, Siraganian RP, Oppenheim JJ (1982) Monoclonal antibodies against human interleukin-2 (IL-2). I. Purification of IL-2 for the production of monoclonal antibodies. J Immunol 128:1620–1624

Stadler BM, Hirai K, Tadokoro K, de Weck AL (1985a) Distinction of the human basophil promoting activity from human interleukin 3. Int Arch Allergy Appl Immunol 77:151–154

Stadler BM, Hirai K, Tadokoro K, de Weck AL (1985b) Distinction of the human basophil promoting activity from a human IL-3 like factor. In: Sorg C, Schimpel A (eds) Cellular and molecular biology of lymphokines. Academic, Orland, pp 479–483

Stadler BM, Hirai K, Brantschen S, Nakajima K, de Weck AL (1987) Biochemical characterization of the human basophil-promoting activity. Int Arch Allergy Appl Immunol 82:338–340

Stellweg EJ, Dahlberg AE (1980) Electrophoretic transfer of DNA, RNA and protein onto diazobenzyloxymethyl (DBM)-paper. Nucl Acids Res 8:290–317

Tadokoro K, Stadler BM, de Weck AL (1983) Factor dependent in vitro growth of human bone marrow derived basophil-like cells. J Exp Med 158:857–871

Taniguchi T, Matsui H, Fugita T, Takaoka C, Kashima N, Yoshimoto RE, Hamuro J (1983) Structure and expression of a cloned cDNA for human interleukin-2. Nature 302:305–310

Tertian G, Yung YP, Guy-Grand D, Moore MAS (1981) Long-term in vitro culture of murine mast cells. I. Description of a growth factor-dependent culture technique. J Immunol 127:788–794

Thomas PS (1980) Hybridization of denatured RNA and small DNA fragments transferred to nitrocellulose. Proc Natl Acad Sci USA 77:5201–5205

Thomas PS (1983) Hybridization of denatured RNA transferred or dotted to nitrocellulose paper. Methods in Enzymology 100:255–266

Timonen T, Ortaldo J, Stadler BM, Bonnard GD, Herberman RB (1982) Cultures of human natural killer cells: growth in the presence of interleukin 2. Cell Immunol 72:178–185

Wahl GM, Stern M, Stark GR (1979) Efficient transfer of large DNA fragments from agarose gels to diazobenzyloxymethyl-paper and rapid hybridization by using dextran sulfate. Proc Natl Acad Sci USA 76:3683–3687

Warner NL, Moore MAS, Metcalf D (1969) A transplantable myelomonocytic leukemia in BALB/c mice: cytology, karyotype and muramidase content. J Natl Cancer Inst 43:963

Warren HS, Hargreaves J, Hapel AJ (1985) Some interleukin-3 dependent mast-cell lines also respond to interleukin-2. Lymphokine Res 4:195–204

Watson J (1979) Continuous proliferation of murine antigen-specific helper T lymphocytes in culture. J Exp Med 150:1510–1519

Watson JD, Crosier PS, March CJ, Conlon PJ, Mochizuki DY, Gillis S, Urdal DL (1986) Purification to homogeneity of a human hematopoietic growth factor that stimulates the growth of a murine interleukin 3-dependent cell line. J Immunol 137:854–857

Weinstein Y (1977) 20-α-hydroxysteroid dehydrogenase: a T lymphocyte-associated enzyme. J Immunol 119:1223–1229

Welte K, Platzer E, Lu L, Gabrilove JL, Levi E, Mertelsmann R, Moore MAS (1985) Purification and biochemical characterization of human pluripotent hematopoietic colony-stimulating factor. Proc Natl Acad Sci USA 82:1526–1530

Wong GG, Witek JA, Temple PA, Wilkens KM, Leary AC, Luxenberg DP, Jones SS, Brown EL, Kay RM, Orr EC, Shoemaker C, Golde DW, Kaufman RJ, Hewick RM, Wang EA, Clark SC (1985) Human GM-CSF: molecular cloning of the complementary DNA and purification of the natural and recombinant proteins. Science 228:810–815

Yang YC, Ciarletta AB, Temple PA, Chung MP, Kovacis S, Witek-Gianotti JS, Leary AC, Kriz R, Donahme RE, Wong GG, Clark SC (1986) Human IL-3 (multi CSF): identification by expression cloning of a novel hematopoietic growth factor related to murine IL-3. Cell 47:3–10

Ymer S, Tucker WQJ, Sanderson CJ, Hapel AJ, Campbell HD, Young IG (1985) Constitutive synthesis of interleukin-3 by leukaemia cell line WEHI-3B is due to retroviral insertion near the gene. Nature 317:255–258

Yokota T, Lee F, Rennick D, Hall C, Arai N, Mosmann T, Nabel G, Cantor H, Arai KI (1984) Isolation and characterization of a mouse cDNA clone that expresses mast-cell growth-factor activity in monkey cells. Proc Natl Acad Sci USA 81:1070–1074

Yung YP, Eger R, Tertian G, Moore MAS (1981) Long-term in vitro culture of murine mast cells. II. Purification of a mast cell growth factor and its dissociation from G-CSF. J Immunol 127:794–799

CHAPTER 9

Production and Measurement of Interferons

S.S. ALKAN

A. An Overview of the Interferon System

I. Introduction

Interferons (IFNs) are a set of protein molecules which can be considered as lymphokines (LKs) in that they are produced by and act upon lymphoid organs and cells. However, one can also regard them as a separate system in view of the fact that some of the IFNs can be produced by and respond to nonlymphoid cells. IFNs are a diverse set of molecules, each of which has unique features. One of the most important properties of the whole IFN family is their ability to induce antiviral activity in target cells. It is this unique ability that led to the discovery of the IFNs nearly three decades ago.

II. Discovery of Interferons

The phenomenon of "viral interference" was first described about five decades ago as "the protective action" of a yellow fever virus against other strains of the same or unrelated viruses (HOSKINS 1935). Numerous reports have since appeared on "viral interference" which was characterized as the ability of one virus to interfere with the replication of another (challenge) virus until ISAACS and LINDENMANN (1957) coined the name interferon. In their original experiments, ISAACS and LINDENMANN (1957) added inactivated influenza virus to pieces of chicken egg chorioallantoic membrane and, after washing unadsorbed virus, incubated the membranes at 37 °C for several hours. They then took the culture fluid and incubated this with fresh membrane fragments overnight. When they added live influenza virus to such cultures, they observed that the viral replication was inhibited. The tissues exposed to inactivated virus had released a "factor" that transferred the "viral resistance" to fresh tissues. This factor was called interferon (IFN). The stages of antiviral action of IFN are illustrated in Fig. 1.

Shortly after this discovery, it was demonstrated that IFN was acid stable and protein in nature. It did not inactivate viruses directly, but rather rendered cells resistant to viruses. Later, it became clear that IFN exhibited some species specificity. Also, it was shown that virtually all types of viruses (as well as other substances) can induce IFN in almost every type of animal cell (both in vitro and in vivo). IFNs were found to inhibit virtually all types of virus replication, although possibly via different mechanisms (STEWART 1979).

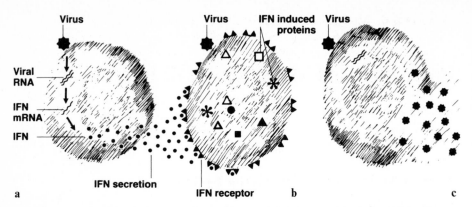

Fig. 1a–c. Stages of antiviral action of interferon. Cell is infected with virus (**a**). Viral RNA triggers the synthesis of IFN mRNA, IFN is synthesized and produced. Secreted IFN binds to specific receptors on the surface of neighboring cell (**b**). IFN-receptor binding triggers a number of changes, including the synthesis of a many new proteins which together render the cell resistant to virus. An unprotected cell (**c**) cannot inhibit the replication of virus, and bursts

III. Heterogeneity of Interferons

There are multiple types of IFNs which can be distinguished by functional, immunologic, and biochemical means. Human IFNs are the most widely studied group of glycoproteins, and they represent a family of closely related gene products with a molecular weight in the range of 17–25000. To date, three major classes of human IFNs have been identified. The current and the old nomenclatures as well as some properties of IFNs are summarized in Table 1. Note that the old definitions were based on the major cell types which produced IFNs. IFN-α and IFN-β are both synthesized in response to virus infections. IFNαs represent a group of proteins that are the products of a multigene family. Comparison of amino acid

Table 1. Some characteristics of human interferons

Nomenclature (new/old)	Molecular weight	Located on chromosome (No. of genes)	No. of subtypes	Resistance to PH 2	Main producing cell
IFNα Leucocyte IFN (type I)	18–20	9 (30)	13–17	+	White blood cells
IFNβ Fibroblast IFN (type I)	20–24	9 (1)	1	+	Fibroblasts
IFN-γ Immune IFN (type II)	20–25	12 (1)	1	−	T lymphocytes, NK cells

and nucleotide sequences shows that there exists about 80% homology between subtypes of IFN-α, and that IFN-αs and IFN-β have relatively similar structures with a 30%–45% homology at the nucleotide level (TANIGUCHI et al. 1980a). However, IFN-γ shows no similarities with the other two (TAVERNIER and FIERS 1984).

Both IFN-α and IFN-β genes are located on chromosome 9, while the IFN-γ gene is located on chromosome 12. The IFN-α family, which represents the most diversified gene pool, can be divided into two groups: IFN-α I. and IFN-α II. The IFN-α I gene group consists of at least 20–30 different sequences while IFN-β exists as a single gene, however some individuals may carry duplicated β genes or variant α genes, indicating concerted gene evolution of the IFN family within the species (VON GABAIN 1986).

The single genome of IFN-γ which is located on chromosome 12 shows no homology to IFN-α or IFN-β, and it possesses several introns while both IFN-α and IFN-β genes are uniquely devoid of introns. The genes of all major human IFN types have now been cloned and expressed in bacteria, yeast, or mammalian cells. Thus, it is now possible to produce large quantities of these IFNs fairly easily.

IV. Multiple Biologic Effects of Interferons

As mentioned, the IFNs were first identified by their ability to protect cells against virus infections. In recent years it has become clear that there exist not only several types (α, β, γ) and subtypes (α-A, B, C etc.) of IFNs, but that all IFN molecules can exert several different biologic effects on target cells, some of which are listed in Table 2. These effects include inhibition of cell growth, replication, regulation and expression of specific genes, modulation of differentiation, and immunomodulation.

Table 2. Multiple biologic effects of interferons

---

1. Induction of antiviral state
     Enzyme induction; protein kinase, inhibition of chain initiation
     $2'$-$5'$-Oligoadenylate synthetase; mRNA, rRNA degradation
     Specific inhibition of viral mRNA; translation
     Inhibition of virus attachment, uncoating, assembly transcription, translation, maturation, and release
2. Regulation of cell growth
     Cell cycle changes; inhibition of G_0–S transition, prolongation of G, S, or G_2
     Inhibition of DNA replication
     Regulation of protein synthesis
3. Modulation of cell differentiation
     Enhancement of effects of inducers; dsRNA, etc.
     Enhanced expression of histocompatibility antigens; HLA class I (A, B, C) and II (Ia)
4. Changes in expression of specific genes
     $2'$-$5'$-Oligoadenylate synthetase (increased)
     HLA-A, β-microglobulin, HLA-D (increased)
     Oncogenes; *ras, myc,* $_{pp}60^{spc}$ (decreased)

The mechanism of the antiviral action of IFNs has been widely studied (for reviews see REVEL 1979; STEWART 1979). It is now established that the crucial step in the activation mechanisms is the presence of double-stranded RNA. This agent activates the enzyme designated 2'-5'-A polymerase which in turn activates an endonuclease, resulting in preferential cleavage of viral mRNA. Information concerning the effects of IFNs on cell proliferation and differentiation has only accumulated during the last decade and is reviewed by CLEMENS and MCNURLAN (1985). The importance of IFNs, in particular IFN-γ, as immunomodulatory molecules has been recognized only recently and the first reviews have started to appear (HOCHKEPPEL and ALKAN 1986; DE MAEYER-GUIGNARD and DE MAEYER 1985; KIRCHNER 1984). Meanwhile, it has become clear that IFNs are released by a variety of cell types on induction, and exert their biologic functions on the target cells through specific membrane receptors. IFN-αs and IFN-β act via the same receptor, but IFN-γ has its own distinct receptor (BRANCA and BAGLIONI 1981; MOGENSEN et al. 1984; LITTMANN et al. 1985; ORCHANSKY et al. 1984; ZOON and ARNHEITER 1984).

B. Interferon Induction/Production

I. Induction

Interferons are produced by cells which are stimulated by agents called "inducers." In addition to the original finding of induction of IFNs by viruses (ISAACS and LINDENMANN 1957), IFN synthesis can be induced by an ever-increasing and impressive range of substances (GORDON and MINKS 1981; MAYER 1980; STEWART 1979). It is perhaps easier to list those substances which do not induce IFNs; nevertheless, Table 3 gives an overall view on the kinds of IFN inducers discovered so far. It should be clear that this classification is only a tentative one. For a complete list of inducers the reader is referred to the reviews already mentioned.

It is important to note at this point that when cells are exposed to various (inducer) substances, they produce not only IFN, but rather a cocktail of LKs. In fact, various cells in response to the same stimulus may produce different LKs as illustrated in Fig. 2. For instance, activated macrophages/monocytes may produce IL-1 and IFN-α in response to mitogens, while mitogens (or antigens) stimulate T lymphocytes to produce IL-2, IL-3, and IFN-γ, but not IL-1.

Recently, it has become more evident that different inducers stimulate the same or different cells to produce different LKs. Furthermore, target cells having various LK receptors will respond to each "LK cocktail" differently. Therefore, despite successful purification of each IFN subtype and other LKs, and identification of their specific receptors, the complex nature of LK interactions, synergistic/antagonistic actions, and regulation of LK-mediated cell functions requires intensive investigation.

Table 3. Classes of interferon inducers

1. Viruses
   Influenza, adenovirus, etc.
2. Nucleic acids
   dsRNA, etc.
3. Bacteria
   Bacterial products, bacteriophages
4. Fungal extracts
   Candida, etc.
5. Other microorganisms
   Chlamydiae (conjunctivitis agents)
   Rickettsiae *(Rickettsia prowazekii)*
   Protozoa *(Toxoplasma gondii, Trypanosoma cruzi)*
6. Mitogens (PHA, PWM, Con A, etc.)
7. Immunologic inducers
   Specific antigens
   Specific antibodies (anti-lymphocyte)
   Alloantigens
   Syngeneic autostimulation
   Lymphokines (IL-2)
8. Synthetic inducers
   a) Anionic polymers (dextran sulfate)
      Polycarboxylates, sulfates, phosphates
      Polynucleotides (poly (I) · poly (C))
   b) Low molecular weight inducers (tilorone, quinacrine)

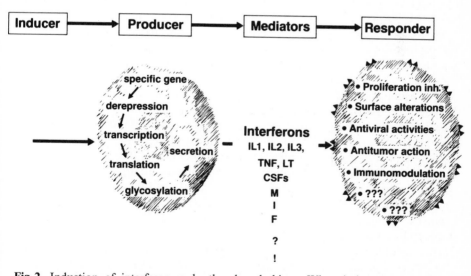

Fig. 2. Induction of interferon and other lymphokines. When inducer agents (virus, dsRNA, antigen, etc., listed in Table 3) meet a producer cell, repressed genes of IFNs (and other LKs) are derepressed, transcribed, and translated. After glycosylation, the proteins are secreted. IFNs (and almost all the other LKs) are paracrine molecules; they act on neighboring cells through specific receptors. Different IFNs exert similar or different effects on various target cells which are listed in Table 2

II. Induction/Production by Cells In Vitro

Despite the diversity of inducers and the possibility of several different IFN inductions mechanisms (GORDON and MINKS 1981), the interaction of any inducer (viral, nonviral) with a producer cell (usually a cell line) results in a similar induction-production curve (STEWART 1979). There is always a lag period after the addition of inducer substance. This "induction phase " usually lasts 1–8 h, depending on the system, followed by the appearance of IFN and a rapid rise to its maximum level within 1 h. This "production phase" can last for a few hours, then rapidly declines. The later phase is sensitive to protein inhibitors while the first phase can be blocked by actinomycin D.

This mechanism of normal induction is different from "superinduction" where metabolic inhibitors can be used to increase the yield of IFN produced. Also, cells pretreated with low doses of IFN make more IFN than untreated cells, and this phenomenon is termed "priming." Another effect of IFN on its own production is seen when cells are pretreated with large doses of IFN for several hours. Such cells, when induced to make IFN, produce less IFN than untreated cells. This phenomenon is referred to as "blocking" (STEWART 1979). It has been demonstrated that the age of culture, temperature, hormones, and many other factors may also influence the rate and degree of IFN production.

III. Production In Vivo

Virus infections are the best tools to study the site of IFN production in vivo. It has been found that in many infections IFN production is highest in the target tissues of the virus (STEWART 1979), such as the lungs of mice infected with influenza viruses, the brains of mice infected with encephalitogenic viruses, and the cerebrospinal fluid of patients with central nervous system diseases (e.g., multiple sclerosis and acute encephalitis). Also, IFN can be found at local viral inoculation sites such as brain, liver, lungs, skin, and the peritoneal cavity. The highest levels of IFN usually coincide with the highest levels of virus in any particular location. However, after viremia, many viruses also induce circulating serum IFNs. Some local infections, such as eye infections with herpes simplex or intranasal infections with influenza virus, stimulate IFN production at those sites.

Nonviral IFN inducers (poly (I) poly (C), poly L-Lys, tilorone, etc.) are also used to study in vivo IFN production. When animals are injected intravenously with endotoxins, IFN is produced within 2 h and large quantities of IFN can be found in the spleen. When low molecular weight inducers are administered intravenously, intraperitoneally, or orally, high levels of IFN can be induced in the serum, lungs, liver, spleen, and lymph nodes of animals.

A considerable amount of work has been carried out to elucidate the cellular origin of IFN production with a variety of different inducers. Macrophages from the peritoneal cavity or spleen of mice have been shown to produce IFNs in response to viruses, dsRNA, polysaccharides, endotoxin, and bacteria (STEWART 1979). The spleen and thymus normally contribute to IFN production; however, splenectomized or thymectomized mice are able to compensate for the lack of these organs. In fact, nu/nu mice treated with certain inducers can make more

IFN than normal mice. Also, there seem to be some inducers (such as myxoviruses) which induce IFN in radiosensitive target cells while others (vesicular stomatitis, vaccinia, and herpes viruses) induce IFN in radioresistant cells in the body (STEWART 1979). Also, there seems to be enough evidence indicating that IFNs are spontaneously produced in the body. The physiologic role of endogeneous IFN is discussed by BOCCI (1981).

It is known that lymphocytes from peripheral blood can produce all forms of IFNs in response to viral/nonviral inducers (KIRCHNER and MARCUCCI 1984). There is now a general belief that both T and B lymphocytes and macrophages can produce type I IFNs while IFN-γ is produced exclusively by T lymphocytes. It should be mentioned here that antigen-specific T cells need the help of antigen-presenting cells (macrophages, dendritic cells, B cells, etc.) in order to recognize antigens and produce IFN (BECKER 1985; KIRCHNER and MARCUCCI 1984; DE MAEYER-GUIGNARD and DE MAEYER 1985).

IV. Mass Production and Purification

1. Natural Interferons

Human leukocyte IFNs are usually produced by the method of CANTELL and TOVEL (1971; CANTELL 1979). Briefly, human leukocytes are incubated with a virus (such as Sendai or Newcastle disease viruses) to induce IFN. The antiviral activity is then found in the culture medium after overnight incubation of white blood cells. The use of casein instead of animal or human serum as a protein source during IFN induction simplifies subsequent purification steps. Leukocytes from patients with chronic myelogenous leukemia can also be used for large-scale production of IFNs (for review see PESTKA et al. 1985). Human IFN-γ is usually produced in lymphocyte cultures stimulated with a phorbol ester (TPA) and a mitogen (PHA, phytohemagglutinin) (YIP et al. 1981). Human cell lines such as Namalva stimulated with mitogens like PHA are another source of leukocyte IFNs (HAVEL et al. 1977).

Recent developments in mammalian cell culture systems have focused interest on the utilization of such systems for the production of IFNs. More recently, however, a better method has become available. This is the use of recombinant DNA technology which now allows the production of almost any class of animal or human IFN on an industrial scale that pre-1980 "interferonologists" could only dream of.

2. Recombinant Interferons

The successful cloning of the genes of human leukocyte IFN (α) (GOEDDEL et al. 1981; NAGATA et al. 1980), fibroblast IFN (β) (TANIGUCHI et al. 1980 b; DERYNCK et al. 1980), and immune IFN (γ) (GRAY et al. 1982), and their expression in bacteria have been reported, and many other reports have followed (for review see PESTKA et al. 1985). In 1 l culture medium from *Escherichia coli* (which carries an IFN gene) there is roughly as much IFN as could have been produced by leukocytes from 100 blood donors. With presently available fermentation techniques and new culture systems, thousands of liters of cells can be grown and grams (or even kilograms) of recombinant IFNs can be produced within a reasonable time.

Recently, genes coding for the murine IFN-α family (4–10 members) (SHAW et al. 1983), mouse IFN-γ (GRAY and GOEDDEL 1983), rat IFN-γ (DIJKEMA et al. 1985), and bovine IFN-α, -β, and -γ have also been cloned (Genentech Patent EP 0088 622, Priority US 355 298 and US 438 128).

3. Purification

Purification of IFN has presented one of the greatest problems in the field. This was partially due to a limited supply and the heterogeneity of IFN molecules. For conventional methods of IFN purification the reader is referred to STEWART (1979). Suffice it to say that, after its discovery, it took about two decades to purify IFN to homogeneity (RUBINSTEIN et al. 1979), and this was finally achieved by applying three high pressure liquid chromatography steps after an initial concentration of human leukocyte IFN. Overall purification was 80 000-fold, and the specific activity of the pure IFN was $2–4 \times 10^8$ units/mg.

At about the time when recombinant IFNs became available in the early 1980s, another new technology, the production of monoclonal antibodies by hybridoma cells, also became available (KOEHLER and MILSTEIN 1975; Chap. 6). Using semipurified (SECHER and BUERKE 1980) highly purified (STAEHELIN et al.

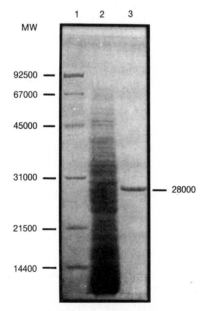

Fig. 3. SDS-PAGE of monoclonal antibody column-purified IFN-α. Human recombinant IFN-α-B (or α-8) was purified by affinity chromatography. Track 1 standard protein mixture; track 2 unpurified; and track 3 purified IFN preparations. SDS-PAGE (12.5%) was performed under reducing conditions and stained with Coomassie blue. This single-step chromatography yielded a single band of IFN of higher molecular weight than other IFN-α subtypes

1981), or crude human leukocyte IFN preparations (ALKAN et al. 1983), several groups have produced monoclonal antibodies and used them for large-scale purification of human IFNs by covalently attaching the antibodies to solid supports such as Sephadex, Affigel, etc., and using them as an immunoadsorbent. With this technique, it is possible to achieve up to 5000-fold purification in a single step. Fig. 3 shows human recombinant IFN-α-B before and after purification with monoclonal antibodies from our laboratory. Several monoclonal antibodies have now been produced and have been used to map the epitopes of several human IFN-α subtypes (ALKAN 1985).

Recently, monoclonal antibodies against human IFN-β (HOCHKEPPEL et al. 1981), and IFN-γ (LIANG et al. 1985; LE et al. 1985) as well as murine IFN-γ (SPITALNY and HAVELL 1984) and rat IFN-γ (H. SCHELLEKENS and P. VAN DER MEIDE 1987, personal communication) have been produced. Since IFN purification by affinity chromatography has become available, we can expect to see several species of IFN molecules in crystalline form in the near future. Also, as will be seen in the following section, these monoclonal antibodies have already been used to develop sensitive immunologic assays for each type of IFN.

C. Interferon Assays

From the discovery of IFN (1975) until recently (i.e., for a quarter of a century) IFN was assayed on the basis of its indirect biologic activities on target cells. In general, this was accomplished by measuring any of a vast number of parameters of virus replication in IFN-treated cells. Table 4 gives an overview of biologic and nonbiologic IFN assays. Since a complete list of biologic assays is reviewed and evaluated in depth by STEWART (1979), I shall discuss only general considerations and describe a few, widely used, IFN assays.

Table 4. Interferon assays

Biologic	Nonbiologic (immunologic)

1. Antiviral assays
    Plaque reduction (S, W)
    Yield reduction (R, S, W, L)
    Cytopathic effect inhibition (R, S, P, W, L)
    Radiochemical (R, S, P, W, L)
    Others (R, P, L)
	1. Radioimmunoassays (RIA)
	    Tandem RIA (R, S, P, W, L)
	    Competitive RIA (R, S, P, L)

2. Antiproliferative assays
 	
    Cell multiplication inhibition (R, S)
    DNA replication inhibition (R, S, P, W, L)
	2. Enzyme-linked immunoassays (ELISA)
	    Tandem ELISA
	    Competitive ELISA (?)

3. Assays detecting induced proteins
    Intracellular proteins; 2′-5′-Oligoadenylate
       synthetase (R, S, L)
    Surface proteins; major histocompatibility
       complex classes I, II (R, S, L)
	3. Immunodotting (?)

R, reproducible; S, sensitive; P, practical; W, widely used; L, large sample size.

I. Biologic Assays

It should first be noted that all biologic IFN assays (be they antiviral, antiprolifer-ative or via induction of proteins) require living tissue culture cells which are markedly heterogeneous. Also, since all these assays are based on an indirect quantitation of an IFN activity, one must always ascertain that the "effect" is really attributable to IFN. Some of the criteria for acceptance of a substance as an IFN have been described previously (McNEILL 1981; STEWART 1979).

1. Antiviral

Just considering the methods based on measuring the antiviral actions of IFNs, there are as many ways to quantitate IFNs as there are ways of measuring virus replication. A typical antiviral assay is performed as follows. An IFN preparation is diluted serially in culture medium (usually two- to threefold) and each dilution is incubated for some hours (or usually overnight) with the test cells which are then infected with selected, pretitrated challenge virus. After appropriate inter-vals (24, 48 h, etc.), the virus growth parameter is measured in each of the culture series. In each assay, appropriate controls must be included (i.e., cells with me-dium alone, cells with or without virus in the absence of IFN, and cells with IFN alone). IFN activity quantitated in terms of each bioassay is referred to as an IFN "unit." If we define "units" of IFN as the reciprocal of end point dilutions of an IFN preparation which protects 50% of the cells, then it is obvious that a "unit" of IFN could vary greatly with the same preparation, depending on the sensitivity of target cells to the IFN and challenge virus. For this reason, international ref-erence IFN preparations have been made available for interested investigators. Each laboratory can equate units of its IFN to these "international reagents" which are accepted by the World Health Organization and can be obtained from the Division of Biological Standards, National Institute for Medical Research, Mill Hill, London NW7 1AA, United Kingdom, or from the Research Resources Branch, Building 31, the National Institutes of Health, Bethesda, MD 20014, United States.

Each IFN assay has to contain an international standard IFN, titrated in parallel with the test IFNs. This is necessary for other reasons as well as those al-ready mentioned. Test IFN preparations may contain factors which influence the assay. In an antiviral assay, end points can be derived by plotting dilutions of the test IFN against percentage function measured in controls. This plot normally produces a semilinear slope over a range corresponding to 50% (25%–75%) of virus growth. In fact, in all IFN bioassays, semisigmoid relationships are found. Virus-induced effect is conventionally expressed as a reciprocal dilution giving a reliable inhibition end point. As a general consideration, it should be emphasized that in any antiviral assay, even with low dilution steps of the IFN sample, a two-fold difference in IFN titer is of marginal significance (50% experimental error). Most of the IFN assays are listed in Table 4. A brief description of some selected, widely used, antiviral assays is given below. An evaluation of assays based on fac-tors such as reproducibility, sensitivity, expense, rapidity, and safety which influ-ence the choice of assays is also indicated in Table 4.

a) Virus Plaque Reduction Assays

The ability of viruses to form plaques offers a convenient method for quantitation of virus (WAGNER 1961; for review see STEWART 1979). Usually, IFN is diluted in two- to threefold steps and added to confluent cell monolayers. After overnight incubation at 37 °C, the cultures are incubated with a convenient number of plaque-forming particles of the challenge virus. After 1 h, the unadsorbed virus is removed, the cells overlaid with a semisolid agar medium, and 1–3 days later virus plaques are counted. The reciprocal dilution of the IFN reducing the plaque count to 50% of that in the virus controls is the titer or end point unit. This assay method is laborious and expensive, but it has been widely used (STEWART 1979).

b) Virus Yield Reduction Assays

Direct measurement of virus yields has advantages over plaque reductions assays in that the test can be performed with challenge viruses which do not form clear plaques and the reduction can be measured in a variety of ways, e.g., measurement of infectious virus particules or viral products (hemagglutinin, or neurominidase). All these methods are sensitive and accurate. Measuring infectious virus directly is laborious, and so it cannot be used for large numbers of IFN samples. The hemagglutinin measurement assay was used by the discoverers of IFN (ISAACS and LINDENMANN 1957) and is a highly sensitive and precise assay. Reduction of hemadsorption with Sendai virus is based on adsorption of erythrocytes to virus-infected cells (STEWART 1979). After washing, the red cells are lysed and the hemoglobin is quantitated by optical density. A modification of this method uses ^{51}Cr-labeled erythrocytes. Measurement of neurominidase yields has been reported to be reproducible, rapid, and sensitive, and is widely used; however, the assay needs a cell system that is a good producer of neurominidase.

c) Cytopathic Effect Inhibition Assays

Some viruses exert cytopathic effects (CPE) on cells that can be visualized either directly under the microscope or indirectly via vital dye uptake by target cells. This method, first introduced by Ho and ENDERS (1959), has been used with slight modifications to assay a variety of IFN types with several different viruses (for review see STEWART 1979). Because of its simplicity, speed, and reproducibility, this latter test has become perhaps the most widely used IFN assay. A full description of the CPE inhibition assay which has been adapted to a "semimicro" system by ARMSTRONG (1971) is given here. We routinely use this assay in our laboratory for human (α, β, γ), mouse, and rat IFN determinations.

Growth medium (50 µl RPMI + 2% fetal calf serum) is distributed into each well of 96-well flat-bottom microtiter plates. The IFN sample (25 µl) is introduced into the first well of the row, and 25-µl aliquots from each well transferred to subsequent wells to provide 1 : 3 serial dilutions. When dilutions are finished (including on each plate a standard IFN as well as cell and virus controls), freshly trypsinized cell suspensions (e.g., Wish or Hep2 cells for human, L929 cells for mouse, Ratec cells for rat) are then introduced into each well (100 µl containing 1–2×10^4 viable cells) and the plates are then incubated overnight at 37 °C in a 5% CO_2 atmosphere.

After incubation a 50-µl suspension of virus (vesicular stomatitis virus for all animal cell types or Mengo virus for human cells) containing 500–1000 plaque-forming units in

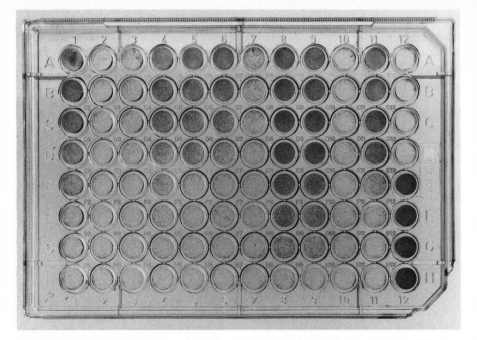

Fig. 4. Standard antiviral (cytopathic effect inhibition) assay for IFNs. Photograph of a dyed microtiter plate in which an IFN assay has been performed as described in the text. The last row (12) shows virus and cell controls (four wells each). Row 11 shows the titration of an IFN standard (500 units/ml). Other rows were treated with several different IFN (test) samples all titrated (threefold) vertically. Sample rows 8 and 9, for instance, contained 4000 units/ml IFN while sample row 1 was like the standard, and rows 2 and 10 contained no IFN activity

serum-free medium, is added to each well, except cell controls. Plates are incubated for further 48 h at 37 °C. When virus control wells show 100% lysis (as judged by microscopic examination), the plates are decanted, and the wells filled with dye fixer solution (0.5% crystal violet, 5% formalin, in 50% ethanol/saline). After 1 min, the dye fixer solution is decanted, the microtiter plates are rinsed copiously with water and allowed to dry at room temperature. As can be seen in Fig. 4, an IFN titer can already be read at this time by visual inspection. (For better quantitation the dye can be eluted and absorbance measured spectrophotometrically.) I believe this method is currently in use in many laboratories for assaying a variety of IFN types. A modification of this assay which utilizes bovine kidney cells (MDBK) requires less time as results can be otained within 24 h (RUBINSTEIN et al. 1981). Our laboratory also uses this assay because the MDBK cells are sensitive to a variety of species of IFN (bovine, human, rat, and mouse).

d) Viral RNA Labeling Assays

Viral RNA can be labeled by incubating radiolabeled RNA precursors with virus in culture medium. This allows detection of IFN-induced virus inhibition by inhibition of radiolabel ([^{3}H] uridine) incorporation (ALLEN and GIRON 1970). This sensitive, precise, and reproducible assay with various modifications has been used in many laboratories.

2. Antiproliferative

IFNs induce a number of changes in cells, one of which is to inhibit cell growth. This can be measured by various parameters such as cell counting or inhibition of [^{3}H] thymidine incorporation into DNA. The use of a number of such assays for the quantitation of IFNs has been described (for review see CLEMENS and MCNURLAN 1985; STEWART 1979) however, they are of limited use as the question of whether all IFNs are identical in their ability to induce growth inhibition has not so far been resolved. It is known that certain cells (such as human Daudi and mouse L1210 cell lines) are more sensitive to IFN's growth inhibitory action than others, and kinetics of growth inhibition vary greatly among different cell lines.

3. Detection of Induced Proteins

One of the enzymes induced by IFN is 2'-5'-oligoadenylate synthetase (also referred to as 2'-5'-A polymerase), levels of which can be detected quantitatively (MINKS et al. 1979; REVEL 1979). Also, certain IFNs induce cell surface antigens such as major histocompatibility complex class I (HLA or H-2) or class II (Ia) which can be detected by labeled specific antibodies. However, all these assays suffer from the fact that not every IFN acts in the same way. For example IFN-γ has been found to be more potent than the others as an Ia inducer (KIRCHNER 1984). Factors which influence the biologic assays (such as IFN incubation time, assay duration, age of cell culture, etc.) are reviewed by STEWART (1979).

II. Nonbiologic (Immunologic) Assays

It is only within the last few years that monoclonal antibodies have become available against various IFN types. Such antibodies not only help in purification of IFNs, but also aid in the development of "nonbiologic" assays for quantitative measurement of IFNs. Biologic assay by their nature are complex, though sensitive, lengthy, laborious, and subject to inherent variability (GIART and FLEISCHAKER 1984). Therefore, the immunoassays described here fulfill a major need for simple, reproducible, direct IFN assays.

1. Radioimmunoassays

The first immunoradiometric assay of human leukocyte IFN was developed by using the first monoclonal antibody in combination with a polyclonal sheep IFN-specific antibody (SECHER 1981), and this test has been made commercially available by Celltech Ltd. (Slough, Berkshire, United Kingdom). More recently, we have analyzed the antigenic structure (epitopes) of human IFN-αs, and found several pairs of monoclonal antibodies which recognize different epitopes of a given IFN-α subtype (ALKAN 1985), and this work has enabled us to develop tandem RIAs as sensitive as the antiviral assays (ALKAN et al. 1985).

A tandem RIA is performed as follows. Monoclonal antibody (it can also be polyclonal) is coupled to polystyrene macrobeads (Spherotech, Zürich, Switzerland; instead of beads 3- to 5-ml tubes or 96-well plates can be used). After blocking the unbound sites on the beads by overnight incubation with 10% horse serum, each sample is incubated with

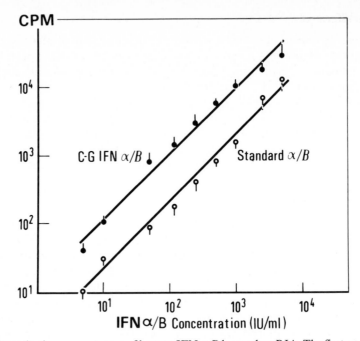

Fig. 5. Quantitative measurement of human IFN-α-B by tandem RIA. The first monoclonal antibody was fixed to macrobeads and the second was labeled with [125]I. The beads were incubated with various doses of IFN, washed, and counted. Parallel but non superimposable curves of standard natural and recombinant IFN-α-B reflect the differences in the bioassay results (units/ml) obtained in two different laboratories

test (and standard) IFN dilutions for 4 h at 4 °C. After washing the beads, an ^{125}I-labeled second monoclonal antibody (which does not cross-react with the first) is added and the beads are incubated overnight at 4 °C. The beads are then washed four times and transferred to a gamma counter.

Results of such an assay are shown in Fig. 5. The binding is linear over a relatively wide range of IFN concentrations, and complete parallelism of the slopes was obtained with standard (natural) and recombinant IFN-α-B. Human IFN-β or IFN-γ and certain other subtypes of human IFN-α are not detected in this RIA. It is not known, however, whether this assay measures only biologically active IFN. A recently developed RIA for human IFN-γ (Centacor, Malvern, PA, United States) seems to detect only the active IFN-γ molecule (Sedmak et al. 1985). Another tandem RIA for human IFN-γ is also available from Celltech.

This type of RIA offers many advantages over bioassays in term of speed (4 h instead of 3 days), reproducibility, simplicity, and determination of IFN type (α, β, γ) and some subtype specificity (α-A, B, etc.) (Alkan et al. 1985). In addition, at least some of the RIAs are equally effective when using either serum or culture media, which is a requirement for use in clinical trials aiming to monitor IFN levels in patient serum.

2. Other Immunologic Assays

a) Tandem ELISA

This assay is essentially the same as the tandem RIA already described, except that a second IFN-specific antibody is labeled with an enzyme in order to avoid using radioactive isotopes. We have labeled a second IFN-specific monoclonal antibody with alkaline phosphatase and obtained similar results to those presented in Fig. 5. However, this tandem ELISA is less reproducible than RIA. Perhaps for this reason ELISA is not yet in general use. When the minor problems, due to enzymes or high backgrounds, are solved tandem ELISA may well replace RIA.

b) Dot Immunobinding

To our knowledge, this method, which has been applied to a wide range of proteins (TOWBIN and GORDON 1984) has not yet been discovered by IFN researchers. As can be seen in Fig. 6, we have demonstrated that very small amounts of natural or recombinant human IFN subtypes applied to nitrocellulose paper can easily be detected by means of IFN-specific antibodies (S. S. ALKAN 1986, unpublished work). The method is sensitive (picogram range), reproducible, rapid, and, in particular, suitable for large sample numbers. However, its potential as a semiquantitative IFN screening assay has not yet been widely recognized.

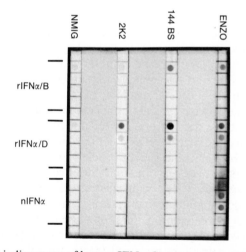

Fig. 6. Dot immunobinding assay of human IFNs. Concentrations of IFNs per 0.5 µl spot were: for IFN-α-B 10–0.01 ng; IFN-α-D 4–0.004 ng; nIFN-α: 1–0.001 ng. After air-drying, the nitrocellulose filter strips are incubated with either normal mouse serum (NMIG), monoclonal antibody 2K2, 144BS, or a polyclonal anti-IFN from ENZO Biochem Inc., New York. Spots were visualized by a peroxidase-labeled rabbit anti-mouse immunoglobulin

c) Combined Immunoprecipitation Bioassay

This assay was originally developed to detect IFN-specific antibodies present in culture supernatants at a time when purified IFN was available neither for immunization nor for testing (Alkan et al. 1983; Eshar et al. 1983).

The principle of combined immunoprecipitation bioassay (Ci-Ba) is to immunoprecipitate IFN by an anti-IFN and a second antibody (e.g., anti-mouse Ig), to dissolve the precipitate with acid (for IFN-αs) or base (for IFN-γ) and to assay the activity of immunoprecipitated IFN in a standard antiviral bioassay, as described previously (Sect. C.I.1). Two points are worth mentioning here. First, Ci-Ba, as has been demonstrated previously (Alkan et al. 1983), can be used for the determination of the relative amounts of IFN subtypes in a given natural leukocyte IFN preparation for which purified IFN preparations are not required. Second, the assay can be useful in searching for antibodies against very impure, novel LK.

D. Interferon in the Clinic and its Future

There is no doubt that IFN is one of the most interesting molecules in biology. Within about three decades of its discovery, many facets of IFN biology have been uncovered, but IFN has still not moved from the laboratory into the clinic. Perhaps this is normal, remembering the journey of penicillin from Fleming's laboratory to the clinic.

IFN, the first LK to be discovered, has suffered from many problems in large-scale production, purification, and assays. With the help of the new developments of genetic engineering and hybridoma technology, these problems have been solved only very recently. With the aid of the latter, immunologic purification and quantitation of IFNs are now becoming easier and more reliable. Large amounts of recombinant, pure IFN became available in the 1980s, and these materials are now being used in large-scale clinical trials. Treatment of many viral diseases and some malignant diseases with natural or recombinant IFN have yielded promising results; however, one cannot yet say that IFN is in use as a routine drug. This is because new problems have arisen during clinical testing. IFN is a potent molecule and does produce toxic reactions and side effects. Apart from inducing severe influenza-like symptoms, IFN can cause several other more serious adverse reactions, including hematologic and nervous system toxicity. For optimal use, the dosage, route of administration, duration of treatment, and last but not least, the type of IFN to be used (IFN-α subtypes, and IFN-β or IFN-γ) have to be studied. Thus, even after solving the major purification problems of LK such as IFN (and more recently IL-2), translation of recent advances into clinical applications is not going to be easy and rapid; it requires considerable effort and perhaps new application methods, e.g., targeting via carrier molecules such as monoclonal antibodies (Alkan et al. 1984; Alkan 1986).

Cantell (1979) recently reviewed the clinical findings with conventionally administered natural IFN-αs. Clinical experience with recombinant IFNs has also been summarized (Merigan 1983; Kirkwood and Ernstoff 1984; Borden 1984). Altogether, current phase I (10% efficacy) and phase II trial results with

IFNs establish their clinical potential. Most encouraging results were obtained in leukemia, multiple myeloma, low grade lymphoma, renal bladder carcinoma, melanoma, Hodgkin's lymphoma, and Kaposi's sarcoma. Very high remission rates of hairy cell leukemia (which has been a difficult disease to treat with cytotoxic drugs) has been reported (QUESADA et al. 1984). In general, response to recombinant IFN as a single agent in solid tumors has been poor.

Immunomodulatory actions of IFNs, in particular IFN-γ, have been recognized only recently (BECKER 1985; HOCHKEPPEL and ALKAN 1986; DE MAEYER-GUIGNARD and DE MAEYER 1985). Therefore, it is too early to discuss the use of IFNs or antagonists in autoimmune diseases such as rheumatoid arthritis or lupus erythematosus.

The great promise of IFN as an antiviral agent was evident from the beginning, primarily because its protective effect is not limited to a single virus. Can we use IFN today to prevent and cure natural viral infections in humans? The answer is – not yet. How about herpetic keratitis, herpes zoster, herpes simplex, cytomegalovirus infections in transplant patients, or hepatitis B infections? In all these viral diseases, and especially in warts, a therapeutic effect of IFN has been reported. Recently, IFN-α has also been shown to have some efficacy in preventing the common cold (JUST et al. 1986). However, in all these indications, no consensus has yet been reached as to the optimal dose or route of administration of IFNs. Although nobody has any doubt about IFN's antiviral action in vivo, the optimal clinical regimen for IFN treatment is proving difficult to determine, and negative results are often obtained if IFN is not used properly (CANTELL 1979). In conclusion, despite the clear antiviral, antitumor, and immunomodulatory actions of IFNs, routine clinical use of these LK as drug therapies (by themselves or in combination with other drugs) will be achieved within the next 5–10 years (indeed, an IFN-α-A(2) is already available to clinicians). I believe that IFNs and other LKs (IL-1–4, TNF, etc.) as natural biologic response modifiers are going to change the face of medicine, provided that new treatment strategies are developed (ALKAN 1986).

References

Alkan SS (1985) Epitope analysis of six human IFN-alpha subtypes by monoclonal antibodies. In: Dianzani F, Rossi GB (eds) The interferon system. Raven, New York, p 237 (Serono symposia, vol 24)

Alkan SS (1986) Specific targeting of interferons by monoclonal antibodies: Potential for targeting other lymphokines. In: Lymphokines, the new super-drugs? Conference, London, 3–4 March 1986. IBC Technical Services, London

Alkan SS, Weideli H-J, Schuerch AR (1983) Monoclonal antibodies against human leucocyte interferons for the definition of subclasses and their affinity purification. Protides Biol Fluids 30:495–498

Alkan SS, Miescher-Granger S, Braun DG, Hochkeppel HK (1984) Antiviral and antiproliferative effects of interferons delivered via monoclonal antibodies. J Interferon Res 4:355–363

Alkan SS, Hochkeppel HK, Küttel L (1985) Epitope analysis by monoclonal antibodies of five human recombinant interferon subtypes. In: Kirchner H, Schellekens H (eds) The biology of the interferon system 1984. Elsevier, Amsterdam, pp 91–98

Allen PT, Giron DJ (1970) A rapid sensitive assay for interferons based on the inhibition of MM virus nucleic acid synthesis. Appl Microbiol 20:317–322

Armstrong JA (1971) Semi-micro, dye-binding assay for rabbit interferon. Appl Microbiol 21:723–725

Becker S (1985) Effect of interferon-gamma on class-II antigen expression and accessory cell function. Surv Immunol Res 4:135–145

Bocci V (1981) Production and role of interferon in physiological conditions. Biol Rev 56:49–85

Borden EC (1984) Interferons and cancer: how the promise is being kept. Interferon 5:43–83

Branca AA, Baglioni C (1981) Evidence that type I and II interferons have different receptors. Nature 294:768–770

Cantell K (1979) Why is interferon not in clinical use today? Interferon 1:1–28

Cantell K, Tovel DR (1971) Substitution of milk for serum in the production of human leucocyte interferon. Appl Microbiol 22:625–628

Clemens MJ, McNurlan MA (1985) Regulation of cell proliferation and differentiation by interferons. Biochem J 226:345–360

De Maeyer-Guignard J, De Maeyer E (1985) Immunomodulation by interferons: recent developments. Interferon 1: 6:69–91

Derynck R, Remaut E, Saman E, Stanssens P, de Clercq E, Content J, Fiers W (1980) Expression of human fibroblast interferon gene in *Escherichia coli*. Nature 287:193–197

Dijkema R, van der Meide PH, Pouwels PH, Caspers M, Dubbeld M, Schellekens H (1985) Cloning and expression of the chromosomal immune interferon gene of the rat. EMBO J 4:761–767

Eshhar Z, Novik D, Gigio O, Marks Z, Friedlander Y, Revel M, Rubinstein M (1983) Monoclonal antibodies to human leukocyte and fibroblast interferon. Protides Biol Fluids 30:491–494

Giard DJ, Fleischaker RT (1984) A study showing a high degree of interlaboratory variation in the assay of human interferons. J Biol Stand 12:265–269

Goeddel DV, Leung DW, Dull TJ, Gross M, Lawn RM, McCandliss R, Seeberg PH et al. (1981) The structure of eight cloned human leukocyte interferon cDNAs. Nature 290:20–26

Gordon J, Minks MA (1981) The interferon renaissance: molecular aspects of induction and action. Microbiol Rev 45:244–266

Gray PW, Goeddel DV (1983) Cloning and expression of murine immune interferon cDNA. Proc Natl Acad Sci USA 80:5842–5846

Gray PW, Leung DW, Pennica D, Yelverton E, Najarian R, Simenson CC, Derynck R et al. (1982) Expression of human immune interferon cDNA in *E. coli* and monkey cells. Nature 295:503–508

Havel EA, Yip YK, Vilcek J (1977) Characteristics of human lymphoblastoid (Namalwa) interferon. J Gen Virol 38:51–59

Ho M, Enders JE (1959) An inhibitor of viral activity appearing in infected cell cultures. Proc Natl Acad Sci USA 45:385–389

Hochkeppel HK, Alkan SS (1986) Immunomodulatory actions of interferons. In: Revel M (ed) Clinical aspects of interferon. Nijhoff, Boston, (Developments in molecular virology) (1987)

Hochkeppel HK, Menge U, Collins J (1981) Monoclonal antibodies against human fibroblast interferon. Eur J Biochem 118:437–442

Hoskins M (1935) A protective action of neurotropic against viscerotropic yellow fever virus in *Macacus rhesus*. Am J Trop Med Hyg 15:675–680

Isaacs A, Lindenmann J (1957) Virus interference I. The interferon. Proc R Soc [B] 147:257–267

Just M, Berger R, Ruuskanen O, Lünd M, Linder S (1986) Intranasal interferon alfa-2a treatment of common cold. A preliminary study. J Interferon Res [Suppl 1] 6:32

Kirchner H (1984) Interferon gamma. Prog Clin Biochem Med 1:169:203

Kirchner H, Marcucci F (1984) Interferon production by leukocytes. In: Vilcek J, de Maeyer E (eds) Interferon and the immune system. Elsevier, Amsterdam, pp 7–34 (Interferon, vol 2)

Kirkwood JM, Ernstoff MS (1984) Interferons in the treatment of human cancer. J Clin Oncol 2:336–352

Köhler G, Milstein C (1975) Continuous culture of fused cells secreting antibody of predefined specificity. Nature 256:495–497

Le J, Chang TW, Lio V, Yip YK, Vilcek J (1985) Monoclonal antibodies as structural probes for oligomeric human interferon-gamma. J Interferon Res 5:445–453

Liang CM, Herren S, Sand A, Jost T (1985) Study of antigenic epitope recognized by monoclonal antibodies to recombinant interferon-gamma. Biochem Biophys Res Commun 128:171–178

Littman SJ, Devos R, Baglioni C (1985) Binding of unglycosylated and glycosylated human recombinant interferon to cellular receptors. J Interferon Res 5:471–476

Mayer U (1980) Structural and biological relationships of low molecular weight interferon inducers. Pharmacol Ther 8:173–192

McNeill TA (1981) Interferon assays. J Immunol Methods 46:121–127

Merigan TC (1983) Human interferon as a therapeutic agent-current status. N Engl J Med 308:1530–1531

Minks AM, Bevin S, Maroney PA, Baglioni C (1979) Synthesis of 2'5-oligo(A) in extracts of interferon-treated HeLa cells. J Biol Chem 254:5058–5064

Mogensen KE, Bandu M-T, Vignaux F, Uze G, Eid P (1984) Receptor mediated pathways for interferon action: in vivo implications. Med Oncol Tumor Pharmacother 1:77–85

Nagata S, Mantei N, Weissmann C (1980) The structure of one of the eight or more distinct chromosomal genes for human interferon. Nature 287:401–408

Orchansky P, Novick D, Fischer DG, Rubinstein M (1984) Type I and type II interferon receptors. J Interferon Res 4:275–282

Pestka S, Langer JA, Fisher PB, Weinsten IB, Ortaldo J, Herberman RB (1985) The human interferons: from the past and into the future. In: Ford RJ, Maizel AL (eds) Mediators in cell growth and differentiation. Raven, New York, pp 261–281

Quesada JR, Reuben J, Manning JT, Hersh EM, Gutterman JU (1984) Alpha interferon for induction of remission in hairy cell leukemia. N Engl J Med 310:15–18

Revel M (1979) Molecular mechanisms involved in antiviral effects of interferons. Interferon 1:101–163

Rubinstein M, Rubinstein S, Familletti PC, Miller RS, Waldman AA, Pestka S (1979) Human leukocyte interferon: production, purification to homogeneity and initial characterization. Proc Natl Acad Sci USA 76:640–644

Rubinstein S, Familetti PC, Pestka S et al. (1981) Convenient assay for interferons. J Virol 37:755–758

Secher DS (1981) Immunoradiometric assay of human leukocyte interferon using monoclonal antibody. Nature 290:501–503

Secher DV, Burke DC (1980) A monoclonal antibody for large scale purification of human leukocyte interferon. Nature 285:446–450

Sedmak JJ, Siebenlist R, Grossberg SE (1985) Human IFN antiviral activity correlates with immunological reactivity in a double-monoclonal antibody radiometric assay. J Interferon Res 5:397–402

Shaw GD, Boll W, Taira H, Mantei N, Lengyel P, Weissmann C (1983) Structure and expression of cloned murine IFN genes. Nucleic Acids Res 11:555–573

Spitalny GL, Havel EA (1984) Monoclonal antibody to murine gamma interferon inhibits lymphokine-induced antiviral and macrophage tumoricidal activity. J Exp Med 159:1560–1565

Staehelin T, Durrer B, Schmidt J, Takacs B, Stocker J, Miggiano V, Stöhle C et al. (1981) Purification and characterization of recombinant human leukocyte interferon (IFNrA) with monoclonal antibodies. J Biol Chem 256:9750–9754

Stewart W II (1979) The interferon system. Springer, Vienna New York

Taniguchi T, Mantai N, Schwarzstein M, Nagata S, Maramatsu M, Weissmann C (1980a) Human leukocyte and fibroblast interferons are structurally related. Nature 285:547–549

Taniguchi T, Ohno S, Fujii-Kuriyama Y, Muramatsu M (1980b) The nucleotide sequence of human fibroblast interferon cDNA. Gene 10:11–15

Tavernier J, Fiers W (1984) The presence of homologous regions between interferon sequences. Carlsberg Res Common 49:359–364

Towbin H, Gordon J (1984) Immunoblotting and dot immunobinding – current status and outlook. J Immunol Methods 72:313–340

Von Gabain A, Ohlsson M, Lindström E, Lundström M, Lundgren E (1986) Polymorphism and gene duplication in the human IFNα and β gene family. In: Jörnvall H (ed) Molecular evolution of life. Chemica Stripta, vol 26B. Cambridge University Press, Cambridge, pp 357–362

Wagner RR (1961) Biological studies of interferon. Suppression of cellular infection with eastern equine encephalomyelitis virus. Virology 13:323–337

Yip YK, Roy H, Pang L, Urban C, Vilcek J (1981) Partial purification and characterization of human (immune) interferon. Proc Natl Acad Sci USA 78:1601–1605

Zoon KC, Arnheiter H (1984) Studies of the interferon receptors. Pharmacol Ther 24:259–278

CHAPTER 10

Factors Regulating IgE Synthesis

C. Gaveriaux, T. Payne, and F. Loor

A. IgE Regulation

IgE antibodies are normally involved in the elimination of parasites, but they are also produced in some individuals against antigens which should normally be eliminated by another class of antibody. Such antigens are called allergens. Structural characteristics of antigens may determine allergenicity to some extent, but dysregulation of the immune response is the major reason for the development of IgE-mediated allergy. Recent studies indicate that the type of antibody produced to a particular antigen is governed by Fc receptor-bearing T cells and class-specific immunoglobulin-binding factors which can suppress, or in some cases enhance, the response of that isotype (Löwy et al. 1983). Of the immunoglobulin-binding factors, those which regulate the initiation of an IgE response have been the best studied and are described in this chapter. Mechanisms involved in maintaining a high level of IgE synthesis long after allergen exposure are more complex, and persisting IgE-secreting cells can be refractory to T cell control (Holt and Turner 1985).

I. Development of an IgE Response

An IgE antibody response is normally initiated by activation of membranous IgE-bearing B lymphocytes (B_ε) which differentiate into cells producing antibody at a high rate (PC_ε). The serum IgE antibody then binds to receptors present on the plasma membrane of various cell types, including blood basophils and tissue mast cells (A cells, cells involved in anaphylaxis). These receptors specifically bind to the Fc portion of native IgE with high affinity, and are thus termed "high affinity $Fc_\varepsilon R$." If the A cells armed with specific IgE antibody then encounter further allergen, activation of the A cells will occur, provided the allergen has caused IgE-mediated clustering of the $Fc_\varepsilon R$. This effector phase of IgE-mediated immunoprotection consists of the release of a variety of mediators stored in the A cell granules. The mediators in turn cause complex tissue responses which result in the elimination of parasites, but can in some cases also lead to inappropriate allergic/anaphylactic responses.

Although there exist some animal models in which the defect in this defense mechanism lies at the level of the A cell (Kitamura et al. 1978; Kitamura and Go 1979), most types of dysregulation of the IgE immune response have their origin at the level of B_ε cell – PC_ε cell differentiation. Results described for IgE synthesis (Sect. A.III), together with recent findings in allergic asthma, suggest that low affinity IgE receptors on cells other than mast cells can play an important role in allergic responses (Capron et al. 1985; Morley et al. 1985).

II. Evidence for a Specific IgE Isotype Regulation

The general outline of specific immunoglobulin isotype regulation which has emerged over the past 5–10 years is most advanced for IgE, owing to the intensive research of the groups led by Ishizaka (1984; Ishizaka et al. 1985), Katz (1982, 1985; Katz et al. 1984), Kishimoto (1982; Suemura and Kishimoto 1985), and Watanabe et al. (1976) and Hirano et al. (1983). The present picture of the control mechanisms for IgE antibody production is one of astonishing complexity, involving a variety of cell types and factors. A few models provide a general concept of how IgE synthesis might be controlled in mice, rats, and humans. However, further dissection of the regulatory mechanisms has led to divergent and sometimes contradictory interpretations by the various groups as to how genetic, antigenic, and environmental factors could affect the outcome of animal exposure to antigen. Since the same variables have no influence on the IgG response, the concept of isotype-specific regulation in addition to the antigen-specific T helper and T suppressor regulatory mechanisms was proposed.

The IgE isotype response may be selectively enhanced under the following conditions (for references see reviews by Ishizaka 1976; Katz 1982): (a) in humans with the hyper-IgE syndrome (Saryan et al. 1983; Thompson et al. 1985); (b) in rodents exposed to a low dose of X-rays or a low dose of cyclophosphamide injected prior to the antigen; (c) in rodents and humans suffering from an intestinal nematode infestation; (d) in humans or rodents immunized with antigens in adjuvants such as aluminum hydroxide and *Bordetella pertussis*; and (e) in rodents immunized with antigens chemically coupled to rutin-like polyphenolic compounds (Francus et al. 1983). By contrast, the IgE response can be selectively depressed: (a) in selected strains of mice, and is even absent in strains such as SJL (Revoltella and Ovary 1969; Pfeiffer et al. 1983); (b) in rodents immunized with antigens in certain adjuvants such as complete Freund's adjuvant (CFA); (c) in rodents repeatedly exposed to CFA components prior to antigen injection; and (d) in rodents immunized with antigens chemically coupled to the active component of CFA, i.e., the *Mycobacterium* (Kishimoto et al. 1976), and possibly even with antigen-conjugated muramyl peptides (Kishimoto et al. 1979).

III. Models of IgE Regulation

It has been proposed that T lymphocytes regulate the key events leading to high or low IgE responsiveness in the models of both Ishizaka and Kishimoto, whereas the Katz group gives this role to B cells. Some unusual features of the Lyt surface phenotype markers have been noted for T cells providing IgE helper or suppressor signals, but recent data indicate that attempts to make strict correlations of such markers with their cellular function may not be relevant.

The two main models of IgE regulation in the murine immune system have been developed by Ishizaka (1984; Ishizaka et al. 1985) and Katz et al. (1984;

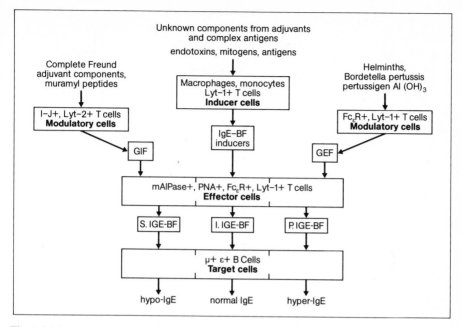

Fig. 1. Ishizaka model of IgE regulation

MARCELLETTI and KATZ 1984; KATZ 1985) (Figs. 1 and 2). We have incorporated some features which were implicit in their models, but not explicitly formulated as such, and have made some extrapolations in order to include related findings.

The key cells in the Ishizaka model of IgE regulation (ISHIZAKA et al. 1985) are $Fc_\varepsilon R^+$, Lyt-1$^+$ T cells. They produce IgE-binding factors (IgE-BF) of similar peptide composition, but with different carbohydrate chains which induce different biologic activities. A suppressor factor (S.IgE-BF), an inactive factor (I.IgE-BF), and a potentiating factor (P.IgE-BF) have been described. All can bind B cell membranous IgE and modulate the ability of the B lymphocytes to be activated to IgE-producing cells (PC_ε), and thus regulate serum IgE production. The key $Fc_\varepsilon R^+$, Lyt-1$^+$ T cells are themselves under the control of other leukocytes, an inducer cell class which includes macrophages, monocytes, and Lyt-1$^+$ T cells, and two modulatory T cell classes: an $Fc_\varepsilon R^-$ T cell with a suppressor phenotype (I-J$^+$, Lyt-2$^+$ T cells) and an $Fc_\varepsilon R^+$ T cell with a helper surface phenotype (Lyt-1$^+$ T cells). The inducer cells are presumed to release interferon-like substances which induce the synthesis of the IgE-BF peptide moiety by the $Fc_\varepsilon R^+$, Lyt-1$^+$ cells that are central to the model. The level of glycosylation of IgE-BF, a post-translational maturation process, appears to be under the control of at least two other factors, a glycosylation-inhibiting factor (GIF) and a glycosylation-enhancing factor (GEF). GIF is released by the $Fc_\varepsilon R^-$, Lyt-2$^+$ modulatory cells as a 16 kdalton phosphorylated, lipomodulin-like molecule, whereas GEF appears to be released by the $Fc_\varepsilon R^+$, Lyt-1$^+$ modulatory T cells as a 25 kdalton galactose-binding, kallikrein-like molecule (i.e., an enzyme targeted through its lectin character).

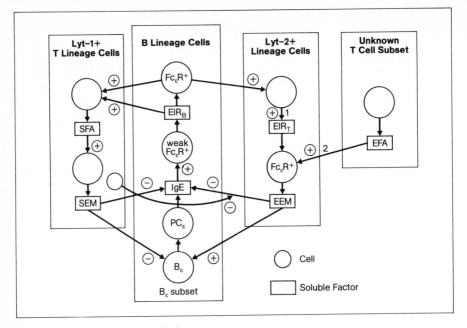

Fig. 2. Katz model of IgE regulation

GIF thus appears to inhibit the N-glycosylation of IgE-BF via inhibition of phospholipase A_2, whereas the reverse appears to be true for GEF. Based on present knowledge of carbohydrate biosynthesis (BERGER et al. 1982), the principal action of GEF might be to increase the trimming of the high mannose carbohydrates and addition of terminal sugars such as sialic acid and fucose. It is known that phosphorylated lipomodulin is inactive (HIRATA et al. 1982) and GIF must also be dephosphorylated to be effective. A given cell will only be a target for GIF if it expresses a membrane-located phosphatase, presumably of the alkaline type (mAlPase), like that found on other cell types such as activated B lineage cells (MOSBACH-OZMEN et al. 1986). This feature is very unusual in T lymphocytes, alkaline phosphatase only being described as a marker of immature cells in the thymus. To be effective, GEF must find binding sites for its peanut agglutinin (PNA)-like activity (binding of terminal galactose residues) on the target cell and a substrate for its proteolytic activity (possibly an unknown kininogen). This could lead to the production of kinin-like molecules (bradykinin also potentiates the glycosylation of IgE-BF), and these peptides could inactivate endogenous lipomodulin via phosphorylation, allowing higher phospholipase A_2 activity, leading to an enhancement of IgE-BF glycosylation. Thus, the IgE-BF-producing cell must simultaneously be a target for both GIF and GEF and could have the rare phenotype Lyt-1[+], mAlPase[+], PNA[+], $Fc_\varepsilon R^+$. Under the normal conditions of the immune response, both GIF and GEF are being produced, but the ratio of the two products depends on a number of factors, such as the type and schedule of antigen administration, the type of adjuvant, chemical alterations of the antigen, and time after injection. As shown in Fig. 1, different adjuvants or components of adjuvant have more or less well-defined cellular targets, particularly as inferred from their ability to induce the production of IgE-BF peptides inducer molecules, GIF, or GEF.

In this scheme of IgE regulation, the function of $Fc_\varepsilon R$ expressed on the different cells is not evident. However, earlier studies by Ishizaka's team have shown an increase of $Fc_\varepsilon R$ expression when lymphoid cells were exposed to IgE in vitro. Since IgE-BF could comprise fragments of $Fc_\varepsilon R$, further characterization of the relevance of $Fc_\varepsilon R$ expression to IgE-BF production and biologic activity will be required.

Ishizaka's model can be adapted to account for IgE antibody-inducing, natural and artificial antigens which contain rutin-like polyphenols (FRANCUS et al. 1983). When such antigens are recognized through the antigen receptor of the $Lyt-1^+$, $mAlPase^+$, PNA^+, $Fc_\varepsilon R^+$ T cells, antigen binding actually targets to the cell surface the rutin-like polyphenols, which have been described as capable of generating kinins independently (BECKER and DUBLIN 1977). Local kinin generation would bypass GEF and directly activate IgE-BF glycosylation. The resulting $P.IgE$-BF would eventually lead to high IgE production in response to such antigens.

The central cells in the Katz model (Fig. 2) are $Fc_\varepsilon R^+$ B cells. According to the original description by MARCELLETTI and KATZ (1984), serum IgE would act on $Fc_\varepsilon R^-$ B cells to induce expression of $Fc_\varepsilon R$. We find it difficult to envisage in molecular terms how a cell could recognize a molecule if not through a receptor of sufficient avidity. It is more reasonable to suggest that IgE is recognized through Fc receptors on the B cells. The B cells described by Katz would in fact be "weak $Fc_\varepsilon R^+$" B cells, the weakness of their Fc-binding capacity resulting either from a low receptor density or receptors of low affinity. Thus, serum IgE would stimulate weak $Fc_\varepsilon R^+$ B cells to produce a factor termed EIR_B (IgE-induced regulant of B cell origin) which would increase the expression of $Fc_\varepsilon R$ by these (or possibly other) B cells. This could be achieved either by increasing receptor density or by switching the weakly IgE-cross-reactive Fc receptor to a truly specific $Fc_\varepsilon R$. These $Fc_\varepsilon R^+$ B cells would then interact with T cells of either the $Lyt-1^+$ subset and stimulate them to produce the suppressive factor of anaphylaxis (SFA), or with the $Lyt-2^+$ subset to produce the IgE-induced regulant of T cell origin (EIR_T). The formation of SFA may require either a direct cell–cell contact between the $Fc_\varepsilon R^+$ B cells and the $Lyt-1^+$ T cells or simple exposure of the T cells to EIR_B. The targets of SFA would also be $Lyt-1^+$ T cells which would be further stimulated to produce the suppressor effector molecule, SEM, which suppresses IgE synthesis both in vitro and in vivo.

The production of EIR_T appears to require intracellular contact between the $Fc_\varepsilon R^+$ B cells and the $Lyt-2^+$ T cells. The targets of this factor are $Lyt-2^+$ cells, and they are stimulated to express Fc_ε receptors. At some point during this process, ill-defined T cells would produce an enhancing factor of anaphylaxis (EFA) which would have the newly induced $Fc_\varepsilon R^+$ cells as its target. This would stimulate the latter cells to produce the enhancing effector molecule (EEM) which enhances IgE synthesis both in vitro and in vivo. Both EEM and SEM are IgE-BFs which might be expected to respectively upregulate or downregulate B cell responsiveness through binding to their membranous IgE. However, both final effector molecules are thought to exert a negative feedback effect on the induction of $Fc_\varepsilon R^+$ B cells by IgE, i.e., the cells which play the central role in initiating the suppressive and enhancing arms of IgE regulation through interaction with Lyt-1^+ and Lyt-2^+ cells, respectively. The inhibition of IgE-induced $Fc_\varepsilon R$ expression on B cells by SEM and EEM could be simply explained by their IgE-binding property, i.e., by preventing the IgE from delivering the induction signal for $Fc_\varepsilon R$ expression. While neither SEM nor EEM interfere with $Fc_\varepsilon R$ expression induction of Lyt-2^+ by EIR_T, SEM appears to be inhibitory for the induction of $Fc_\varepsilon R$ on B cells by EIR_B, whereas EEM has no effect. Until the biochemical properties of EIR_B, EIR_T, and their congeners have been characterized in molecular terms, these findings will remain difficult to understand. A further complexity comes from the need for a regulated positive feedback on IgE production. This might be provided by the competition of ill-defined Lyt-1^+ T cells with the inhibitory effects of EEM on $Fc_\varepsilon R$ expression by the key B cells of the Katz model. It has not been explained how these Lyt-1^+ cells can have a negative influence on EEM when it acts on $Fc_\varepsilon R^+$ B cells, but no influence when it acts on B_ε cells: both cell types have surface-expressed IgE (through which EEM would probably bind), either bound through a receptor in the first case or acting as an endogenous membrane receptor for antigen in the second case.

Despite their differences, the two models show some common features:

1. Neither the antigen nor the modulatory treatment act uniquely or directly on the IgE-bearing B cells to bring about their final differentiation into IgE-secreting plasma cells, but act through a cascade of positive and negative regulatory cells and factors. Various dysregulations of IgE antibody responses, both over- and under-responsiveness, could be provoked at several steps of the cascade.

2. Under normal conditions, i.e., when IgE and/or other Ig classes develop as appropriate, there is a regulated balance of positive and negative signals for B_ε cell activation or the capacity of B_ε cells to be activated via antigen binding to their membranous IgE. Both models allow for an early positive feedback and a later negative feedback to produce IgE when and where it is needed. This may depend on the serum concentration of IgE and feedback effects on the regulatory cells, but the details are still unclear.

3. Cells expressing $Fc_\varepsilon R$ of low affinity (at least an order of magnitude lower than the affinity of A cell $Fc_\varepsilon R$; Spiegelberg 1984), are intimately involved in the key steps of IgE production, although the phenotype attributed to those cells, and the steps at which they act, differ in the two models (e.g., B cells and Lyt-2^+ T cells according to Katz and Lyt-1^+ cells according to Ishizaka). Incubation of the $Fc_\varepsilon R^+$ cells concerned with high IgE concentrations leads to an upregulation of $Fc_\varepsilon R$ expression, which contrasts with the downregulation phenomena usually observed for glycoprotein and other hormones interacting with their receptors. The functional significance of $Fc_\varepsilon R$ expression remains elusive in both models.

4. An important common feature now recognized for the different models is that factors which eventually modulate the responsiveness of B_ε cells are IgE-BFs. The existence of such factors has been central to the models of the Kishimoto – Yamamura team, and of the Ishizaka team, for whom further research concentrated on events which regulated the production of IgE-BF. The research of the Katz team developed after the initial identification of an SFA and they only re-

cently recognized IgE-BFs as the factors which modulate B_ε cell activity. Curiously enough, although the events in the cascade in both models are often described in great detail, the problem of explaining the mechanism by which an IgE-BF might modulate B_ε cell responsiveness to antigen has not been tackled.

IV. Methods for Measuring IgE-Specific Immunoregulation

An important limitation on studies of the regulation of IgE production in vivo or in vitro comes from the very low levels of IgE found in serum. Detection requires very sensitive methods, thus increasing the risk of artifactual results due to insufficient specificity of the antibody reagents used. The IgE-specific antibodies generally available are usually considered to have poor specificity, but this is all relative since they are required to detect IgE specifically in the presence of immunoglobulins of other classes at concentrations which are several orders of magnitude higher. Very few antibody reagents successfully fulfill these demands. The measurement of IgE is usually performed by radioimmunoassays (LIU et al. 1980) or enzyme immunoassays (DE WECK et al. 1985), which, with few exceptions, measure both native and denatured IgE. The only relevant test commonly employed for measuring native IgE is the passive cutaneous anaphylaxis reaction (BROCKLEHURST 1978), an in vivo test which requires the use of many animals, but is very sensitive, highly specific, and physiologic since the IgE is recognized by $Fc_\varepsilon R$ on the effector A cells.

In vitro assays of IgE antibody production are also hampered by the low IgE titers and by the fact that, in the tissues such as spleen and lymph nodes which are commonly used for in vitro immunology, IgE-producing cells are present at a very low frequency. IgE-specific reverse plaque assays (DEGUCHI et al. 1983) have been generally used for measuring IgE-producing cells, but because of the variability of the assay (SUEMURA and KISHIMOTO 1985), they were later replaced by either immunofluorescent detection of cytoplasmic IgE-containing cells or an enzyme-linked immunosorbent assay of the IgE released into the supernatant (DE WECK et al. 1985).

IgE-binding factors (IgE-BF and IgE-TsF, IgE-T-suppressive factor) are measured through their capacity to bind to insolubilized polyclonal or monoclonal IgE (YODOI et al. 1981), their inhibitory action on the formation of rosettes between low affinity $Fc_\varepsilon R^+$ cells and IgE coated red cells (YODOI et al. 1981), or their capacity to upregulate or downregulate IgE production in vitro by normal or hybridoma cells (SUEMURA et al. 1983). Discrimination between S.IgE-BF and P.IgE-BF is made not only through their different in vitro modulatory action on IgE production (UEDE et al. 1984), but also through their specific carbohydrate composition (YODOI et al. 1982). GEF and GIF are essentially identified by their capacity to induce IgE-BFs with carbohydrate structures characteristic of P.IgE-BF and S.IgE-BF, respectively (IWATA et al. 1983 a,b).

SFA is evaluated indirectly through its capacity to downregulate IgE production in vitro or in vivo (ZURAW et al. 1981). All other factors reported in the preceding sections, including some IgE-BFs, have been too poorly characterized (e.g., activity reported in a crude cell culture supernatant) or depend on isolated descriptions. For these reasons, the methods for their characterization have not been described.

In the following section, we will first describe the preparation and characterization of SFA and of the IgE-BF-like products obtained by various groups; IgE-TsF characterized by the Kishimoto-Yamamura group, the two types of IgE-BFs obtained by Ishizaka's group in rats, mice, and humans, and finally the GIF and GEF identified by the same group.

B. Production and Measurement of IgE-Regulating Factors

Factors regulating IgE production in the mouse and the rat can be isolated from serum, from in vitro cultures of lymphocytes from treated animals, or from the supernatants of specific hybridomas. Factors regulating human IgE have been obtained from culture supernatants of peripheral blood lymphocytes from normal or "atopic" patients.

I. Suppressive Factor of Allergy (SFA)

The suppressive factor of allergy defined by KATZ (1982) was obtained from the serum of low responder mice (SJL) following intraperitoneal injection of complete Freund's adjuvant (CFA) (TUNG et al. 1978) or from the ascitic fluid produced in these animals by weekly intraperitoneal injection of CFA in saline. On passing unfractionated ascites fluid from SJL mice over a concanavalin A(Con A)–Sepharose column, the nonabsorbed fraction suppressed the enhanced IgE response of SJL mice induced by 250 rad X-irradiation before antigen challenge. By contrast, the fraction which was absorbed onto the Con A–Sepharose and which could be eluted by α-methylmannoside, showed clear enhancing effects (TUNG et al. 1978). Moreover, CFA could induce both enhancing and suppressive activities detectable in the serum of high and low responder mice (KATZ et al. 1979). In all these experiments, animals were immunized with dinitrophenyl (DNP)–*Ascaris*, DNP–bovine serum albumin, or DNP–keyhole limpet hemocyanin, and the anti-DNP IgE production was measured by the passive cutaneous anaphylaxis (PCA) reaction after injection of DNP–bovine serum albumin in Evans blue (HAMAOKA et al. 1974).

ZURAW et al. (1981) showed that the in vitro induction by pokeweed mitogen of spontaneous IgE synthesis by mononuclear cells from human peripheral blood can also be selectively suppressed by human SFA recovered from the culture supernatant of a two-way human mixed lymphocyte reaction. IgE was measured by a solid phase radioimmunoassay system (ZURAW et al. 1981), the IgE specificity of which was later reconfirmed (CHEN et al. 1984). A human T cell hybridoma (1C1) which constitutively produces large amounts of SFA has been constructed (KATZ 1985). SFA from this hybridoma was effective in inhibiting both murine and human IgE synthesis in vitro.

II. Human IgE-Binding Factors (IgE-BF)

Human IgE-BF have been reported by several groups. An IgE-BF was produced by RPMI 8866 cells, a B cell line expressing Fc receptors and releasing IgE-potentiating factor (SARFATI et al. 1984a,b). The factor released by cells treated with tunicamycin, an inhibitor of protein glycosylation, suppressed IgE secretion by human U266 myeloma cells and completely inhibited the activity of IgE-potentiating factors on B lymphocytes from allergic individuals. IgE, IgG, IgM, and IgA levels in the culture supernatant were measured by a solid phase sandwich radioimmunoassay.

DE WECK et al. (1985) examined the action of an IgE-BF secreted by T cell hybridomas on the in vitro spontaneous IgE synthesis by cells from different atopic individuals. The IgE was detected with an enzyme-linked immunosorbent assay system (ELISA) with a tandem of monoclonal IgE-specific antibodies directed against different IgE-specific Fc epitopes.

Supernatants of cultures of T cells derived from patients with elevated serum IgE levels were shown by SARYAN et al. (1983) to induce significant IgE synthesis in 7-day cultures of normal B cells isolated from peripheral blood. A subsequent publication from this group (LEUNG et al. 1985) reported the isolation of $Fc_\varepsilon R^+$ and $Fc_\varepsilon R^-$ T cells from patients with the hyper-IgE syndrome, and indicated that the cells could be maintained in long-term culture by use of interleukin 2. The supernatants from the $Fc_\varepsilon R^+$ T cell lines specifically enhanced IgE synthesis in B cells derived from patients with allergic rhinitis, but not from normal individuals. IgE was detected in these experiments by a paper immunosorbent test (PRIST) assay.

III. IgE Class-Specific Suppressive Factors of T Cell Origin (IgE-TsF)

1. Mouse IgE-TsF

A mouse IgE-suppressive factor, IgE-TsF, was defined by KISHIMOTO (1982). It was produced by injecting mice intraperitoneally with 100 µg DNP–*Mycobacterium* in incomplete Freund's adjuvant, removing the spleen cells 2 weeks after immunization, and incubating 5×10^7 cells with 2×10^6 DNP–human serum albumin pulsed macrophages. The cell-free supernatant was then used as a source of IgE-TsF, which in turn was detected in an in vitro culture system: DNP–ovalbumin-primed cells were cultured for 24 h with 0.1 µg/ml DNP–ovalbumin, then washed and cultivated for 6 days with the cell-free supernatant which had been dialyzed against culture medium. For in vivo experiments, 1 ml cell-free supernatant was administered intravenously to normal mice before challenging with 5 µg DNP–ovalbumin in aluminum hydroxide gel (alum), and sera were collected on days 7, 10, and 14. IgE against DNP and against an unrelated antigen, benzylpenicilloyl, in sera or the culture supernatants were measured with the PCA reaction (KISHIMOTO et al. 1978). IgE-producing cells were also measured by the plaque-forming cell (PFC) assay (SUEMURA et al. 1981).

IgE-TsF has also been produced by T cell hybridomas (SUGIMURA et al. 1982; WATANABE et al. 1978). Incubation of IgE-TsF from these sources with IgE-producing hybridomas for 1 h at 37 °C resulted in both a reduction of the number of IgE-secreting cells, as determined in a reverse plaque assay, and of the number of cytoplasmic IgE-positive cells detected by immunofluorescence (SUEMURA et al. 1983).

2. Human IgE-TsF

A human IgE-TsF similar to that found in the mouse has been detected in culture supernatants of T cells from patients with pulmonary tuberculosis (SUEMURA and KISHIMOTO 1985). After activation with 10 µg/ml purified protein derivative and/ or 2.5 µg/ml human IgE for 6–7 days, these T cells showed a suppressive effect on the polyclonal IgE response induced by 2.5 µg/ml pokeweed mitogen together with *Staphylococcus aureus* strain Cowan I. The cell-free supernatant from these T cell populations was effective in suppressing both spontaneous IgE production and mitogen- or antigen-induced IgE responses in cultures of peripheral blood lymphocytes obtained from atopic or normal patients. The IgE response was first assessed with a reverse plaque assay (DEGUCHI et al. 1983) and then with a sensitive IgE-specific ELISA (GOLDSMITH 1981), using rabbit anti-IgE as a coating and a mixture of monoclonal IgE-specific antibodies with different epitope specificities for detection.

IV. IgE-Binding Factors (IgE-BF)

1. Rat IgE-BF

The suppressive IgE-BF (S.IgE-BF) is spontaneously released when mesenteric lymph node cells from rats treated repeatedly with CFA are cultured for 24 h (HIRASHIMA et al. 1980 b). Serum from rats treated with CFA and culture filtrates of their spleen cells also induced normal mesenteric lymph node cells to form S.IgE-BF (HIRASHIMA et al. 1981 b). Alternatively, this IgE-BF could be produced by infecting rats for 8 days with 2500 larvae of *Nippostrongylus brasiliensis* and then incubating their mesenteric lymph node cells for 24 h with rat IgE. On the other hand, potentiating IgE-BF (P.IgE-BF) is released by rat mesenteric lymph node cells obtained 2–4 weeks after subcutaneous injection of *Nippostrongylus brasiliensis* larvae and cultured for 24 h without IgE (SUEMURA et al. 1980). The suppressive and potentiating factors can be purified from cell-free culture supernatants and serum samples by gel filtration through a Sephadex G-75 column and by binding to IgE-Sepharose, followed by elution at pH 3. They can be separated from each other by fractionation on lentil lectin Sepharose (YODOI et al. 1980), PNA, or Con A–Sepharose (YODOI et al. 1982). UEDE et al. (1984) prepared a rat–mouse T cell hybridoma, 23B6, which, on incubation with rat IgE, produces two species of IgE-BF (15 and 30 kdalton). The 15 kdalton factor selectively suppresses the IgE response of BALB/c-primed spleen cells in vitro to homologous antigen. P.IgE-BF has been produced by transfection of COS 7 monkey kidney cells with a cDNA clone obtained with mRNA of 23B6 hybridoma cells incubated with IgE (ISHIZAKA et al. 1985). These cells, when cultivated in the presence of glycosylation-inhibiting factor (GIF), produced S.IgE-BF instead of P.IgE-BF, confirming that both products share a common gene. In fact, transfection with a single cDNA clone (8.3) resulted in IgE-BFs of various sizes (60, 30, 14, and 11 kdalton), the smallest resulting from post-translational modifications of the 60 kdalton, single polypeptide chain IgE-BF (JARDIEU et al. 1985). The coding sequence of that IgE-BF cDNA revealed homogolies to a polymerase gene (MARTENS et al. 1985), but more dramatically a 72% homology of the 3' terminal two-thirds with the *gag* and *pol* genes of Syrian hamster intracisternal A particles (IAP), an endogenous retrovirus (TOH et al. 1985). Finally, both nucleic acid data (blot analyses, DNA sequence comparisons, and heteroduplex analyses) and encoded protein data (immunochemical cross-reactivity) suggested that this IgE-BF is a member of the endogenous retrovirus-like IAP gene family in the mouse (MOORE et al. 1986). Up to 97% of the coding sequence of this IgE-BF gene could be accounted for by recombination of the *gag* and *pol* genes from two mouse IAP genomes (IAP-IL3 and MIARN) (YMER and YOUNG 1986). Four other IgE-BF cDNAs were all found to represent structural variants of the full-size IAP genome (KUFF et al. 1986). Since it now appears that the IgE-BF genetic material is an integral part of the murine IAP retrotransposon genome, a definite demonstration of the biologic activity of these IAP-IgE-BF cDNA-encoded proteins is awaited with interest.

Some 5–7 days after rats were given a single intraperitoneal injection of *Bordetella pertussis* vaccine containing 10^{10} organisms, P.IgE-BF was detected in sera of the treated animals (HIRASHIMA et al. 1981a). Their circulating lymphocytes and spleen cells spontaneously release an IgE-BF with affinity for lentil lectin and which potentiates IgE responses. In order to assesss the suppressive or potentiating effect of an IgE-BF, a suspension of DNP–ovalbumin-primed rat spleen cells was mixed with a sample of the factor and cultivated with 1 μg/ml DNP–ovalbumin for 5 days (HIRASHIMA et al. 1980b; SUEMURA et al. 1980). The number of IgE- and IgG2-containing cells which developed from 10^6 nucleated cells placed in culture were counted by indirect immunofluorescence, with fluorescein-labeled goat anti-rabbit IgG and rabbit antibodies specific for rat IgE (HIRASHIMA et al. 1980a). Possible IgE-regulating factors were also mixed with mouse plasma cells together with antigen or mouse IgE-secreting hybridoma cells, and IgE production was measured by the PCA reaction (BROCKLEHURST 1978), PFCs (UEDE et al. 1984), or surface or cytoplasmic IgE-containing cells (UEDE et al. 1984; SUEMURA et al. 1980).

2. Mouse IgE-BF

Mouse IgE-BF was obtained by incubation of normal spleen cells with 10 μg/ml homologous IgE, 2 μg/ml polyinosinic–polycytidylic acid, or 200 units/ml beta interferon for 24 h (UEDE et al. 1983). These factors were also found in the culture filtrates of antigen-primed spleen cells which had been stimulated with 10 μg/ml homologous antigen for 24 h (UEDE and ISHIZAKA 1984). Characterization of these IgE-BFs with respect to their IgE suppressive or potentiating activities was the same as for the rat IgE-BFs. The suppressive IgE-BF could easily be obtained from SJL mice, whereas BDF_1 strain mice served as a better source of the potentiating IgE-BF.

3. Human IgE-BF

The group led by Ishizaka also developed systems for the production of human IgE-BFs. Peripheral blood mononuclear cells from ragweed-sensitive patients formed IgE-BFs when incubated with 10 μg/ml ragweed antigen E and 10 μg/ml human IgE for 4 days. IgE-BFs were also formed in a mixed lymphocyte culture of cells from normal individuals when the activated lymphocytes were cultured for a further 2 days in the presence of 10 µg/ml IgE (Ishizaka and Sandberg 1981). In addition, normal cells that proliferated in the presence of interleukin 2 formed IgE-BF when incubated with human IgE for 2 days. Based on these findings, Huff and Ishizaka (1984) constructed a human hybridoma, which, on incubation with human IgE, produces IgE-BF with affinity for Con A. The IgE-BFs were characterized by their selective binding to human IgE–Sepharose, but not to human IgG- or rat IgE-Sepharose, and their ability to inhibit rosette formation of a human cell line (RPMI 8866) having receptors for IgE, with fixed bovine red cells coated with human IgE. A purified IgE-BF obtained from the 166A2 clone selectively potentiated the IgE-forming response of rat mesenteric lymph node cells (Huff and Ishizaka 1984). The effect of this IgE-BF on human IgE production is currently being studied.

V. Glycosylation-Enhancing and -Inhibiting Factors (GEF and GIF)

1. Rat GEF and GIF

GIF can be produced in supernatants of mesenteric lymph node cells obtained from 8-day *Nippostrongylus brasiliensis*-infected rats (Iwata et al. 1984a) and from 24-h culture of spleen cells (10^7 cells/ml) collected from keyhole limpet hemocyanin–CFA-primed rats (Iwata et al. 1984a; Uede and Ishizaka 1982). Culture filtrates of 23A4 hybridoma cells incubated for 24 h with IgE have also been employed as a source of GIF (Iwata et al. 1984a). GEF and bradykinin induced both 23A4 hybridoma cells and normal mesenteric lymph node cells to release GIF (Iwata et al. 1984b).

Measurement of GIF was performed as follows. Aliquots of normal mesenteric lymph node cells were cultured for 24 h with an equal volume of the culture filtrate to be tested, together with 10 µg/ml rat IgE. After filtration and concentration, the culture supernatants were fractionated on lentil lectin–Sepharose, as described for IgE-BF. Normal mesenteric lymph node cells cultured with IgE alone formed IgE-BF that distributed approximately equally between the effluent and eluate fractions. The majority of IgE-BF formed in the presence of GIF failed to bind to the lentil lectin (Iwata et al. 1984a,b). 23A4 cells can replace normal mesenteric lymph node cells for the detection of GIF (Iwata et al. 1983a).

GEF can be induced by incubation of normal rat spleen cells for 48 h with 0.2 µg/ml pertussigen (leukocytosis-promoting factor) from *Bordetella pertussis* (Iwata et al. 1983a), or with 5 µg/ml Con A for 24 h (Iwata et al. 1983b). The factor was also detected in a 24-h culture supernatant of rat mesenteric lymph node cells obtained 14 days after infection with *Nippostrongylus brasiliensis*, or released on stimulation of keyhole limpet hemocyanin–alum-primed spleen cells (Iwata et al. 1984a). To detect GEF, 23A4 cells were incubated for 24 h in the presence or absence of the sample to be tested. The presence of GEF was assayed by the distribution of IgE-BF formed between the eluate and effluent fraction of a lentil lectin and a PNA–Sepharose column. The IgE-BF formed in the presence of GEF bound to lentil lectin and not to PNA (Iwata et al. 1984a,b). Normal mesenteric lymph node cells could be substituted for 23A4 cells (Uede and Ishizaka 1982).

2. Mouse GIF

GIF was released by Lyt-2^+, I-J$^+$ T cells following antigenic stimulation of spleen cells from mice treated with three intravenous injections of ovalbumin (JARDIEU et al. 1984). The factor was characterized by its ability to induce S.IgE-BF when added to normal BALB/c mouse spleen cells incubated with 10 µg/ml monoclonal mouse IgE, as well as by its ability to inhibit the Fc$_\varepsilon$R expression on rat lymphocytes. The GIF released spontaneously from antigen-specific suppressor T cells binds to I-J-specific antibodies, to a monoclonal antibody against lipomodulin, and has affinity for specific antigen and therefore appears related to antigen-specific suppressor factor (JARDIEU et al. 1984).

C. Future Developments

Several laboratories are at present engaged in finding practical routes to prepare the factors which regulate IgE synthesis. Sufficient pure material is likely to be available in the next few years to allow determination of the role of each of these factors in both primary and ongoing responses, and also in allergic conditions in humans. Mechanisms for modifying the immunoglobulin isotype formed to a given antigen clearly do exist and practical routes to achieving specific isotype regulation are likely to become research topics in an increasing number of laboratories over the next decade.

References

Becker CG, Dublin T (1977) Activation of factor XII by tobacco glycoprotein. J Exp Med 146:457–467

Berger EG, Buddecke E, Kamerling JP, Kobata A, Paulson JC, Vliegenthart JFG (1982) Structure, biosynthesis and functions of glycoprotein glycans. Experientia 38:1129–1162

Brocklehurst WE (1978) Passive cutaneous anaphylaxis. In: Weir DM (ed) Immunochemistry. Blackwell, Oxford, pp 21.1–21.6 (Handbook of experimental immunology, vol 1, 3rd edn)

Capron A, Ameisen JC, Joseph M, Auriault C, Tonnel AB, Caen J (1985) New functions for platelets and their pathological implications. Int Arch Allergy Appl Immunol 77:107–114

Chen PP, Nonaka M, O'Hair CH, Cohen PA, Zuraw BL, Katz DH (1984) Human IgE synthesis in vitro by pokeweed mitogen-stimulated human lymphoid cells: verification with a reconfirmed ε specific radioimmunoassay. J Immunol 133:1909–1913

Deguchi H, Suemura M, Ishizaka A, Ozaki Y, Kishimoto S, Yamamura Y, Kishimoto T (1983) IgE class-specific suppressor T cells and factors in humans. J Immunol 131:2751–2756

De Weck AL, Stadler BM, Knutti-Müller J, Ruff P, Hofstetter H, Ludin C, Heusser C (1985) Factors influencing human IgE synthesis in vitro and in vivo. Int Arch Allergy Appl Immunol 77:38–44

Francus T, Siskind GW, Becker CG (1983) Role of antigen structure in the regulation of IgE isotype expression. Proc Natl Acad Sci USA 80:3430–3434

Goldsmith PK (1981) A highly sensitive enzyme linked immunosorbent assay for human immunoglobulin E: comparison of microtiter plates and dishes methodologies. Anal Biochem 117:53–60

Hamaoka T, Newburger PE, Katz DH, Benacerraf B (1974) Hapten-specific IgE antibody responses in mice. III. Establishment of parameters for generation of helper T cell function regulating the primary and secondary response of IgE and IgG B lymphocytes. J Immunol 113:958–973

Hirano T, Kumagai Y, Okumura K, Ovary Z (1983) Regulation of murine IgE production: importance of a not-yet-described T cell for IgE secretion demonstrated in SJA9 mice. Proc Natl Acad Sci USA 80:3435–3438

Hirashima M, Yodoi J, Ishizaka K (1980 a) Regulatory of IgE-binding factors from rat T lymphocytes. IV. Formation of IgE-binding factors in rats treated with complete Freund's adjuvant. J Immunol 125:2154–2160

Hirashima M, Yodoi J, Ishizaka K (1980 b) Regulatory role of IgE-binding factors from rat T lymphocytes. III. IgE-specific suppressive factor with IgE-binding activity. J Immunol 125:1442–1448

Hirashima M, Yodoi J, Huff TF, Ishizaka K (1981 a) Formation of IgE-binding factors by rat T lymphocytes. III. Mechanisms of selective formation of IgE-suppressive factors by treatment with complete Freund's adjuvant. J Immunol 127:1810–1816

Hirashima M, Yodoi J, Ishizaka K (1981 b) Regulatory role of IgE-binding factors from rat T lymphocytes. V. Formation of IgE-potentiating factor by T lymphocytes from rats treated with Bordetella pertussis vaccine. J Immunol 126:838–842

Hirata F, Notsu Y, Iwata M, Parente L, DiRosa M, Flower RJ (1982) Identification of several species of phospholipase inhibitory proteins by radioimmunoassay for lipomodulin. Biochem Biophys Res Commun 109:223–230

Holt PG, Turner KJ (1985) Persistent IgE-secreting cells which are refractory to T-cell control. Int Arch Allergy Appl Immunol 77:45–46

Huff TF, Ishizaka K (1984) Formation of IgE-binding factors by human T-cell hybridomas. Proc Natl Acad Sci USA 81:1514–1518

Ishizaka K (1976) Cellular events in the IgE antibody response. Adv Immunol 23:1–75

Ishizaka K (1984) Regulation of IgE synthesis. Annu Rev Immunol 2:159–182

Ishizaka K, Sandberg K (1981) Formation of IgE-binding factors by human T lymphocytes. J Immunol 126:1692–1696

Ishizaka K, Huff TF, Jardieu P, Moore KW, Martens CL (1985) IgE-binding factors. Selective regulation of the IgE responses by T cell factors. Int Arch Allergy Appl Immunol 77:13–20

Iwata M, Huff TF, Uede T, Munoz JJ, Ishizaka K (1983 a) Modulation of the biological activities of IgE-binding factor. II. Physicochemical properties and cell sources of glycosylation-enhancing factor. J Immunol 130:1802–1808

Iwata M, Munoz JJ, Ishizaka K (1983 b) Modulation of the biological activities of IgE-binding factor. IV. Identification of glycosylation-enhancing factor as a kallikrein-like enzyme. J Immunol 131:1954–1960

Iwata M, Akasaki M, Ishizaka K (1984 a) Modulation of the biologic activities of IgE binding factor. VI. The activation of phospholipase by glycosylation enhancing factor. J Immunol 133:1505–1512

Iwata M, Huff TF, Ishizaka K (1984 b) Modulation of the biological activities of IgE-binding factor. V. The role of glycosylation-enhancing factor and glycosylation-inhibiting factor in determining the nature of IgE-binding factors. J Immunol 132:1286–1293

Jardieu P, Uede T, Ishizaka K (1984) IgE-binding factors from mouse T lymphocytes. III. Role of antigen-specific suppressor T cells in the formation of IgE-suppressive factor. J Immunol 133:3266–3273

Jardieu P, Moore K, Martens C, Ishizaka K (1985) Relationship among IgE-binding factors with various molecular weights. J Immunol 135:2727–2734

Katz DH (1982) IgE antibody response in vitro: from rodents to man. Prog Allergy 32:105–160

Katz DH (1985) The IgE antibody system is coordinately regulated by FcR epsilon positive lymphoid cells and IgE-selective soluble factors. Int Arch Allergy Appl Immunol 77:21–25

Katz DH, Bargatze RF, Bogowitz CA, Katz LR (1979) Regulation of IgE antibody production by serum molecules. IV. Complete Freund's adjuvant induces both enhancing and suppressive activities detectable in the serum of low and high responder mice. J Immunol 122:2184–2190

Katz DH, Bogowitz CA, Katz LR (1984) The IgE antibody system: mature, peripheral B lymphocytes exert regulatory influences on the IgE systems of self-reconstituting, sublethally irradiated mice. J Mol Cell Immunol 1:83–89

Kishimoto T (1982) IgE class specific suppressor T cells and regulation of the IgE response. Proc Allergy 32:265–317

Kishimoto T, Hirai Y, Suemura M, Yamamura Y (1976) Regulation of antibody response in different immunoglobulin classes. I. Selective suppression of anti-DNP IgE antibody response by preadministration of DNP-coupled mycobacterium. J Immunol 117:396–404

Kishimoto T, Hirai Y, Suemura M, Nakanishi K, Yamamura Y (1978) Regulation of antibody response in different immunoglobulin classes. IV. Properties and function of "IgE class-specific" suppressor factor(s) released from DNP-*Mycobacterium*-primed T cells, J Immunol 121:2106–2112

Kishimoto T, Hirai Y, Nakanishi K, Azuma I, Nagamatsu A, Yamamura Y (1979) Regulation of antibody response in different immunoglobulin classes. VI. Selective suppression of IgE response by administration of antigen-conjugated muramylpeptides. J Immunol 123:2709–2715

Kitamura Y, Go S (1979) Decreased production of mast cells in S1/S1^d anemic mice. Blood 53:492–497

Kitamura Y, Go S, Hatanaka K (1978) Decrease of mast cells in W/W^v mice and their increase by bone marrow transplantation. Blood 52:447–452

Kuff EL, Mietz JA, Trounstine ML, Moore KW, Martens CL (1986) cDNA clones encoding murine IgE-binding factors represent multiple structural variants of intracisternal A-particle genes. Proc Natl Acad Sci USA 83:6583–6587

Leung DYM, Young MC, Geha RS (1985) Secretion of IgE-specific potentiating factors by human Fc R$^+$ T cell lines. Int Arch Allergy Appl Immunol 77:232–234

Liu FT, Bohn JW, Ferry EL, Yamamoto H, Molinaro CA, Sherman LA, Klinman NR, Katz DH (1980) Monoclonal dinitrophenyl-specific murine IgE antibody: preparation, isolation and characterization. J Immunol 124:2728–2737

Löwy I, Brezin C, Neauport-Sautes C, Theze J, Fridman WH (1983) Isotype regulation of antibody production: T-cell hybrids can be selectively induced to produce IgG1 and IgG2 subclass-specific suppressive immunoglobulin-binding factors. Proc Natl Acad Sci USA 80:2323–2327

Marcelletti JF, Katz DH (1984) FcR$_\varepsilon$$^+$ lymphocytes and regulation of the IgE antibody system. III. Suppressive factor of allergy (SFA) is produced during the in vitro FcR$_\varepsilon$ expression cascade and displays corollary physiologic activity in vivo. J Immunol 133:2837–2844

Martens CL, Huff TF, Jardieu P, Trounstine ML, Coffman RL, Ishizaka K, Moore KW (1985) cDNA clones encoding IgE-binding factors from a rat-mouse T cell hybridoma. Proc Natl Acad Sci USA 82:2460–2464

Moore KW, Jardieu P, Mietz JA, Trounstine ML, Kuff EL, Ishizaka K, Martens CL (1986) Rodent IgE-binding factor genes are members of an endogenous retrovirus-like gene family. J Immunol 136:4283–4290

Morley J, Page CP, Sanjar S (1985) Pharmacology of the late response and its relevance to asthma prophylaxis. Int Arch Allergy Appl Immunol 77:73–78

Mosbach-Ozmen L, Lehuen-Renard A, Gaveriaux C, Loor F (1986) Membrane alkaline phosphatase activity: an enzymatic marker of B-cell activation. Ann Inst Pasteur Immunol 137D:109–125

Pfeiffer P, König W, Bohn A (1983) Genetic dependence of IgE antibody production in mice infected with the nematode *Nippostrongylus brasiliensis*. I. Modulation of the IgE antibody response in vivo by serum factors. Int Arch Allergy Appl Immunol 72:347–355

Revoltella R, Ovary Z (1969) Reaginic antibody production in different mouse strains. Immunology 17:45–54

Sarfati M, Rector E, Sehon AH, Delespesse G (1984a) In vitro synthesis of IgE by human lymphocytes. IV. Suppression of the spontaneous IgE synthesis by IgE-binding factors secreted by tunicamycin-treated RPMI 8866 cells. Immunology 53:783–790

Sarfati M, Rector E, Wong M, Rubio-Trujillo M, Sehon AH, Delespesse G (1984b) In vitro synthesis of IgE by human lymphocytes. II. Enhancement of the spontaneous IgE synthesis by IgE-binding factors secreted by RPMI 8866 lymphoblastoid B cells. Immunology 53:197–205

Saryan JA, Leung DYM, Geha RS (1983) Induction of human IgE synthesis by a factor derived from T cells of patients with hyper-IgE states. J Immunol 130:242–247

Spiegelberg HL (1984) Structure and function of Fc receptors for IgE on lymphocytes, monocytes and macrophages. Adv Immunol 35:61–88

Suemura M, Kishimoto T (1985) Regulation of human IgE response by T cells and their products. Int Arch Allergy Appl Immunol 77:26–31

Suemura M, Yodoi J, Hirashima M, Ishizaka K (1980) Regulatory role of IgE-binding factors from rat T lymphocytes. I. Mechanism of enhancement of IgE response by IgE potentiating factor. J Immunol 125:148–154

Suemura M, Shiho O, Deguchi H, Yamamura Y, Böttcher I, Kishimoto T (1981) Characterization and isolation of IgE class-specific suppressor factor (IgE-TsF). I. The presence of the binding site(s) for IgE and of the H-2 gene products in IgE-TsF. J Immunol 127:465–471

Suemura M, Ishizaka A, Kobatake S, Sugimura K, Maeda K, Nakanishi K, Kishimoto S, Yamamura Y, Kishomoto T (1983) Inhibition of IgE production in B hybridomas by IgE class-specific suppressor factor from T hybridomas. J Immunol 130:1056–1060

Sugimura K, Nakanishi K, Maeda K, Kashiwamura SI, Suemura M, Shiho O, Yamamura Y, Kishimoto T (1982) The involvement of two distinct subsets of T cells for the expression of the IgE class specific suppression: establishment and characterization of PC-specific, T15 idiotype-positive T hybridomas and IgE class-specific, antigen-nonspecific T hybridomas. J Immunol 128:1637–1644

Thompson LF, Spiegelberg HL, Buckley RH (1985) IgE Fc receptor positive T and B lymphocytes in patients with the hyper IgE syndrome. Clin Exp Immunol 59:77–84

Toh H, Ono M, Miyata T (1985) Retroviral gag and DNA endonuclease coding sequences in IgE-binding factor gene. Nature 318:388–389

Tung AS, Chiorazzi N, Katz DH (1978) Regulation of IgE antibody production by serum molecules. I. Serum from complete Freund's adjuvant-immune donors suppresses irradiation-enhanced IgE production on low responder mouse strains. J Immunol 120:2050–2059

Uede T, Ishizaka K (1982) Formation of IgE-binding factors by rat T lymphocytes. VI. Cellular mechanisms for the formation of IgE-potentiating factor and IgE-suppressive factor by antigenic stimulation of antigen-primed spleen cells. J Immunol 129:1391–1397

Uede T, Ishizaka K (1984) IgE-binding factors from mouse T lymphocytes. II. Strain differences in the nature of IgE-binding factor. J Immunol 133:359–367

Uede T, Sandberg K, Bloom BR, Ishizaka K (1983) IgE-binding factors from mouse T lymphocytes. I. Formation of IgE-binding factors by stimulation with homologous IgE and interferon. J Immunol 130:649–654

Uede T, Huff TF, Ishizaka K (1984) Suppression of IgE synthesis in mouse plasma cells and B cells by rat IgE-suppressive factor. J Immunol 133:803–808

Watanabe N, Kojima S, Ovary Z (1976) Suppression of IgE antibody production in SJL mice. I. Nonspecific suppressor T cells. J Exp Med 143:833–845

Watanabe T, Kimoto M, Maruyama S, Kishimoto T, Yamamura Y (1978) Regulation of antibody response in different antibody classes. V. Establishment of T hybrid cell lines secreting IgE class-specific suppressor factor. J Immunol 121:2113–2117

Ymer S, Young IG (1986) Homology between IgE-binding factor gene and endogenous retroviruses. Nature 323:186–188

Yodoi J, Hirashima M, Ishizaka K (1980) Regulatory role of IgE-binding factors from rat T lymphocytes. II. Glycoprotein nature and source of IgE-potentiating factor. J Immunol 125:1436–1442

Yodoi J, Hirashima M, Bloom BR, Ishizaka K (1981) Formation of IgE-binding factors by rat T lymphocytes. I. Induction of IgE-binding factors by poly I:C and interferon. J Immunol 127:1579–1585

Yodoi J, Hirashima M, Ishizaka K (1982) Regulatory role of IgE-binding factors from rat T lymphocytes. V. The carbohydrate moieties in IgE-potentiating and IgE-suppressive factors. J Immunol 128:289–295

Zuraw BL, Nonaka M, O'Hair CH, Katz DH (1981) Human IgE antibody synthesis in vitro: stimulation of IgE responses by pokeweed mitogen and selective inhibition of such responses by human suppressive factor of allergy (SFA). J Immunol 127:1169–1177

CHAPTER 11

Generation, Biology, and Assay of Efferent Lymphokines

D. Gemsa

A. Introduction

To the novice, the immune system presents itself as an extremely complex network of cellular and humoral interactions. This inherent complexity is a reflection of the external world that, by a large variety of attack systems, constantly threatens the integrity of the body. In order to cope with a diverse group of invaders and nonself agents, the immune system had to adapt accordingly and was forced to develop efficient recognition and defense systems (Chap. 1). Among these immunologically specific and nonspecific reactions in both the cellular and humoral compartments, there is a considerable degree of cooperation that requires precise regulation. Beside the well-studied generation of help and suppression in the T and B lymphocyte compartments, it has only recently been fully recognized that non-antibody products of lymphocytes (lymphokines) and macrophages (monokines) may play a prominent role during the induction, maintenance, and effector phases of an immune response. Although lymphokines were first detected in lymphocyte culture supernatants only 20 years ago, this field of immunology has suffered until recently from the lack of a clear biochemical definition of the materials that were generated and employed in a variety of test systems. Usually, a certain lymphokine was named according to a functional response that it generated in a particular in vitro assay. This resulted in a multitude of different names and postulated factors. With the advent of gene technology, it has been possible to improve the characterization of some lymphokines in biochemical terms. This progress has permitted a better study of lymphokine effects in various stages of the immune response.

Fortunately, it may turn out that the large number of functionally characterized lymphokines may be reduced to a more realistic number of factors. This conclusion is based on recent observations that the use of a purified lymphokine in various assay systems may produce different effects previously attributed to different lymphokines. A notable example is gamma interferon (IFN-γ) which has been called "a lymphokine for all seasons" (Vilcek et al. 1985; Chap. 9). As Smith (1984) pointed out, there is a certain parallel between antibody and lymphokine research. Antibodies were initially classified according to the functions that they exerted in certain test systems, and only the elucidation of their molecular structure finally permitted their assignment to distinct classes of immunoglobulins. It is apparent that the field of lymphokine research has now reached a similar respectable position, aided by genetic engineering and subsequent molecular identification of some of the major lymphokines.

In this chapter, the molecular and biologic characteristics of some antigen-nonspecific factors will be described in detail. The selection of these cytokines has been made on the basis of the following criteria: the availability of "hard" biochemical data; proven importance in mediating effector or regulator functions in the immune response; and possible implications for therapeutic procedures. This does not preclude the possibility that, in the future, other lymphokines, which are not described here, may be of equal or greater biologic importance.

B. Migration-Inhibitory Factor (MIF)

I. Original Observations and Biologic Characteristics

When lymphocytes from animals with cellular hypersensitivity reactions are incubated with specific antigens or with mitogens, a plethora of lymphokines with different biologic activities are released. Among these soluble factors, one finds the migration-inhibitory factor (MIF); in fact, it was the first lymphokine to be described (Bloom and Bennett 1966; David 1966). This factor prevents the random migration of macrophages out of capillary tubes. Inhibition of macrophage migration, however, does not imply that the cells exhibit a reduced activity. In contrast, MIF-stimulated macrophages display enhanced functions such as metabolism, adherence, ruffled membrane motility, and spreading (David 1975). Furthermore, it has been demonstrated that MIF may be a signal to induce differentiation of macrophages from precursors (Sorg 1982; Sorg et al. 1984). MIF production by lymphoid cells could be correlated to the state of cellular immunity and was, for many years, considered to be a molecular equivalent of the delayed-type hypersensitivity state. MIF displays little species restriction and, thus, can be tested across species barriers. MIF selectively inhibits the migration of monocytes and macrophages. A companion factor, named leukocyte-inhibitory factor (LIF), has been detected which inhibits the random movement of neutrophils (Rocklin et al. 1980; Borish and Rocklin 1985). No biochemical relationship between the two factors has as yet been established. More than with other lymphokines, the interaction of MIF with receptors on macrophages has been the focus of intensive biochemical studies. It has been demonstrated that glycolipids, containing L-fucose and sialic acid, function as cell surface receptors for MIF (Liu et al. 1980, 1984).

II. Cellular Source

In the analysis of the cellular sources of MIF, it has become apparent that several cell types are involved. In the murine system, MIF release in response to soluble antigen seemed to be restricted to helper T cells of the Lyt-1$^+$ subset, whereas the Lyt-2$^+$,3$^+$ subpopulation with cytotoxic/suppressor activities produced little if any of the lymphokine (Adelman et al. 1980). Interestingly, MIF production by T cells was strictly dependent on the presence of macrophages from syngeneic or allogeneic sources (Sharma et al. 1979). The role of helper macrophages, however, was not related to antigen processing or presentation, since unknown soluble products (possibly interleukin 1) were capable of restoring MIF release from macrophage-depleted spleen cells. Also, B lymphocytes have been shown to be a source of MIF, but, in contrast to T lymphocytes, only polyclonal stimulants such as endotoxin appeared to be effective, whereas specific antigens remained inactive (ADELMAN et al. 1980). It is unclear at present whether nonlymphoid cells could represent a source of MIF. More recently, a report has furnished evidence that macrophages as well as endothelial cells may produce MIF in chronic inflammatory lesions as tissue sections bind a monoclonal MIF-specific antibody (BURMEISTER et al. 1985).

III. Molecular Characteristics

It appears that several molecular entities with MIF activity may exist. In the guinea pig, the species which has been preferentially used for many studies, two distinct compounds with molecular weights of 25000–40000, and 65000 have been characterized (REMOLD and MEDNIS 1979). In the human system, three distinct MIF compounds have been described that differ in molecular weight, buoyant density, isoelectric point, and kinetics of production. From the distinct sensitivities to trypsin and neuraminidase, it appears that the earlier produced MIF (1st-day MIF) is a protein, whereas the two later produced species of MIF (2nd-day MIF) may be the glycosylated forms of the earlier released protein (WEISER et al. 1981). In another study, SORG (1980) characterized MIF activities associated with molecular weights of 60000, 45000, 30000, and 15000, suggesting structurally related molecules which may be oligomers of a common low molecular weight monomer. Unfortunately, in contrast to other lymphokines, no information is presently available on the amino acid composition of MIF, and the cloning of the MIF gene has not been achieved so far.

In view of the many biochemical similarities of different lymphokines, it still cannot be definitely established that all MIFs are separate entities, distinct from other cytokines. Although MIF has been shown to be clearly different from macrophage-activating factor (MAF) (KNIEP et al. 1981), a functional and biochemical overlap with IFN-γ has frequently been suggested (NETA and SALVIN 1982). Indeed, one report has substantiated this possibility, since it could be clearly demonstrated that natural as well as recombinant IFN-γ displayed strong MIF activity. Furthermore, MIF activity in mitogen-induced blood lymphocyte cultures could be neutralized with a monoclonal IFN-γ-specific antibody (THURMAN et al. 1985). These findings do not exclude the possibility of other MIF-like cytokines without antiviral activity, but such possible coidentities require that a definite biochemical analysis of the MIFs should be undertaken with modern biotechnology techniques, involving gene cloning and expression. Retrospectively, it is particularly disappointing that the first lymphokine ever to be described still lacks definite characterization at the molecular level.

IV. Measurement

MIF activity may be measured by two related, but different bioassays. One method determines the degree of MIF-mediated inhibition of random migration of peritoneal exudate macrophages from capillary tubes (BLOOM and BENNETT

1966; DAVID 1966). Hematocrit tubes, filled with macrophages, are centrifuged at 100 g, cut at the cell-fluid interface, and placed in culture chambers, with or without MIF-containing supernatants. After 24 or 48 h incubation, the area of migration is projected and measured by planimetry. The other assay employs peritoneal macrophages suspended in 0.2% agarose droplets in microtiter plates. Migration of macrophages is measured at 24 or 48 h incubation by determining the distance of migration from the edge of the agarose droplet to the periphery by using a micrometer grid eyepiece in an inverted microscope (HARRINGTON and STASTNY 1973). As bioassays, both methods have their limitations and should eventually be replaced by immunoassays which will, however, require the availability of pure MIF and the development of highly specific antibodies.

C. Macrophage-Activating Factor (MAF)

I. Original Observations and Biologic Characteristics

The term macrophage activation was introduced by MACKANESS (1969) to characterize the enhanced microbicidal functions of macrophages in animals with acquired immunity to *Listeria monocytogenes*. The animals not only acquired resistance against the immunizing agent, but also against antigenically unrelated microorganisms. These findings led to the concept that macrophages become activated during a specific immune response, but as effector cells they are immunologically nonspecific. With regard to the underlying mechanism, it became clear that activation of macrophages is the outcome of an exclusive interaction with T lymphocytes. Activation does not require close macrophage–T cell contact, but is mediated by a lymphokine released from antigenically stimulated T lymphocytes. It was soon discovered that this lymphokine, named macrophage-activating factor (MAF), induced not only microbicidal, but also tumoricidal activity in macrophages (for review see NORTH 1978; COHN 1978; KARNOVSKY and LAZDINS 1978; SCHREIBER and CELADA 1985; GEMSA et al. 1985). In addition, numerous reports have appeared over the last 15 years, demonstrating that MAF enhances a broad spectrum of other functional and biochemical activities of macrophages. These changes include a stimulation of metabolism, secretion, and functions such as endocytosis or adherence (for review see GEMSA et al. 1985). However, the latter functional changes may also be induced by compounds unrelated to MAF. This caused a certain dilemma in defining the term macrophage activation. For clarity, it may be advisable to define macrophage activation in a strict sense as the expression of an enhanced antimicrobial and antitumor activity, regardless of whether or not it is accompanied by an augmentation of other biochemical or functional parameters.

For many years, the molecular identity of MAF evaded detection, and it remained unknown whether the broad spectrum of MAF-enhanced activities was due to one or more types of MAF. Various attempts to purify MAF, to establish its molecular weight, and to separate its activity from other lymphokines were rather unrewarding (for review see SCHREIBER and CELADA 1985). However, the valid concept evolved that macrophage activation is a two-step process in which MAF primes macrophages for reception of a second triggering signal which may be, among others, a bacterial product such as lipopolysaccharide (WEINBERG et al. 1978). The limiting factor in all efforts to identify MAF was the lack of sufficient amounts of material to permit purification. This problem was partially overcome when long-term T cell clones and T cell hybridomas were established which released large amounts of MAF (KELSO et al. 1982; PRYSTOWSKI et al. 1982; GEMSA et al. 1983, 1984; KRAMMER et al. 1983). With these studies, it became possible to separate MAF from other lymphokine activities. The most rewarding progress was the demonstration that (at least in the murine system) MAF could not be separated from IFN-γ.

II. Molecular Characteristics

The identity of IFN-γ and MAF has been postulated on the basis of physico-chemical properties, molecular characteristics, and biology activity (KLEIN-SCHMIDT and SCHULTZ 1982; ROBERTS and VASIL 1982). A scientific breakthrough took place when it became possible to express cDNA of human IFN-γ in *Escherichia coli* and other host cells (Chap. 9). The secreted protein had biologic properties similar to the purified natural IFN-γ (GRAY et al. 1982). The 143 amino acid sequence of mature IFN-γ was found to be unrelated to other types of interferon. There is evidence for only one IFN-γ gene which is located on the long arm of the human chromosome 12. Human IFN-γ consists of two components, of molecular weight 20 and 25 000 which are formed by post-translational glycosylation of a 15 500 protein (for review see VILCEK et al. 1985). Carbohydrates are absent from the recombinant IFN-γ molecules produced in *E. coli*, but this does not affect the biologic activity. Although murine IFN-γ is rather similar in molecular weight to human IFN-γ, it shows only 40% homology with the human compound, which could explain the tendency of IFN-γ to be species specific (GRAY and GOEDDEL 1983).

Recombinant IFN-γ has been found to induce the priming step for macrophage activation efficiently (PAGE et al. 1983). However, IFN-γ alone was incapable of macrophage activation, emphasizing the requirement for a second triggering signal such as lipopolysaccharide. The involvement of IFN-γ as an important MAF component was underlined further by the observation that monoclonal antibodies to IFN-γ inhibited the induction of activated macrophages by the usual MAF-containing T lymphocyte supernatants (MÄNNEL and FALK 1983; SPITALNY and HAVELL 1984).

Although this evidence clearly suggests that IFN-γ can function as an MAF for induction of tumor cytotoxicity, and that it may constitute the major MAF in lymphokine preparations, this conclusion does not rule out the existence of other lymphokines with MAF activity that are unrelated to IFN-γ. In support of this notion, it has been reported that some T cell hybridomas secrete MAF without the concomitant release of IFN-γ (RATLIFF et al. 1982; ERICKSON et al. 1982; KRAMMER et al. 1983, 1985). It is difficult to explain these findings simply on the basis that the MAF assays appear to be several times more sensitive than the usual antiviral bioassays for IFN-γ and, therefore, small but sufficient IFN-γ concentrations may have evaded detection. Also in the human system, it has been difficult to prove that IFN-γ is the predominant, or even the only MAF (ANDREW et al. 1984).

III. Several MAFs and Steps in Macrophage Activation

Based on our current information, several MAFs and macrophage activation sequences may be envisaged (Gemsa et al. 1985):

1. IFN-γ as a priming signal and lipopolysaccharide or another microbial product as a triggering signal. This possibility has been well established over the last few years. Such a sequence may be of predominant importance for the activation of macrophages directed against microorganisms, since sufficient microbial products are present to serve as triggering signals.

2. Modified IFN-γ molecules and microbial products as triggering signals. This assumption finds support in the forthcoming evidence that the IFN-γ molecule may contain at least two different functional domains, one mediating antiviral activity, and another inducing tumoricidal activity (Schreiber and Celada 1985). Incomplete synthesis or partial proteolysis of the IFN-γ molecule may result in biologically active compounds that selectively express MAF, but no antiviral activity.

3. IFN-γ as a priming signal and another lymphokines as a triggering signal. Evidence for such a second-signal lymphokine has been presented by our own group (Krammer et al. 1985; Gemsa et al. 1985). A lymphokine, termed macrophage cytotoxicity-inducing factor (MCIF), has been functionally dissected from IFN-γ by employing macrophages from C3H/HeJ mice which are genetically unresponsive to the triggering signal lipopolysaccharide. This triggering lymphokine may be particularly important for macrophage antitumor activity, as under these conditions sufficient microbial products may not be available for triggering IFN-γ-primed macrophages.

4. MAF entirely distinct from IFN-γ and active with or without triggering signals. The evidence for such a lymphokine is presently scarce, although such activities may be found in supernatants of stimulated human lymphocytes (Andrew et al. 1984; Lohmann-Matthes and Kreutzer 1984) or continuous T cell lines (Meltzer et al. 1982).

5. Interleukin 2 as an activating signal. This classical lymphokine, available as a recombinant product, has recently been shown to bind to interleukin 2 receptors on human monocytes (Holter et al. 1986). Furthermore, the first reports have appeared that interleukin 2 may induce cytotoxic macrophages (Malkovsky et al. 1986; Kniep and Lohmann-Matthes 1986). Thus, interleukin 2, which was originally thought to be a lymphokine exclusively affecting lymphocytes, may display a much broader activity spectrum, including macrophage activation (Chap. 8).

6. Colony-stimulating factors (CSFs) as MAF-like compounds. These cytokines, previously thought to cause only proliferation and differentiation of progenitor cells, have recently been shown to affect mature cells as well (Grabstein et al. 1986; Warren and Ralph 1986; Ralph et al. 1986). Two highly purified or recombinant types, CSF-1 and GM-CSF, activated macrophages to tumor cytotoxicity, apparently without the help of additional triggering signals.

7. MAF which induces activated macrophages that only inhibit growth of tumor cells without lysing them. Strong evidence for the existence of such a tumor cytostasis-inducing lymphokine has been reported by our group (Gemsa et al. 1983, 1984, 1985). This lymphokine has been detected in the supernatants of a T

cell line and several T cell hybridomas (KRAMER et al. 1983); it bears no physico-chemical resemblance to IFN-γ, and stimulates metabolic parameters of macro-phages in a manner entirely different from IFN-γ and other MAFs. It is feasible that this type of cytostasis-inducing MAF may mediate its action by a release of interleukin 1 which has been shown to be antiproliferative toward certain tumor cells (LOVETT et al. 1986; ENDO et al. 1986).

Taken together, the present evidence clearly points to IFN-γ as a major MAF that induces the priming step in macrophage activation. With regard to all other MAFs not displaying IFN-γ activity, the final proof of their existence must be based on biochemical and not only on functional data (PICK 1985). However, the initial functional characterization of a MAF represents an essential prerequisite to biochemical characterization. This approach has been successful in the case of IFN-γ, resulting in a cloned gene and definition of the complete amino acid se-quence, and similar progress may be achieved with other types of MAF or factors cooperating with IFN-γ.

One question still remains unanswered. What happens to a macrophage fol-lowing activation to cytotoxicity? Does it return to the former nonactivated state? Our recent results suggest that activation, i.e., differentiation to a highly special-ized function, may rapidly terminate the cells's life (GONG et al. 1986).

IV. Measurement

Several assay methods exist for the presence of MAF in a T lymphocyte-derived culture supernatant. As a screening assay, one may employ a tumor growth in-hibition assay (GEMSA et al. 1981, 1983, 1984). Either resident or elicited perito-neal macrophages are incubated with tumor cells in a ratio of 2:1 in a total vol-ume of 0.2 ml in flat-bottom microtiter plates, with or without the addition of MAF. This assay is terminated after 48 h incubation with a 4-h pulse of [^{3}H] thy-midine which is only incorporated into tumor DNA, and can be measured by liq-uid scintillation spectroscopy. The amount of [^{3}H] thymidine incorporation re-flects the number tumor cells and is a measure of the antitumor activity of acti-vated macrophages. The MAF unit may be defined as the amount that activates macrophages to inhibit tumor growth by 50%. A more laborious, but more exact modification employs direct enumeration of tumor cells. A growth inhibition as-say does not differentiate between tumor cytostatic and tumor cytolytic macro-phages. Therefore, it is advisable to use, in parallel, an assay determining the cy-tolytic activity of macrophages (GEMSA et al. 1983). Macrophages are incubated in microtiter plates with or without MAF-containing solutions for 12–16 h, and thereafter, radiolabeled tumor cells are added at an effector: target cell ratio of 5:1 to 10:1. After a further incubation of 18–24 h (in the case of ^{51}Cr-labeling of tumor cells) or 48 h (when using [^{3}H] thymidine as label), the amount of iso-tope which is released in the culture supernatant is determined. The unit of MAF may be defined as that amount producing 50% of maximal, specific, isotope re-lease from tumor cells. Nowadays, a MAF assay has to be correlated with an IFN-assay (Chap. 9) in order to estimate the contribution of IFN-γ to the MAF activity. MAF activity may also be determined in antimicrobial assay systems; however, these tests are cumbersome and often prone to unacceptable varia-tions.

D. Tumor Necrosis Factor (TNF-α)

I. Original Observations

Tumor necrosis factor (TNF-α) was originally detected in the serum of bacille Calmette–Guérin-infected mice which were subsequently challenged with endotoxin (CARSWELL et al. 1975). The name TNF characterizes an endotoxin-elicited serum factor that causes a hemorrhagic necrosis in transplanted tumors after systemic administration.

Retrospectively, it is interesting that the antitumor effects of bacteria and their products had been known for 120 years (BUSCH 1866). In 1888, BRUNS summarized previous findings and reported that tumors could spontaneously regress when patients were infected by bacteria causing erysipelas. Shortly thereafter, COLEY (1891) described similar findings and started to use filtrates of bacterial cultures (Coley's toxins) to treat cancer patients. Today, it is difficult to decide whether the previously observed, occasional regression of tumors was actually due to a tumor-toxic action of bacterial products or to the generation of TNF-α.

II. Biologic Characteristics

The agents used for priming rodents to TNF-α release, such as bacille Calmette–Guerin, *Corynebacterium parvum*, or zymosan, cause activation of macrophages in various lymphoid organs. Extensive studies have demonstrated that activated macrophages are the cellular source of TNF-α (MATTHEWS 1978, 1981; MÄNNEL et al. 1980 a,b). Therefore, TNF-α should be referred to as a monokine and not a lymphokine.

TNF-α has shown remarkable in vivo and in vitro activity. In classical experiments, a hemorrhagic necrosis was induced in transplanted methylcholanthrene-induced sarcomas when the mice were treated with serum derived from other animals infected with bacille Calmette–Guérin and challenged with endotoxin (CARSWELL et al. 1975; GREEN et al. 1976). During maximum response, a large portion of the tumor mass was destroyed. However, as pointed out by BERENDT et al. (1978 a,b), a dramatic destruction of the central tumor mass may no always be followed by a complete regression of the tumor. Thus, hemorrhagic necrosis may only cause a temporal halt in tumor growth by reducing blood flow to solid tumors and by killing many, but not all, tumor cells. Extensive in vivo studies are still required to establish the long-term effect of TNF-α on tumor regression.

A large body of information has been collected with regard to in vitro effects of TNF-α on tumor cells. The immediate effect of TNF-α is cytostasis as manifested in cell arrest in G_2. Thereafter, cytolysis ensues, and extensive killing can be observed after 7 h exposure to TNF-α (RUFF and GIFFORD 1981; DARZYN-KIEWCS et al. 1984). Cells undergo lysis preferentially during late stages of mitosis, indicating that hitherto unknown metabolic disturbances occur which may interfere with synthesis or assembly of cell membranes. It is of particular interest that TNF-α induced a sixfold stimulation of RNA synthesis in sensitive target cells that reached a maximum when the cells started to die (OSTROVE and GIFFORD 1979). It has been speculated that TNF-attacked cells may actively resist destruction, and the increased RNA synthesis may represent a compensatory repair mechanism. This notion finds support in the observation that actinomycin D markedly enhances sensitivity to TNF-α (RUFF and GIFFORD 1981).

TNF-α exclusively kills transformed cell lines and leaves normal cells unaffected (MÄNNEL et al. 1980 a,b). However, not all tumor cell lines display in vitro sensitivity to TNF-α. For example, in a test panel of 23 human cancer cell lines, TNF-α was cytolotic for 7 cell types, cytostatic for 5, and had no effect on 11 (WILLIAMSON et al. 1983). In another study (SUGARMAN et al. 1985), cell lines could be subdivided into three groups which either displayed an antiproliferative response to TNF-α (only tumor cells), showed no response, or even showed a growth enhancement (only normal cells). Thus, it remains questionable whether evolution had cancer in mind when designing TNF (OLD 1985); other regulatory or protective actions of TNF may be equally or more important.

Along this line, it has recently been reported that TNF-α may represent a differentiation-inducing factor that, in synergy with IFN-γ, may drive immature myeloid cells into fully differentiated monocytes (TRINCHIERI et al. 1986). Furthermore, TNF-α has been shown to be intrinsically pyrogenic and, in addition, to stimulate the release of interleukin 1 from macrophages and endothelial cells (DINARELLO et al. 1986; NAWROTH et al. 1986; Chap. 7). Thus, TNF-α may set in motion a chain of events leading to diverse biologic activities such as differentiation, immunoregulation, fever, and cytotoxicity. The spectrum of activities has recently been further expanded by the discovery that TNF-α possesses strong antiviral activity (MESTAN et al. 1986; WONG and GOEDDEL 1986; NAIN and GEMSA, in preparation), suggesting that one of its major functions may be to combat viral infection.

III. Molecular Characteristics

Only very recently, has it been possible to differentiate TNF-α clearly from other cytokines such as interferons, interleukin 1 and 2, or CSF. Depending on the species studied, several forms of TNF had been reported, ranging in molecular weight from 18 to 150000. Further progress was hampered until 1984, since only crude or partially purified TNF preparations were available for biologic studies. This disappointing picture was immediately changed when the gene coding for human TNF-α was cloned and expressed (PENNICA et al. 1984; WANG et al. 1985). The amino acid sequence was established, a molecular weight of 17100 was found, and the gene product exhibited a 50% homology with lymphotoxin (TNF-β) (AGGARWAL et al. 1985a). While TNF research was formerly carried out by a small group of investigators, there is now a general interest in studying a compound which at one time gave rise to more skepticism than belief. In retrospect, it is reassuring that use of the currently available, pure recombinant TNF-α has confirmed many previous findings obtained with crude material.

In biologic studies, no species specificity has been found for TNF-α activities prepared from such diverse sources as mice, rabbits, rats, and humans. When the amino acid sequences of murine and human TNF-α were compared, a 79% homology was found between both compounds, which indicates that TNF molecules have been highly conserved during evolution (PENNICA et al. 1985).

IV. TNF Receptors

TNF-sensitive tumor cells have cell surface receptors with a high affinity to TNF. An average of 2000 receptor sites per cell have been calculated and, interestingly, cells display a common receptor for both TNF-α and TNF-β (lymphotoxin), since the binding of one compound could be inhibited by the other and vice versa (Aggarwal et al. 1985 b). This finding established on a biochemical basis the previously observed, similar biologic activities of both types of TNF. Cell lines that were rendered resistant to TNF lose their specific receptors and this has led to the notion that determination of TNF receptors on tumor biopsies may be of predictive value in assessing therapeutic approaches with TNF (Rubin et al. 1985). Unfortunately, no information is presently available on TNF-α receptors on normal cells. As mentioned already, TNF may affect not only transformed, but also normal cells. Thus, therapeutic TNF-α applications may be ambiguous; TNF-α may kill tumor cells and may stimulate immune defense systems, but it may also produce unwanted side effects such as an undesirably high release of inflammatory mediators, severe metabolic acidosis, and hypertriglyceridemia.

TNF apparently cooperates with other cytokines, most notably IFN-γ. Treatment of tumor cells with IFN-γ enhanced the antiproliferative effect of TNF-α (Sugarman et al. 1985), possibly mediated by a two- to threefold increase of TNF receptors (Aggarwal et al. 1985 b). Furthermore, IFN-γ facilitates the endotoxin-induced production of TNF-α, possibly by enhancing TNF-α synthesis at both the transcriptional and translational level (Beutler et al. 1986). Synergistic effects of TNF-α or TNF-β with IFN-γ have recently been reported for neutrophil activities such as phagocytosis and antibody-dependent cellular cytotoxicity. An enhancement of functions occurred which was greater than that caused by the same dose of cytokine alone (Shalaby et al. 1985).

V. Identity of TNF-α with Cachectin

A different aspect of TNF-α activity was recently revealed when it was shown that TNF-α was identical with a factor called cachectin (Beutler et al. 1985 a). Cachectin is produced by endotoxin-treated macrophages; it inhibits the activity of fat-producing enzymes in adipocytes (Beutler et al. 1985 b) and thus mobilizes energy reserves required by an infected host. A persistent production of cachectin/TNF-α may ultimately result in cachexia typically associated with chronic infections and malignancies. Thus, a physiologic response leading to TNF-α release may, in the long run, damage the host during chronic infections and malignancies by depleting energy stores. Furthermore, it has recently been shown that cachectin/TNF-α was a potent stimulus of PGE_2 and collagenase production by human synovial cells and dermal fibroblasts (Dayer et al. 1986), suggesting that this monokine may play an important role in tissue destruction and remodeling during chronic inflammatory diseases. In conclusion, a great deal of effort must still be invested in TNF-α research before experimental observations can be translated into clinical applications.

VI. Measurement

The presence of TNF-α in serum or cell culture supernatants may be assayed either by the more laborious in vivo tests or by standardizable in vitro systems. In the in vivo bioassay, mice with 7 day-old subcutaneous transplants of methylcholanthrene-induced fibrosarcoma 7–8 mm in diameter are intravenously injected with a test sample. At 24 h after TNF treatment, the tumors are visually and histologically examined and scored for hemorrhagic necrosis (CARSWELL et al. 1975). In a maximum response, 50%–70% and in a moderate response, 25%–50% of the tumor mass is necrotic. In the bioassay, the unit of TNF activity has been defined as the lowest concentration that will induce massive tumor necrosis.

In vitro tests are based on the survival of TNF-exposed target cells. One may either count the number of treated cells and compare it with control cultures after 48 h (CARSWELL et al. 1975), or estimate cytotoxicity by measuring [³H] thymidine release from prelabeled tumor cells (MÄNNEL et al. 1980a,b). Although several other methods have been proposed (RUFF and GIFFORD 1981; KULL and CUATRECASAS 1981), the following assay system has gained the widest acceptance, owing to its reproducibility and convenience (RUFF and GIFFORD 1980; AGGARWAL et al. 1985a).

Mouse L929 fibroblast cells are plated in 96-well flat-bottom microtiter plates at 6×10^4 cells in 0.1 ml, to establish a dense monolayer. Serial dilutions of TNF-α and actinomycin D at a final concentration of 1 µg/ml are added. In the presence of actinomycin D, the killing of L929 cells by TNF-α is greatly enhanced (OSTROVE and GIFFORD 1979). After 18 h incubation, the plates are washed, and cell lysis is assessed by staining with 0.5% crystal violet. Dye uptake may be directly read in an ELISA plate reader or after elution with Sorensen's buffer. Controls that are run in parallel should include a TNF-resistant L929 cell line (OLD 1985) and serial dilutions of recombinant TNF-α for calibration. The unit of TNF-α is usually defined as the amount required for 50% cell lysis.

Although the in vitro assay system is relatively uncomplicated, it can be anticipated that easier test systems will become available, since the production of recombinant TNF-α and appropriate antibodies will allow the development of specific ELISAs and RIAs.

E. Lymphotoxin (TNF-β)

I. Original Observations

Lymphotoxin is a lymphokine released from lymphocytes following antigen or mitogen stimulation. Owing to its resemblance to the macrophage product tumor necrosis factor (TNF-α), it has been suggested that it should be renamed tumor necrosis factor-β (AGGARWAL et al. 1985c). Originally, it was observed by RUDDLE and WAKSMAN (1967) that antigen-sensitized lymphocytes were capable of lysing bystander fibroblasts in the presence of specific antigen. Shortly thereafter, it was shown that this lysis was due to the release of a lymphokine named lymphotoxin (GRANGER and KOLB 1968; GRANGER and WILLIAMS 1968). Although lymphotoxin release was antigen specific, its action against target cells lacked antigen specificity (RUDDLE and WAKSMAN 1968).

II. Biologic Characteristics

Lymphotoxin preferentially displays anticellular activities against neoplastic cells, whereas there is little or no effect on normal cells. Its action against neoplastic cells is primarily cytostatic rather than cytolytic (Evans and Heinbaugh 1981). Lymphotoxin has been implicated as one of several effector mechanisms in T lymphocyte-mediated cytotoxicity (Ware and Granger 1981), antibody-dependent, cell-mediated cytotoxicity (Kondo et al. 1981), and natural killer cell cytotoxicity (Wright and Bonavida 1981). However, as cytotoxic effects of lymphotoxin are not apparent before 24 h incubation, it may not be involved in those rapid killing mechanisms that are frequently seen within 4–8 h of incubation (Eardley et al. 1980).

The precise mechanism by which lymphotoxin arrests cell growth or kills target cells is not known. After binding to receptors, an early decrease in the number of polysomes and an increase of RNA synthesis, but no alteration of glycolysis, oxidative phosphorylation, or Na^+, K^+ pump were observed (Rosenau et al. 1973). An extensive reduction of plasma membrane protein was found, although a direct proteolytic activity of lymphotoxin could not be detected (Rosenau et al. 1979). A final stage of lymphotoxin action was shown to be a decrease of DNA synthesis and release of low molecular weight DNA fragments (Williams and Granger 1973; Ruddle 1985). At present, the primary lesion induced by lymphotoxin remains unknown, and it is likely that the cellular defects reported represent only one link in the chain of events leading to cell death.

In general, it has been maintained that lymphotoxin preferentially kills tumor target cells, although similar to TNF-α's activity, not all neoplastic cells are sensitive. It is entirely feasible that lymphotoxin did not appear during evolution with the primary task of fighting tumor cells, but of keeping other undesirable cells under control. In line with this suggestion, it has been shown that virus-infected cells display an enhanced lytic susceptibility to lymphotoxin (Eifel et al. 1979). This finding suggests a role for lymphotoxin as an effective mediator that counteracts microbial invasion; however, additional reports are lacking to support this conclusion.

III. Producer Cells

Lymphotoxin is produced by lymphocytes, usually T lymphocytes, following antigen or mitogen stimulation. It appears that, in the murine system, Lyt-1$^+$ T lymphocytes secrete more lymphotoxin than do Lyt-2$^+$ cells (Eardely et al. 1980). In the human system, lymphotoxin production was not restricted to a particular T cell subset and, in particular, OKT4$^+$ as well as OKT8$^+$ cells were equally efficient producers (Leopardi and Rosenau 1984). Thus, contrary to expectations, lymphotoxin secretion was not confined to cytotoxic T lymphocytes. Interestingly, several B lymphoblastoid cell lines have been reported to produce lymphotoxin (Aggarwal et al. 1984; Granger et al. 1984), a finding which raises doubt whether T lymphocytes are the exclusive lymphotoxin producers. However, purified normal B cells have so far been found to be incapable of secreting lymphotoxin.

IV. Molecular Characteristics

Until recently, lymphotoxin research was impeded by the availability of only crude preparations from lymphocyte cultures. Difficulties in purifying the minute quantities of lymphotoxin in primary lymphocyte cultures have been overcome by using lymphoblastoid cell lines which, either constitutively or after stimulation, produce sufficient amounts for biochemical analysis (GRANGER et al. 1984; AGGARWAL et al. 1984). Previously, it was claimed that lymphotoxin represents a multicomponent family of related growth inhibitory and cytotoxic glycoproteins (GRANGER et al. 1984), ranging in molecular weight from 12 to 200000. According to apparent molecular weight, different subclasses of α, β, and γ lymphotoxin have been described (GRANGER et al. 1978). Whether this heterogeneity of lymphotoxin may actually represent aggregates or breakdown products derived from a single molecular species has recently been tackled by amino acid sequence analysis and, in addition, cloning and expression of DNA for human lymphotoxin (AGGARWAL et al. 1984; GRAY et al. 1984; NEDWIN et al. 1985). Protein sequencing and cDNA cloning have shown that fully active, recombinant lymphotoxin contains 171 residues with a molecular weight of 18600, and that natural lymphotoxin is glycosylated, which increases its molecular weight to 25000. Hybridization studies suggested that lymphotoxin is encoded by a single gene and, furthermore, various lymphotoxin-specific antibodies are capable of neutralizing all the differently sized lymphotoxins. Thus, it appears that the previously described heterogeneity of the lymphotoxin family is most likely due to aggregates that may easily form, both in vivo and in vitro. It remains to be determined whether differently sized aggregates may have physiologic relevance. As mentioned already, it was of particular interest that lymphotoxin displayed a 50% homology with TNF-α (AGGARWAL et al. 1985a), although it was antigenically different. Since cells carry a common receptor for TNF-α and lymphotoxin (AGGARWAL et al. 1985b), it appears justified to assign the term TNF-β to lymphotoxin.

V. Synergism with Other Cytokines and Effects on Lymphocytes

An attractive aspect of lymphotoxin activity is its synergism with interferons. Treatment of target cells with IFN-α as well as with IFN-β results in a potent augmentation of the cytostatic and cytolytic effects of lymphotoxin (WILLIAMS and BELLANTI 1983; LEE et al. 1984; STONE-WOLFF et al. 1984). These observations suggest that interferons may prime target cells for lymphotoxin cytotoxicity, possibly by increasing the number of lymphotoxin receptors on susceptible cells. One may deduce from these findings that nature has composed a cooperative network of lymphokines in which small amounts of different cytokines are more efficient than large doses of a single compound. Following nature's lead, one may eventually design therapeutic lymphokine applications that are more rational than today's single-component trials and less burdened with undesirable side effects.

A further clue to the multifaceted action of lymphotoxin has been given in a report by CONTA et al. (1985). These authors clearly demonstrated that lymphotoxin not only killed transformed fibroblasts, but also produced a suicidal inhibition of proliferation and cell death of those T cells that produce lymphotoxin. Thus, lymphotoxin-producing cells may be ultimately removed by their own product which may represent a self-regulatory mechanism to limit an unrestricted T cell response during the immune response. It remains to be investigated further whether lymphotoxin may be a suppressor molecule of other immunoregulatory circuits.

VI. Anticarcinogenic Activity

As shown by EVANS (1982), lymphotoxin may not only display cytotoxic actions toward tumor cells, but it may also prevent a carcinogen-induced morphological transformation of normal cells. The anticarcinogenic activity of lymphotoxin appeared to be more potent than its tumor growth inhibitory activity. Induction of an anticarcinogenic state in normal cells was associated with increased membrane glycoprotein synthesis, whereas inhibition of tumor growth was accompanied by a reduced glycoprotein synthesis (FUHRER and EVANS 1983). These profound, lymphotoxin-induced alterations in the cell membrane of neoplastic cells may explain, at least in part, the enhanced susceptibility to natural killer cells (RANSOM and EVANS 1982).

VII. Measurement

The in vitro assays for the presence of lymphotoxin do not differ essentially from those described for TNF-α. They include measurements of radionucleotide uptake and release (GRANGER and WILLIAMS 1968; SMITH et al. 1977; EVANS and HEINBAUGH 1981), enumeration of surviving cells by direct counting of unlysed cells (KOLB and GRANGER 1968; CONTA et al. 1985), or staining of residual cells with neutral red or crystal violet (STONE-WOLFF et al. 1984; AGGARWAL et al. 1984). The most sensitive target cell is the mouse fibroblast L929 cell, pretreated with actinomycin D to enhance the sensitivity. Similar to TNF-α determinations, the unit of lymphotoxin is defined as the amount required for 50% cell lysis of plated cells. In vivo assays for lymphotoxin may also be performed by using the same necrosis assay described for TNF-α (GRAY et al. 1984). If it is uncertain whether the cellular source of lymphotoxin, the lymphocyte, is the producer cell in an incubation system, difficulties may arise in differentiating the lymphotoxin activity from TNF-α. This problem will be resolved in the near future by the availability of highly specific immunoassays which can now be developed on the basis of immunization with recombinant lymphotoxin.

F. Osteoclast-Activating Factor (OAF)

I. Biologic Characteristics

Recently, evidence has accumulated which indicates that there are close interactions between the immune system and bone metabolism. The activation of osteoclasts to resorb bone during chronic inflammation, as seen in rheumatoid arthritis and periodontal disease, or during malignancies such as myeloma, was found to be due to soluble products released from stimulated leukocytes (HORTON et al. 1972; MUNDY et al. 1974a,b; MUNDY 1981). These biologically active effector molecules have been named osteoclast-activating factor (OAF) (HORTON et al. 1972). OAF was released in vitro when mononuclear leukocytes were stimulated with mitogens or specific antigens. OAF could be clearly distinguished from other bone-resorbing factors such as parathyroid hormone, vitamin D metabolites, and prostaglandins by different physicochemical characteristics (RAISZ et al. 1975). Despite its presence in only minute quantities in leukocyte culture supernatants, a partial purification of the active compounds has been attempted and has yielded factors that differ markedly in molecular weight (MUNDY and RAISZ 1977; HORTON et al. 1979). Until recently, all the available evidence has indicated that OAF was a lymphokine released from stimulated lymphocytes.

At the light microscopic level, the major morphological change caused by OAF is an increase in the size and number of osteoclasts (MUNDY 1981). In locally restricted inflammatory foci, intense osteoclastic bone resorption frequently occurs in those areas that are adjacent to inflammatory cells. It is plausible to attribute bone resorption to leukocyte-derived OAF, although it remains unknown whether local osteolysis may serve to prevent further spread of an infection. OAF appears also to be responsible for the hypercalcemia frequently observed during hematologic malignancies. It has been hypothesized that bone resorption and concomitant hypercalcemia in myelomas were due to OAF released by myeloma cells (MUNDY 1981). In contrast to parathyroid hormone, OAF is only locally active and, therefore, an apparent hypercalcemia could only occur in patients with a large tumor cell burden. Little information has been obtained with regard to the biochemical mechanisms that lead to increased activities of osteoclasts in response to OAF, except for experiments demonstrating a dependence on prostaglandins (YONEDA and MUNDY 1979; Chaps. 14, 15).

II. Molecular Characteristics

Recently, significant progress in the further identification of OAF has been achieved by assaying various recombinant cytokines for OAF activity. It has become clear that the bone-resorbing activity in the culture supernatant of activated leukocytes represents a multicomponent family rather than one distinct factor (MUNDY et al. 1985). On the one hand, it has been shown that interleukin 1 possesses OAF activity (GOWEN et al. 1983; Chap. 7), while on the other hand, OAF activity has been attributed to the monocyte product, tumor necrosis factor (TNF-α) and to the lymphocyte product, lymphotoxin (TNF-β) (BERTOLIBI et al. 1986a). Thus, OAF is at best a descriptive term coined when cytokines could only be identified by more or less specific biologic assays. Although substantial OAF activity could be blocked by a monoclonal antibody against lymphotoxin (BERTOLINI et al. 1986b), it was also found that OAF activity produced in short-term cultures of less than 24 h was not lymphotoxin. From our current knowledge, it seems that activation of osteoclasts may be achieved by various compounds, and further studies will be required to delineate the contribution of each of these factors. In a recent report, evidence has been presented that interleukin 1 may not stimulate osteoclasts directly, but may primarily affect osteoblasts which then are induced to transmit a short-range signal that activates osteoclastic bone resorption (Thompson et al. 1986). Furthermore, it has been reported that IFN-γ may represent an opposing factor capable of abolishing the bone resorption stimulated by interleukin 1 and recombinant lymphotoxin (Gowen et al. 1986). This demonstrates, once again, the existence of a well-balanced network among the cytokines, in which some factors stimulate, while others suppress certain cell functions. Based on these findings, complications may arise when selected cytokines are employed for therapeutic procedures. Because of the apparent interactions between the immune system and bone metabolism, the deliberate stimulation of one system by a single cytokine may help that system, but may harm the other.

III. Measurement

OAF activity is determined in time-consuming bioassays on bone explants (Trummel et al. 1975). Pregnant rats are injected at day 18 of gestation with ^{45}Ca, and on the following day the fetal bone is explanted and cultured for 48 h in the presence or absence of OAF. Release of ^{45}Ca from prelabeled bone is taken as an indication of OAF activity. Now that OAF has been found to consist of the well-known cytokines interleukin 1, TNF-α, and lymphotoxin, a determination of these compounds may be more informative than the laborious bioassay.

G. Soluble Immune Response Suppressor (SIRS)

I. Biologic Characteristics

An immune response consists of complex interactions between antigens, various leukocytes, and their soluble products. In this response, T lymphocytes of the helper or suppressor type are regulatory cells. Populations of suppressor T cells may be either antigen specific or antigen nonspecific. It has been shown that most suppressor T cells release soluble mediators that carry the same antigen specificity as the cells from which they are derived. Among suppressor T cell factors, the soluble immune response suppressor (SIRS) is entirely antigen nonspecific, and may arise later than the more antigen specific and genetically restricted suppressor factors (Aune et al. 1982). SIRS has been extensively studied over the last few years, and some details of its biologic function and biochemistry are now known.

SIRS is a lymphokine released from mitogen- or interferon-activated suppressor T lymphocytes in both murine and human cell systems (Aune et al. 1983; Schnaper et al. 1984). It suppresses a variety of immune activites, including antibody synthesis, mixed lymphocyte and cytotoxic lymphocyte responses to alloantigens, DNA synthesis to T and B cell mitogens, and division of both normal and tumor cells (Tadakuma and Pierce 1978; Aune and Pierce 1981 a, 1982; Aune et al. 1982). A first clinical study in patients has indicated that the suppressed immune response frequently found in nephrotic syndrome is most likely due to enhanced release of SIRS (Schnaper and Aune 1985). The primary target cell of SIRS is the macrophage which oxidizes the lymphokine in a H_2O_2-dependent reaction to the biologically active form, $SIRS_{ox}$ (Aune and Pierce 1981 b, 1982).

By biochemical analysis, it has been found that $SIRS_{ox}$ caused an oxidation of 35%–45% of total cullular sulfhydryls, suggesting a catalytic action in which $SIRS_{ox}$ is reduced back to SIRS and sulfhydryls are oxidized to sulfenyl derivatives (AUNE 1984). Thus, cellular components essential for cell division are oxidized, which may cause an antigen-nonspecific immunosuppression. In many aspects, the effects of $SIRS_{ox}$ resemble those described for the action of cytoskeletal disrupting agents. $SIRS_{ox}$ has been reported to inhibit microtubule assembly without affecting other cell structures such as microfilaments, or functions such as protein synthesis and enzyme activities (IRONS et al. 1984). This finding was not unexpected, since microtubule integrity has been known to be sensitive to sulfhydril-modifying agents. It is evident that regular microtubule assembly is critical for an immune response which leads to blastogenesis, cell division, and secretion (see Chap. 4). On the basis of these results, it has been suggested that microtubules may represent the primary target structure for the action of SIRS. At present, it is unknown whether SIRS interferes only with microtubules of immunologically relevant cells or whether it displays a much broader spectrum of activity directed toward other cells. In the search for factors opposing SIRS activity, it seems reasonable to examine various growth-enhancing factors and, indeed, interleukin 1, interleukin 2, and epidermal growth factor are capable of reversing SIRS effects (AUNE 1985a).

II. Molecular Characteristics

Only recently has it been possible to purify and characterize SIRS. By using supernatants of a T cell hybridoma that constitutively produces SIRS, the existence of two molecular weight forms (21 and 14000 by SDS–PAGE analysis) have been found (AUNE et al. 1983). Slight differences between both forms were detected, and it was found that the larger lymphokine was biologically more active than the smaller one. Further progress has led to a cell-free translation of SIRS and a characterization of its mRNA (NOWOWIEJSKI-WIEDER et al. 1984). However, current research has not yet achieved cloning and expression of the SIRS gene (or genes) in order to identify its composition exactly and to compare it with other, already sequenced, lymphokines. Current information indicates that SIRS is distinguishable from TNF-α and TNF-β by differences in target cell susceptibility, and it is apparently different from interleukin 1 and 2 and interferons, since they do not bind to SIRS-specific antibodies (T. M. AUNE 1986, personal communication).

III. Measurement

SIRS and its oxidized derivative $SIRS_{ox}$ are usually assayed in a plaque-forming cell (PFC) test in which the in vitro immunoglobulin production in response to sheep erythrocytes is determined (AUNE and PIERCE 1981a; Chap. 5). Single spleen cell cultures (5×10^6 per 0.5 ml) are incubated with sheep erythrocytes (2.5×10^6 per 0.5 ml) for 5 days in the presence or absence of SIRS-containing test samples. IgM PFC responses are determined by a hemolytic plaque assay, with sheep erythrocytes as indicator cells. The unit of SIRS activity has been arbitrarily defined as the amount that suppresses an antibody response by 50% (AUNE and PIERCE 1982). Recently, after generation of monoclonal SIRS-specific antibodies, an ELISA has been developed that is capable of detecting picogram quantities of SIRS (AUNE 1985 b). This test system may facilitate the detection of SIRS in serum or urine of patients with abnormal activation of suppressor T cells (SCHNAPER and AUNE 1985).

H. Chemotactic Cytokines

I. Biologic Characteristics

Leukocytes are mobile cells that need to accumulate at sites of antigenic challenge and inflammation. The capacity of leukocytes to migrate to areas of immune reactivity is triggered by a variety of chemotactic factors. By definition, chemotaxis is a unidirectional migration of leukocytes along an increasing gradient of a chemoattractant. In contrast, chemokinesis is an enhanced, but undirected cellular mobility to biologically active compounds which are not present in a gradient. A large variety of chemotactic factors for different leukocytes exist, and all serve to focus cells at sites of immune and/or inflammatory reactions. Among these are factors derived from bacteria, from the activated complement system (C3a, C5a), or from arachidonic acid metabolism (leukoktriene B_4). This chapter will only deal with cytokines (lymphokines and monokines) released from and active on lymphocytes and macrophages.

Delayed-type hypersensitivity reactions and other localized, chronic immune reactions are characterized by a heavy mononuclear cell infiltration, consisting of lymphocytes and macrophages. It has been shown that only a very small percentage of lymphocytes in such lesions have actually recognized the antigen, while the majority are not specifically sensitized to the eliciting antigen. Thus, it has been concluded that antigen might initially attract some antigen-specific T lymphocytes which then, upon antigen stimulation, might recruit a large number of additional leukocytes by release of chemotactic factors (CENTER and CRUIKSHANK 1982).

In earlier reports, it was demonstrated that, after antigen or mitogen stimulation, lymphocytes from lymph nodes or from peripheral blood released a factor which was chemotactic for mononuclear phagocytes (WARD et al. 1970; ALTMAN et al. 1973). Also, extracts obtained from skin sites of delayed-type hypersensitivity reactions contained chemotactic activity for monocytes and lymphocytes, but not for neutrophils (COHEN et al. 1973). Similarly, during local graft-versus-host reactions, chemotactic factors for monocytes were produced which displayed no activity toward neutrophils (WARD and VOLKMAN 1975). A further analysis revealed that several different stimuli could induce chemotactic activity from different producer cells. B lymphocytes responded with chemotactic factor secretion following stimulation with polymeric mitogens, antigen-antibody complexes, anti-Ig, and C3b (WAHL et al. 1974; SANDBERG et al. 1975; KOOPMAN et al. 1976; WARD et al. 1977). T lymphocytes, on the other hand, responded to antigens and classical T cell mitogens (ALTMAN et al. 1975). Thus, it appears to be well established that stimulated B and T lymphocytes produce some factors, among a variety of other lymphokines, that chemotactically attract mononuclear leuko-cytes. Finally, two recent reports have demonstrated that monocytes are capable of releasing a chemotactic factor for neutrophils (KOWNATZKI et al. 1986; YOSHI-MURA et al. 1987).

II. The Search for Molecular Characterization

Some progress has been made in the biochemical characterization of chemotactic lymphokines. A factor selectively chemotactic for T lymphocytes has an apparent molecular weight of 56000 and consists of four similar 14000 dalton sialoprotein compounds (CRUIKSHANK and CENTER 1982). Unfortunately, no determination of the amino acid composition has been performed as yet, and therefore, a resemblance to other cloned lymphokines has not been established. It appears that production is limited to histamine type 2 receptor-bearing human T cells (BERMAN et al. 1984). In another study, it was demonstrated that a lymphocyte chemotactic factor is produced by suppressor/cytolytic T cells, and that it selectively attracts T lymphocytes of the helper/inducer phenotype (VAN EPPS et al. 1983 a,b; POTTER and VAN EPPS 1986). This finding indicates a close lymphokine-mediated interaction between both T cell subpopulations in which the suppressor/cytolytic T cell subset is the driving force to recruit, unexpectedly, more helper cells. There is sufficient evidence for the existence of chemotactic factors for monocytes. However, the presently available information is insufficient for biochemical characterization of such chemotactic lymphokines for monocytes, although it appears that they may have molecular weights similar to those of lymphocyte chemotactic factors.

Of the well-characterized cytokines, the monokine interleukin 1 has recently been shown to be chemotactically active for monocytes and lymphocytes (see Chap. 7). LUGER et al. (1983) reported that the interleukin 2-like epidermal cell thymocyte-activating factor (ETAF) and purified interleukin 1 were capable of attracting monocytes. Release of, and chemotactic response to, interleukin 1 may suggest an autocrine cell regulation. The chemotactic response of B lymphocytes to interleukin 1 is more pronounced than the T lymphocyte response (MIOSSEC et al. 1984). Furthermore, interleukin 2 has recently been shown to be chemotactically active toward lymphocytes, with a predominant activity toward helper cells (KORNFELD et al. 1985). It remains to be elucidated to what extent the chemotactic factors, which have been functionally characterized in bioassays, differ biochemically from the better-characterized, cloned cytokines.

Brief mention should be made of distinct lymphokines which inhibit lymphocyte migration (MCFADDEN et al. 1984; BERMAN et al. 1984). These MIFs have been shown to be produced simultaneously with chemotactic lymphokines, and it has been proposed that they immobilize chemoattracted lymphocytes after arrival at sites of antigen deposition.

III. Measurement

The usual chemotaxis assays are performed in Boyden chambers in which leuko-cytes are allowed to migrate through micropore filters separating an upper chamber containing leukocytes from a lower chamber containing the chemotactic compound. After incubation periods of 2–4 h, the filters are fixed with formaldehyde, stained, dehydrated, and cleared with xylene. The distance in micrometers that the leading cells migrate into the membrane is microscopically determined by examining five high power (400 ×) fields on each of two filter membranes. Values may be expressed as a migration index, i.e., the difference between migration to a chemotactically positive sample and to a control sample (Miossec et al. 1984).

J. Concluding Remarks

The lymphokines discussed in this chapter are involved in the efferent limb of the immune response, and may be regarded as typical examples of how, formerly obscure, biochemically undefined factors are leaving the dark ages and entering a more enlightened era of respectability. Most important in this development has been the exploitation of advanced biotechnology, such as the establishment of high producer cell lines and hybridomas, modern purification procedures aided by the availability of polyclonal or monoclonal antibodies, and last but not least, the successful cloning and expression of lymphokines in bacteria and other host cells. As exemplified by TNF-α, TNF-β, and IFN-γ, the use of recombinant products has helped to clarify formerly disputed or unknown physiologic functions of lymphokines. This has contributed enormously to the understanding of how the immune response interacts and which regulatory circuits are involved.

From these investigations, it will soon be possible to transfer knowledge from basic research to clinical applications. A large number of immunologic diseases occur in which a deficiency or dysregulation of lymphokine production may exist. It is, therefore, obvious that clinical trials aimed at substituting the organs defects by external replacement therapy should be considered. At the present preliminary stage of clinical research, it has turned out that natural or recombinant lymphokines certainly are not miracle drugs, without side effects but, undoubtedly, they are extremely promising – with the proviso that conditions for their use are optimized (summarized in Kalden and Röllinghoff 1986; Chap. 27). One aspect of the action of lymphokines deserves a particular comment: their range of activity is not solely restricted to the immune system, but they affect other organ system, sometimes in quite unexpected ways. The "unwanted side effects" during clinical applications of lymphokines just illustrate that the immune system cannot be considered in isolation, and lymphokines and other cytokines may provide interconnecting links to other organ systems.

When planning clinical applications of lymphokines, several important aspects are worth taking into consideration:

1. Substitution therapy requires a diagnostic test of an existing underproduction. Only then may replacement therapy restore the interacting network system of the immune response.
2. The effect of lymphokines depends on the response of receptors on target cells; if they are missing, other receptor-bearing cells may still be affected and produce undesired side effects.

3. Lymphokines often act in combination, for example, one lymphokine may induce the expression of receptors for a second lymphokine. Under these conditions, low doses of several lymphokines may be more efficient than a high single-dose lymphokine.

4. The route of lymphokine administration may be important in determining whether a lymphokine reaches the preferred target cells, or other cells, and whether it is rapidly removed and metabolized. Similarly, the use of single large or multiple small, short-term or long-term applications must be studied in detail.

5. To avoid systemic effects or rapid metabolism, it may be preferable to "educate" the patient's leukocytes extracorporeally with lymphokines, and thereafter reconstitute an immune response by reinfusion of these cells.

6. Since many lymphokines appear to carry different functional domains within their molecular structure, genetic bioengineering may aid in construction of compounds with a higher target cell specificity and less side effects. Furthermore, it is feasible that hybrid lymphokines may be designed that carry "custom-made" functional domains.

7. Overproduction of a lymphokine may lead, just like deficient production, to a derangement of the immune response. Application of opposing lymphokines or receptor-blocking analogs may represent a possible therapeutic approach.

These considerations are only a few that relate to the imminent question of how to deal clinically with biologically highly potent compounds that are on the one hand "natural," but on the other hand not free from side effects (see also Chap. 27). Basic research, coupled with clinical "trials and errors," will help to clarify the potential therapeutic value inherent in this rapidly expanding field of immunology.

References

Adelman NE, Ksiazek J, Yoshida T, Cohen S (1980) Lymphoid sources of murine migration inhibition factor. J Immunol 124:825–830

Aggarwal BB, Moffat B, Harkins RN (1984) Human lymphotoxin. Production by a lymphoblastoid cell line, purification and initial characterization. J Biol Chem 259:686–691

Aggarwal BB, Kohr WJ, Hass PE, Moffat B, Spencer SA, Henzel WJ, Bringman TS et al. (1985a) Human tumor necrosis factor. Production, purification, and characterization. J Biol Chem 260:2345–2354

Aggarwal BB, Eessaln TE, Hass PE (1985b) Characterization of receptors for human tumour necrosis factor and their regulation by γ-interferon. Nature 318:665–667

Aggarwal BB, Kohr WJ, Henzel WJ, Moffat B, Hass PE (1985c) Comparative biochemistry of human lymphotoxin and tumor necrosis factor. In: Sorg C, Schimpl A (eds) Cellular and molecular biology of lymphokines. Academic, New York, pp 665–673

Altman LC, Snyderman R, Oppenheim JJ, Mergenhagen SE (1973) A human mononuclear leukocyte chemotactic factor: characterization, specificity and kinetics of production by homologous leukocytes. J Immunol 110:801–810

Altman LC, Chaccy B, Mackler BF (1975) Physicochemical characterization of chemotactic lymphokines produced by human T and B lymphocytes. J Immunol 115:18–21

Andrew PW, Rees ADM, Scoging A, Dobson N, Matthews R, Whittall JT, Coates ARM, Lowrie DB (1984) Secretion of a macrophage-activating factor distinct from interferon-γ by human T cell clones. Eur J Immunol 14:962–964

Aune TM (1984) Modification of cellular protein sulfhydryl groups by activated soluble immune response suppressor. J Immunol 133:899–906

Aune TM (1985a) Inhibition of soluble immune response suppressor activity by growth factors. Proc Natl Acad Sci USA 82:6260–6264

Aune TM (1985b) ELISA for the detection of the lymphokine soluble immune response suppressor. J Immunol Methods 84:33–44

Aune TM, Pierce CW (1981a) Mechanisms of action of macrophage-derived suppressor factor produced by soluble immune response suppressor-treated macrophages. J Immunol 127:368–372

Aune TM, Pierce CW (1981b) Conversion of soluble immune response suppressor to macrophage derived factor by peroxide. Proc Natl Acad Sci USA 78:5099–5103

Aune TM, Pierce CW (1982) Preparation of soluble immune response suppressor and macrophage-derived suppressor factor. J Immunol Methods 53:1–14

Aune TM, Sorensen CM, Pierce CW (1982) Non-antigen-specific suppressor T cell mediators: structure and action. In: Pick E (ed) Lymphokines, vol 5. Academic, New York, pp 387–410

Aune TM, Webb DR, Pierce CW (1983) Purification and initial characterization of the lymphokine soluble immune response suppressor. J Immunol 131:2848–2852

Berendt MJ, North RJ, Kirstein DP (1978a) The immunological basis of endotoxin-induced tumor regression. Requirement for T-cell-mediated immunity. J Exp Med 148:1550–1559

Berendt MJ, North RJ, Kirstein DP (1978b) The immunological basis of endotoxin-induced tumor regression. J Exp Med 148:1560–1569

Berman JS, McFadden RG, Cruikshank WW, Center DM, Beer DJ (1984) Functional characteristics of histamine-bearing mononuclear cells. II. Identification and characterization of two histamine-induced human lymphokines that inhibit lymphocyte migration. J Immunol 133:1495–1504

Bertolini DR, Nedwin GE, Bringman TS, Smith DD, Mundy GR (1986a) Stimulation of bone resorption and inhibition of bone formation in vitro by human tumour necrosis factor. Nature 319:516–518

Bertolini DR, Nedwin G, Bringman T, Mundy GR (1986b) Evidence that recombinant human lymphotoxin possesses OAF activity. J Bone Miner Res (in press)

Beutler B, Mahoney J, Le Trang N, Pekala P, Cerami A (1985a) Purification of cachectin, a lipoprotein lipase-suppressing hormone secreted by endotoxin-induced RAW 264.7 cells. J Exp Med 161:984–995

Beutler B, Milsark IW, Cerami AC (1985b) Passive immunization against cachectin/tumor necrosis factor protects mice from lethal effect of endotoxin. Science 229:869–871

Beutler B, Tkacenko V, Milsark I, Krochin N, Cerami A (1986) Effect of γ-interferon on cachectin expression by mononuclear phagocytes. Reversal of the 1ps^d (endotoxin resistance) phenotype. J Exp Med 164:1791–1796

Bloom BR, Bennett B (1966) Mechanism of a reaction in vitro associated with delayed-type hypersensitivity. Science 153:80–82

Borish LC, Rocklin RE (1985) Human leukocyte inhibitory factor (LIF)-induced potentiation of antibody-dependent cellular cytotoxicity (ADCC) by human neutrophils. In: Sorg C, Schimpl A (eds) Cellular and molecular biology of lymphokines. Academic, New York, pp 561–565

Bruns P (1888) Die Heilwirkung des Erysipels auf Geschwülste. Beitr Klin Chir 3:443–446

Burmeister G, Zwadlo G, Michels E, Bröcker EB, Malorny U, Sorg C, Flad HD (1985) Use of a monoclonal antibody for the detection of human migration inhibitory factor (MIF) in isolated cells and tissues. In: Sorg C, Schimpl A (eds) Cellular and molecular biology of lymphokines. Academic, New York, pp 797–802

Busch (1866) Verhandlungen ärztlicher Gesellschaften. Berl Klin Wochenschr 3:245–246

Carswell EA, Old LJ, Kassel RL, Green S, Fiore N, Williamson B (1975) An endotoxin-induced serum factor that causes necrosis of tumors. Proc Natl Acad Sci USA 72:3666–3670

Center DM, Cruikshank W (1982) Modulation of lymphocyte migration by human lymphokines. I. Identification and characterization of chemoattractant activity for lymphocytes from mitogen-stimulated mononuclear cells. J Immunol 128:2563–2568

Cohen S, Ward PA, Yoshida T, Burek CL (1973) Biologic activity of extracts of delayed hypersensitivity skin reaction sites. Cell Immunol 9:363–376

Cohn ZA (1978) The activation of mononuclear phagocytes: fact, fancy and future. J Immunol 121:813–816

Coley WB (1891) Contribution to the knowledge of sarcoma. Ann Surg 14:199–220

Conta BS, Powell MB, Ruddle NH (1985) Activation of Lyt-1$^+$ and Lyt-2$^+$ T cell cloned lines: stimulation of proliferation, lymphokine production, and self-destruction. J Immunol 134:2185–2190

Cruikshank W, Center DM (1982) Modulation of lymphocyte migration by human lymphokines. II. Purification of a lymphotactic factor (LCF). J Immunol 128:2569–2574

Darzynkiewicz Z, Williamson B, Carswell EA, Old LJ (1984) Cell cycle-specific effects of tumor necrosis factor. Cancer Res 44:83–90

David JR (1966) Delayed hypersensitivity in vitro. Its mediation by cell-free substances formed by lymphoid cell-antigen interaction. Proc Natl Acad Sci USA 56:72–77

David JR (1975) Macrophage activation by lymphocyte mediators. Fed Proc 34:1730–1736

Dayer JM, Beutler B, Cerami A (1986) Cachectin/tumor necrosis factor stimulates collagenase and prostaglandin E_2 production by human synovial cells and dermal fibroblasts. J Exp Med 162:2163–2168

Dinarello CA, Cannon JG, Wolff SM, Bernheim HA, Beutler B, Cerami A, Figari IS, Palladino MA, O'Connor JV (1986) Tumor necrosis factor (cachectin) is an endogenous pyrogen and induces production of interleukin 1. J Exp Med 163:1433–1450

Eardley DD, Shen FW, Gershon RK, Ruddle NH (1980) Lymphotoxin production by subsets of T cells. J Immunol 124:1199–1202

Eifel P, Billingsley A, Lucas ZJ (1979) Rapid killing of viral-infected L cells by α-lymphotoxin. Cell Immunol 47:197–203

Endo Y, Matsushima K, Oppenheim JJ (1986) Mechanism of in vitro antitumor effects of interleukin 1. Immunobiology 172:316–322

Erickson KL, Cicurel L, Gruys E, Fidler IJ (1982) Murine T-cell hybridomas that produce lymphokine with macrophage-activating factor activity as a constitutive product. Cell Immunol 72:195–201

Evans CH (1982) Lymphotoxin – an immunologic hormone with anticarcinogenic and antitumor activity. Cancer Immunol Immunother 12:181–190

Evans CH, Heinbaugh JA (1981) Lymphotoxin cytotoxicity, a combination of cytolytic and cytostatic responses. Immunopharmacology 3:347–359

Fuhrer JP, Evans CH (1983) The anticarcinogenic and tumor growth inhibitory activities of lymphotoxin are associated with altered membrane glycoprotein synthesis. Cancer Lett 19:283–292

Gemsa D, Kramer W, Napierski I, Bärlin E, Till G, Resch K (1981) Potentiation of macrophage tumor cytostasis by tumor-induced ascites. J Immunol 126:2143–2150

Gemsa D, Debatin KM, Kramer W, Kubelka C, Deimann W, Kees U, Krammer PH (1983) Macrophage-activating factors from different T cell clones induce distinct macrophage functions. J Immunol 131:833–844

Gemsa D, Kubelka C, Debatin KM, Krammer PH (1984) Activation of macrophages by lymphokines from T-cell clones: evidence for different macrophage-activating factors. Mol Immunol 21:1267–1276

Gemsa D, Kozan B, Kubelka C, Debatin KM, Krammer PH (1985) T cell clones secrete lymphokines that activate different macrophage functions. In: Pick E (ed) Lymphokines, vol 11. Academic, New York, pp 119–156

Gong JH, Sprenger H, Gemsa D (1986) Lymphokine-induced activation of the macrophage cell line PU5-1.8 is associated with reduction of DNA- and RNA-synthesis. Immunobiology 173:386

Gowen M, Wood DD, Ihrie EJ, McGuire MKB, Russel RGG (1983) An interleukin 1 like factor stimulates bone resorption in vitro. Nature 306:378–380

Gowen M, Nedwin G, Mundy GR (1986) Preferential inhibition of cytokine-stimulated bone resorption by recombinant interferon gamma. J Bone Miner Res 1:75

Grabstein KH, Urdal DL, Tushinski RJ, Mochizuki DY, Price VL, Cantrell MA, Gillis S, Conlon PJ (1986) Induction of macrophage tumoricidal activity by granulocyte-macrophage colony-stimulating factor. Science 232:506–508

Granger GA, Kolb WP (1968) Lymphocyte in vitro cytotoxicity: mechanisms of immune and non-immune small lymphocyte mediated target L cell destruction. J Immunol 101:111–120

Granger GA, Williams TW (1968) Lymphocyte cytotoxicity in vitro: activation and release of a cytotoxic factor. Nature 218:1253–1254

Granger GA, Yamamoto RS, Fair DS, Hiserodt JC (1978) The human LT system. I. Physical-chemical heterogeneity of LT molecules released by mitogen-activated human lymphocytes in vitro. Cell Immunol 38:388–402

Granger GA, Johnson DL, Plunkett JM, Masunaka JK, Orr SL, Yamamoto RS (1984) Lymphotoxins, a multicomponent family of effector molecules. In: Goldstein AL (ed) Thymic hormones and lymphokines. Plenum, New York, pp 223–233

Gray PW, Goeddel DV (1983) Cloning and expression of murine immune interferon cDNA. Proc Natl Acad Sci USA 80:5842–5846

Gray PW, Leung DW, Pennica D, Yelverton E, Najarian R, Simonsen CC, Derynck R, Sherwood PJ, Wallace DM, Berger SL, Levinson AD, Goeddel DV (1982) Expression of human immune interferon cDNA in *E. coli* and monkey cells. Nature 295:503–508

Gray PW, Aggarwal BB, Benton CV, Bringman TS, Henzel WJ, Jarett JA, Leung DW et al. (1984) Cloning and expression of cDNA for human lymphotoxin, a lymphokine with tumour necrosis activity. Nature 312:721–724

Green S, Dobrjansky A, Carswell EA, Kassel RL, Old LJ, Fiore N, Schwartz MK (1976) Partial purification of a serum factor that causes necrosis of tumors. Proc Natl Acad Sci USA 73:381–385

Harrington JT, Stastny P (1973) Macrophage migration from an agarose droplet: development of a micromethod for assay of delayed hypersensitivity. J Immunol 110:752–759

Holter W, Grunow R, Stockinger H, Knapp W (1986) Recombinant interferon-γ induces interleukin 2 receptors on human peripheral blood monocytes. J Immunol 136:2171–2175

Horton JE, Raisz LG, Simmons HA, Oppenheim JJ, Mergenhagen SE (1972) Bone resorbing activity in supernatant fluid from cultured human peripheral blood leukocytes. Science 177:793–795

Horton JE, Koopman WJ, Farrar JJ, Fuller-Bonar J, Mergenhagen SE (1979) Partial purification of a bone-resorbing factor elaborated from human allogeneic cultures. Cell Immunol 43:1–10

Irons RD, Pfeifer RW, Aune TM, Pierce CW (1984) Soluble immune response suppressor (SIRS) inhibits microtubule function in vivo an microtubule activity in vitro. J Immunol 133:2032–2036

Kalden JR, Röllinghoff M (eds) (1986) Clinical application of lymphokines and cytokines. Immunobiology 172:157–460

Karnovsky ML, Lazdins JK (1978) Biochemical criteria for activated macrophages. J Immunol 121:809–813

Kelso A, Glasebrook AL, Kanagawa O, Brunner KT (1982) Production of macrophage-activating factor by T lymphocyte clones and correlation with other lymphokine activities. J Immunol 129:550–556

Kleinschmidt WJ, Schultz RM (1982) Similarities of murine gamma interferon and the lymphokine that renders macrophages cytotoxic. J Interferon Res 2:291–299

Kniep EM, Lohmann-Matthes ML (1986) Interleukin 2 activates human monocytes to cytotoxicity. Immunobiology 173:122

Kniep EM, Domzig W, Lohmann-Matthes M-L., Kickhöfen B (1981) Partial purification and chemical characterization of macrophage cytotoxicity factor (MCF, MAF) and its separation from migration inhibitory factor (MIF). J Immunol 127:417–422

Kolb WP, Granger GA (1968) Lymphocyte in vitro cytotoxicity: characterization of human lymphotoxin. Proc Natl Acad Sci USA 61:1250–1255

Kondo LL, Rosenau W, Wara DW (1981) Role of lymphotoxin in antibody-dependent cell-mediated cytotoxicity (ADCC). J Immunol 126:1131–1133

Koopman WJ, Sandberg AL, Wahl SM, Mergenhagen SE (1976) Interaction of soluble C3 fragments with guinea pig lymphocytes. Comparison of effects of C3a, C3b, C3c, and C3d on lymphokine production and lymphocyte proliferation. J Immunol 117:331–336

Kornfeld H, Berman JS, Beer DJ, Center DM (1985) Interleukin-2 stimulated lymphocyte migration. In: Sorg C, Schimpl A (eds) Cellular and molecular biology of lymphokines. Academic, New York, pp 533–537

Kownatzki E, Kapp A, Uhrich S (1986) Novel neutrophil chemotactic factor derived from human peripheral blood mononuclear leucocytes. Clin Exp Immunol 64:214–222

Krammer PH, Echtenacher B, Gemsa D, Hamann U, Hültner L, Kaltmann B, Kees U, Kubelka C, Marcucci F (1983) Immune-interferon (IFN-γ), macrophage activating factors (MAFs), and colony-stimulating factors (CSFs) secreted by T cell clones in limiting dilution microcultures, long-term cultures, and T cell hybridomas. Immunol Rev 76:5–28

Krammer PH, Echtenacher B, Hamann U, Kaltmann B, Kees U, Kubelka C, Gemsa D (1985) The role of T cell-clone and hybridoma-derived lymphokines in macrophage activation. In: van Furth R (ed) Mononuclear phagocytes. Characteristics, physiology and function. Nijhoff, Amsterdam, pp 533–540

Kull FC, Cuatrecasas P (1981) Preliminary characterization of the tumor cell cytotoxin in tumor necrosis serum. J Immunol 126:1279–1283

Lee SL, Aggarwal BB, Rinderknecht E, Assisi F, Chiu H (1984) The synergistic anti-proliferative effect of γ-interferon and human lymphotoxin. J Immunol 133:1083–1086

Leopardi E, Rosenau W (1984) Production of α-lymphotoxin by human T-cell subsets. Cell Immunol 83:73–82

Liu DY, Petschek KD, Remold HG, David JR (1980) Role of sialic acid in the macrophage glycolipid receptor for MIF. J Immunol 124:2042–2047

Liu DY, Yu SF, Miller PA, Remold HG, David JR (1984) Glycolipid-dependent interaction between human migration inhibitory factor and mononuclear phagocytes. Cell Immunol 88:350–360

Lohmann-Matthes M-L, Kreutzer H-P (1984) Human macrophage activating factor activates macrophages across species barrier. Lymphokine Res 3:256

Lovett D, Kozan B, Hadam M, Resch K, Gemsa D (1986) Macrophage cytotoxicity: interleukin 1 as a mediator of tumor cytostasis. J Immunol 136:340–347

Luger TA, Charon JA, Colat M, Micksche M, Oppenheim JJ (1983) Chemotactic properties of partially purified human epidermal cell-derived thymocyte-activation factor (ETAF) for polymorphonuclear and mononuclear cells. J Immunol 131:816–820

Mackaness GB (1969) The influence of immunologically committed lymphoid cells on macrophage activity in vivo. J Exp Med 129:973–992

Malkovsky M, North ME, Loveland B, Asherson GL, Fiers W (1986) Augmentation of monocyte cytotoxicity by recombinant interleukin-2. 6th international congress of immunology, Toronto, Canada, p 164

Männel D, Falk W (1983) Interferon-γ is required in activation of macrophages for tumor cytotoxicity. Cell Immunol 79:396–402

Männel DN, Meltzer MD, Mergenhagen SE (1980a) Generation and characterization of a lipopolysaccharide-induced and serum-derived cytotoxic factor for tumor cells. Infect Immun 28:204–211

Männel DN, Moore RN, Mergenhagen SE (1980b) Macrophages as a source of tumoricidal activity (tumor-necrotizing factor). Infect Immun 30:523–530

Matthews N (1978) Tumour necrosis factor from the rabbit. I. Mode of action, specificity and physicochemical properties. Br J Cancer 38:310–315

Matthews N (1981) Production of an anti-tumour cytotoxin by human monocytes. Immunology 44:135–142

McFadden RG, Cruikshank WW, Center DM (1984) Modulation of lymphocyte migration by human lymphokines. III. Characterization of a lymphocyte migration inhibitory factor (LyMIF$_{35K}$). Cell Immunol 85:154–167

Meltzer MS, Benjamin WR, Farrar JJ (1982) Macrophage activation for tumor cytotoxicity: induction of macrophage tumoricidal activity by lymphokines from EL-4, a continuous T cell line. J Immunol 129:2802–2807

Mestan J, Digel W, Mittnacht S, Hillen H, Blohm D, Möller A, Jacobsen H, Kirchner H (1986) Antiviral effects of recombinant tumour necrosis factor in vitro. Nature 323:816–819

Miossec P, Yu C-L, Ziff M (1984) Lymphocyte chemotactic activity of human interleukin 1. J Immunol 133:2007–2011

Mundy GR (1981) Control of osteoclast function by lymphokines in health and disease. In: Pick E (ed) Lymphokines, vol 4. Academic, New York, pp 395–408

Mundy GR, Raisz LG (1977) Big and little forms of osteoclast activating factor. J Clin Invest 60:122–128

Mundy GR, Luben RA, Raisz LG, Oppenheim JJ, Buell DN (1974a) Bone-resorbing activity in supernatants from lymphoid cell lines. N Engl J Med 290:867–871

Mundy GR, Raisz LG, Cooper RA, Schechter GP, Salmon SE (1974b) Evidence for the secretion of an osteoclast stimulating factor in myeloma. N Engl J Med 291:1041–1046

Mundy GR, Ibbotson KJ, D'Souza SM (1985) Tumor products and the hypercalcemia of malignancy. J Clin Invest 76:391–394

Nawroth PP, Bank I, Handley D, Cassimeris J, Chess L, Stern D (1986) Tumor necrosis factor/cachectin interacts with endothelial cell receptors to induce release of interleukin 1. J Exp Med 163:1363–1375

Nedwin GE, Jarett-Nedwin JA, Leung DW, Gray PW (1985) Cloning and expression of the cDNA for human lymphotoxin. In: Sorg C, Schimpl A (eds) Cellular and molecular biology of lymphokines. Academic, New York, pp 675–684

Neta R, Salvin SB (1982) Lymphokines and interferon: similarities and differences. In: Pick E (ed) Lymphokines, vol 7. Academic, New York, pp 137–163

North RJ (1978) The concept of the activated macrophage. J Immunol 121:806–809

Nowowiejski-Wieder I, Aune TM, Pierce CW, Webb DR (1984) Cell free translation of the lymphokine soluble immune response suppressor (SIRS) and characterization of its mRNA. J Immunol 132:556–558

Old LJ (1985) Tumor necrosis factor (TNF). Science 230:630–632

Ostrove JM, Gifford GE (1979) Stimulation of RNA synthesis in L-929 cells by rabbit tumor necrosis factor. Proc Soc Exp Biol Med 160:354–358

Pace JL, Russell SW, Torres BA, Johnson HM, Gray PW (1983) Recombinant mouse γ-interferon induces the priming step in macrophage activation for tumor cell killing. J Immunol 130:2011–2013

Pennica D, Nedwin GE, Hayflick JS, Seeburg PH, Derynck R, Palladino MA, Kohr WJ, Aggarwal BB, Goeddel DV (1984) Human tumour necrosis factor: precursor structure, expression and homology to lymphotoxin. Nature 312:724–729

Pennica D, Hayflick JS, Bringman TS, Palladino MA, Goeddel DV (1985) Cloning and expression in Escherichia coli of the cDNA for murine tumor necrosis factor. Proc Natl Acad Sci USA 82:6060–6064

Pick E (1985) Preface. Lymphokines 11:XII–XVI

Potter JW, van Epps DE (1986) Human T-lymphocyte chemotactic activity: nature and production in response to antigen. Cell Immunol 97:59–66

Prystowsky MB, Ely JM, Beller DI, Eisenberg L, Goldman J, Goldman M, Goldwasser E et al. (1982) Alloreactive cloned T cell lines. VI. Multiple lymphokine activities secreted by helper and cytolytic cloned T lymphocytes. J Immunol 129:2337–2344

Raisz LG, Luben RA, Mundy GR, Dietrich HW, Horton JE, Trummel CL (1975) Effect of osteoclast activating factor from human leukocytes on bone metabolism. J Clin Invest 56:408–413

Ralph P, Warren MK, Nakoinz I, Lee M-T, Brindley L, Sampson-Johannes A, Kawasaki ED et al. (1986) Biological properties and molecular biology of the human macrophage growth factor, CSF-1. Immunobiology 172:194–204

Ransom HG, Evans CH (1982) Lymphotoxin enhances the susceptibility of neoplastic and preneoplastic cells to natural killer cell mediated destruction. Int J Cancer 29:451–458

Ratliff TL, Thomasson DL, McCool RE, Catalona WJ (1982) T-cell hybridoma production of macrophage activating factor (MAF). I. Separation of MAF from interferon gamma. J Reticuloendothel Soc 393:397

Remold HG, Mednis AD (1979) Two migration inhibitory factors differ in density and susceptibility to neuraminidase and proteinase. J Immunol 122:1920–1925

Roberts WK, Vasil A (1982) Evidence for the identity of murine gamma interferon and macrophage activating factor. J Interferon Res 2:519–532

Rocklin RE, Bendtzen K, Greineder D (1980) Mediators of immunity: lymphokines and monokines. Adv Immunol 29:56–136

Rosenau W, Goldberg ML, Burke GC (1973) Early biochemical alterations induced by lymphotoxin in target cells. J Immunol 111:1128–1135

Rosenau W, Burke GC Moy J (1979) Lymphotoxin-induced loss of plasma-membrane protein. Am J Pathol 94:473–482

Rubin BY, Anderson SL, Sullivan SA, Williamson BD, Carswell EA, Old LJ (1985) High affinity binding of ^{125}I-labeled human tumor necrosis factor (LuKII) to specific cell surface receptors. J Exp Med 162:1099–1104

Ruddle NH (1985) Lymphotoxin redux. Immunol Today 6:156–159

Ruddle NH, Waksman BH (1967) Cytotoxic of lymphocyte-antigen interaction in delayed hypersensitivity. Science 157:1060–1062

Ruddle NH, Waksman BH (1968) Cytotoxicity mediated by soluble antigen and lymphocytes in delayed hypersensitivity. III. Analysis of mechanisms. J Exp Med 128:1267–1279

Ruff MR, Gifford GE (1980) Purification and physico-chemical characterization of rabbit tumor necrosis factor. J Immunol 25:1671–1677

Ruff MR, Gifford GE (1981) Tumor necrosis factor. Lymphokines 2:235–272

Sandberg AL, Wahl SM, Mergenhagen SE (1975) Lymphokine production by C3b-stimulated B cells. J Immunol 115:139–144

Schnaper HW, Aune TM (1985) Identification of lymphokine soluble immune response suppressor in urine of nephrotic children. J Clin Invest 76:341–349

Schnaper HW, Pierce CW, Aune TM (1984) Identification and initial characterization of concanavalin A- and interferon-induced human suppressor factors: evidence for a human equivalent of murine soluble immune response suppressor (SIRS). J Immunol 132:2429–2435

Schreiber RD, Celada A (1985) Molecular characterization of interferon as a macrophage activating factor. In: Pick E (ed) Lymphokines, vol 11. Academic, New York, pp 87–118

Shalaby MR, Aggarwal BB, Rinderknecht E, Svedersky LP, Finkle BS, Palladino MA (1985) Activation of human polymorphonuclear neutrophil functions by interferon-γ and tumor necrosis factors. J Immunol 135:2069–2073

Sharma JM, Herberman RB, Djeu JY, Nunn ME (1979) Production of migration inhibition factor by spleen cells of normal rats upon culture in vitro with tumor cells and cells expressing endogenous virus. J Immunol 123:222–231

Smith KA (1984) Lymphokine regulation of T cell and B cell function. In: Paul WE (ed) Fundamental immunology. Raven, New York, pp 559–576

Smith ME, Laudico R, Papermaster BW (1977) A rapid quantitative assay for lymphotoxin. J Immunol Methods 14:243–251

Sorg C (1980) Characterization of murine macrophage migration inhibitory activities (MIF) released by concanavalin A stimulated thymus or spleen cells. Mol Immunol 17:565–569

Sorg C (1982) Modulation of macrophage functions by lymphokines. Immunobiology 161:352–360

Sorg C, Michels E, Marlorny U, Neumann C (1984) Migration inhibitory factors and macrophage differentiation. Springer Semin Immunopathol 7:311–320

Spitalny GL, Havell EA (1984) Monoclonal antibody to murine gamma interferon inhibits lymphokine-induced antiviral and macrophage tumoricidal activities. J Exp Med 159:1560–1565

Stone-Wolff DS, Yip YK, Kelker HC, Le H, Henriksen-Destefano D, Rubin BY, Rinderknecht E, Aggarwal BB, Vilcek J (1984) Interrelationships of human interferon-gamma with lymphotoxin and monocyte cytotoxin. J Exp Med 159:828–843

Sugarman BJ, Aggarwal BB, Hass PE, Figari JS, Palladino MA, Shepard HM (1985) Recombinant human tumor necrosis factor-α: effects on proliferation of normal and transformed cells in vitro. Science 230:943–945

Tadakuma T, Pierce CW (1978) Mode of action of a soluble immune response suppressor (SIRS) produced by concanavalin A-activated spleen cells. J Immunol 120:481–486

Thompson BM, Saklatvala J, Chamber TJ (1986) Osteoblasts mediate interleukin 1 stimulation of bone resorption by rat osteoclasts. J Exp Med 164:104–112

Thurman GB, Braude IA, Gray PW, Oldham RK, Stevenson HC (1985) MIF-like activity of natural and recombinant human interferon-γ and their neutralization by monoclonal antibody. J Immunol 134:305–309

Trinchieri G, Kobayashi M, Rosen M, Loudon R, Murphy M, Perussia B (1986) Tumor necrosis factor and lymphotoxin induce differentiation of human myeloid cell lines in synergy with immune interferon. J Exp Med 164:1206–1225

Trummel CL, Mundy GR, Raisz LG (1975) Release of osteoclast activating factor by normal peripheral blood leukocytes. J Lab Clin Med 85:1001–1007

Van Epps DE, Potter JW, Durant DA (1983a) Production of a human T lymphocyte chemotactic factor by T cell subpopulations. J Immunol 130:2727–2731

Van Epps DE, Durant DA, Potter JW (1983b) Migration of human helper/inducer T cells in response to supernatants from Con A-stimulated suppressor/cytotoxic T cells. J Immunol 131:697–700

Vilcek J, Gray PW, Rinderknecht E, Sevastopoulos CG (1985) Interferon-γ: a lymphokine for all seasons. In: Pick E (ed) Lymphokines, vol 11. Academic, New York, pp 1–32

Wahl SM, Iverson GM, Oppenheim JJ (1974) Induction of guinea pig B-cell lymphokine synthesis by mitogenic and nonmitogenic signals to Fc, Ig, and C3 receptors. J Exp Med 140:1631–1645

Wang AM, Creasey AA, Ladner MB, Lin LS, Strickler J, van Arsdell JN, Yamamoto R, Mark DF (1985) Molecular cloning of the complementary DNA for human tumor necrosis factor. Science 228:149–154

Ward PA, Volkman A (1975) The elaboration of leukotactic mediators during the interaction between parental-type lymphocytes and F_1 hybrid cells. J Immunol 115:1394–1399

Ward PA, Remold HG, David JR (1970) The production by antigen-stimulated lymphocytes of a leukotactic factor distinct from migration inhibitory factor. Cell Immunol 1:162–174

Ward PA, Unanue ER, Goralnick SJ, Schreiner GF (1977) Chemotaxis of rat lymphocytes. J Immunol 119:416–421

Ware CF, Granger GA (1981) Mechanisms of lymphocyte-mediated cytotoxicity. The effects of anti-human lymphotoxin antisera on the cytolysis of allogenic B cell lines by MLC-sensitized human lymphocytes in vitro. J Immunol 126:1919–1926

Warren MK, Ralph P (1986) Macrophage growth factor CSF-1 stimulates human monocyte production of interferon, tumor necrosis factor, and colony stimulating activity. J Immunol 137:2281–2285

Weinberg JB, Chapman HA, Hibbs JB (1978) Characterization of the effects of endotoxin on macrophage tumor cell killing. J Immunol 12:72–80

Weiser WY, Greineder DK, Remold HG, David JR (1981) Studies on human migration inhibitory factor: characterization of three molecular species. J Immunol 126:1958–1962

Williams TW, Bellanti JA (1983) In vitro synergism between interferons and human lymphotoxin: enhancement of lymphotoxin-induced target cell killing. J Immunol 130:518–520

Williams TW, Granger GA (1973) Lymphocyte in vitro cytotoxicity: mechanisms of human lymphotoxin-induced target cell destruction. Cell Immunol 6:171–185

Williamson BD, Carswell EA, Rubin BY, Prendergast JS, Old LJ (1983) Human tumor necrosis factor produced by human B-cell lines: synergistic cytotoxic interaction with human interferon. Proc Natl Acad Sci USA 80:5397–5401

Wong GHW, Goeddel DV (1986) Tumor necrosis factors-α and -β inhibit virus replication and synergize with interferons. Nature 323:819–822

Wright SC, Bonavida B (1981) Selective lysis of NK-sensitive target cells by a soluble mediator released from murine spleen cells and human peripheral blood lymphocytes. J Immunol 126:1516–1521

Yoneda T, Mundy GR (1979) Prostaglandins are necessary for osteoclast-activating factor production by activated peripheral blood leucocytes. J Exp Med 149:279–283

Yoshimura T, Matsushima K, Oppenheim JJ, Leonard EJ (1987) Neutrophil chemotactic factor produced by lipopolysaccharide (LPS)-stimulated human blood mononuclear leukocytes: Partial characterization and separation from interleukin 1. J Immunol 139:788–793

CHAPTER 12

Lymphocyte Purification, Growth, Cloning and Functional Assays

M. J. H. RATCLIFFE and J. R. LAMB

A. Introduction

Lymphocytes comprise an extremely heterogeneous mixture of cells, differing in both specificity and function. Thus the immune system can recognise and respond to an enormous range of antigens and can mount functionally distinct types of responses to different forms of antigen (Chap. 1). The classical reductionalist approach to the problem of lymphocyte heterogeneity has been to obtain homogeneous populations of cells. In this way the signals acting on different populations of cells and the consequences of such signals can be determined. Homogeneous populations of cells have been prepared by either the extensive purification of mixed populations of cells or, more rigorously, by the growth and cloning of single cells from a mixed population.

Lymphocyte heterogeneity is apparent at two levels, one of which is represented by the specificity of the lymphoid cell. Lymphocytes express receptors on their surface which allow an individual cell to recognise and respond to a particular antigenic determinant. These receptors are therefore variable from one cell to another within the same lymphoid subset. Homogeneous populations of cells have been extensively used to provide a source of material to study the sequence and structure of the antigen receptors on lymphocytes, the nature of the interaction of these receptors with antigen and the repertoire of antigen receptors expressed as a consequence of antigenic challenge (Chap. 2).

The second level of lymphocyte heterogeneity relates to the different functions of the immune system which are mediated by different classes or subsets of lymphocytes. Thus B cells which produce antibodies and T cells which are responsible for a variety of cell-mediated immune functions form the major lymphoid compartments and represent distinct lineages of cells. Within each of these lineages further subsets of cells can be functionally defined, T cells being either helper, cytotoxic or suppressor cells and B cells segregating into virgin B cells, memory cells or plasma cells. In addition, within each of these subsets further functional heterogeneity may occur.

From the pharmacological viewpoint, there is already considerable evidence that different lymphoid subsets show markedly different responses to a variety of pharmacological mediators. However, by the antigen-nonspecific nature of the interaction of pharmacological mediators with lymphoid cells, it is apparent that the precise specificity of a cell within a particular lymphoid subset will not influence its pharmacological response. Therefore, although antigen is frequently used to stimulate lymphocyte growth, in this chapter we will consider antigen as a means to trigger the antigen receptor, rather than going into detail about the properties of any particular antigen.

Broadly speaking there are three main strategies for the preparation of homogeneous populations of cells. The most rigorous of these depends on the ability to grow the cell of interest in tissue culture for extended periods of time. When this is possible, it becomes practical to obtain clones of cells, each derived from a single precursor, resulting in a population of cells homogenous with respect to both antigen specificity and lymphocyte function. However techniques are not yet available for the long-term growth of some lymphocyte subsets and alternative approaches have been used with success. Lymphocyte transformation makes it possible to derive long-term lines of immortalised cells which can subsequently be cloned. Alternatively, functionally homogeneous populations of cells can be prepared by purification of a lymphoid subset from a functionally heterogeneous mixture of normal cells.

I. Tissue Culture

For obvious reasons, the tissue culture requirements for long-term growth and cloning of lymphoid cells are much more stringent than those required for short-term assays. Therefore some of the important aspects of long-term lymphocyte tissue culture have been outlined.

All the tissue culture described in this chapter is performed at 37 °C in a maximally humidified incubator with an atmosphere of 5% CO_2 in air. The choice of tissue culture medium is fairly wide, but RPMI 1640, Dulbecco's modified Eagle's medium (DMEM) or Iscove's modified Dulbecco's medium (IMDM) will usually be appropriate in most circumstances. These media can be obtained from a variety of commercial sources in either liquid or powdered form. If they are obtained in powdered form, the distilled water used to reconstitute the medium should be of high quality. Commercial media usually need to be supplemented with 2-mercaptoethanol (5×10^{-5} M), antibiotics (e.g. penicillin 100 IU/ml and streptomycin 100 µg/ml or alternatively gentamicin 50 µg/ml) and buffering such as HEPES and/or sodium hydrogen carbonate to enable the medium to equilibrate to pH 7.4 in 5% CO_2. Routinely, we use IMDM with penicillin/streptomycin, 2-mercaptoethanol and 3.025 g/l sodium hydrogen carbonate.

In addition, the major supplement for tissue culture is a source of serum. For murine cell culture, fetal calf serum (FCS) is most frequently used at 5%–10%. There is considerable variation in batches of commercial FCS and several batches should therefore be screened. A batch which supports good positive responses without inducing high background responses can then be selected. Having selected a suitable batch, enough of that lot should be obtained to last as long as possible. FCS needs to be heat inactivated at 56 °C for 30 min prior to use in tissue culture after which it can be stored for extended periods at −70 °C.

Human cells can be cultured in FCS although better responses are frequently obtained with normal human serum. AB serum is usually prepared by heat inactivation, screened, selected and stored in the same way as FCS. A variety of commercial replacements for serum are now available which, while frequently not resulting in a "defined" medium, may allow reproducible replacement of FCS.

For short-term tissue culture, when using IMDM, serum can be replaced with iron-saturated transferrin (5 µg/ml), bovine serum albumin (500 µg/ml) and soybean lipids (20 µg/ml) (Iscove and Melchers 1978) (all of which can be obtained from Boehringer Mannheim GmbH, Mannheim) specially selected for tissue culture. Long-term growth of normal cells in such serum-free medium has proved more difficult to obtain and may put inappropriate selective pressure on the responding cells.

Cell preparations can be prepared in a variety of media or Dulbecco's phosphate-buffered saline (0.1 g/l $CaCl_2$, 0.2 g/l KH_2PO_4, 0.2 g/l KCl, 0.1 g/l $MgCl_2 \cdot 6 H_2O$, 8 g/l NaCl, 1.15 g/l $Na_2HPO_4 \cdot 2 H_2O$) (PBS). Routinely we use minimum essential medium buffered with 2 g/l sodium hydrogen carbonate and 20 mM HEPES buffer in order to maintain pH 7.4 in atmospheric air (0%, CO_2).

II. Freezing and Thawing of Cells

There are several reasons for the cryopreservation of cells. Apart from the obvious use as a means of storage, cell freezing provides insurance against stocks of cells becoming contaminated or losing activity.

Cells are resuspended in ice-cold freezing medium (70% RPMI, 20 % FCS, 10% dimethylsulphoxide) and loaded into sterile liquid nitrogen ampoules. The ampoules are placed inside a polystyrene box which is sealed and placed in a -70 °C freezer. This allows the cells to cool down to -70 °C slowly. After leaving the cells at -70 °C overnight, they can be transferred to liquid nitrogen storage.

Cells are thawed by removing the ampoule from liquid nitrogen and placing it in a 37 °C water bath until the ice has just melted. The cells are then washed immediately in tissue culture medium to remove the dimethylsulphoxide and placed in tissue culture. The cells are examined for viability after 24 h.

B. T Cell Growth and Cloning

I. Introduction

The regulatory and effector functions of the cellular arm of the immune system are mediated by highly specialised and functionally heterogeneous populations of T lymphocytes which, like B lymphocytes, have a diverse repertoire of specificities that are clonally distributed (Chap. 1). The isolation of monoclonal T lymphocytes is therefore important, since a comprehensive understanding of the immune system and how it can be manipulated will depend on a detailed knowledge of the structure and function of individual clones of cells.

The cloning of T lymphocytes has become possible over the last decade for two main reasons. The first lies in the increasing understanding of how T cells interact with antigen and the demonstration that this interaction depends on the presence of accessory cells whose function is to "present" antigen to the T cell. The second major advance was the realisation that interleukin 2 (IL-2, previously known as T cell growth factor or TCGF) could maintain T cells in long-term culture (MORGAN et al. 1976; GILLIS and SMITH 1977). This allowed the isolation and expansion of monoclonal populations of both murine (FATHMAN and HENGARTNER 1978; NABHOLZ et al. 1978; SCHREIER and TEES 1980) and human T cells (BACH et al. 1979; SREDNI et al. 1981 a,b; LAMB et al. 1982).

Exploitation of the IL-2 dependence of activated T cells is not the only method of isolating T cell clones and alternative approaches such as hybridisation (KONTIAINEN et al. 1978; KAPPLER et al. 1981; OKADA et al. 1981) and viral transformation (FINN et al. 1979; POPOVIC et al. 1983) have been used with success.

II. In Vivo Generation of Antigen-Primed T Cells

Mice are usually primed with protein or cellular antigen emulsified in an equal volume of complete Freund's adjuvant by injecting about 50 µl emulsion containing 100 µg protein antigen or 2×10^7 cells subcutaneously at the base of the tail or in the footpads. Some 5–8 days later the draining lymph nodes contain antigen-responsive cells which can be grown in vitro (CORRADIN et al. 1977). Spleen or lymph nodes taken from mice sublethally infected with live virus 7–14 days earlier will contain T cells responsive to viral antigens.

Murine T cells are usually purified by passage of spleen or lymph node cells through nylon wool columns (JULIUS et al. 1973). Nylon wool columns (1 g dry weight prewashed nylon wool for 5×10^7 cells packed in a 10-ml syringe or 4 g for 2×10^8 cells in a 35-ml syringe) are filled with PBS and 5% FCS and incubated at 37 °C for 1 h. The column is then washed with 2 column volumes warm PBS/FCS and cells (2×10^7/ml) in warm PBS/ FCS are loaded onto the column dropwise. After incubating at 37 °C for 1 h, T cells are eluted with 2 column volumes warm (37 °C) PBS/FCS dropwise.

For ethical reasons, generating primed populations of human T cells is more difficult. The commonest source of primed human T cells is peripheral blood lymphocytes taken from volunteers about a week after vaccination with tetanus toxoid, influenza virus or BCG. Alternatively, peripheral blood lymphocytes taken from patients with viral infections such as influenza will contain virus-specific T cells.

Human peripheral blood lymphocytes are prepared by drawing human blood by sterile venipuncture into preservative-free heparin to a concentration of about 5 units per millilitre. Then, 1 volume blood is diluted with an equal volume of minimum essential medium and layered over 1 volume Ficoll-Hypaque (density 1.077). After centrifugation at 1500 g for 15 min at room temperature mononuclear cells are harvested from the interface and washed twice. The proportion of T cells in human peripheral blood lymphocytes is high, about 75%, and so T cells, prior to growth, are not usually prepared away from the other cells in the suspension. For some strong antigens such as alloantigens, in both mice and humans, priming in vivo may not be required.

III. Feeder Cells

T lymphocytes recognise and are activated by antigen in the context of polymorphic proteins encoded in the major histocompatibility complex (Mhc). Antigen has therefore to be presented to T cells by specialised antigen-presenting cells and so the initial stage of T lymphocyte growth requires the presence of both antigen and antigen-presenting cells or feeders. For mouse T cell growth, the commonest sources of feeders are red blood cell-depleted (Sect. C.VII.1) spleen cells (5×10^6/ml) or peritoneal exudate cells ($0.5–1.0 \times 10^6$/ml). For human T cell growth, peripheral blood leukocytes ($0.5–1.0 \times 10^6$/ml) which can be depleted of T cells (see Sect. C.VII.2) are used.

Feeder cells do not need to divide to exert their function and are therefore treated by either irradiation with 2–3000 rad (from a γ-emitting source such as ^{60}Co or ^{137}Cs or from an X-ray source). Alternatively, cell division is blocked by incubation of cells with mitomycin C 100 µg/ml at 37 °C for 1 h. Mitomycin C has to be carefully removed from the feeder cells (four washes) to prevent carryover into the T cell activation cultures.

Transformed B cell lines have been successfully used as feeders in short-term assays (McKEAN et al. 1981; RATCLIFFE et al. 1984). However long-term growth of T cells has not been supported by transformed cells. Transformed cells are usually more radioresistant than normal cells and therefore should be treated with mitomycin C as described rather than by irradiation prior to use in tissue culture.

Since T cells recognise antigen in the context of polymorphic determinants on the Mhc antigens, feeder cells have to be syngeneic to the responding T cells. In mouse tissue culture this is not a problem, owing to the availability of inbred strains of mice. For human T cell growth this is more of a problem and a constant source of Mhc identical feeder cells must be ensured. One way round this problem is to obtain feeder cells from the same volunteer who provided the T cells.

IV. Antigen In Vitro

If the antigen used to stimulate the T cells is expressed on antigen-presenting cells themselves, e.g. responses to alloantigens, then feeders expressing that antigen can be used instead of syngeneic feeders. Similarly, for viral antigens, syngeneic feeder cells can be infected with live virus at 37 °C for a few hours before irradiation and washing. Soluble proteins are usually included at 10–100 µg/ml. Particulate antigens such as foreign red blood cells are usually included at about 0.2%. Optimal in vitro antigen doses vary depending on the antigen used and should be evaluated by titration.

V. Sources of Interleukin 2

T cell growth and cloning requires IL-2 and so a routine source of IL-2 is a requirement for this work. Mouse, rat, human and gibbon IL-2 all support the growth of mouse T cells. However mouse and rat IL-2 do not support the growth of human T cells (see also Chap. 8).

1. EL4 T Cell Lymphoma

The mouse EL4 cell line was subcloned by Dr. J Farrar to generate a subline which secretes high levels of IL-2 when seeded at $1-2 \times 10^6$/ml in medium without FCS supplemented with 1% horse serum and 10 ng/ml phorbol myristate acetate (FARRAR et al. 1980). After 16 h, the cells are removed by centrifugation and the supernatant filtered through 0.22-µm filters and stored at −20 °C. The drawback with this supernatant is the presence of phorbol myristate acetate which is difficult to remove completely and may exert a pharmacological effect on the responding cells.

2. Lectin-Stimulated Rat Spleen Cells

Rat spleen cells depleted of red blood cells (Sect. C.VII.1) are cultured at 5×10^6/ml in tissue culture medium with 5% FCS and 2 µg/ml concanavalin A. After 24 h, the supernatant is harvested and stored as in Sect. B.V.1. The activity of the concanavalin A in the supernatant can be inhibited with methyl-α-D-mannopyrannoside (0.05 M final concentration, grade III, Sigma Chemical Co., St. Louis) when the supernatant is used.

3. MLA-144

This gibbon cell line constitutively secretes IL-2 which supports the growth of human or murine T cells and so the supernatant of MLA-144 cells grown to about $1-2 \times 10^6$/ml can be harvested and stored as in Sect. B.V.1. Obtaining a stock of MLA-144 cells which is free of mycoplasma is important since some stocks of MLA-144 contain mycoplasma which can be highly inhibitory for T cell growth and cloning.

4. Lectin-Stimulated Human T Cells

Human peripheral blood leukocytes (Sect. B.II) are cultured at 10^6/ml in medium supplemented with 2.5% normal human serum and phytohemagglutinin 0.1 µg/ml (or 1/1000) for 48 h. IL-2-containing supernatant is harvested and stored as in Sect. B.V.1.

5. Recombinant IL-2

The sources of IL-2 mentioned so far have all successfully supported T lymphocyte growth and cloning. However all contain contaminants such as the molecules used to stimulate IL-2 production and/or other biological mediators produced by the stimulated cells. The purest source of IL-2 is therefore recombinant human IL-2 produced by gene cloning in bacteria (Taniguchi et al. 1983) and commercially available from several sources. Because bacterially produced IL-2 is not glycosylated it may not be as stable as the fully glycosylated molecule although it supports long-term T cell growth in vitro. In addition, recombinant IL-2 may sometimes contain low levels of bacterial products.

6. Assay for IL-2

Test supernatants are serially diluted in tissue culture medium and cultured with 5000 cells of an IL-2-addicted cell line such as CTL (Gillis and Smith 1977) or HT2 (Watson 1979) in 200 µl per well of a 96-well tissue culture plate. Wells are pulsed with 1 µCi [^{3}H] thymidine in 10 µl after 16–24 h and harvested 8 h later for counting incorporated radioactivity on a scintillation counter (see also Chap. 8). For T cell growth and cloning, mammalian cell-derived IL-2 supernatants are routinely used at 5%–20% and bacterially produced recombinant IL-2 at about 5 ng/ml.

VI. Antigen-Independent Growth and Cloning

Some T cells, after stimulation with antigen and feeders, are induced to express receptors for IL-2 constitutively. Such cells are usually of the cytotoxic phenotype (L3T4$^-$,Ly2$^+$ in mice, T4$^-$,T8$^+$ in humans).

1. Antigen-Independent Growth

T cells (10^6/ml) are stimulated in the presence of antigen and feeders for 3–4 days. Viable T cell blasts are prepared by centrifugation over Ficoll-Hypaque (density

1.077) for 15 min at 1400 g and reseeded at 10^5/ml in the presence of IL-2. Viable cells are prepared and reseeded with IL-2 every 2–3 days, gradually decreasing the input T cell number to 10^4/ml. After a few passages, cells which do not constitutively express IL-2 receptors will have stopped growing allowing those which do express receptors constitutively to grow out (NABHOLZ et al. 1978; WATSON 1979).

2. Antigen-Independent Cloning

Once a cell line is established that requires IL-2 alone for continued growth the cells can be cloned without the addition of antigen or feeders. The cells are diluted to 30/ml in medium supplemented with IL-2 and aliquots of 10 µl are distributed in the wells of a 60-well Terasaki tissue culture plate. The wells are examined for growth after 5–7 days using an inverted microscope and when the wells begin to fill up the contents are transferred to a well of a 96-well tissue culture plate containing 200 µl medium with IL-2. As this well begins to fill up, the cells can be transferred to a 2-ml culture in a 24-well plate and from there into larger cultures, always in the presence of IL-2. Alternatively, cells can be diluted to 2/ml in IL-2 containing medium and seeded at 200 µl per well in a 96-well tissue culture plate. Again, when the well begins to fill up the cells are transferred to 2-ml cultures as before. Such clones are usually very sensitive to a lack of IL-2 and will die rapidly if they consume all the available IL-2.

3. Assay for Cytotoxic T Cell Activity

Target cells expressing the cellular or viral antigen to which the T cells were primed are labelled with ^{51}Cr by incubating target cells (10^7/ml) with 500 µCi ^{51}Cr (fresh sodium chromate, specific activity 10 mCi/ml) for 1 h at 37 °C. Transformed cell lines or lymphocytes activated by lectin for 2–3 days usually make the best targets and can be infected with virus if required. After three washes, 10^4 targets are cocultured with titrated numbers of test T cells in 200 µl tissue culture medium in a V-bottomed microtiter plate for 4 h at 37 °C. Before and after culture the plate is centrifuged at 1000 rpm for 1 min. Then, 100 µl supernatant is removed for counting of released ^{51}Cr.

The positive control represents the counts released by detergent lysis of the targets and the negative control represents the counts spontaneously released by the targets in the absence of T cells. The percentage cytotoxicity is calculated as

$$\frac{\text{Test sample (cpm)} - \text{spontaneous release (cpm)}}{\text{Detergent lysis (cpm)} - \text{spontaneous release (cpm)}} \times 100$$

To demonstrate cytotoxic T cell specificity, target cells must express the appropriate antigen and Mhc antigens before they are lysed.

VII. Antigen-Dependent T Cell Lines

Most T cells after stimulation with antigen express IL-2 receptors for a few days during which they are responsive to IL-2. Continued growth of such cells requires a further exposure to antigen and feeders in order to induce re-expression of the

IL-2 receptor. Generally such cells fall into the T helper cell category (L3T4$^+$,Ly2$^-$ in mice, T4$^+$T8$^-$ in humans). Within this population of cells, some T cells produce IL-2 when stimulated with antigen and others do not.

1. Growth of T Cell Lines

A wide variety of techniques have been used to grow T cells which do not express IL-2 receptors continuously. In vivo primed T cells (10^6/ml) are stimulated with antigen and feeders for 10–14 days. Viable cells, prepared by centrifugation over Ficoll-Hypaque (Sect. B.VI.1), are reseeded at 3×10^5/ml with fresh antigen and feeders. Every 14 days thereafter viable cells are prepared and seeded at 10^5/ml with fresh antigen and feeders.

The principle of this approach is that some T cells are stimulated by antigen to produce a burst of IL-2. This IL-2 is consumed by cells expressing IL-2 receptors which are thereby induced to divide. Cells constitutively expressing IL-2 receptors will die when the IL-2 is exhausted, however, helper T cells lose the expression of IL-2 receptors and stop growing, but remain viable. Subsequent exposure to antigen and feeders will produce another burst of IL-2 production and induce IL-2 receptors which drives further rounds of cell proliferation. This procedure clearly selects for the maintenance of T cells which can produce IL-2 in the culture.

A variant of this procedure which has been used successfully is to stimulate primed T cells (10^6/ml) as before with antigen and feeders for 3–4 days and then culture the viable cells (10^6/ml) for 7–14 days in the presence of feeders alone (Kimoto and Fathman 1980). This resting period performs the same function as allowing the culture with antigen and feeders to run for 10–14 days. Viable cells can then be reseeded as before at 3×10^5/ml with antigen and feeders for 3–4 days before another resting period with feeders alone. This procedure also selects for the maintenance of T cells which can produce IL-2 in culture and has been used to generate both mouse (Kimoto and Fathman 1980) and human T cell lines (Volkman et al. 1984).

Long-term T cell lines can also be generated by stimulating primed T cells with antigen and feeders and then alternating with growth in the presence of IL-2 (Lanzavecchia et al. 1983). After an initial culture of T cells ($1–2 \times 10^6$/ml) with antigen and feeders for 7 days, viable cells are reseeded at 2×10^5/ml with IL-2 every 2–3 days thereafter. After 3–5 weeks, viable cells are reseeded at 5×10^4/ml with feeders and antigen for 7 days before returning to further growth with IL-2 alone. This approach enhances the rate of growth of the T cell line both because of the constant presence of IL-2 and also because it removes the requirement that there must be IL-2-producing cells in the culture.

A further approach is to provide the activated T cells with fresh antigen and fillers every 4–5 days. In vivo primed T cells are seeded at 10^6/ml in the presence of antigen and feeders. After 4–5 days viable cells are prepared by Ficoll-Hypaque centrifugation and reseeded at 3×10^5/ml with antigen and feeders. After 4–5 days viable cells are again prepared and reseeded at 10^5/ml. Subsequently viable cells are reseeded every 4–5 days at 4×10^4/ml with fresh antigen and feeders (Ratcliffe and Julius 1982). This approach proves successful when the feeders are irradiated with an X-ray source, but not when the feeders are irradiated with a γ-emitting ^{60}Co source. Triggering of the T cell antigen receptor can downregulate the functional expression of the receptor. A likely reason why this final approach may work is that X-irradiated feeders lyse fairly rapidly in culture whereas γ-irradiated cells may persist in culture for longer periods of time maintaining the presence of appropriately presented antigen, thereby downregulating the functional expression of the T cell antigen receptor for longer periods of time.

2. Assay of Antigen-Dependent T Cell Lines

The commonest assay for T cell lines (or clones derived from them) are antigen-driven proliferation and IL-2 release. To assay for proliferation, T cells after one or more rounds of in vitro growth are cultured at $2\text{--}10 \times 10^4$/ml with titrated antigen and syngeneic or allogeneic feeder cells ($1\text{--}5 \times 10^6$/ml). IL-2 may be added into the assay if growth of the T cell line depends on exogenous IL-2 as well as antigen and feeder cells. Proliferation is assessed after 2–4 days by the addition of 1 μCi [^{3}H] thymidine for the final 8–16 h of culture, after which the cells are harvested for scintillation counting of incorporated radioactivity.

To assay for IL-2 release, T cells are cocultured at up to 10^6/ml in the presence of antigen and syngeneic or allogeneic feeders for 16–24 h. Aliquots of supernatant are then assayed for IL-2 content (Sect. B.V.6). A T cell line can be considered specific (i.e. enriched in the cells of interest) if positive responses in either assay show a complete dependence on antigen and syngeneic feeders expressing the appropriate Mhc antigens.

VIII. Cloning from Antigen-Dependent T Cell Lines

1. When to clone

The first decision to be made is the stage at which clones should be derived from a T cell line. Generally, the longer a line has been in tissue culture the higher the cloning efficiency. However, since the growth rate of individual clones within a population is variable, long-term T cell cultures can become oligoclonal with time (NABHOLZ et al. 1980 a,b). Thus the cloning of long-term T cell lines may isolate a very selective and unrepresentative proportion of the T cell repertoire. For this reason cloning of T cells from shorter-term cultures may be preferable and short-term cultures of T cells induced with viral, soluble and alloantigen have been successfully used to generate clones representative of the T cell repertoire.

2. Limiting Dilution Cloning

Establishing monoclonal T cells by limiting dilution cloning is the most commonly used of the IL-2-dependent cloning techniques (Chap. 6). Basically it involves the plating of an enriched population of activated T cells at a titrated or known limiting number of cells per well of a microtitre plate in the presence of feeder cells, specific antigen and IL-2. The plating efficiency in IL-2-dependent limiting dilution cloning can be as high as 25% and may approach 100% (LUTZ et al. 1980; LAMB et al. 1982) as compared with 1% observed with soft agar cloning (Sect. B.VIII.4) (Sredni et al. 1981 b). Limiting dilution cultures with evidence of T cell growth between 6 and 14 days observed using an inverted microscope are expanded with the addition of fresh feeder cells, antigen and IL-2 into larger wells and then into tissue culture flasks, transferring about every 10 days. As soon as possible, cells should be checked for their IL-2 dependence by splitting into wells with antigen, feeders and no IL-2. "Clones" should be harvested under conditions where the Poisson distribution predicts the probability of a culture being derived from a single cell to be >95%, usually when fewer than 10% of the wells are positive for growth. However, at this stage "clones" are frequently derived from an input of more than one cell per well. Putative clones, once they have been screened for their ability to respond to the inducing antigen (Sect. B.VII.2), must therefore be subcloned by limiting dilution to establish that they are truly monoclonal. Ideally, the cloning efficiency at this stage should be high enough to allow cloning from an average of 0.3 cells per well.

3. Micromanipulation

An approach which immediately overcomes the problem of ensuring clonality is micromanipulation (Zagury et al. 1975) where individual cells are seeded mechanically, using a drawn-out sterile capillary tube to pick up single cells observed in very dilute cell suspensions with an inverted microscope into a well prepared with antigen, feeders and IL-2. A modification of the fluorescence-activated cell sorter can be used to do this automatically.

4. Semisolid Agar Cloning

Activated T cells after a cycle of in vitro stimulation are suspended with feeders (10^5–10^6/ml) and antigen in soft agar (0.2%–0.5% in culture medium at 45 °C) and plated onto a preformed feeder layer of 0.5% agar in tissue culture medium. In some, but not all protocols, a source of IL-2 is added at this stage. After a variable interval of 4–7 days, colonies of cells appear near the top surface of the agar (Fathman and Hengartner 1978). These colonies are extracted from the soft agar with a fine capillary tube and transferred to liquid culture in 0.2 ml culture medium with antigen, feeders and antigen for expansion. The concentration of activated T cells plated should be titrated in such a way as to allow T cell growth to appear as discrete colonies in the agar.

Both human (Sredni et al. 1981 a) and murine (Fathman and Hengartner 1978) colonies have been isolated in this way. Small colonies of lymphocytes of differing morphology develop within the agar layer itself (type I colonies), while smaller type II colonies appear later on the surface of the agar. For any colony formation to occur the continuous presence of antigen is required and its concentration is critical since the amount of antigen required for type II colonies is twice that which induces optimal development of the type I colonies.

The distinction between T cell colonies and clones must be clearly made in terms of their probability of being derived from a single cell. The term colony refers to a cell population usually picked from agar and it is difficult, particularly for type II colonies, to estimate the probability of this being clonal. This is further hampered by the ability of T cells to migrate through the semisolid agar and therefore recruitable cells may be activated and proliferate. After removal from the agar, the colonies are expanded in liquid culture in microtitre plates in the presence of irradiated feeder cells, antigen and IL-2. When the colonies have expanded to sufficient numbers they can be assayed for antigen dependence by their ability to proliferate to specific antigen in the presence of feeder cells (Sect. B.VII.2). Once colonies of interest have been established multiple recloning at high plating efficiency is necessary using either limiting dilution or semisolid agar to secure clonality.

5. Summary

IL-2-dependent cloning has facilitated the isolation of individual cells reactive with a variety of soluble and particulate antigens and which function as helper, cytotoxic and suppressor T cells. The approach of choice will often depend on the frequency of clonally responding precursors. If the cloning efficiency is low, as is often the case when cloning from T cell populations which have not been grown for extended periods of time in vitro, micromanipulation may not be suitable. Under these circumstances, limiting dilution cloning is frequently used as a first step, followed by micromanipulation to ensure clonality of the limiting dilution "clone".

IX. Use of Transformed Cell Lines

In the remainder of this section we will consider the use of transformed cells generated by either spontaneous transformation, viral transformation or cell hybridisation. The major advantage of such cells is the ease of cell growth, making it possible to obtain large amounts of material. In addition, the adaptation of in vivo tumours to in vitro growth as cell lines makes it possible to obtain completely homogeneous populations of cells. The disadvantage of transformed cell lines is that by nature of their immortalised status, the control over their proliferation is abnormal and so transformed cell lines have limited suitability for studies on the physiology of cell growth control. In addition, many tumours are refractory to signals which may activate normal cells (the reverse can also be true). Despite these drawbacks however, many transformed cells have been of use in shedding light on the physiology of lymphocyte activation and maturation.

X. T Cell Hybridisation

The use of somatic cell hybridisation to establish monoclonal T cells is based on the success of generating monoclonal antibodies resulting from the fusion of normal B cells and nonsecreting myelomas (KOHLER and MILSTEIN 1975; see Chap. 6). Although this technique has proven to be highly successful in generating murine T cell clones, for human T cells it remains as yet unreliable. The first murine T–T hybrids were generated by fusing suppressor T cells with the AKR thymoma BW5147 (KONTIAINEN et al. 1978; KAPP et al. 1980), and more recently T cell hybridomas of the helper/inducer subset (L3T4$^+$,Lyt-2$^-$) have been constructed (KAPPLER et al. 1981).

T cells (10^6/ml) from lymph nodes of primed mice are restimulated in vitro with the relevant antigen and feeder cells. The resulting viable cells are isolated by centrifugation over Ficoll-Hypaque (Sect. B.VI.1) and fused to azaguanine-resistant BW5147. Alternatively the fusion partner, F56-14.13.AG2 which has the property of antigen-inducible IL-2 release can be used (Kappler et al. 1981). This is advantageous if antigen-dependent IL-2 release is to be used as the assay system (Sect. B.VII.2). The fusion protocol using polyethylene glycol is essentially identical to that described in Chap. 6, selecting fused cells in medium containing hypoxanthine, aminopterin and thymidine. As soon as the hybrids have expanded to a sufficient number of cells they are assayed for antigen specificity by IL-2 production following stimulation with the appropriate antigen in the presence of syngeneic antigen-presenting cells. T cell hybrids of interest are then cloned by limiting dilution.

Cytolytic hybrids have been obtained by the fusion of IL-2-dependent cytotoxic T cell clones with BW5147 (Nabholz et al. 1980b). The resultant hybrids, although specific in effector function like the parent cells from which they were derived, only grew in the presence of exogenous IL-2. Initially from these hybrids IL-2-independent variants were isolated, but they had lost specific cytolytic activity (Nabholz et al. 1980b). However more recently, cytolytic, IL-2-independent, antigen-specific variants have been reported (Haas and Kisielow 1985).

For the generation of human T cell hybrids the approach is somewhat similar. Normal peripheral blood leukocytes activated in vitro with antigen or mitogen have been fused to human T lymphoblastoid cells by means of polyethylene glycol and stable lines cloned by limiting dilution (Okada et al. 1981; Butler et al. 1983). Antigen-specific human T cell hybrids resulting from the fusion of antigen-specific, IL-2-dependent T cell lines with the T cell lymphoma Jurkat have been produced (DeFreitas et al. 1982). These T cell hybridomas, when stimulated with antigen-pulsed histocompatible monocytes, released IL-2 and furthermore induced antigen-specific antibody production when cocultured with human B cells in the presence of specific antigen.

Attempts to fuse human IL-2-dependent, antigen-specific cytolytic T cells to a lymphoblastoid line (Lakow et al. 1983; Gallagher and Stimson 1984) have been less successful. None of the resultant hybridomas displayed specific cytolytic activity although their proliferative response could be increased after exposure to antigen. The loss of chromosomes from these hybrids resulted in alterations in phenotype and the loss of function and so maintaining stability of function of human T–T hybrids appears to remain a major problem (Gallagher and Stimson 1984).

XI. Viral Transformation

The final methodology of generating immortal monoclonal T cells is that of viral transformation. This method has no immediate advantages over that of somatic cell hybridisation and for that reason we will not go into much technical detail. However as with T cell hybridisation the approach does negate the requirement for growing the cells in the presence of IL-2 and feeder cells. Murine T lymphocytes have been successfully transformed with the RNA tumour virus, radiation leukemia virus (RadLV) (Finn et al. 1979). T cells from immunised mice are infected in vitro with RadLV and then introduced intrathymically into irradiated (500 rad) congeneic recipients. The resulting lymphomas which develop after several months can then be re-established in vitro, maintained in long-term culture and cloned. Such T lymphoma cells have been able to provide antigen-specific T cell help in vivo when adoptively transferred into syngeneic, antigen-primed mice. In addition, the functional properties of the transformed T cell appeared to be unaltered as compared with the original population. However T cell transformation by RadLV is limited to certain strains of mice since viral replication is genetically restricted both by the *H-2* complex, such that only *H-2^b* and *H-2^d* haplotypes are readily infected, and also by *Fv-1*, a gene unrelated to the *H-2* complex. Suppressor T cells primed in vivo and enriched in vitro by binding to antigen have also been immortalised in this way (RICCIARDI-CASTAGNOLI et al. 1981).

Human T lymphocytes have been transformed by cocultivation with neoplastic T cell lines producing the RNA retrovirus human T cell leukaemia/lymphoma virus (HTLV-I) which is tropic for the helper/inducer (T4) T cell subset (POPOVIC et al. 1983). While numerous HTLV-infected T cell lines have been isolated, the functional characteristics and specificity of the parent cells have not been determined. More recently, antigen-specific T cell clones have been infected with HTLV (POPOVIC et al. 1984; SUCIU-FOCA et al. 1984; VOLKMAN et al. 1985). However, detailed analysis of the activation requirements of lymphokine release and B cell help demonstrated that after HTLV infection the T cells had become dysregulated (VOLKMAN et al. 1985; SUCIU-FOCA et al. 1984). Thus while HTLV-I can immortalise human T4 cells the resulting dysregulation of activation requirements and function suggests that such an approach may be of limited value in the analysis of normal T cell physiology.

XII. Summary

The isolation and expansion of T lymphocyte clones can be achieved by several methodologies each of which has its own advantages. IL-2-dependent cloning provides T cells most closely approximated to their normal physiologic condition (nontransformed) and the analysis of such clones has revealed detailed information on the activation requirements and effector function of helper and cytotoxic T cells (for reviews see FATHMAN and FITCH 1982; FELDMANN et al. 1986). Although IL-2-dependent suppressor T cells have been cloned (FRESNO et al. 1981; BENSUSSAN et al. 1984) reports of such cells are infrequent, suggesting that optimal growth conditions for this lymphoid subset still require definition.

T cell hybridomas free of the restrictive growth requirements of IL-2-dependent clones have been of critical importance in facilitating the biochemical and molecular analysis of T cell antigen recognition (for reviews see DAVIS 1985; Chap. 2) and of lymphokine production (FATHMAN and FITCH 1982). Finally, although transformation of T cells with oncogenic viruses may not be effective on all T cell subsets and in addition may induce functional abnormality, they may nonetheless be of particular use in evaluating the potential of pharmacological agents in the management of adult T cell lymphomas. It must always be considered, however, that the way in which the T cells are grown and cloned or immortalised may influence their subsequent biological properties.

C. B Cell Growth and Cloning

I. Introduction

In contrast to T cells, there is to date no well-characterised method for the long-term growth and cloning of normal, nontransformed B cells. For this reason we will consider two approaches to preparing functionally homogeneous populations of cells, both of which have proved useful in studying the physiology of B cells and are therefore suitable for study of the effects of pharmacological mediators. The first approach is immortalisation by either viral transformation, the use of tumour cell lines or by cell hybridisation. However, since such cell populations are transformed and therefore not subject to normal growth control, we will also consider some of the methods available for purifying homogeneous populations of normal B cells in order to study the control of B cell growth and activation.

B cells, like T cells comprise a heterogeneous lineage of lymphocytes. It remains unclear as to how many subsets of B cells exist and how these subsets are related. For example, B cell populations can be subdivided on the basis of the presence or absence of various cell surface antigens. Human B cells can be segregated into Leu-1$^+$ and Leu-1$^-$ populations (CALIGARIS-CAPPIO et al. 1982), a discrimination which has an equivalent in the mouse where B cells segregate into Ly1$^+$ and Ly1$^-$ cells (HAZAKAWA et al. 1984). Mouse B cells also differ in the expression of Lyb-5 cell surface antigen (AHMED et al. 1977). It remains controversial as to whether the heterogeneous expression of such cell surface antigens reflects different lineages of B cells or whether various surface antigens are expressed at different stages of maturation along the same B cell lineage.

Maturation of B cells along a lineage from pre-B cell to plasma cell is closely regulated and different signals are required to move a cell from one stage of maturation to the next. In addition, different signals likely control maturation and cell division (see for example *Immunol Rev*, vol 78, 1984). B cells are therefore functionally heterogeneous with regard to their stage of maturation and/or lineage.

II. Spontaneously Transformed Cells

We will first consider some of the cell lines available as a consequence of usually undefined transformation events in vivo. Such cells have usually arisen as tumours in vivo and have been maintained either as in vivo tumours or by adaptation to in vitro growth as transformed cell lines. Although the following list is by no means exhaustive, the cell lines described here are interesting in that they can be moved from one stage of maturation to another and have therefore contributed to our understanding of B lymphocyte physiology. Again the nature of transformed cells is such that the caveat in Sect. B.IX applies.

1. 70Z3

The mouse pre-B in vitro cell line 70Z3 expresses cytoplasmic Igμ chains, but not light chains in an analogous fashion to pre-B cells, although the κ light chain gene is rearranged. This cell has been used as a model for the pre-B–B cell transition in B cell ontogeny, although the observation that normal pre-B cells do not have rearranged light chain genes means that 70Z3 probably represents a late-stage pre-B cell (MAKI et al. 1980). The 70Z3 cell can be stimulated by a variety of mediators including lipopolysaccharide (SAKAGUCHI et al. 1980; PAIGE et al. 1978) and B cell maturation factor (or factors) (SIDMAN et al. 1984a) to express B cell surface Ig (sIg) detected by immunofluorescence as a consequence of light chain gene expression. These cells are routinely grown in medium with 5%–10% FCS, however some batches of FCS can activate 70Z3 to sIg expression, possibly owing to the presence of bacterial lipopolysaccharides.

2. WEHI-279

The mouse B cell lymphoma WEHI-279 appears to represent an early B cell in that it expresses sIgM, but secretes very little immunoglobulin. In the presence of B cell maturation activities, this cell is induced to secrete IgM as a result of a shift in the levels of the secretory type of IgM from the surface type of IgM (PAIGE et al. 1982). This transition is also seen in the presence of low levels of gamma interferon (γ-IFN). However, γ-IFN also induces mortality in the cell such that after 48–60 h in the presence of γ-IFN the great majority of cells are dead (SIDMAN et al. 1984a,b). As with the 70Z3 cell line, these cells are routinely grown in tissue culture medium with 5%–10% FCS.

3. CH12

The CH12 cell lymphoma appears to represent a resting B cell, expressing surface IgM, but secreting little antibody. This cell is routinely grown as a transplantable in vivo tumour in B10.H-2^aH-2^bp/Wts mice and has limited growth potential in vitro. It may however be possible to adapt the cell to in vitro long-term growth. CH12 cells appear to be refractory to soluble B cell maturation factors. However culture of this cell line in the presence of its specific antigen (sheep red blood cells) and Mhc-restricted, antigen-specific helper T cells induces a proportion of the CH12 cells to secrete antibody, measured by plaque formation (LOCASCIO et al. 1984a). In addition, this cell can be activated by antigen and Mhc class II-specific antibodies (replacing T cell help) (LOCASCIO et al. 1984b). However normal resting B cells are not induced to secrete antibody when stimulated by anti-immunoglobulin and anti-class II reagents. Thus the parallel between the CH12 lymphoma and the normal resting B cell is not complete.

4. BCL.1

The BCL.1 murine cell line is again an in vivo passaged tumour cell grown in BALB/c mice by intravenous injection of about 5×10^6 cells. The cells taken from the spleen of tumour-bearing mice have limited growth potential in vitro (SLAVIN and STROBER 1977). In the presence of soluble activities corresponding to one of the B cell growth factors, however, the BCL.1 cell is stimulated to take up increased levels of radioactive thymidine (SWAIN et al. 1983) in a standard proliferation assay. This response has been used as a measure of B cell growth factor activity. Again the drawback with this cell line is the lack of a parallel to a clearly defined stage in normal B cell ontogeny.

5. CESS

The human in vitro line CESS expresses surface IgG and secretes low levels of IgG. Secretion of IgG can be enhanced in the presence of B cell differentiation activities (MURAGUCHI et al. 1981). This antibody is detected either by reverse plaque formation on protein A red blood cells (GRONOWICZ et al. 1976) or by detection of soluble IgG in culture supernatants by radioimmunoassay or enzyme-linked assays. As with the BCL.1 cell it is not clear whether there is a parallel with a clearly defined stage of B cell development.

III. Epstein–Barr Virus Transformation of Human B Cells

1. Viral Infection

Human B cells can be transformed into immortalised cell lines and cloned by infection with the Epstein–Barr virus EBV. The target B cells for EBV transformation are the dense B cells corresponding to the completely nonactivated B cell population with the activated B cell being resistant to infection and transformation (AMAN et al. 1984). The commonest source of EBV is the cell line B95-8. This cell line is derived from cotton-topped marmoset peripheral blood mononuclear cells infected with EBV obtained from a cell line in turn derived from an infectious mononucleosis patient (MILLER and LIPMAN 1973). The cell line contains 10%–20% of cells undergoing lytic viral infection at any one time.

B95-8 cells are grown to 10^6/ml, the cells are removed by centrifugation at 400 g for 10 min followed by filtering the medium through a 0.45-μm filter which allows the infectious encapsulated virus to pass through. To concentrate the virus, the culture supernatant is centrifuged at 13 000 g for 2 h at 4 °C. The pellet is resuspended in culture medium and stored. For long-term storage, the virus is suspended in tissue culture medium with 20% FCS and frozen at or below -70 °C.

Infection of B cells is carried out by suspending up to 10^7 peripheral blood leukocytes in 1 ml B95-8 culture supernatant, or more concentrated virus, in culture medium for 1 h at 37 °C with gentle agitation. The cells are then pelleted, the supernatant removed and the cells cultured.

2. Culture of EBV Lines

T cells in the human peripheral blood population frequently suppress the generation of immortal lines from EBV-infected B cells. This problem can be circumvented by the addition of cyclosporin A (1 μg/ml) for the first 2–3 weeks of culture to prevent T cell activation (see Chap. 21). Thus immortalised lines can be obtained from infected cells seeded at about 5×10^5/ml in the presence of cyclosporin A. Cultures are incubated at 37 °C in a humidified incubator containing 5% CO_2 and are fed by weekly replacement of half the medium without disturbing the cell layer. Cultures visualised with an inverted microscope will contain foci or proliferating transformed B cells after 1–2 weeks. EBV-transformed cells generally grow to about 10^6/ml and as they approach this concentration they should be diluted to about 10^5/ml. The normal cell doubling time is 48–72 h, but each line or clone will have slightly different characteristics.

Infection of normal human B cells with EBV can induce a proportion of cells to mature to antibody secretion (ROSEN et al. 1977). Clones with relatively stable characteristics can however be derived from a homogeneous transformed population.

IV. Abelson Virus Transformation of Murine B Cells

Abelson murine leukemia virus, in conjunction with Moloney murine leukaemia virus, causes in vitro transformation of murine B lineage cells (ROSENBERG et al. 1975). Stock Abelson virus is derived by the infection of the NIH/3T3 cell line ANN-1 (SCHER and SIEGLER 1975) with Moloney murine leukemia virus (itself derived from the supernatant of confluent JLS-VII cells; FAN and PASKIND 1974).

After 16 h incubation with Moloney virus, ANN-1 supernatant is harvested, filtered through 0.45-μm filters and stored at -70 °C. Target cells are infected with Abelson virus by culturing equal volumes of cell (10^6/ml) with 1 ml virus stock and 4 μg/ml Polybrene for 2.5 h at 37 °C, resuspending the cells every 15 min. Infected cells are washed once and cultured at 5×10^5/ml. Foci of proliferating cells appear at 1–2 weeks incubation and can be expanded and cloned by standard techniques (Sect. C.VI).

The majority of cells transformed under these conditions are of B lineage, especially when the target cells are derived from the bone marrow or fetal liver, and include both pre-B and mature, but early stage, B cells. One advantage of Abelson-transformed lines is that they frequently retain characteristics of the cell from which they were derived, including responsiveness to maturational activities and many Abelson lines can be induced to undergo Ig gene rearrangement (ALT et al. 1986).

V. B Cell Hybridisation

A range of B cell lymphomas at various different stages of maturation have been characterised. Although B cell hybridisation is most frequently used to generate monoclonal antibody-secreting cells (KOHLER and MILSTEIN 1975), hybridisation of spleen B cells with other types of fusion partner will often yield hybrids which do not secrete antibody. If a fusion partner is selected for growth in the presence of 20 μg/ml 8-azaguanine and will subsequently die in the presence of hypoxanthine, aminopterin and thymidine, it can be used to generate B cell hybrids. Frequently there is no great advantage in using a B cell hybrid rather than using the transformed B cell fusion partner itself. Occasionally however, one may fuse with the intention of including within the hybrid properties derived from the spleen cell, such as alloantigen expression or an antigen-specific surface immunoglobulin.

VI. Growth and Cloning of Transformed Cells

1. In Vivo Growth

Many murine lymphoid tumours will grow in the ascites of syngeneic mice. Usually cells will grow to a much higher concentration in vivo than they do in vitro although the presence of other cells in the ascites means that the tumour cell preparations are not pure. Frequently, higher yields of cells are obtained in mice which have been given an injection of 0.5 ml pristane (2,6,10,14-tetramethyl-pentadecane) intraperitoneally 7 days to 6 weeks before inoculation of the tumour. If syngeneic or congeneic mice which have the same Mhc alleles as the tumour are not available, nu/nu mice of any Mhc haplotype can be used. These mice are genetically T cell deficient and therefore do not reject the tumour. Tumour cells are harvested for passage or use by killing the mouse and removing ascites fluid with a syringe for tumours which grow in suspension or surgically excising solid tumours. Alternatively for tumours passaged by intravenous injection, most tumour cells will be found in the spleen.

4. In Vitro Growth

In vitro adapted lymphomas will generally grow in most media in the presence of 5%–10% inactivated FCS. Cells will usually grow to 1–2×10^6/ml and can be diluted down to 0.5–1×10^5/ml. Some care must be taken to ensure that the batch of FCS used does not induce changes in the phenotype of the cells being grown (e.g. the 70Z3 cell line). When changing cells from one medium to another it is usually best to do it gradually by progressively diluting out the cells from the old medium into new medium.

3. In Vitro Cloning

Some transformed cells are very easy to clone by simply diluting the cells to about 2/ml in medium and distributing 0.2-ml aliquots into 96-well sterile flat-bottom tissue culture plates. Alternatively, cells can be diluted to 30/ml and 10 µl per well distributed into the wells of a 60-well Terasaki plate. If the cloning efficiency is high then statistically most wells in which there is growth should contain cells derived from a single input cell. Occasionally, if cells are clumpy or if a more rigorous cloning procedure is required micromanipulation can be used (Sect. B.VIII.3).

Many cell lines fail to grow from single cells or from very low concentrations, frequently because they require autocrine factors, i.e. factors produced by the cells which are required for their own proliferation (DUPREZ et al. 1985). At limiting dilution there is simply not enough of the autocrine factors produced to support the growth of the cell. This problem can often be obviated by cloning the cells in the presence of 10%–20% of a supernatant derived from the cell line itself when growing at fairly high concentrations (10^6/ml). Such a supernatant will contain any autocrine factors the cell may be producing. Alternatively, cloning efficiency may frequently be improved by culturing the cells in the presence of irradiated, syngeneic feeders at (0.2–1×10^6/ml).

4. Mycoplasma Contamination

Many in vitro grown lines and clones of cells contain mycoplasma. Because of the possible effects of mycoplasma products in B cell activation (SITIA et al. 1985) it is obviously important to obtain mycoplasma-free cells. Cell lines can sometimes be cleared of mycoplasma by several serial passages as an in vivo tumor followed by readaptation to in vitro growth. When mycoplasma contamination is a potential problem, cell lines should be tested regularly.

VII. Purification of Normal B Cells

Frequently there is no convenient transformed cell line model for the assay of a particular activity. In addition, it is always important to relate biological activities back to normal cells. There are two main reasons for purifying B cells from a homogeneous population. The first is that the presence of other cells may mask the response (or lack of response) of the B cells to a given stimulus. Second, it is important to know whether a stimulus operates directly on the B cell rather than indirectly by stimulating a contaminating cell to produce activities which may then act on the B cell. The main contaminating cells in lymphoid tissues are red blood cells, T cells and cells of the monocyte/macrophage lineage.

1. Red Blood Cell Depletion

Human peripheral blood leukocytes can be freed of red blood cells as in Sect. B.II. Murine spleen cells are freed of red cells by incubation of cells washed in protein-free medium (e.g. MEM or PBS) with about 3 ml per spleen 0.85% ammonium chloride buffered to pH 7.4. After lysis, which usually takes about 1 min, the cells are washed three times.

2. T Cell Depletion

Human T cells express receptors which bind to sheep red blood cells (SRBC) (KAPLAN and CLARK 1974). SRBC stored in Alsever's solution are washed three times in saline. Then 1 volume SRBC is mixed with 5 volumes 40.2 mg/ml S-2-aminoethylisothiouronium bromide in distilled water (pH 9) and incubated at 37 °C for 20 min. After three washes in PBS, the coupled SRBC are stored at 4 °C. Equal volumes of coupled SRBC (4%) and mononuclear cells (10^7/ml) are mixed together with 0.5 volumes FCS. After centrifugation at 300 g for 10 min, the cells are incubated on ice for 1 h. The mixture is resuspended and layered onto Percoll (density 1.08, about 65%, see Sect. C.VII.5) and centrifuged at 1500 g for 20 min at room temperature. The interface containing the T-depleted non-rosette-forming [E-rosette ($-$)] mononuclear cells is washed three times. This procedure can be repeated for more rigorous depletion.

Mouse T cells express the Thy-1 antigen, either Thy-1.1 or Thy-1.2, depending on the strain of mouse. A wide variety of monoclonal Thy-1-specific antibodies are available both commercially and in many laboratories, which in conjunction with guinea pig complement will kill T cells.

Lymphocytes (2×10^7/ml) are incubated with a titrated amount of anti-Thy-1 for 45 min on ice. The cells are pelleted and resuspended in the same volume of guinea pig complement (guinea pig serum absorbed with an equal volume of packed sheep red blood cells for 60 min on ice, followed by absorption with agarose and storage at $-70\,°C$) and incubated at $37\,°C$ for 45 min to 1 h. The procedure can be repeated if necessary for more rigorous depletion.

Nu/nu mice are congenitally athymic and so have very low levels of mature T cells. Such mice provide a good source of T-depleted lymphocytes.

3. Monocyte/Macrophage Depletion

Purifying B cells away from cells of the monocyte/macrophage lineage is difficult and the most stringent depletion will require more than one of the following most frequently used techniques (CORBEL and MELCHERS 1983).

Monocyte/macrophages are more adherent than B cells and so one approach is to suspend the cells to 5–10×10^6/ml in tissue culture medium with FCS or serum substitute and to add 5 ml to a tissue culture Petri dish (100 mm diameter). The plate is placed in a $37\,°C$ incubator for 3–4 h. Nonadherent cells are resuspended by gently swirling the plate, and harvested.

A second method involves the use of beads as an adherent surface. Sterile Sephadex G-10 beads are swollen for 2 h in sterile medium. The Sephadex is loaded into a sterile 30-ml plastic syringe plugged with sterile glass wool. Then, 10^8 cells in 1 ml are passed through the column and eluted with 25 ml medium. Cells eluting between 5 and 15 ml are collected and washed (LY and MISHELL 1974; CORBEL and MELCHERS 1983).

A third approach is to purify small, high density B cells (Sect. C.VII.5), since monocyte/macrophages tend to be larger, less dense cells. This approach clearly subfractionates B cells and for this reason may not be appropriate in all cases.

4. Positive Selection of B Cells

Whereas the previous approaches purify B cells by depletion of non-B cells, this procedure purifies B cells in a positive fashion by binding the B cells to anti-Ig-coated Petri dishes (MAGE et al. 1977). First, 5 ml PBS containing affinity-purified anti-immunoglobulin (100 µg/ml) and bovine serum albumin (300 µg/ml) is added to 100-mm tissue culture Petri dishes and incubated overnight at $4\,°C$. The coating mixture is harvested and stored for reuse and the plates washed five times in PBS. Then, 5×10^7 cells in 5 ml PBS are added to the plate and allowed to settle for 1 h, the plate being swirled half way through the incubation at $4\,°C$. The nonadherent cells are removed by swirling the plate with several washes of PBS and the adherent, B cell-enriched, population can then be harvested by vigorous pipetting of PBS onto the plate.

5. Subfractionation of B Cells

Two general approaches have been used most widely. If the B cell population is heterogeneous with regard to the expression of a cell surface alloantigen, antibody to that antigen can be used, in conjunction with complement, to deplete antigen-positive cells by protocols similar to the T cell depletion described earlier (Sect. C.VII.2).

The other common subfractionation of B cells is based on their density. Percoll (Pharmacia) is diluted with five-fold concentrated MEM, 20 mM HEPES, and 2 g/l sodium hydrogen carbonate to yield a stock solution of 80% Percoll which is isotonic, pH 7.4. The stock 80% Percoll can then be diluted with MEM to the desired densities (which may vary from batch to batch of Percoll and should therefore be tested). Stepwise gradients can then be formed and cells (up to 2×10^8 in 2 ml MEM for a 15-ml tube) layered on top of the gradient. The tube is centrifuged at 1500 g for 30 min at room temperature and the bands of cells formed at the interfaces between the Percoll layers harvested and washed three times. Small, high density, resting B cells usually band at the interface between 70% and 63% Percoll, while large, activated B cell blasts usually band at the interface between the 46% and 40% Percoll layers (RATCLIFFE and JULIUS 1982).

VIII. Summary

Cloning normal, nontransformed B cells in numbers sufficient for biochemical and pharmacological use is not, at present, possible as a consequence of the lack of a defined system for the long-term growth of B cells in tissue culture. Thus, of necessity, alternative approaches have been used. The use of transformed cell lines provides a plentiful and pure supply of material for studying the effects of pharmacological mediators, but it must always be remembered that the target cells are, in at least some respects, abnormal. The alternative approach of B cell purification provides normal B cell populations, but leaves open the possibility that the response measured depends on the presence of contaminating cells. A combination of the two approaches such that any effects demonstrated on a transformed B cell line can be reproduced on normal B cells is generally most convincing.

D. Concluding Remarks

The immune system can be viewed as a network of interacting cells of a variety of different lineages and subtypes, communicating with each other by a combination of cellular interactions and soluble mediators. Signals received by membrane receptors are transduced into the responding cell, resulting in biochemical changes within the cell, ultimately leading to the activation or inactivation of specific genes. Thus there are many potential stages in an immune response which are susceptible to modulation by pharmacological mediators. The major contribution of the growth and cloning of lymphoid cells in pharmacology is to help sort out the precise stage in the immune response at which a biologically active molecule is operating.

This principle is well illustrated by the analysis of the effects of cyclosporin A on the immune system (see also Chap. 21). Early in vivo experiments revealed that one of its many immunosuppressive effects was to prolong skin allograft survival. This correlated with the in vitro finding that cyclosporin A inhibited alloantigen-induced (HESS and TUTSCHKA 1980) and mitogen-induced (BOREL et al.

1977) T cell proliferative responses. However the target for cyclosporin A was only evaluated with the advent of T lymphocyte clones. With IL-2-dependent alloreactive T cell clones, the biological effects of cyclosporin A on mixed lymphocyte reactions was demonstrated on helper T cells, causing inhibition of IL-2 release and blocking antigen-dependent activation of the cytotoxic T cell population. Similarly, cyclosporin A inhibited antigen-induced IL-2 secretion, as well as the specific and nonspecific lytic activity of cytotoxic T cell hybridomas (KAUFMANN and ROSENBERG 1984).

Our understanding of the physiological activity of another group of widely used immunosuppressive agents, glucocorticosteroids, has also been enhanced by the use of monoclonal T cell populations (see also Chap. 17). Thus it was observed that hydrocortisone had minimal inhibitory effects on the proliferative response of murine cytolytic T cell clones to exogenous IL-2, but had a profound effect on IL-2 secretion (GILLIS et al. 1979), similar effects being seen on human T lymphocyte clones (MOSS et al. 1984).

In vitro grown and cloned lymphoid cells therefore represent a powerful tool in the discovery and characterisation of pharmacological mediators designed to modulate the immune response.

References

Ahmed A, Scher I, Sharrow SO, Smith AH, Paul WE, Sachs DH, Sell KW (1977) B lymphocyte heterogeneity: development of an allo-antiserum which distinguishes B lymphocyte differentiation alloantigens. J Exp Med 145:101–110

Alt FW, Blackwell TK, DePinho RA, Reth MG, Yancopoulos GD (1986) Regulation of genome rearrangement events during lymphocyte differentiation. Immunol Rev 89: 1–30

Aman P, Ehlin-Henriksson B, Klein G (1984) Epstein-Barr virus susceptibility of normal human B lymphocyte populations. J Exp Med 159:208–220

Bach FH, Inouye H, Hank JA, Alter BJ (1979) Human T lymphocyte clones reactive in primed lymphocyte typing in cytotoxicity. Nature 281:307–310

Bensussan A, Acuto O, Hussey RE, Milanese C, Reinherz EL (1984) T3-Ti receptor triggering of T8$^+$ suppressor T cells leads to unresponsiveness to interleukin-2. Nature 311:565–567

Borel JF, Feurer C, Gubler HU, Stahelin H (1977) Effects of the new anti-lymphocyte peptide cyclosporin A in animals. Immunology 32:1017–1025

Butler JL, Muraguchi A, Lane HC, Fauci AS (1983) Development of a human T-T cell hybridoma secreting B cell growth factor. J Exp Med 157:60–67

Caligaris-Cappio F, Gobbi M, Bofill M, Janossy G (1982) Infrequent normal B lymphocytes express features of B-chronic lymphocytic leukemia. J Exp Med 155:623–628

Corbel C, Melchers F (1983) Requirements for macrophages or for macrophage- or T cell-derived factors in the mitogenic stimulation of murine B lymphocytes by lipopolysaccharide. Eur J Immunol 13:528–533

Corradin G, Etlinger HM, Chiller JM (1977) Lymphocyte specificity to protein antigens. I. Characterisation of the antigen induced in vitro T-cell dependent proliferative response with lymph node cells from primed mice. J Immunol 119:1048–1053

Davis MM (1985) Molecular genetics of the T cell receptor beta chain. Annu Rev Immunol 3:537–560

DeFreitas EC, Vella S, Linnenbach A, Zimijewski C, Koprowski H, Croce CM (1982) Antigen-specific human T cell hybrids with helper activity. Proc Natl Acad Sci USA 79:6646–6650

Duprez V, Lenoir G, Dautry-Varsat A (1985) Autocrine growth stimulation of a human T cell lymphoma line by interleukin 2. Proc Natl Acad Sci USA 82:6932–6936

Fan H, Paskind M (1974) Measurement of the sequence complexity of cloned Moloney murine leukemia virus 60 to 70S RNA: evidence for a haploid genome. J Virol 14:421–429

Farrar JJ, Fuller-Farrar J, Simon PL, Hilfiker ML, Stadler BM, Farrar WL (1980) Thymoma production of T cell growth factor (interleukin 2). J Immunol 125:2555–2558

Fathman CG, Fitch FW (1982) Isolation, characterisation and utilisation of T lymphocyte clones. Academic, New York

Fathman CG, Hengartner H (1978) Clones of alloreactive T cells. Nature 272:617–618

Feldman M, Lamb JR, Woody JN (1986) Human T cell clones: a new approach to immunoregulation. Humana, New York

Finn OJ, Boniver J, Kaplan HS (1979) Induction, establishment in vitro and characterisation of functional, antigen-specific, carrier primed murine T cell lymphomas. Proc Natl Acad Sci USA 76:4033–4037

Fresno M, Nabel S, McVay-Bondreau L, Furthmayer H, Cantor H (1981) Antigen-specific T lymphocyte clones. I. Characterisation of a T lymphocyte clone expressing antigen specific suppressive activity. J Exp Med 153:1246–1259

Gallagher G, Stimson WH (1984) Human T cell hybrids with HLA-restricted proliferative response to Epstein-Barr virus infected B cells. Immunology 53:611–621

Gillis S, Smith KA (1977) Long term culture of tumour specific cytotoxic T cells. Nature 268:154–156

Gillis S, Crabtree GR, Smith KA (1979) Glucocorticoid-induced inhibition of T cell growth factor II. The effect on the in vitro generation of cytolytic T cells. J Immunol 123:1632–1637

Gronowicz E, Coutinho A, Melchers F (1976) A plaque assay for all cells secreting Ig of a given type or class. Eur J Immunol 6:588–590

Haas W, Kisielow P (1985) Cytolytic T cell hybridomas. II. Interleukin-2-independent cytolytic variants. Eur J Immunol 15:755–760

Hazakawa K, Hardy RR, Honda M, Herzenberg LA, Steinberg AD, Herzenberg LA (1984) Ly-1 B cells: functionally distinct lymphocytes that secrete IgM autoantibodies. Proc Natl Acad Sci USA 81:2494–2498

Hess AD, Tutschka PJ (1980) Effect of cyclosporin A on human lymphocyte responses in vitro. I. CsA allows for the expression of alloantigen-activated suppressor cells while preferentially inhibiting the induction of cytolytic effector cells in MLR. J Immunol 124:2601–2608

Iscove NN, Melchers M (1978) Complete replacement of serum by albumin, transferrin and soybean lipid in cultures of lipopolysaccharide-reactive B lymphocytes. J Exp Med 147:923–933

Julius MH, Simpson E, Herzenberg LA (1973) A rapid method for the isolation of functional thymus-derived murine lymphocytes. Eur J Immunol 3:645–649

Kaplan ME, Clark C (1974) An improved rosetting assay for detection of human T lymphocytes. J Immunol Methods 5:131–135

Kapp JA, Araneo BA, Clevinger BL (1980) Suppression of antibody and T cell proliferative responses to L-glutamic and ^{60}-L-alanine-^{30}-L-tyrosine^{10} (GAT) by a specific monoclonal T cell factor. J Exp Med 152:235–240

Kappler JW, Skidmore B, White J, Marrack P (1981) Antigen-inducible, H-2 restricted, interleukin-2 producing T cell hybridomas. Lack of independent antigen and H-2 recognition. J Exp Med 153:1198–1214

Kaufmann Y, Rosenberg SA (1984) Blocking by cyclosporin of antigen induced maturation and lymphokine secretion by cytotoxic T lymphocyte hybridomas. Transplantation 38:148–151

Kimoto M, Fathman CG (1980) Antigen reactive T cell clones. I. Transcomplementing hybrid I-A region gene products function effectively in antigen presentation. J Exp Med 152:759–770

Kohler G, Milstein C (1975) Continuous cultures of fused cells secreting antibody of predefined specificity. Nature 256:495–497

Kontiainen S, Simpson E, Bohrer E, Beverly PCL, Herzenberg LA, Fitzpatrick WC, Vogt T et al. (1978) T cell lines producing antigen specific suppressor factors. Nature 274:477–480

Lakow E, Tsoukas CD, Vaughan JH, Altman A, Carson DA (1983) Human T cell hybrids specific for Epstein-Barr virus infected B lymphocytes. J Immunol 130:169–172

Lamb JR, Eckels DD, Lake P, Johnson AH, Hartzman RJ, Woody JN (1982) Antigen specific human T lymphocyte clones; induction antigen specificity and MHC restriction of influenza virus immune clones. J Immunol 128:233–238

Lanzavecchia A, Ferrarini M, Celada F (1983) Human T cell lines with antigen specificity and helper activity. Eur J Immunol 13:733–738

LoCascio NJ, Haughton G, Arnold LW, Corley RB (1984 a) Role of cell surface immunoglobulin in B lymphocyte activation. Proc Natl Acad Sci USA 81:2466–2469

LoCascio NJ, Corley RB, Arnold LW, Haughton G (1984 b) Monoclonal antibody against I-E antigens can substitute for T helper cells in the differentiation of a B cell lymphoma. Immunobiol 167:10

Lutz CT, Glasebrook AL, Fitch FW (1980) Alloreactive cloned T cell lines. III. Accessory cell requirements for the growth of cloned cytolytic T lymphocytes. J Immunol 126:1404–1408

Ly LA, Mishell RI (1974) Separation of mouse spleen cells by passage through columns of Sephadex G-10. J Immunol Methods 5:239–247

Mage MG, McHugh LL, Rothstein TL (1977) Mouse lymphocytes with and without surface immunoglobulin: preparative scale separation in polystyrene tissue culture dishes coated with specifically purified anti-immunoglobulins. J Immunol Methods 15:47–56

Maki R, Kearney J, Paige C, Tonegawa S (1980) Immunoglobulin gene rearrangement in immature B cells. Science 209:1366–1369

McKean D, Infante A, Nilson A, Kimoto M, Fathman CG, Walker E, Warner N (1981) Major histocompatibility complex-restricted antigen presentation to antigen-reactive T cells by B lymphocyte tumour cells. J Exp Med 154:1419–1431

Miller G, Lipman M (1973) Release of infectious Epstein-Barr virus by transformed marmoset leukocytes. Proc Natl Acad Sci USA 69:383–387

Morgan DA, Ruscetti FW, Gallo RC (1976) Selective in vitro growth of T lymphocytes from normal human bone marrow. Science 193:1007–1008

Moss FM, Knight J, Lamb JR (1984) The differential effects of hydrocortisone on activation and tolerance induction in human lymphocyte clones. Hum Immunol 11:259–270

Muraguchi A, Kishimoto T, Miki Y, Kuritani T, Kaieda T, Yoshizaki K, Yamamura Y (1981) T cell replacing factor-induced IgG secretion in a human B blastoid cell line and demonstration of acceptors for TRF. J Immunol 127:412–416

Nabholz M, Engers HD, Collaro D, North M (1978) Cloned T cell lines with specific cytolytic activity. Curr Top Microbiol Immunol 81:176–187

Nabholz M, Conzelmann A, Acuto O, North M, Haas W, Pohlit H, von Boehmer H et al. (1980 a) Established murine cytolytic T cell lines as tools for a somatic cell genetic analysis of T cell functions. Immunol Rev 51:125–156

Nabholz M, Cianfriglia M, Acuto O, Conzelmann A, Haas W, von Boehmer H, MacDonald HR, Pohlit H, Johnson JP (1980 b) Cytolytically active murine T cell hybrids. Nature 287:437–440

Okada M, Yoshimura N, Kaieda T, Yamamura Y, Kishimoto T (1981) Establishment and characterisation of human T hybrid cells secreting immunoregulatory molecules. Proc Natl Acad Sci USA 78:7717–7721

Paige CJ, Kincade PW, Ralph P (1978) Murine B cell leukaemia cell line with inducible surface immunoglobulin expression. J Immunol 121:641–647

Paige CJ, Schreier MH, Sidman CL (1982) Mediators from cloned helper T cell lines affect immunoglobulin expression by B cells. Proc Natl Acad Sci USA 79:4756–4760

Popovic M, Lange-Wantzin G, Sarin PS, Mann D, Gallo RC (1983) Transformation of human umbilical cord blood T cells by human T cell leukaemia/lymphoma virus. Proc Natl Acad Sci USA 80:5402–5406

Popovic M, Flomenberg N, Volkman DJ, Mann D, Fauci AS, Dupont B, Gallo RC (1984) Alteration of T cell functions by infection with HTLV-I or HTLV-II. Science 226:459–462

Ratcliffe MJH, Julius MH (1982) H-2 restricted T-B cell interactions involved in polyclonal B cell responses mediated by soluble antigen. Eur J Immunol 12:847–852

Ratcliffe MJH, Julius MH, Kim K-J (1984) Heterogeneity in the response of T cells to antigens presented by B lymphoma cells. Cell Immunol 88:49–60

Ricciardi-Castagnoli P, Doria G, Adorini L (1981) Production of antigen specific suppressor T cell factor by radiation leukemia virus-transformed suppressor T cells. Proc Natl Acad Sci USA 78:3804–3808

Rosen A, Gergely P, Jondal M, Klein G, Britton S (1977) Polyclonal Ig production after Epstein-Barr virus infection of human lymphocytes in vitro. Nature 267:52–54

Rosenberg N, Baltimore D, Scher CD (1975) In vitro transformation of lymphoid cells by Abelson murine leukaemia virus. Proc Natl Acad Sci USA 72:1932–1936

Sakaguchi N, Kishimoto T, Kikutani H, Watanabe T, Yoshida N, Shimizu A, Yamawaki-Kataoka Y, Honjo T, Yamamura Y (1980) Induction and regulation of immunoglobulin expression in a murine pre-B cell line 70Z/3. I. Cell cycle-associated induction of sIgM expression and κ chain synthesis in 70Z/3 cells by LPS stimulation. J Immunol 125:2654–2659

Scher CD, Siegler R (1975) Direct transformation of 3T3 cells by Abelson murine leukaemia virus. Nature 253:729–731

Schreier MH, Tees T (1980) Clonal induction of helper T cells. Conversion of specific signals to non-specific signals. Int Arch Allergy Appl Immunol 61:227–237

Sidman CL, Paige CJ, Schreier MH (1984a) B cell maturation factor (BMF): a lymphokine or family of lymphokines promoting the maturation of B lymphocytes. J Immunol 132:209–222

Sidman CL, Marshall JD, Mariello NC, Roths JB, Schultz LD (1984b) Novel B-cell maturation factor from spontaneously autoimmune viable motheaten mice. Proc Natl Acad Sci USA 81:7199–7202

Sitia R, Rubartelli A, Deambrosis S, Pozzi D, Hammerling U (1985) Differentiation in the murine B cell lymphoma I.29: inductive capacities of lipopolysaccharide and *Mycoplasma fermentans* products. Eur J Immunol 15:570–575

Slavin S, Strober S (1977) Spontaneous murine B cell leukaemia. Nature 272:624–626

Sredni B, Yolkman D, Schwartz RH, Fauci AS (1981a) Antigen specific human T cell clones: development of clones requiring HLA-DR compatible presenting cells for stimulation in the presence of antigen. Proc Natl Acad Sci USA 78:1858–1862

Sredni B, Tse HY, Chen C, Schwartz RH (1981b) Antigen specific clones of proliferating T lymphocytes. I. Methodology, specificity and MHC restriction. J Immunol 126:341–347

Suciu-Foca N, Rubenstein P, Popovic M, Gallo RC (1984) Reactivity of HTLV-transformed human T cell lines to MHC class II antigens. Nature 312:275–277

Swain SL, Howard M, Kappler J, Marrack P, Watson J, Booth R, Wetzel GD, Dutton RW (1983) Evidence for two distinct classes of murine B cell growth factors with activities in different functional assays. J Exp Med 158:822–835

Taniguchi T, Matsui H, Fujita T, Takaoka C, Kashima N, Yoshimoto R, Hamuro J (1983) Structure and expression of a cloned cDNA for human interleukin-2. Nature 302:305–310

Volkman DJ, Matis LA, Fauci AS (1984) Development and characterisation of interleukin-2 independent antigen specific human T cell clones that produce multiple lymphokines. Cell Immunol 88:323–335

Volkman DJ, Popovic M, Gallo RC, Fauci AS (1985) Human T cell leukaemia/lymphoma virus-infected antigen specific T cell clones: indiscriminant helper function and lymphokine production. J Immunol 134:4237–4243

Watson J (1979) Continuous proliferation of murine antigen-specific helper T lymphocytes in culture. J Exp Med 150:1510–1519

Zagury D, Bernard J, Thiemesse N, Foldman M, Berke G (1975) Isolation and characterisation of individual functionally reactive cytotoxic T lymphocytes. Conjugation, killing and recycling at the single cell level. Eur J Immunol 5:818–822

CHAPTER 13

Screening Strategies for Detecting Immunotherapeutic Agents

S. C. GILMAN, R. T. MAGUIRE, and A. J. LEWIS

A. Introduction

Immunotherapeutics are empirically defined as natural or synthetic pharmacologic agents which mediate therapeutic benefit through their ability to modulate some aspect of immune function. Recently, interest in immunotherapeutic agents has increased, primarily owing to a rapidly expanding knowledge of the immune system and to an awareness that many important human diseases are associated with abnormal immune function of pathologic significance (AIUTI et al. 1986). This has led to the emergence of immunopharmacology as a recognized scientific discipline. This field encompasses the pharmacologic regulation of immune responses, the development of immunologically based assays and their research and development applications, the preparation and utilization of monoclonal antibodies and cytokines as pharmacologic tools and therapeutic agents, and the discovery and development of immunotherapeutic agents. The immunopharmacologist must conjoin fundamental pharmacology with modern immunology in an attempt to determine the biologic and biochemical effects of synthetic and natural products on immune responsiveness, elucidate the mechanism (or mechanisms) through which such effects are mediated, and evaluate the clinical potential of such agents (CHIRIGOS and TALMADGE 1985).

In this chapter, we will discuss current approaches to the discovery of immunotherapeutic agents with the aim of developing a rational strategy for development of such agents. Rather than describing in detail the immunopharmacologic activities of various agents under development, it is our intent to take a conceptual approach, using selected experimental data to highlight salient points. For more detailed information regarding specific immunotherapeutic agents, the reader is referred to other chapters in Part 4 of this volume.

B. General Principles of Immunotherapeutic Drug Development

A generalized scheme for the development of immunotherapeutic agents is illustrated in Fig. 1. The major steps in the development process for these agents are not remarkably different from those of agents with other therapeutic indications (antidepressants, antihypertensives, vaccines, etc.). Following a decision to attack a given therapeutic area, screening procedures are then implemented to identify agents which fit established criteria for significant activity (TALMADGE et al.

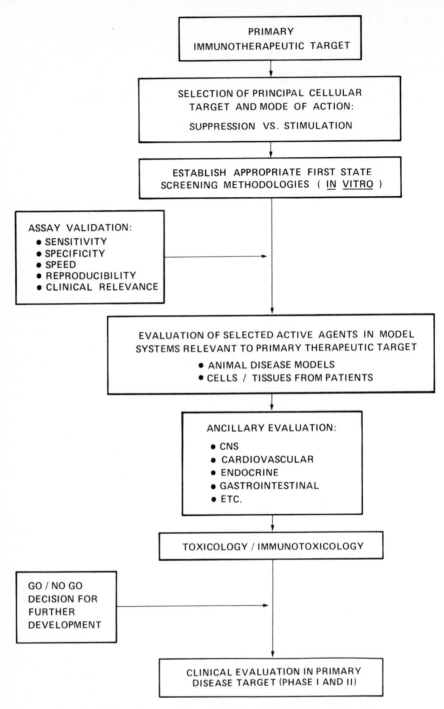

Fig. 1. Developmental scheme for immunotherapeutic agents

1984 b; TALMADGE and HERBERMAN 1986). Interesting compounds are then more critically evaluated for their profile of activity, potency, mechanism of action, and potential for side effects, using secondary animal models of human disease and/or cells and tissues from patients. Toxicologic evaluation follows for the few compounds with documented efficacy and a likelihood of clinical success which is ultimately proven (or disproven) in controlled clinical studies in the primary therapeutic area. Alternative (secondary) therapeutic indications may also arise for particular agents. For example, cytotoxic drugs (methotrexate, cyclophosphamide, etc.), primarily designed as antitumor agents, have also shown clinical utility in the treatment of autoimmune diseases (STEINBERG 1973).

Designing a "rational strategy" for discovering novel immunotherapeutic agents implies that a precise, logical decision-making process follows an in-depth analysis of complete and detailed information concerning a therapeutic target disease. Obviously, owing to insufficient or conflicting data on the etiology and pathophysiology of many diseases, and a lack of definitive correlation between preclinical activity and clinical efficacy, this is a scenario which is more ideal than real. Nonetheless, there are several fundamental considerations that must be addressed prior to initiating drug development programs in the immunotherapeutic area.

I. Target Diseases

The rationale for developing immunotherapeutic agents is based on the premise that: (a) normal and appropriate immune function is necessary for homeostasis – either an insufficient immune response or a misdirected immune response can result in severe and life-threatening disease; and (b) abnormal immune function is a feature of pathologic significance in certain human disease, including various forms of cancer, autoimmune diseases such as rheumatoid arthritis and systemic lupus erythematosus, aging, as well as primary and acquired immunodeficiency diseases (ZVAIFLER 1973; SISKIND et al. 1975; GILMAN 1984; GILMAN and LEWIS 1985, 1986; AIUTI et al. 1986). Increased or decreased function of virtually all hematologic cell types, including polymorphonuclear leukocytes (PMN), macrophages, T cells and their subsets, B cells and natural killer (NK) cells, has been well documented in these disorders (Table 1; PARKER 1973; ROITT et al. 1982; DILLMAN and KOZIOL 1983; GILMAN and LEWIS 1985; AIUTI et al. 1986). While, in most instances, the precise pathophysiologic significance of such immune dysfunction has not been clearly elucidated, improvements in such abnormalities may be clinically beneficial (CHIRIGOS and TALMADGE 1985). Indeed, clinical trials have demonstrated that some of the immunologic aberrations observed in cancer patients and patients with autoimmune or immunodeficiency diseases can be corrected by administration of immunotherapeutic agents, for example, levamisole (Chap. 18) and thymic peptides (Chap. 16; SCHEINBERG et al. 1978; GOLDSTEIN et al. 1982). Moreover, in several instances, this improvement in immune function has been linked to a beneficial clinical response and improved prognosis (EILBER et al. 1975). Since current therapies are inadequate, owing to poor efficacy or toxicity of agents used, all of the diseases listed in Table 1 are reasonable potential clinical targets for immunotherapeutic agents.

Table 1. Potential therapeutic targets for immunotherapeutic agents. (Modified from GILMAN and LEWIS, 1986)

Category	Example	Putative cellular target
Cancer	Leukemia, lymphoma melanomas, etc.	NK, Mϕ, T
Autoimmune diseases	Rheumatoid arthritis	Mϕ, PMN, T, B
	Systemic lupus erythematosus	T, B, other?
	Type I diabetes	T
	Pemphigus	B
Immunodeficiency		
Primary	SCID (several combined immunodeficiency diseases)	T, B
	Purine nucleoside phosphorylase (PNP) deficiency	T
	Adenosine deaminase deficiency	T, B
	Ataxia-telangiectasia	T
	DiGeorge's syndrome	T
	X-linked agammaglobulinemia	B
	IgA deficiency	B
	Common variable immune deficiency	B
Acquired	Due to cancer (see above)	Mϕ, NK, T
	Viral infection	Mϕ, NK, T
	Bacterial infection	T, Mϕ, PMN
	Fungal infection	Mϕ, T
	Aging	T, B, Mϕ
	Miscellaneous Postsurgical	T
	Burns	T
Allergy	Asthma	Mast cell, B
	Dermatitis	Mast cell, T
	Insect sting allergy	Mast cell
	Systemic anaphylaxis	Mast cell, B

B B cell; Mϕ monocyte/macrophage; NK natural killer cell; PMN polymorphonuclear leucocyte; T T cell.

II. Cellular Targets for Immunotherapeutic Agents

The immune system consists of a heterogeneous group of lymphoid cells whose collective function is to provide adequate host defense mechanisms against potentially harmful foreign substances (bacteria, viruses) and prevent or limit the abnormal growth of host tissues (malignant cells). The immune response results from an interacting network of lymphoid cells and their products. Cells of immunologic importance include PMN, granulocytes (basophils, eosinophils, mast cells), monocytes/macrophages, and lymphocytes, and substantial heterogeneity exists within each cell type. Over 100 soluble mediators (cytokines) been described in the literature, based on activity of supernatant fluids from activated lymphoid cells in one or another bioassay procedure (HANSEN et al. 1982; DINARELLO 1984; ROBB 1984).

Two general types of immunologic defense mechanisms can be distinguished, depending on whether or not antigen stimulation is required for the particular mechanism to operate efficiently. Nonspecific or "natural" cellular defense mechanisms are those which do not require prior antigen exposure. Important nonspecific defense include phagocytosis and intracellular killing of infectious agents, PMNs, granulocytes, macrophages, and NK cells, which are able to lyse a variety of tumor cells and virus-infected cells without prior activation (HERBERMAN and HOLDEN 1978). Antigen-specific cellular immune reactions are those in which immune cells specifically recognize antigenic determinants through membrane receptors and evoke immunologic memory which is responsible for the more rapid and vigorous nature of secondary (anamnestic) responses to the same antigen. These cellular immune reactions involve numerous cell types which interact with each other in a complex, but ordered sequence, ultimately resulting in cellular activation and the generation of effector cells or molecules capable of eliminating the invading agent. The magnitude and duration of the immune response are determined by numerous factors, including the antigen dose, prior exposure to antigen, nutritional status of the host, magnitude of T cell help and suppression, and modulation by feedback mechanisms (FATHMAN 1982).

Several immune-mediated diseases are characterized by abnormalities in particular cellular elements in the immune network (Table 1) and, thus, immunotherapeutic agents with specific actions on distinct cells and cellular functions could correct these abnormalities (GILMAN and LEWIS 1986). However, because of the interactive nature of the immune network, even if highly specific agents were developed, they might display effects contrary to those desired or expected. Thus, immunostimulatory drugs may actually suppress some immune reactions, for example, if they activate suppressor rather than helper cells (RENOUX 1980). Conversely, immunosuppressive agents might potentiate certain immune reactions if they preferentially inhibit suppressor cell activity (SIGEL et al. 1982). Thus, immunotherapeutic agents must be considered in the context of their global effects on the immune system.

Having determined, at least on a theoretical basis, the proposed therapeutic area, principal cellular target, and primary mode of action (positive or negative modulation) of a desired immunotherapeutic agent, one must then set up appropriate screening methodologies to identify compounds which would satisfy these criteria.

C. Screening Methodology

The selection of appropriate screening model systems is based on several considerations (TALMADGE et al. 1984b; RENOUX 1986). Ideally, the assays used should be predictive of the ability of the agent to modulate the immune response specifically, in a manner consistent with the desired therapeutic target (i.e., enhancement of interferon production for antiviral agents, increased NK cell or macrophage cytotoxic activity for antitumor agents, etc.). The assay system must be able to evaluate a wide range of chemical entities and biologic materials. Since most immunomodulatory agents show condition-dependent immunostimulation or immunosuppression, the assay used must be carefully standardized and well controlled within individual laboratories. The ideal assay system should also be rapid, sensitive, convenient to operate, and capable of handling numerous

Table 2. Commonly used assays to identify and characterize immunotherapeutic agents. (Modified from GILMAN and LEWIS, 1986)

	Immune function tests (in vitro/in vivo)	Disease models
T cells	T cell cytotoxicity	Organ transplantation Skin graft survival
	Blastogenesis (Con A, PHA, alloantigen)	Graft-versus-host disease (popliteal lymph node assay)
	Lymphokine production (IL-1, IL-2) T_h:T_s ratios	Autoimmune diseases Experimental allergic encephalomyelitis
	Delayed-type hypersensitivity (SRBC, MBSA, oxazolone)	Murine lupus (MRL/1, NZB) Murine immune complex nephritis (DBA/2 into C57B1/6 × DBA/2F)
		Inflammation Rat carrageenan edema/pleurisy Rat adjuvant arthritis Rat collagen arthritis
B cells	Blastogenesis (PWM, LPS)	Infection Viral prophylaxis (herpes simplex, etc.)
	Plaque-forming cells to sheep red blood cells	Bacterial and fungal *(Salmonella typhimurin, Escherichia coli, Candida albicans, Listeria monocytogenes)*
Nonspecific	NK cytotoxicity	Tumor Primary and metastatic (Lewis lung; lymphoma)
	Macrophages (phagocytosis; pinocytosis; chemotaxis; cytotoxicity; release of O_2 radicals, lysosomal enzymes, arachidonate metabolites, and monokines, Ia and C3 expression)	Madison lung, M109 Mammary adenocarcinoma, fibrosarcoma, L1210 Leukemia
	Antibody-dependent cell-mediated cytotoxicity	
	Neutrophils (chemotaxis; release of O_2 radicals, lysosomal enzymes)	

samples. The experimental response measured should be easily quantifiable by objective rather than subjective criteria, and the data obtained must withstand rigorous statistical evaluation and validation. Since most, if not all, currently available immunopharmacologic assays are not satisfactory in all respects (URBANIAK et al. 1979), the use of several assays is recommended, particularly in the early screening phases (Table 2). Practical considerations (convenience, speed, ease of operation and data interpretation) dictate the use of in vitro assays for most primary screening programs. This is then followed by evaluation of "ex vivo" effects in protocols in which in vitro immunologic activity is assessed after in vivo drug exposure, and ultimately, whole-animal studies (RENOUX 1986).

I. Quantification of Lymphocytes

The effects of a drug on the numerical and functional activities of lymphocytes can yield valuable information regarding the agent's selectivity and mode of action. T lymphocyte enumeration is usually performed with peripheral blood samples using surface marker methods that distinguish between T and B lymphocytes and their subsets that are morphologically indistinguishable (Chaps. 6 and 12). Spontaneous binding of lymphocytes to sheep erythrocytes (rosetting) and staining with immunoglobulin-specific antisera is routinely used to identify and separate T and B cells, respectively (URBANIAK et al. 1979). Monoclonal antibodies to surface antigens present on individual cell subsets (OKT3, OKT4, OKT8, etc.) are a powerful tool and can be used to identify cellular elements by rosetting, fluorescence methods, or complement-mediated lysis (REINHERZ and SCHLOSSMAN 1980). More precise and detailed information about lymphocyte numbers, cell size, state of activation, and relative proportion of different cell types can be obtained by cytofluorography, which has, again, been accentuated by the development of monoclonal antibodies to surface antigens (REINHERZ and SCHLOSSMAN 1980).

One pitfall in studies which measure only cell numbers and relative proportions of subsets is an inability to correlate such changes to the functional capacity of the lymphocyte population or whole animal (BACH and CHATENOUD 1982). Thus, following enumeration of OKT4 and OKT8 cells, one must ask "OK, so what?" and measure the functional capacity of the lymphoid population examined.

II. Functional Assays

1. T Cells

The source of lymphocytes utilized for functional assays may include human and animal peripheral blood and lymphoid tissue (e.g., lymph nodes, spleen cells, thymus). The use of "normal" or "diseased" cells/tissue, and optimal or suboptimal concentrations of stimulant clearly affect the quantitative and, often, qualitative response to the drug under examination. For example, immunostimulation is best achieved under suboptimal culture conditions (TALMADGE et al. 1984a).

a) Proliferation

Stimulation of T lymphocytes results in proliferation and transformation of the cells into activated blast-like cells which synthesize DNA de novo. This can be easily quantitated by incorporation of radioactive DNA precursors, usually [³H] thymidine, into the cells. Routine stimulating substances include such polyclonal mitogens as phytohemagglutinin (PHA), concanavalin A (Con A), pokeweed mitogen (PWM), lipopolysaccharide (LPS), and autologous or allogeneic stimulator cells (URBANIAK et al. 1979). In some cases, soluble antigens are used to measure antigen-specific responses, which, in humans, involves routine skin test antigens (purified protein derivative, streptokinase–streptodornase, etc.) to which most individuals are normally exposed. In experimental animals, the antigens used can be any of a number of proteins, such as ovalbumin and keyhole limpet hemocyanin, toward which the animals have been deliberately immunized.

Lymphocyte proliferative assays are widely used as a first screen for immunomodulatory agents. While this is a useful approach, caution must be used in interpreting the significance of such results as many disparate substances, for example, tricyclic antidepressants and histamine type 2 receptor antagonists, show activity in this assay, presumably because lymphocytes express a variety of surface receptors, including those for β-adrenergic, dopaminergic, cholinergic, H_2-histamine, and opiate agonists (SORKIN et al. 1981).

b) T Cell Cytotoxicity

Cytotoxicity represents another functional aspect of T lymphocytes which has immunotherapeutic relevance, particularly with respect to immunostimulatory antitumor agents or immunosuppressive agents used in transplant recipients. Models designed to detect agents which affect the generation of cytolytic cells are the most useful in this regard; few agents have been shown to affect the cytolytic activity of activated effector cells directly.

c) Regulatory T Cells

Modulation of helper (Th) and/or suppressor (Ts) cell functions by immunotherapeutic agents represents an important potential mode of action which has not been fully explored for most agents. Regulatory cell functions are assessed by the ability of various cell populations to increase or decrease humoral (e.g., immunoglobulin secretion) or cellular (e.g., cytotoxic T cell activity) immunity in reconstitution experiments which are generally performed in vitro. Since these assays require the use of cell separation/purification techniques and a two-stage culture system (generation of Th/Ts in first culture and assay for function in a second culture), these are not particularly amenable to rapid screening use. Experimental systems used to generate Ts and Th cells include dinitrochlorobenzene (DNCB), poly(L-glutamic acid-L-lysine-L-tyrosine) (GAT), hydroxy-3-nitrophenylacetyl or azobenzenarsonate haptens, mitogens (Con A, PHA, PWM), allogeneic cells, tumor cells, and bacterial products such as staphylococcal entertoxin B (DORF and BENACERRAF 1984; ROGERS et al. 1985). Unfortunately, there have been few studies which have attempted to characterize the effects of immunotherapeutic agents in these systems and this remains an important area for future research.

d) Natural Killer Cells

Natural killer (NK) cells are large granule-containing lymphocytes (LGL) which are able to lyse a wide variety of target cells in cytotoxicity assays. NK cells are thought to play a significant role in host resistance against tumor growth and metastasis (HERBERMAN and HOLDEN 1978). NK cells can be further activated in vitro by culture with lymphokines; e.g., interferon (IFN) or interleukin 2 (IL-2), to generate "lymphokine-activated" killer cells (LAK). NK cells can be conveniently measured by ^{51}Cr-release assays using labeled target cells (YAC-1, K-562). In vitro culture of the test compounds with circulating or tissue NK cells for 24 h usually precedes the cytotoxicity assay, although alternatively drugs can be incorporated directly into the assay itself. In vivo, the drug can be administered and NK activity measured as described. Circulating IFN levels should also be assessed because elevations of these by the test agent can augment NK activity.

e) In Vivo Assays

Numerous delayed-type hypersensitivity assays have been developed in order to assess T cell activation in vivo (Table 2). These assays often involve sensitization of mice with a T cell-dependent antigen such as methylated bovine serum albumin (MBSA) or SRBC followed by intradermal challenge of the antigen into the footpad (LEWIS et al. 1981–2, 1985). Increase in footpad swelling or thickness can be utilized to quantitate the response. Similarly, contact hypersensitivity to oxazolone and DNCB with the ear as the site of challenge has been used successfully to achieve the same goal in mice and guinea pigs. These responses to antigen are complex and involve many aspects of the immune response, including helper, suppressor, and effector T cell functions, as well as macrophage activation and inflammatory mediator release. Skin graft rejection and graft-versus-host responses are also useful in vivo models (Table 2).

2. B Cells

Immunoglobulin secretion is the hallmark for measuring B cell function. This frequently involves the measurement of antibodies to specific antigens administered (e.g., SRBC, EL4 cells). Antibody responses to T-dependent and T-independent antigens should both be evaluated. Plaque-forming cell (PFC) assays based on the original Jerne technique (CUNNINGHAM and SZENBURG 1968) are regularly used to enumerate antibody-secreting cells (Chap. 5). Mice are sensitized to antigen (SRBC, LPS, etc.) and spleen cells are then assayed directly for PFC formation, or first restimulated in vitro with the same antigen in Mishell–Dutton cultures. To a lesser extent, enzyme-linked and radioimmunoassay procedures have been used to measure immunoglobulin secretion. As in the case of T cells, B cell proliferation can also be evaluated by means of selected B cell mitogens (dextran sulfate, LPS, etc.) which can be quantitated by incorporation of $[^3H]$ thymidine into the cells.

3. Phagocytes

a) Neutrophils

Alterations in circulating neutrophils or monocytes are some of the earliest indications of immune deficiency. Quantitative methods for enumerating such cells include phagocytosis (zymosan or latex particles) and histochemical stains such as myeloperoxidase. Chemotaxis to appropriate chemoattractants (C5a, formyl-Met-Leu-Phe, leukotriene B_4) and random motion are useful functional assays performed in vitro and in vivo, and the release of several soluble mediators, such as hydrolytic lysosomal enzymes, oxygen-reactive species, and arachidonic acid metabolites can also be conveniently measured.

b) Monocytes

Human peripheral blood monocytes and mouse peritoneal macrophages are frequently used for evaluation of the effects of immunotherapeutic agents. Drug-induced activation of human and murine monocytes can be determined by measuring pinocytosis of labeled colloidal gold, phagocytosis of particles (zymosan, *Candida albicans*), enhancement of oxidative metabolism (chemiluminescence), secretion of lysosomal enzymes (acid hydrolases), arachidonic acid metabolites (prostaglandins and leukotrienes), superoxide radicals, and induction of cytotoxic activity against tumor cells (HURST and NUKI 1981; ADAMS and HAMILTON 1984). Clearance rates of carbon particles or ^{125}I-labeled triolein from serum can be examined to assess in vivo reticuloendothelial cell function.

4. Cytokines

A variety of leukocyte-derived soluble factors or cytokines are produced during lymphocyte activation processes, and these mediators possess numerous biologic activities (see Chaps. 7–9 and 11). Cytokines include such mediators as the IFNs, interleukins, colony-stimulating factors, cytotoxic factors (e.g., tumor necrosis factor TNF) as well as over 100 ill-defined biologically active substances (HANSEN et al. 1982; GEARING et al. 1985).

The use of cytokines as immunotherapeutics has been enthusiastically pursued, but based on the current clinical experience with IFNs and IL-2, it has not been overwhelmingly successful (STRANDER and EINHORN 1982; MERLUZZI and LAST-BARNEY 1985). The evaluation of purified recombinant cytokines (i.e., IL-1, IL-2, IFNs) should definitively resolve the clinical utility of these cytokines within a shord period. Moreover, identification and characterization of agents which augment or mimic cytokine action/secretion (agonists) as well as agents which inhibit the binding and/or biologic response of cells to cytokines (antagonists) may overcome some of the problems encountered with cytokine therapy (e.g., the rapid in vivo clearance of these agents) (FARRAR et al. 1984; LEWIS and GILMAN 1987).

D. Future Developments in Screening Methodology

I. Biochemical Assays of Lymphocyte Activation

One of the main limitations of immunopharmacologic studies aimed at identifying and developing novel immunotherapeutic agents is that most assay systems are based on complex biologic responses (e.g., cellular proliferation) rather than more quantitative and reliable biochemical or immunochemical techniques. Thus, increased knowledge of the relevant biochemical events in lymphocyte activation processes should lead to the development of more rapid and specific screening procedures, for example, based on phospholipase A_2, protein kinase C, or calcium/calmodulin alterations accompanying activation signals (CHANG et al. 1986; FARRAR and TAGUCHI 1985; Chaps. 3 and 4). Similarly, the development of immunoassays (enzyme-based or radiolabeled) for measuring cytokine concentrations would facilitate screening assays which detect drug-induced alterations in cytokine secretion/utilization.

II. Radioreceptor Assays

The use of radioligand-binding assays permits the evaluation of compounds for their direct interaction with cell surface recognition sites (receptors). Structure–activity relationships generated by these binding assays may help improve specificity and potency of compounds. However, these assays do not take into account those compounds requiring metabolic activation, and generally measure only relative potency rather than efficacy, so that it is difficult to assess whether a compound interacting with a ligand-binding site functions as an agonist or an antagonist.

Radioligand-binding assays have not as yet been utilized extensively in the development of novel immunotherapeutics. This can be ascribed partly to the lack of ideal drugs from which to model new agents, but perhaps it is largely due to ignorance concerning the specific mechanisms of action of many immunomodulators. Receptors for IL-2 have been identified and characterized, and inhibition of IL-2 binding could be used as a screen to detect IL-2 receptor antagonists as potential immunosuppressive agents (ROBB 1984). Receptors for IL-1 have been identified which may also be amenable to screening systems to detect IL-1 antagonists as putative antirheumatic agents (AURON et al. 1984; MARCH 1985). Specific receptors for TNF have also been reported (RUBIN et al. 1985). However, primarily because of difficulty in purifying suitable quantities of these cytokines from culture supernatant fluids, these assays are not yet in general use. The availability of large quantities of recombinant molecules should alleviate supply problems and allow agonists and antagonists to be rapidly screened for activity by overcoming the more laborious and less specific biologic assays currently in use. For example, a specific cytosolic binding protein for cyclosporin A, referred to as cyclophilin, was recently described with [^{3}H] cyclosporin A as ligand (see Chap. 21). This may allow the development of new cyclosporin A analogs, much as isolation of benzodiazepine receptors facilitated development of new benzodiazepine anxiolytic drugs (SORKIN et al. 1981).

III. Monoclonal Antibodies

Monoclonal antibodies have already led to rapid advances in the understanding of immune regulation and how the normal immunoregulatory balance is perturbed in patients with autoimmune and immunodeficiency disorders, cancer, etc. (MORIMOTO et al. 1983; Chap. 6).

Monoclonal antibodies have at least four major applications in the development of new immunotherapeutic agents (OLSSON 1983; ZALCBERG 1985). First, their continued use in the study of immunologic defects in various human diseases may reveal additional therapeutic applications for immunotherapeutics. Second, the use of monoclonals as reagents to purify and characterize cytokines and their receptors, and to develop immunochemical assays for these soluble mediators, should reveal additional cellular and humoral targets for immunomodulatory action of immunotherapeutic agents. Third, monoclonal antibodies themselves, used either alone or coupled to a toxin or other agent, could constitute an important class of new immunotherapeutics (WOFSY 1985). However, certain obstacles must first be overcome, including rapid metabolism and clearance of the antibodies, development of antibody-specific and idiotype-specific antibodies, and hypersensitivity reactions which occur after multiple injections (REISFIELD and SELL 1985). Finally, monoclonal antibodies will be important tools to measure the specificity and magnitude of immunologic responses elicited in patients in clinical studies utilizing new immunotherapeutic agents.

E. Clinical Trials of Immunotherapeutic Agents

The ultimate screening test of any promising immunotherapeutic agent occurs during phase I and II clinical trials in humans. It is becoming increasingly clear that the design of phase I clinical trials with immunotherapeutic agents and other biologic response modifiers is considerably different from those of other agents. The concept of a two-stage phase I program for such agents has recently been espoused, especially by investigators in the cancer field (HERBERMAN 1985; PINSKY 1985). The first aim of a phase I trial should be to determine toxicity, and if possible, a maximal tolerated dose in normal volunteers or in patients. Initial studies are designed to establish a safe dose range in which to perform, in the appropriate patient populations, the second stage of phase I testing, i.e., the establishment of the optimal dose and schedule for obtaining the desired immunologic effects. An important question to address concerns exactly what immunologic assays should be measured in the various patient populations (AMERY 1981). The temptation to monitor tests which are easy to perform, but which are not appropriate for the patients under study should be resisted, as these are unlikely to yield useful information. Skin tests for delayed-type hypersensitivity are probably the most overutilized tests in this regard. Certainly, if an agent has specific immunomodulatory properties identified in preclinical models, these should be monitored. Similarly, if the patient populations studied have known specific immunologic deficits, the ability of the immunotherapeutic to correct these deficiencies should be evaluated. For example, patients with rheumatoid arthritis have been reported to have increased helper:suppressor T cell ratios in the peripheral blood (DUKE et al. 1983), whereas these values may be decreased in patients with systemic lupus erythematosus (BAKKE et al. 1983). The T helper:suppressor ratio could be studied in these patient populations during administration of an immunotherapeutic agent, and correlations could be discovered between changes in this ratio and in disease activity, as demonstrated in studies with fanetizole (ROCKLIN et al. 1984), levamisole (SCHEINBERG et al. 1978), and thymic peptides (VEYS et al. 1982). In all studies, the patients enrolled in these trials should be capable of a response, which generally means that they should be studied as early in their disease process as possible.

Since the dose–response curve for the desired immunologic effect may not be known, pharmacokinetic assays for serum availability should be performed with various routes of administration. It is possible that an immunologic effect may persist long after serum levels of the agent in question become undetectable. Therefore, the time course of these effects in single- and multiple-dose studies should be determined.

Another aspect of immunotherapy which must be considered in phase I and II trials is the ability of the agent under investigation to produce an effect near the target tissue. Thus, a monoclonal antibody against a specific tumor tissue must be delivered to that tissue in large enough quantities to produce a biologically significant effect. The therapeutic efficacy of agents which activate NK cell function will be questionable if the NK cells are incapable of migrating into metastatic tumor deposits. Likewise, in rheumatoid arthritis patients, it is important to demonstrate that the investigational agent has effects in the joints and not just in the peripheral blood.

The purpose of phase II testing is to demonstrate the clinical efficacy and safety of the experimental immunotherapeutic agent. Studies utilizing the investigational drug as a single agent or in the adjuvant setting are undertaken utilizing the optimal immunomodulatory dose, schedule, and route of administration, as determined in phase I.

Furthermore, immunotherapeutics with additive or synergistic activities can be combined in an effort to improve the clinical response. For example, it has been demonstrated that infusions of IL-2 and LAK cells are more beneficial for cancer patients than infusions of either agent alone (ROSENBERG et al. 1985).

In summary, the early clinical trials with promising immunotherapeutic agents should ascertain the toxicitiy of the agent and confirm the ability of the drug to modify immune responses in a manner appropriate to the patient population under study. The optimal dose, schedule, and route of administration for this effect should be determined, and pharmacokinetic data should be obtained. Finally, phase II studies should be performed to demonstrate the clinical efficacy in relation to the immune response elicited.

References

Adams DO, Hamilton TA (1984) The cell biology macrophage activation. Ann Rev Immunol 2:283–318

Aiuti F, Rosen F, Cooper MD (1986) Recent advances in primary and acquired immunodeficiencies. Serono Symp Ser 28:1–434

Amery WK (1981) Cancer immunotherapy: some critical comments regarding immunological monitoring. Int J Immunopharmacol 3:339–348

Auron PE, Webb A, Rosenwasser LJ, Mucci SF, Rich A, Wolff S, Dinarello CA (1984) Nucleotide sequence of human monocyte interleukin 1 precursor DNA. Proc Natl Acad Sci USA 81:7907–7911

Bach JF, Chatenoud L (1982) The significance of T cell subsets defined by monoclonal antibodies in human diseases. Ann Immunol 133:131–136

Bakke A, Kinkland PA, Kitridou RC, Quismorio FP, Rea T, Ehresmann GR, Horowitz DA (1983) T-lymphocyte subsets in systemic lupus erythematosus. Arthritis Rheum 26:745–750

Chang J, Gilman SC, Lewis AJ (1986) Interleukin 1 activates phospholipase A_2 in rabbit chondrocytes: a possible signal for IL 1 action. J Immunol 136:1283–1287

Chirigos MA, Talmadge JE (1985) Immunotherapeutic agents: their role in cellular immunity and their therapeutic potential. Springer Semin Immunopathol 8:327–346

Cunningham AJ, Szenberg A (1968) Further improvements in the plaque technique for detecting single antibody-forming cells. Immunology 14:599–600

Dillman RO, Koziol JA (1983) Statistical approach to immunosuppression classification using lymphocyte surface markers and functional assays. Cancer Res 43:417–421

Dinarello CA (1984) Interleukin 1. Rev Infect Dis 6:51–95

Dorf ME, Benacerraf B (1984) Suppressor cells and immunoregulation. Ann Rev Immunol 2:127–158

Duke O, Panayi GS, Janossy G, Poulter LW, Tidman N (1983) Analysis of T-cell subsets in the peripheral blood and synovial fluid of patients with rheumatoid arthritis by means of monoclonal antibodies. Ann Rheum Dis 42:357–361

Eilber FR, Nizze JA, Morton DL (1975) Sequential evaluation of general immune competence in cancer patients: correlation with clinical course. Cancer 55:660–665

Farrar JJ, Benjamin WR, Cheng L, Pawson BA (1984) Interleukin 2. Ann Rep Med Chem 19:191–200

Farrar WL, Taguchi M (1985) Interleukin 2 stimulation of protein kinase C membrane association: evidence for IL-2 receptor phosphorylation. Lymphokine Res 4:87–93

Fathman CG (1982) Regulation of the immune response. In: Luderer AA, Weetal HH (eds) Clinical cellular immunology – molecular and therapeutic reviews. Humana, New Jersey, pp 31–66

Gearing AJH, Johnstone AP, Thorpe R (1985) Production and assay of the interleukins. J Immunol Methods 83:1–27

Gilman SC (1984) Lymphokines in immunological aging. Lymphokine Res 3:117–123

Gilman SC, Lewis AJ (1985) Immunomodulatory drugs in the treatment of rheumatoid arthritis. In: Rainsford KD (ed) Antiinflammatory and antirheumatic drugs, vol 3. CRC Press, Florida, pp 127–154

Gilman SC, Lewis AJ (1986) Immunopharmacological approaches to drug development. In: Williams M, Malick JB (eds) Drug discovery and development. Humana, New Jersey, pp 227–256

Goldstein AL, Low TLK, Thurman GB, Zatz M, Hall NR, McClure JE, Hu SK, Schulof RS (1982) Thymosins and other hormone-like factors of the thymus gland. In: Mihich E (ed) Immunological approaches to cancer therapeutics. Wiley, New York, pp 137–190

Hansen JM, Rumjanek VM, Morley J (1982) Mediators of cellular immune reactions. Pharmacol Ther 17:165–198

Herberman RB (1985) Design of clinical trials with biological response modifiers. Cancer Treat Rep 69:1161–1164

Herberman RB, Holden HT (1978) Natural cell-mediated immunity. Adv Cancer Res 27:305–377

Hurst N, Nuki G (1981) The macrophage – origins, functions, and role in the rheumatoid diseases. In: Dick WC (ed) Immunological aspects of rheumatology. Elsevier/North-Holland, New York, pp 183–207

Lewis AJ, Gilman SC (1987) Actions of novel immunoregulants useful in the treatment of rheumatoid arthritis as may be relevant to their toxicity. In: Rainsford KD, Velo GP (eds) Toxicity of antiinflammatory and antirheumatic drugs. Part II. Studies in major organ systems. MTP Press, Lancaster, VK, pp 253–269, CRC Press, Florida

Lewis AJ, Parker H, Diluigi J, Datko L, Carlson RP (1981–82) Immunomodulation of delayed hypersensitivity to methylated bovine serum albumin in mice using subliminal and normal sensitization procedures. J Immunopharmacol 3:289–307

Lewis AJ, Carlson RP, Chang J (1985) Experimental models of inflammation. In: Bonta IL, Bray MA, Parnham MJ (eds) The pharmacology of inflammation. Elsevier, New York, pp 371–397 (Handbook of inflammation, vol 5)

March CB, Mosley B, Larsen A, Cerretti P, Braedt V, Prive V, Gillis S, Henney CS, Kronheim SR, Grabstein K, Conlon PJ, Hopp TP, Cosman D (1985) Cloning, sequence, and expression of two distinct human interleukin 1 complementary DNAs. Nature 315:641–647

Merluzzi VJ, Last-Barney K (1985) Potential use of human interleukin 2 as an adjunct for the therapy of neoplasia, immunodeficiency and infections disease. J Biol Response Mod 7:31–39

Morimoto C, Schlossman SF, Reinherz EL (1983) Use of monoclonal antibodies in the study of autoimmunity and immunodeficiency. In: Haynes BF, Eisenbath GS (eds) Monoclonal antibodies. Academic, Florida, pp 1–21

Olsson L (1983) Monoclonal antibodies in clinical immunobiology. Derivation, potential and limitations. Allergy 38:145–154

Parker CW (1973) The immunotherapy of cancer. Pharmacol Rev 25:325–342

Pinskey CM (1985) Applicability of phase I trial results in the design of phase II and III biological response modifier trials. Cancer Treat Rep 69:1171–1173

Reinherz EL, Schlossman SF (1980) The differentiation and function of human T lymphocytes. Cell 19:821–827

Reisfeld RA, Sell S (1985) Monoclonal antibodies and cancer therapy. Liss, New York, pp 1–585

Renoux G (1980) Trends in immunopotentiation. Int J Immunopharmacol 2:1–6

Renoux G (1986) Characterization of immunotherapeutic agents: the example of imuthiol. Methods Find Exp Clin Pharmacol 8:45–50

Robb RJ (1984) Interleukin 2: the molecule and its function. Immunol Today 5:203–209

Rocklin RE, Hemady Z, Matloff S, Kiselis I, Lima M (1984) Correction of an *in vitro* immunoregulatory defect in atopic subjects by the immunostimulatory drug fanetizole mesylate (CP-48,410). Int J Immunopharmacol 6:1–8

Rogers CM, Rogers TJ, Gilman SC (1985) Effects of Wy-18,251 (3-*p*-chlorophenyl)-thiazolo[3,2-*a*]benzimidazole-2-acetic acid), levamisole and indomethacin on the generation of murine T suppressor cells *in vitro*. J Immunopharmacol 7:479–488

Roitt IM, Male D, Young A, Jones M, Nivehaus L, Corbett M, Hay FC (1982) Autoimmune phenomena in rheumatoid arthritis. Adv Inflammation Res 3:49–58

Rosenberg SA, Lotze MT, Murl LM, Leitman S, Chang AE, Ettinghauser SE, Matory YL, Skibbe JM, Shiloni E, Vetto JT (1985) Observations on the administration of autologous lymphokine-activated killer cells and recombinant interleukin-2 to patients with metastatic cancer. N Engl J Med 313:1485–1492

Rubin BY, Anderson SL, Sullivan SA, Williamson BD, Carswell EA, Old LJ (1985) High affinity binding of ^{125}I-labeled human tumor necrosis factor (LuKII) to specific cell surface receptors. J Exp Med 162:1099–1104

Scheinberg MA, Santos L, Mendes N, Musatti C (1978) Decreased lymphocyte response to PHA, Con-A, and calcium ionophore (A23187) in patients with RA and SLE, and reversal with levamisole in rheumatoid arthritis. Arthritis Rheum 21:326–329

Sigel MM, Ghaffer A, Paul R, Licher W, Wellham L, McCumber LJ, Huggins EM Jr (1982) Immunosuppressive agents – their action on inductive and regulatory pathways. The differential effects of agents used clinically and experimentally in the treatment of cancer. In: Luderer AA, Weetal HH (eds) Clinical cellular immunology – molecular and therapeutic reviews. Humana, New Jersey, pp 145–211

Siskind GW, Christian CL, Litwin SD (1975) Immune depression and cancer. Grune and Stratton, New York, pp 1–209

Sorkin E, Del Ray A, Besedovsky HO (1981) Neuroendocrine control of the immune response. In: Steinberg CM, Lefkovits I (eds) The immune system, vol 1. Karger, Basel, pp 340–357

Steinberg AD (1973) Efficacy of immunosuppressive drugs in rheumatic diseases. Arthritis Rheum 16:92–96

Strander H, Einhorn S (1982) Interferon and cancer: faith, hope and reality. Am J Clin Oncol 5:297–301

Talmadge JE, Herberman (1986) The preclinical screening laboratory: evaluation of immunomodulatory and therapeutic properties of biological response modifiers. Cancer Treat Rep 70:171–182

Talmadge JE, Benedict KL, Uithoven KA, Lenz BF (1984a) The effect of experimental conditions on the assessment of T cell immunomodulation by biological response modifiers (thymosin fraction five). Immunopharmacology 7:17–26

Talmadge JE, Oldham RK, Fidler IJ (1984b) Practical considerations for the establishment of a screening procedure for the assessment of biological response modifiers. J Biol Response Mod 3:88–102

Urbaniak SJ, White AG, Barclay GR, Wood SM, Kay AB (1979) Tests of immune function. In: Weir DM (ed) Application of immunological methods. Blackwell, Oxford, pp 47.1–47.3 (Handbook of experimental immunology, vol 3)

Veys E, Hermanns P, Goldstein G, Kung PC, Schindler J, Symoens J, Van Wauve J (1982) T-cell subpopulations determined by monoclonal antibodies in RA. Influence of immunomodulating agents. Adv Inflammation Res 3:155–164

Wofsy D (1985) Strategies for treating autoimmune disease with monoclonal antibodies. West J Med 143:804–809

Zalcberg JR (1985) Monoclonal antibodies to drugs: novel diagnostic and therapeutic reagents. Pharmacol Ther 28:273–285

Zvaifler NJ (1973) The immunopathology of joint inflammation in rheumatoid arthritis. Adv Immunol 16:265–301

Part 3

CHAPTER 14

Selected Autacoids as Modulators of Lymphocyte Function

M. M. KHAN and K. L. MELMON

A. Introduction

Autacoids are biologic mediators of increasing importance. Their name derives from the Greek *autos* meaning self and *akos* meaning medicinal agent. They are ubiquitously distributed, that is, they are found in most tissues and body fluids, and they regulate a variety of major physiologic functions and participate in some well-defined pathologic processes. Although autacoids have been defined as auto-hormones, they differ from hormones in that they are made, play their role, and are destroyed at the same sites. Many tissues make, respond to, and metabolize autacoids. The substances ordinarily are not transported for their physiologic effects; they usually regulate the function of a tissue system in the vicinity of their synthesis and are also metabolized in the same region. But in some pathologic states, excessive amounts of autacoids can reach the systemic circulation and account for many of the symptoms of the disorder (e.g., in the carcinoid syndrome and in patients with pheochromocytoma syndrome; MELMON 1981). With this definition of autacoids, it is not surprising that histamine, catecholamines, and prostaglandins can be included in this class of mediator. Biologically active peptides and lymphokines will no doubt be subsumed in future textbook classifications of autacoids (Fig. 1).

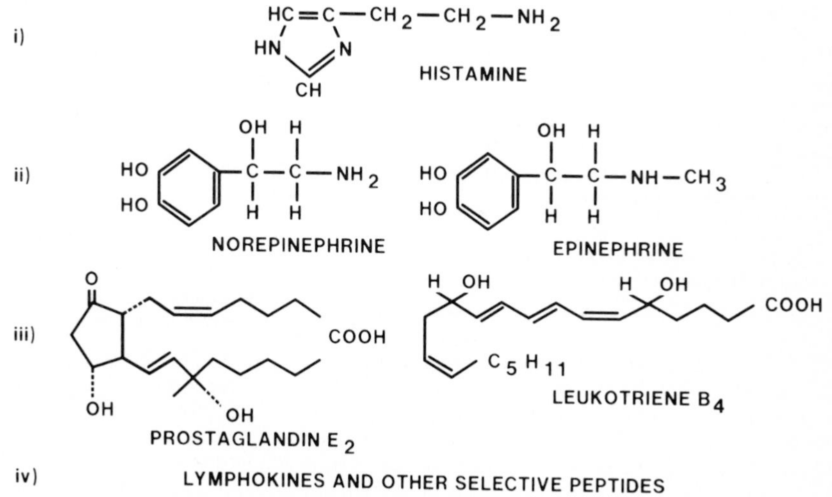

Fig. 1. Autacoids

The role of autacoids as major modulators of immunity has been developing over the past few years and will be the major focus of this chapter. The substances are synthesized and secreted by lymphocytes and other cells involved in the antigen recognition phase. They can also affect physiologic and pathologic mechanisms that determine the response to antigen. Autacoids are capable of modifying the functions of various subsets of lymphoid cells which are regulators of either humoral or cellular immunity. It is becoming quite clear that autacoids may even play a major role in the intercommunication of phenotypically and functionally distinct subsets of lymphoid cells. Although most experimental evidence of the autacoid role as immune modulators comes from in vitro experiments, in vivo data are beginning to appear. These data, so far, are consistent with in vitro data and even coordinate with the clinical hints that autacoids may be important immune modulators in humans (KHAN and MELMON 1985). It even seems reasonable to suggest that anomalies in autacoid-mediated immune events ultimately may explain some diseases of the immune system.

In this chapter, we will focus on how histamine, β-adrenergic agonists, prostaglandins (PGE), and leukotriene B_4 alter the function of individual lymphocytes and perhaps the overall immune response. This focus is used to present examples of autacoid-induced lymphocyte effects. This presentation should help to

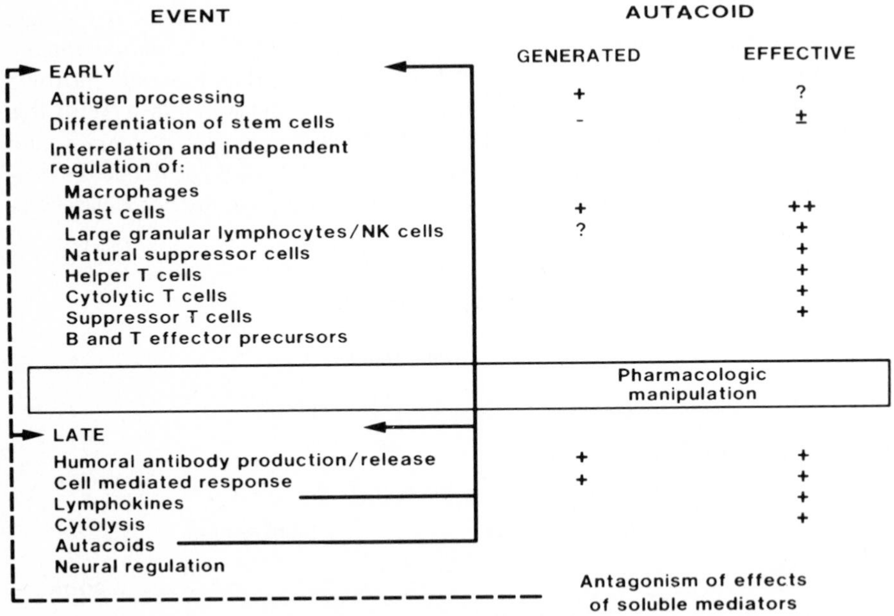

Fig. 2. Possible sites for the regulation of immunity by autacoids. The phases of immune response which could be independently studied experimentally are shown. Pharmacologic manipulations can include radiation, immunosuppressive drugs, cytotoxic drugs, steroids, and monoclonal antibodies. The subsets of cells can be separated and their individual effects evaluated. The *boxed-in area* divides the early from the late phase. It represents the shading of one phase into another and the drugs that can affect both phases. The *question marks* indicate that the results are inconclusive. (Modified from MELMON et al. 1981)

set the stage for the interested scientist (a) to incorporate new data about auta-coids and lymphocytes into a coherent picture of immune modulation; and (b) to allow clear thinking about where the investigative field will lead (Fig. 2).

B. Histamine

Histamine was identified by Kutscher as an active component of ergot. The imad-izole was synthesized by Windaus and Vogt almost simultaneously. Dale and Schultz first reported a role for histamine as a mediator of immediate hypersen-sitivity. Histamine was found to be a ubiquitous amine in every mammalian tissue investigated, but was mainly concentrated in the skin, the lung, and the gastroin-testinal tract. Later, using a model of immediate hypersensitivity, Bartosch and colleagues showed that histamine was released from tissue involved in the im-mune-related response. Some of the major in vivo pharmacologic effects of his-tamine include increased vascular permeability, contraction of bronchial muscle, and the classical triple response of hypersensitivity (DALE and FOREMAN 1984; DOUGLAS 1985).

The study of Riley and West demonstrated that mast cells were a principal storage site for the histamine that was released during inflammatory and immune processes. The histamine that is involved in the inflammatory and immune re-sponses has also been detected in basophils and, in some species, in platelets. It is likely that, as the role of the amine in immunity is more closely defined, other sources of storage and release may be found.

The histamine that is synthesized, stored, and released from mast cells is lo-cated in unusually provocative locations for a role in immune modulation. Usually, we think of mast cells as being closely associated with blood vessels. There, they are not only major effector cells in immediate hypersensitivity, but they can also be activated to release inflammatory mediators during expressions of cell-mediated (delayed-type) hypersensitivity. Mast cells have also been shown to concentrate in lymph nodes and thymus (RAZIN et al. 1984; BURNET 1965), but since a physiologic role for mast cells had not been surmised in these sites, their presence was largely overlooked or considered anomalous. Recent data, however, seem to indicate that their locus is not coincidental, and the hints provided by their presence at sites of immunologic relevance are now being followed up in ex-periments that define the role of mast cells in primary immune modulation. It should not be surprising ultimately to find that these cells are intimately and physiologically associated with lymphocytes that are involved in the immune re-sponse.

Mammalian mast cells are derived from T lymphocytes, monocytes, and mes-enchymal, myeloid, and lymph node sources. Growth and maintenance of the mast cells are dependent on T cell growth factor (BURNET 1965; KITAMURE et al. 1977, 1979; GINSBURG and LAGUNOFF 1967). Furthermore, several lines of evi-dence suggest that increases in the numbers of mast cells and their histamine con-tent may be governed by immunologic events (BEFUS and BIENENSTOCK 1979; YOO et al. 1978; MIMH et al. 1976; WYNNE-ROBERTS et al. 1978). Thus, the fate of the mast cell seems to be intimately connected with the function of other lymphocytes (KHAN et al. 1986d).

Several investigators have shown that the release of histamine from mast cells can be important for the expression of immediate hypersensitivity and the changes in the microvasculature occurring during such events. Lewis and Mangham (1978) have demonstrated that the histamine content of both allografts and autografts increased during the "healing in" of grafts, even though histamine did not contribute to the initial vasodilation. However, at the onset of rejection, the histamine content of the allografts (but not of the autografts) increased to concentrations which, in the rabbit, cause vasoconstriction. The vascular effects were delayed by the use of antihistamines that competitively blocked the histamine-induced vasoconstriction. The initial increase in histamine in allografts and autografts may have been the result of an increase in newly synthesized histamine. The later increase in histamine content that was coincident with the onset of rejection of allografts was probably released from basophils.

The first indication that histamine could affect the immune response was reported by Pepys (1955). He observed that injection of histamine with an antigen into the site of a tuberculin skin test reduced the subsequent expression of the delayed-type hypersensitivity reaction. These findings were not what had been expected from a mediator of inflammation, and indeed the observation was not fully appreciated until recently. Now several other laboratories have helped to accumulate data that support the immune modulating role of histamine. In spite of these data, however, physicians continue to ignore the inhibitory role that histamine plays, and blithely use antihistamines to "prevent" the clinical effects of hypersensitivity!

Histamine modulates the activity of immunocompetent cells via cell surface receptors. Adenylate cyclase, which is responsible for a number of intracellular functions, is usually linked to histamine type 2 receptors. However, in some instances, stimulation of histamine type 2 receptors on the lymphoid cell, and the subsequent intracellular accumulation of cAMP may not regulate the function of the cell (Khan et al. 1985a). Some subsets of immunocompetent cells also possess histamine type 1 receptors on their cell surface which are not linked to adenylate cyclase (Cameron et al. 1986; Khan et al. 1987). While some investigators have proposed a linkage of guanylate cyclase to histamine type 1 receptors, the second messenger associated with lymphocyte H_1 receptors is not fully defined.

During the past 10 years, several investigators have explored the role of cAMP as a mediator of immune regulation. In general, most investigators have proposed an overall suppressive effect of cAMP on immune function, regardless of the stimulus that induces accumulation of the intracellular cAMP. Several investigators have shown a concomitant increase in intracellular concentrations of cAMP and histamine-induced suppression of a number of in vitro models of immunity (Bourne et al. 1974). Histamine-induced inhibition of neutrophil chemotaxis is associated with increased intracellular cAMP and is inhibited by the H_2 antagonist cimetidine (Hill et al. 1975). Histamine inhibits lysosomal enzyme release from granulocytes; the inhibition is directly correlated with the accumulation of cAMP and is blocked by the H_2 receptor antagonist metiamide. Not surprisingly, other autacoids, (e.g., isoproterenol or prostaglandins), and dibutyryl cAMP produce equivalent effects, and inhibitors of phosphodiesterase potentiate the effects of the agonists.

Some concentrations (3×10^{-7} M) of histamine increase eosinophil chemotaxis which is not blocked either by an H_1 or H_2 antagonist. At higher concentrations of histamine (10^{-3} M), inhibition of chemotaxis occurs and can be competitively blocked by H_2 receptor antagonists. Histamine can inhibit the in vitro chemotactic responses of basophils and can inhibit secretion from human basophils. The inhibitory effects of histamine on both basophil secretion and migration are mediated via H_2 receptors.

COFFEY and HADDEN (1985) have shown that cAMP accumulation promotes the differentiation of immature lymphocytes, and that cGMP promotes both clonal proliferation and enhancement of the function of mature lymphocytes. Their approach to this hypothesis has not been tested on phenotypically distinct subsets of lymphoid cells, nor have the biochemical pathways mediating these processes been elucidated.

Histamine can suppress the proliferative response of guinea pig and human lymphoid cells to mitogen. These effects are most convincing when PHA rather than ConA is used as a mitogen. The effects are best demonstrated when mononuclear cells taken from atopic individuals are used in the experiment. During the past several years, it has been suggested that suppression of mitogen-induced proliferation by histamine may be mediated by histamine type 2 receptors. However, the H_2 antagonist cimetidine can itself induce mitogenesis, independent of its histamine-blocking activity.

Histamine suppresses mitogen-induced B lymphocyte proliferation only when the amine is present in high concentrations, and in the presence of T cells with an Fc receptor for IgG (LIMA and ROCKLIN 1981). In contrast, BROSTOFF et al. (1980) have reported that at low concentrations, histamine can augment the proliferation of lymphoid cells to mitogenic stimuli. These apparently opposite effects of histamine illustrate an interesting and important point. Multiple cells involved with some stage of the immune response can respond to a given stimulus both independently and in concert with other cells. Thus, the net effect of histamine (and probably other autacoids) will not only be dependent on the concentration of agonist, but also on the timing of its effect in relation to antigen presentation, the type of antigen presented, and the composition of the mix of cells present during stimulation with autacoid and/or antigen. Seeing opposite effects caused by the same agent does not invalidate the observation, but highlights the need to define the conditions under which the effect has been demonstrated. Indeed, it appears that one explanation of the opposite effects of histamine is the presence of more than one cell population responsive to the autacoid. At least one of these populations may be other than T cells (null cells, natural killer cells, B cells, and/or monocytes bearing histamine receptors have been suggested).

If receptors for histamine were randomly distributed on all lymphoid cells, one certainly could question the likelihood of histamine's physiologic importance as an orderly modifier of lymphocyte function. But is has now become very clear that histamine receptors are nonrandomly distributed on lymphoid cells (KHAN et al. 1985 a–c). For example, thymocytes do not respond to histamine until they are exposed to corticosteroids (ROSZOKOWSKI et al. 1977). T effector cells become increasingly responsive to histamine as a function of the length of time that they are exposed to allogeneic target cells (LICHTENSTEIN 1976). In fact, the action of cytolytic T cells can be inhibited consistently by compounds such as dibutyryl cAMP, cholera toxin, and prostaglandins at any stage of their generation or function, but histamine can suppress only at a given time after immunization. Furthermore, affinity chromatographic techniques have been used to delineate those cells with histamine receptors (MELMON et al. 1974 a,b). Subsequent studies with such cells were among the earliest to demonstrate the role of histamine as an immune modulator. Thus, it was found that precursors of B cells did not possess histamine receptors, but immunologically committed B cells secreting antibodies did. Histamine had no effect on the precursors, but suppressed the production and/or release of antibodies from mature antibody-producing cells. Finally, only a small fraction of suppressor T cells bear histamine receptors, providing another demonstration of the nonrandom distribution of histamine receptors on lymphoid cells. As stated already, this nonrandom distribution of receptor expression helps to explain how histamine can regulate various phases of immune responses in an orderly way.

However, the affinity chromatography technique for cell separation, based on the cell's receptor complement, was neither quantitative in terms of cell separation, nor did it allow reliable recovery of adherent cells (those with histamine receptors) for subsequent study of their physiologic function and the effects of pharmacologic manipulation. Recently, the availability of monoclonal antibodies to antigenic markers on human lymphoid cells has made it possible to separate the subsets of T cells on the basis of these markers (see Chap. 6). Initial studies in a number of laboratories defined two mutually exclusive subsets of human T cells. The suppressor and cytotoxic subsets of T cells ($CD8^+$) can be identified by anti-Leu-2 or OKT8 antibodies. The monoclonal antibody can be used in panning experiments to isolate the subset that comprises approximately 30% of peripheral T cells in healthy individuals. The $CD8^+$ subset, containing both cytotoxic and suppressor cells, interacts with their targets in a class I (HLA-A,B)-restricted manner. A reciprocal subset (designated $CD4^+$), isolated by the use of anti-Leu-3 or OKT4 antibodies, contains approximately 60% of the peripheral T cell in healthy individuals and is designated the helper/inducer subset. Signals from this subset, in conjunction with foreign antigen, are required for B cells to differentiate into plasma cells and secrete immunoglobulin. $CD4^+$ cells also induce the differentiation of other functional subsets of T cells such as cytotoxic and suppressor cells. Helper/inducer cells are activated by antigen-presenting accessory cells only if the latter cells express class II HLA antigens (for example, HLA-DR) that are identical to that of the helper cells. Moreover, recent studies indicate that some $CD4^+$ cells can differentiate into cytolytic T cells, but unlike $CD8^+$ cells, such $CD4^+$ cells kill with specificity for class II HLA molecules of the target cells. Thus, $CD4^+$ helper/inducer cells and cytolytic cells from the $CD8^+$ subset of cells must recognize both foreign antigen and self-HLA determinants. Unlike $CD8^+$ cells, $CD4^+$ cells respond to antigen in association with class II HLA determinants.

We have recently studied the responses of precursors and mitogen-stimulated subsets of human T cells to histamine. The basal cAMP levels varied widely between the subsets of fresh T cells. The helper/inducer $CD4^+/Leu-3^+$ cells had lower basal cAMP than any other subset, including the mixtures of $CD8^+/Leu$-

2^+ cells. When CD8$^+$/Leu-2$^+$ cells were fractionated with 9.3 antibody into separate subpopulations of cytolytic T and suppressor T cells, the basal cAMP levels of the cytolytic T cells (CD8$^+$, 9.3$^+$) increased significantly. However, the basal cAMP concentration of the purified suppressor T cells (CD8$^+$, 9.3$^-$) did not differ from the mixture of cytolytic and suppressor T cells. Thus, suppressor T cells were controlling the basal concentration of cAMP in the cytolytic T cells. Furthermore, responses of the separated subsets to histamine could not be predicted from their basal cAMP levels.

The precursors of helper, cytolytic, and suppressor T cells responded to histamine by intracellular accumulation of cAMP, implying the presence of histamine receptors on each subset. The dose-response curves to the amine and the agonists' maximal efficacy in each subset were different and characteristic for each subset. The precursors of suppressor T cells were most responsive to histamine, and the degree of responsiveness decreased when tested in helper and cytolytic T cells, respectively. Activation of subsets of T cells with mitogen (PHA or Con A) did not produce a significant change in the basal levels of cAMP. Postmitogenic responses to histamine were enhanced only in isolated helper T cells (CD4$^+$) and isolated cytolytic T cells (CD8$^+$, 9.3$^+$). Thus, suppressor T cells (CD8$^+$, 9.3$^-$) may regulate both the basal and postmitogen-stimulated autacoid responses in helper (CD4$^+$) and cytolytic (CD8$^+$, 9.3$^+$) T cells. The altered responses to histamine were blocked by H$_2$, but not by H$_1$ antagonists. The enhanced response to histamine after stimulation with mitogen was not simply due to increased availability of adenylate cyclase (KHAN et al. 1985a).

The enhanced responsiveness of helpers and cytolytic T cells to histamine is likely to be mediated by an increase in the actual number of histamine receptors on each subset of cells, although mechanisms associated with the receptor–cyclase coupling could also be playing a role. Unfortunately, no ligand is available to quantitate the H$_2$ receptors on lymphoid cells, so the mitogen-induced and cell-cell-induced mechanisms of change of responsiveness to histamine cannot be completely defined. Our data do show that there is interdependence of (a) immunologically uncommitted subsets in their response to selected drugs; (b) control of basal and autacoid-induced cAMP production by cell–cell interactions and by mitogenesis; and (c) increased qualitative and quantitative selectivity caused by mitogen in cellular response to autacoids. These experiments confirm the impression that receptors for autacoids are nonrandomly distributed (KHAN and MELMON 1985; KHAN et al. 1985a,b, 1986a,b). The results also help to elucidate the interactions by which systems of cells can create a diversified yet orderly and predictable response to what was thought to have been a ubiquitous and haphazard presence of autacoids.

The pharmacologic effects of histamine on the biologic immune functions of suppressor T cells have been a major focus of many investigators. Clearly, the suppressor cells play a central role in the regulation of the immune response, and much attention has been paid to the effects of autacoids on them. For example, the modulating effects that suppressor T cells have on T cell proliferation, lymphokine production, and cytotoxicity by T cells, as well as antibody production by B cells, can be modified by autacoids, primarily histamine.

Rocklin et al. (1979) have reported that histamine can activate suppressor cells in vitro over a 24- to 48-h incubation period. The effects of histamine on suppressor cell activity are twofold:

1. Histamine decreases the activation of antigen-induced suppressor cells which regulate antibody production. This effect is mediated by H_1 receptors and generally results in enhanced antibody production to specific antigen stimulation by B cells (Mozes et al. 1974).

2. Histamine can also activate suppressor T cells, resulting in the inhibition of proliferation of lymphocytes, production of lymphokines, and production of IgG (Rocklin et al. 1979; Lima and Rocklin 1981; Rocklin 1977).

These processes may in part be mediated by release of a suppressor lymphokine, histamine-induced suppressor factor (HSF). This factor reversibly inhibits production or release of migration-inhibitory factor (MIF) and directly inhibits proliferation of lymphocytes in response to a specific antigen. HSF is secreted by T lymphocytes which are from the $CD8^+$ subset and bear Fc receptors for IgG (T_γ) (Rocklin et al. 1979; Lima and Rocklin 1981; Rocklin 1977). These T lymphocytes have a complement of histamine receptors that are predominantly H_2. The histamine-induced release of HSF is inhibited by H_2 antagonists and not by H_1 antagonists (Rocklin and Beer 1983; Rocklin and Habarek-Davidson 1984).

HSF has been biochemically characterized. It consists of two species of acidic glycoproteins of molecular weight 25–40000. The activation and expression of HSF involves cell-cell interactions between lymphoid cells, macrophages, and their soluble products, including interleukin 1 (IL-1) (Beer et al. 1982a,b; Rocklin et al. 1983). The release of HSF by T cells in response to histamine does not appear to be mediated by cAMP as other agonists, such as isoproterenol, prostaglandin E_1, and cholera toxin, which stimulate accumulation of cAMP, do not cause the release of HSF. Furthermore, dibutyryl cAMP and phosphodiesterase inhibitors do not alter histamine-induced HSF secretion. Once again, these experiments highlight the complex situations required for the expression of the effects of histamine. They also show how the mere presence of the free agonist does not predict a biologic effect unless circumstances of cell mix, commitment to antigen response, and the presence of interleukins are correct.

The $CD8^+$ (Leu-2^+, 9.3^-) suppressor subset includes all the histamine-activated suppressor cells (Sansoni et al. 1985). Histamine at 10^{-4} M is the optimal concentration for induction of suppressor cell function. Treatment of the $CD8^+$, 9.3^- subset for only 30 s is sufficient to initiate the activation process that leads to the full biologic immune modulatory response seen days later. The histamine-treated subset of suppressor cells inhibits phytohemagglutinin-induced T cell proliferation and pokeweed mitogen-induced B cell proliferation. This induction of suppression is mediated by H_2 receptors (Figs. 3 and 4).

In addition to regulating the activity of suppressor T cells, histamine has interesting modulating effects on the secretion of IL-2. When cloned helper T cells are pretreated with histamine and the amine is subsequently removed from the test system, the IL-2-secreting capacity of these cells is enhanced. In contrast, if histamine is added to the same test system that contains cells and antigen, the amine inhibits the IL-2 secretion. It is possible that the latter effect may be me-

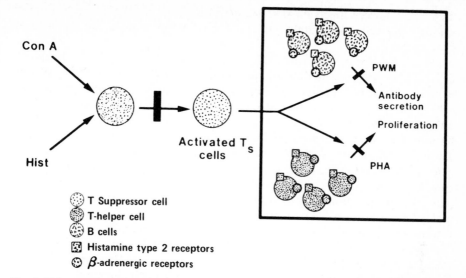

Con A

Hist

Activated T$_s$ cells

PWM

Antibody secretion

Proliferation

PHA

- T Suppressor cell
- T-helper cell
- B cells
- Histamine type 2 receptors
- β-adrenergic receptors

Fig. 3. This scheme shows the activation of the precursors of the suppressor T cells into activated suppressor cells by either histamine or concanavalin A. Activated suppressor cells can then inhibit the phytohemagglutinin-induced proliferation of helper T cells or pokeweed mitogen-induced antibody secretion by B cells. The activation, either by histamine or by concanavalin A, could be blocked by the histamine type 2 receptor antagonist, cimetidine

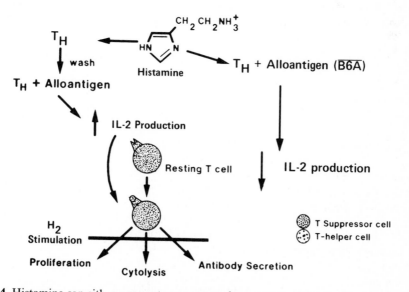

T$_H$

wash

$CH_2 CH_2 NH_3^+$

Histamine

T$_H$ + Alloantigen ($\overline{B6A}$)

T$_H$ + Alloantigen

IL-2 Production

Resting T cell

IL-2 production

H$_2$ Stimulation

Proliferation

Cytolysis

Antibody Secretion

- T Suppressor cell
- T-helper cell

Fig. 4. Histamine can either augment or suppress the secretion of interleukin 2 by T cells, depending on the immune circumstances. The brief exposure of histamine to T cells and subsequent washing results in enhanced IL-2 secretion, whereas if histamine is present with the cells at all times, the IL-2 secretion is suppressed

diated via indirect effects on IL-2 secretion (KHAN et al. 1985a). Activation of suppressor T cells and inhibition of IL-2 secretion by histamine are mediated by H_2 receptors.

Recently, a prominent role of H_1 receptors in the modulation of lymphoid cells with an apparent null phenotype has emerged (KHAN et al. 1985b, 1986c). STROBER (1984) has reported the appearance of naturally occurring suppressor cells in the spleens of neonatal or irradiated mice that may have a key role in the induction of immune tolerance. These cells are related to natural killer cells in terms of their surface phenotype, but differ in function from natural killer cells. The natural suppressor cells have the unique feature of inhibiting the antigen-specific cytolytic arm of the alloreactive immune response, but leaving the antigen-specific suppressive arm intact. It appears that such natural suppressor cells may play an important role in preventing the development of host-versus-graft and graft-versus-host diseases in allogeneic bone marrow chimeras, and in immune tolerance in the neonate and total lymphoid irradiated mice.

Natural suppressor cells possess both H_1 and H_2 receptors (KHAN et al. 1985a; KHAN et al. 1987). Only recently have we found that H_1 activity enhances the function of the natural suppressor cells, whereas the biologic role for H_2 receptors remains to be determined. The stimulation of H_2 receptors enhances the intracellular accumulation of cAMP, whereas the second messenger associated with H_1 receptors has not yet been found (KHAN et al. 1986c). Thus, it now appears that histamine's immune modulatory role can range through both early signal responses to antigen (e.g., stimulation of natural suppressors or T suppressor cells) and late phenotypic expression (e.g., inhibition of T cytolytic effects or lymphokine production) of the immune response (Tables 1 and 2).

Several investigators have reported direct effects of histamine agonists and antagonists on the function of B cells. The precise mechanisms of these observations

Table 1. Effects of histamine on cells and factors important in the immune response

Cell function	Effect	Subtype of histamine receptor involved	
		H_1	H_2
T cell proliferation	Inhibition	?	+
	Augmentation	?	
Suppressor T cell activity	Augmentation		+
Natural suppressor cell activity	Augmentation	+	
Interleukin 2 secretion	Augmentation	?	?
	Suppression	?	?
Cytotoxic T cells	Suppression of cytolysis		+
Histamine-induced suppressor factor	Release		+
Macrophages	Increased respiratory burst	+	
	Suppression of complement synthesis		+
Mast cell	Inhibition of release		+
Neutrophils	Chemotaxis		+

Table 2. Effect of histamine on the cell surface markers of lymphoid cell

Receptor	Effect
SRBC	↑
CD8	↓
CD4	↑
Fc portion of IgG (μ)	↓
Fc portion of IgG (γ)	↑

have not been defined, but they include inhibition of production and/or release of antibody in direct relationship to cAMP accumulation (BOURNE et al. 1974). In addition, H_1 receptor agonists inhibit pokeweed mitogen-induced proliferation of B cells. Finally, it has been suggested that histamine regulates the expression of many cell surface antigens. A partial list includes the Fc portion of IgG (T_γ), OKT8, and OKT4 (BIRCH et al. 1982; NAIR and SCHWARTZ 1983; WHITE and BALLOW 1985). Some of the effects are shown in Table 2.

C. Catecholamines

The naturally occurring catecholamines include epinephrine, norepinephrine, and dopamine. The active principle from suprarenal extracts exhibiting pressor effects was named adrenaline (epinephrine) by Abel in 1899. Ahlquist proposed that the discrete effects of epinephrine, norepinephrine, and isoproterenol on various tissues were mediated by two distinct receptors which were designated as α and β. LANDS et al. (1967 a,b) proposed the presence of two distinct populations of β receptors denoted β_1 and β_2. The α receptors also have been subclassified into α_1 and α_2 categories.

Like imidazoles, β-adrenergic agents can alter various elements of the immune response. Under appropriate conditions (analogous to the varied effects histamine can have in immune regulation), catecholamines can inhibit or augment antibody production. They can inhibit mitogen-induced lymphocyte proliferation, T cell-mediated cytolysis, release of lysosomal hydrolases from human neutrophils, and the release of mediators from mast cells.

A majority of the actions of catecholamines via their β-adrenergic receptors are mediated by activation of adenylate cyclase and subsequent accumulation of intracellular cAMP. The intracellular accumulation of cAMP in response to β-adrenergic agonists has been widely used to study the presence and possible function of β receptors on lymphoid tissues. In one group of early studies of the β-adrenergic effects on B cells, plaque-forming cells, but not precursor B cells, appeared to respond to isoproterenol. The response of the plaque formers to the β agonist was an inhibition of antibody release analogous to the effect of histamine. The conclusion that B cell precursors had no functional β receptor was indirect and based on their inability to bind to affinity labels made of insolubilized conjugates of isoproterenol (MELMON et al. 1974a,b). That impression still stands in spite of the recent availability of more sensitive and specific radioligand markers for β receptors.

Ligands that mark the β receptors have made it possible to identify and quantitate the β-adrenergic receptors on lymphoid cells directly. With [^{3}H] alprenolol and a mixture of immunologically uncommitted precursor human lymphoid cells, approximately 2000 β receptors per average cell can be assayed. We reconfirmed the observation that at least some precursors of immunologically uncommitted lymphoid cells and separated subsets of human T cells, helper cells, cytolytic cells, and suppressor cells, possessed β-adrenergic receptors on their cell surface. (Khan et al. 1986b) In addition, the number of receptors per cell on each subset was proportional to the maximal cAMP generated by a given subset when stimulated by a β-adrenergic agonist. Suppressor T cells possessed approximately 2900 receptors per cell, cytolytic T cells had about 1800 receptors per cell, and helper T cells had about 750 receptors per cell. These data demonstrate that β-adrenergic receptors for autacoids are nonrandomly distributed on human lymphoid tissue. Recently, β-adrenergic receptors have also been found on natural killer cells.

The role of β-adrenergic stimulation of classical receptors in modulating the function of T cells, B cells, and natural killer cells has been studied in several laboratories (Hadden et al. 1970; Melmon et al. 1974a,b; Johnson et al. 1981; Hellstrand et al. 1985). The responsiveness of lymphocytes to mitogen is sensitive to the concentration and timing of the addition of a β-adrenergic agonist as well as the concentration of mitogen in the lymphoid cell culture. Apparently, the effects of concentrations of mitogen that are either above or below the optimum for mitogenic stimulation of lymphocytes are quite readily inhibited by β-adrenergic agents.

Norepinephrine and β-adrenergic agents can augment the murine primary antibody response, and the effects of norepinephrine are mediated via β-adrenergic receptors. In fact, stimulation of β-adrenergic receptors both enhances the peak quantitative antibody production and prolongs the kinetics of the antibody response to antigen. β_1 Adrenergic stimulation simply prolongs the response of the antibody production (Sanders and Munson 1984a,b). The intracellular mechanisms of the adrenergic effects are not clear. It is likely that elevation (up to 12 h) of cAMP concentrations in response to the β-adrenergic agonists is required to enhance the response in terms of the production of antibody. But the magnitude of antibody production is not predicted by the absolute levels of cAMP. It has been postulated that the magnitude of the response is dependent on the early and late ratios of cAMP to cGMP levels.

There may also be a role for α-adrenergic receptors in the modulation of antibody production. Stimulation of α_1 receptors seems to alter the kinetics of antibody production so that it peaks 1 day earlier than in nonstimulated controls. Besedovsky et al. (1981) have reported that α_2 agonists suppress the magnitude of the peak antibody response in a concentration-dependent manner. The inhibition of adenylate cyclase by activation of α_2 receptors and the activation of adenylate cyclase by β_2 agonists has been established in various tissues. It seems feasible that selective regulation of the α or β receptors can modulate the humoral immune response predictably via augmentation or inhibition, respectively.

Isoproterenol and other β agonists inhibit natural killer cell activity, while epinephrine exhibits a dual influence on their function. The preincubation of some sources of human natural killer cells with low concentrations of epinephrine (10^{-8} M) can augment their activity, whereas addition of the drug (10^{-6} M) in lymphocyte target cell cultures consistently suppresses their activity in terms of chromium release from target cells. This dichotomy of effects is yet another illustration that the effects of autacoids on immune functions are dependent not only on the concentration and timing of the addition of the drug, but also on the nature of the cellular mix (immune circumstance) that the drugs encounter.

Investigations of catecholamine effects on immune modulation are in an earlier stage of development than imidazoles, but it is already becoming apparent that some of the immune-related events that have a graded influence on responsiveness to histamine do not affect the responses to catecholamines. That is, T suppressor cells regulate histamine receptors on T cytolytic cells but do not regulate the expression of catecholamine receptors on the same cells. Incubation of T cytolytic cells with allogeneic targets, increases their histamine responsiveness as a function of time of incubation, but responsiveness to catecholamines remains constant. Mitogens affect the responsiveness of T helper cells to histamine, but not to catecholamines.

D. Prostaglandins and Leukotrienes

Several textbooks contain detailed descriptions of the synthetic and metabolic pathways of the prostaglandins (PG) and leukotrienes (SAMUELSSON 1983; SAMUELSSON and PAOLETTI 1981; SAMUELSSON et al. 1980) and the major metabolic pathways are briefly illustrated in Figs. 5 and 6 (see also Chap. 15). Numerous studies have implicated a modulatory role for prostaglandins on immune function. For example, low concentrations of PGE_2 can alter responses to mitogens

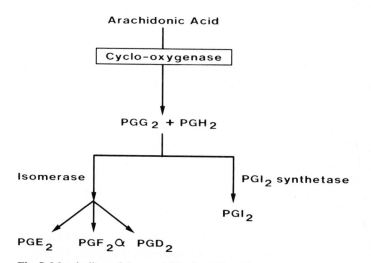

Fig. 5. Metabolites of the arachidonic acid: cyclooxygenase pathway

or antigens (Goodwin et al. 1978; Novagrodsky et al. 1980), E-rosette formation (Erten et al. 1980), the generation/function of cytolytic T cells (Leung and Mihich 1980), and lymphokine production (Rappaport and Dodge 1983).

Smith et al. (1971) demonstrated that some prostaglandins enhanced intracellular cAMP concentrations and suppressed PHA-induced lymphocyte transformation. Because some prostaglandins altered cAMP levels in lymphoid cells, they became candidates as potential immune modulators. However, the data from experiments testing their immune modulatory role are somewhat confusing. The effects are variable and sometimes directly conflicting. PGE_2, for example, blocks mast cell degranulation by increasing intracellular cAMP concentrations (Kaliner and Austen 1974), whereas $PGF_2\alpha$ enhances stimulated mast cell degranulation via its ability to increase cGMP concentrations (Kaliner 1977).

Undoubtedly, as we have seen with histamine and catecholamines, the experimental design *may be* unavoidably complex and inconsistent. Usually, prostaglandin function in vitro has been tested on mixtures of immunocompetent cells. Not only is the mixture of cells quite complex and probably not reproducible, but we are not sure which of the lymphocytes respond to prostaglandins, which metabolize them, and what cells are able to produce them. The heterogeneous sets of cells involved in immune regulation, which include T cells, B cells, null cells, natural killer (N cells K), monocytes, and macrophages, can synthesize and respond to a variety of arachidonic acid metabolites, and the mixture of these metabolites is likely to vary from experiment to experiment. Numerous cell-cell interactions between various subsets of lymphoid cells and various negative and positive feedback signals make it difficult to evaluate the specific function of a given prostaglandin on individual phases of humoral and cellular immunity. Nevertheless, we do have some valuable information on some of their capabilities to modify immunity. One of the commonest models employed to study the effects of prostaglandins on lymphoid cells has been their effect on proliferation caused by mitogens and/or antigens. The prostaglandins can inhibit the proliferation of lymphoid cells, but, as was discussed with catecholamines, the degree of suppression is dependent on the concentration of mitogen (Lewis 1983). The mechanism involved in suppression of lymphocyte proliferation by prostaglandins is not clear, although several possibilities have been proposed. Some forms of suppression may be mediated by macrophages, which store and secrete prostaglandins. In fact, removal of macrophages from lymphoid cell populations augments the lymphocyte response to mitogens.

The effects of prostaglandins on the secretion of lymphokines are also hard to understand. While they inhibit the production of migration-inhibitory factor (MIF), their effects on osteoclast-activating factors do not appear to be substantial. PGE can suppress the functions of both cytotoxic T cells and NK cells. But, once again, it is not hard to find contradictory data, which probably reflects differences in experimental design. Kendall and Targan (1980) and Targan (1981) have suggested that PGE can either inhibit or augment NK cell function, depending on the circumstances of testing.

Apparently, PGE can suppress many functions of lymphoid cells. Morley (1974) has proposed that PGE, derived from macrophages, may be an extracellular modulator of lymphoid cell function and, as PGE release from these cells

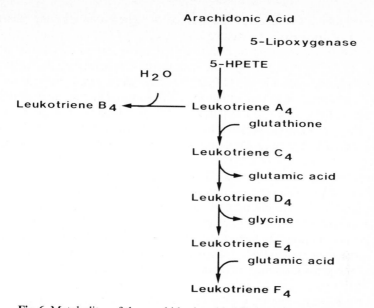

Fig. 6. Metabolites of the arachidonic acid: 5-lipoxygenase pathway

can be stimulated by lymphokines, a PGE_2-dependent negative feedback loop on lymphoid cell function can be postulated. Antigenic stimuli activate macrophage-lymphocyte interaction via production of interleukin 1 (IL-1) (WEBB and NOWO-WIEJSKI 1981). IL-1 stimulates T cells to release interleukin 2 (IL-2), and the cascade of autacoid effects proceeds. GOODWIN and WEBB (1981) have suggested that PGE may also augment the generation of suppressor cells by a negative feedback mechanism. Again, timing and circumstances seem key determinants of the net effect of an agonist. These data are discussed in more detail in Chap. 15.

The leukotrienes (LT) are derived from arachidonic acid by lipoxygenase enzymes (Fig. 6). Three lipoxygenase enzymes produce 5-, 12-, or 15-hydroperoxy-eicosatetraenoic acids (HPETEs). The HPETEs are then converted to either the corresponding HETE or to the unstable epoxide intermediates $5,6\text{-}LTA_4$, $11,12\text{-}LTA_4$, and $14,15\text{-}LTA_4$, which in turn can be converted to a number of dihydroxyeicosatetraenoic acids (di-HETEs). The latter two products (from 12- and 15-HPETEs) are relatively biologically inactive. In contrast, the metabolic products of $5,6\text{-}LTA_4$, which include LTB_4, LTC_4, LTD_4, and LTE_4, are very active biologically. LTC_4, LTD_4, and LTE_4 are responsible for the activity previously described as slow-reacting substances of anaphylaxis (SRS-A). LTF_4 can also be biochemically synthesized in vitro from LTE_4. These complex pathways and factors that alter the availability of leukotrienes are described in standard textbooks and reviews (SAMUELSSON 1983).

Leukotrienes are released by cells in the lungs and by leukocytes during inflammatory and hypersensitivity reactions. The cysteinyl-containing leukotrienes are potent bronchoconstrictors that increase vascular permeability in postcapillary venules and stimulate mucus secretion. LTB_4 causes adhesion and chemotactic movement of leukocytes and stimulates aggregation, enzyme release, and generation of superoxide by neutrophils. LTC_4, LTD_4, and LTE_4 that are released from the lung tissue of asthmatic subjects exposed to specific allergens seem to play a pathophysiologic role in immediate hypersensitivity reactions.

ROLA-PLESZCZYNSKI et al. (1983a, b) have investigated the role of leukotrienes as potential immunomodulators. LTB_4 induced human suppressor cell activity. The induced suppressor cell was a T cell, but it required the presence of adherent cells to exert its suppressive activity. In addition, LTB_4 at very low concentrations enhances the cytotoxic activity of human peripheral blood lymphocytes (PBL).

With the exception of cytotoxic T cell activity, the predominant in vitro effect of LTB_4 on T lymphocytes is suppressive. LTB_4 can suppress the T lymphocyte generation of leukocyte-inhibitory factor (LIF) and mitogen-stimulated proliferation of human PBL. Other leukotrienes, including LTC_4, LTD_4, LTE_4, or $12(s)$-LTB_4, do not suppress the generation of LIF activity nor the proliferation of mitogen-stimulated human PBL. PAYAN and GOETZL (1983) have shown that LTB_4 prevents the generation and/or release of LIF, but does not alter the expression of LIF activity.

Leukotrienes (primarily LTB_4) increase IL-1 production by human monocytes, macrophages, and neutrophils. IL-1 is a 15 kdalton polypeptide and is a regulator of several subsets of lymphoid cells (see Chap. 7). The leukotriene augmentation of IL-1 production by monocytes is nonspecific as a variety of stimuli that initiate the IL-1 response will be augmented by the leukotriene (ROLA-PLESZCZYNSKI and LEMAIRE 1985).

LTB_4 can help to generate active suppressor cells by two pathways: (a) the substance directly activates Leu-2$^+$ suppressor/effector cells in the absence of accessory cells and (b) the substance also interacts with Leu-2$^-$ cells (probably the Leu-3$^+$ subset) from which a fraction is induced to become Leu-2$^+$ cells. This induction by LTB_4 of a predominantly Leu-2$^+$ suppressor cell population appears to require monocytes as a "second signal." The ability of monocytes to synthesize cyclooxygenase products (e.g., thromboxane and prostaglandins) is essential to the activating process. In fact, prostaglandins could actually be the second signal and replace the requirement for monocytes. Inhibition of cyclooxygenase reverses the LTB_4-induced suppression and creates a "helper" effect. Perhaps in such circumstances LTB_4 interacts predominantly with Leu-3$^+$ cells, activating them to exert a helper effect via IL-2 secretion. Finally, LTB_4 may stimulate both IL-1 and IL-2 production.

E. Concluding Remarks

Until a few years ago, autacoids were not considered as even minor contributors to the function of lymphocytes. When it turned out that release of autacoids could be initiated by immune-related events, investigators accepted the role of the autacoids as contributors to inflammation associated with the immune process. Yet, little attention was paid to the possibility that autacoids could substantially affect the immune response itself.

Teleologically, it may be assumed that elements involved in an inflammatory process should regulate the immune response that would otherwise probably be evoked by inflammation. Certainly, inflammation generates immunogens; peptides appear and proteins are conformationally altered as the pH in tissues drops and macrophages process potential immunogens that in no way resemble self. What better candidate for immune modulators than substances that are almost always present at the inflammatory site?

Such a possibility gained credence when it was found that lymphocytes responsible for the immune response expressed receptors for selected autacoids. The function of the autacoids was difficult to pin down, but, as seen in this chapter, a good deal is now known about the chemical and biologic effects that autacoids have on lymphocyte-immunocyte function. Such interactions also sug-

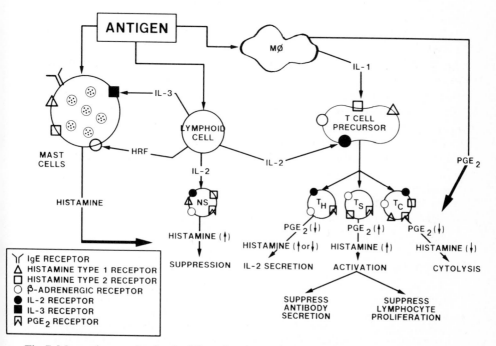

Fig. 7. Macrophage activation by T lymphocyte products or antigen results in the secretion of macrophage factors, e.g., interleukin 1. Interleukin 1 is needed for the secretion of a second lymphokine, interleukin 2. Interleukin 2 causes the clonal expansion of the subsets of T cells (T_S, T_H, T_C). T cells also secrete a third growth factor, interleukin 3, which is required for the proliferation of mucosal mast cells. Mast cells are the primary storage site of histamine and possess cell surface receptors for IgE, histamine, β agonists, and some prostaglandins. Mast cells release histamine in response to an antigen. T cells also secrete a histamine-releasing factor (HRF) which causes the secretion of histamine. Histamine can augment the suppressive capacity of natural suppressor and suppressor T cells, and can suppress the function of helper and cytolytic T cells. Histamine is also the feedback stimulus to inhibit further release of histamine from mast cells via histamine type 2 receptors. PGE_2, produced either by the activated macrophages or by other cells at the site of the inflammation, suppresses the secretion of IL-1 and IL-2, and enhances the suppressive capacity of suppressor T cells. The *arrows* indicate an increase or decrease in the function by histamine and PGE_2

gest a role for cells such as mast cells which generate autacoids and which are widely distributed at the sites of generation of the immune response. They are present in the lymph nodes, thymus, and sites of graft and tumor rejection (Fig. 7). What is their role if not to carry mediators of inflammation and modulators of immunity?

Further work has shown that the receptors for autacoids are not randomly distributed on lymphocytes. The receptors for histamine are present on natural suppressor cells, and emerge and disappear selectively on T cytolytic cells as a function of their environment and the presence or absence of mitogenic transformation. A variety of ways for finely tuned immunologic responses to autacoids, regardless of their concentration or persistence, thus become possible. Many more will become apparent as we continue to upgrade our focus on the nonoverlapping activities of histamine, catecholamines, prostaglandins, and the leukotrienes as immune modulators.

This is an exciting time for the field of immune modulation by autacoids. Many studies have already been carried out in both experimental animals and humans to test the capacity of autacoids to act as important immune modulators. However, the message has not been widely appreciated as the antihistamines, prostaglandins, nonsteroidal anti-inflammatory agents, etc., have been used for purposes other than immune modulation. It will probably not be long before we see experiments in animals, including humans, designed to test the effects of cimetidine, ranitidine, naproxen, aspirin, or indomethacin on the potentiation of IL-2 effects, or in other settings when augmentation of immunity is desirable. It may not even be too long before we see autacoids or their derivatives used as immune modulators.

Acknowledgment. This work was in part supported by NIH grant HL26340.

References

Beer DJ, Dinarello CA, Rosenwasser LJ, Rocklin RE (1982a) Human monocyte-derived soluble product(s) has an accessory function in the generation of histamine and concanavalin A-induced suppressor T cells. J Clin Invest 70:393–400

Beer DJ, Rosenwasser LJ, Dinarello CA, Rocklin RE (1982b) Cellular interactions in the generation and expression of histamine-induced suppressor activity. Cell Immunol 69:101–112

Befus AD, Bienenstock J (1979) Immunologically mediated intestinal mastocytosis in *Nippestrongylus brasiliensis* infected rats. Immunology 38:95–101

Besedovsky HO, DaPrada M, del Rey A, Sorkin E (1981) Immunoregulation by sympathetic nervous system. Trans Pharmacol Sci 2:236–238

Birch RE, Rosenthal AK, Polmer SH (1982) Pharmacological modification of immunoregulatory T lymphocytes. II. Modulation of T lymphocyte cell surface characteristics. Clin Exp Immunol 48:231–238

Bourne HR, Lichtenstein LM, Melmon KL, Henney CS, Weinstein Y, Shearer GM (1974) Modulation of inflammation and immunity by cyclic AMP. Science 184:19–28

Brostoff J, Pack S, Lydyard PM (1980) Histamine suppression of lymphocyte activation in normal subjects and atopics. Clin Exp Immunol 39:739–745

Burnet FM (1965) Mast cells in the thymus of NZB mice. J Pathol Bacteriol 89:271–284

Cameron W, Doyle K, Rocklin RE (1986) Histamine type 1 (H₁) receptor radioligand binding studies on normal T cell subsets, B cells and monocytes. J Immunol 136:2116–2120

Coffey RG, Hadden JW (1985) Neurotransmitter hormones and cyclic nucleotide in lymphocyte regulation. Fed Proc Exp Biol 44:112–117

Dale MM, Foreman JC (1984) Histamine as a mediator of allergic and inflammatory reactions. In: Dale MM, Foreman JC (eds) Textbook of immunopharmacology. Blackwell, Oxford, p 115

Douglas WW (1985) Histamine and 5-hydroxy tryptamine (serotonin) and their antagonists. In: Gilman AG, Goodman LS, Gilman A (eds) The pharmacological basis of therapeutics. Macmillan, New York

Erten U, Emre T, Cavdar AO, Turner RK (1980) In vitro study on the effect of prostaglandin E_2 and F_2 alpha on E-rosette forming activity of normal lymphocytes. Prostaglandins Med 5:255–258

Ginsberg H, Lagunoff D (1967) The in vitro differentiation of mast cells. J Cell Biol 35:685–697

Goodwin JS, Webb DR (1981) Regulation of immune response by prostaglandins. In: Goodwin JS (ed) Suppressor cells in human disease. Dekker, New York, pp 99–135

Goodwin JS, Messner RP, Peake GT (1978) Prostaglandin suppression of mitogen stimulated lymphocytes in vitro. Changes with mitogen dose and preincubation. J Clin Invest 62:753–760

Hadden JW, Hadden EM, Middleton EJ (1970) Lymphocyte blast formation. I. Demonstration of adrenergic receptors in human peripheral lymphocytes. Cell Immunol 1:583–595

Hellstrand K, Hermodsson S, Strannengrad O (1985) Evidence for a β-adrenoceptor mediated regulation of human natural killer cells. J Immunol 134:4095–4099

Hill HR, Estensen RD, Quie PG (1975) Modulation of human neutrophil chemotactic responses by cyclic 3'5'-guanosine monophosphate and cyclic 3'5'-adenosine monophosphate. Metabolism 24:447–456

Johnson DL, Ashmore RC, Gordon MA (1981) Effects of β-adrenergic agents on the murine lymphocyte response to mitogen stimulation. J Immunopharmacol 3:205–219

Kaliner M (1977) Human lung tissue and anaphylaxis. I. The role of cyclic GMP as a modulator of the immunologically induced secretion process. J Allerg Clin Immunol 60:204–211

Kaliner M, Austen F (1974) Cyclic AMP, ATP and reversed anaphylactic histamine release from rat mast cells. J Immunol 112:664–674

Kendall R, Targan S (1980) The dual effect of prostaglandin (PGE_2) and ethanol on the natural killer cytolytic process: effector activation and NK cell-target cell conjugate lytic inhibition. J Immunol 125:2770–2777

Khan MM, Melmon KL (1985) Are autacoids more than theoretic modulators of immunity? Clin Immunol Rev 4:1–30

Khan MM, Melmon KL, Fathman CG, Hertel-Walff B, Strober S (1985a) The effects of autacoids on cloned murine lymphoid cells: modulation of IL-2 secretion and the activity of natural suppressor cells. J Immunol 134:4100–4106

Khan MM, Sansoni P, Engleman EG, Melmon KL (1985b) The pharmacologic effects of autacoids on subsets of human T cells. Regulation of expression/function of H_2 receptors by a subset of suppressor cells. J Clin Invest 75:1578–1583

Khan MM, Silverman ED, Engleman EG, Melmon KL (1985c) Responses of autacoids in subsets of human helper T cells. Proc West Pharmacol Soc 28:225–228

Khan MM, Keaney KM, Krensky AM, Melmon KL (1986a) The modulation of generation/function of human cytotoxic lymphocytes by autacoids: unusually compartmentalized cAMP? Proc West Pharmacol Soc 29:31–34

Khan MM, Sansoni P, Silverman ED, Engleman EG, Melmon KL (1986b) Beta adrenergic receptors on human suppressor helper and cytolytic lymphocytes. Biochem Pharmacol 35:1137–1142

Khan MM, Marr-Leisy D, Verlander MS, Bristow MR, Strober S, Goodman M, Melmon KL (1986c) The effects of derivatives of histamine on natural suppressor cells. J Immunol 137:308–314

Khan MM, Strober S, Melmon KL (1986d) Regulatory effects of mast cells on lymphoid cells: the role of histamine type 1 receptors in the interactions between mast cells, helper T cells and natural suppressor cells. Cell Immunol 103:41–53

Khan MM, Wilson AL, Melmon KL (1987) Characterization of histamine type 1 receptors on natural suppressor lymphoid cells. Biochem Pharmacol 36:3867–3871

Kitamura Y, Shimada M, Hatanaka K, Miyano Y (1977) Development of mast cells from grafted bone marrow cells in irradiated mice. Nature 268:442–443

Kitamura YM, Shimada M, Go S, Matsuda H, Hatanaka K, Seki M (1979) Distribution of mast cell precursors in hematopoietic and lymphopoietic tissues of mice. J Exp Med 150:482–490

Lands AM, Arnold A, McAuliff JP, Luduena FP, Brown TG (1967a) Differentiation of receptor systems activated by sympathomimetic amines. Nature 214:597–598

Lands AM, Luduena FP, Buzzo HJ (1967b) Differentiation of receptors responsive to iso-proterenol. Life Sci 6:2241–2249

Leung KH, Mihich E (1980) Prostaglandin modulation of development of cell mediated immunity in culture. Nature 288:597

Lewis GP (1983) Immunoregulatory activity of metabolites of arachidonic acid and their role in inflammation. Br Med Bull 39:243–248

Lewis GP, Mangham BA (1978) Changes in blood flow and mediator content of rabbit skin grafts. Br J Pharmacol 64:123–128

Lichtenstein LM (1976) The interdependence of allergic and inflammatory processes. In: Johansson SGO, Standberg K, Uvnas B (eds) Molecular and biological aspects of the acute allergic reaction. Plenum, New York, p 233

Lima M, Rocklin RE (1981) Histamine modulates in vitro IgG production by human mononuclear cells. Cell Immunol 64:324–336

Melmon KL (1981) The endocrinologic function of selected autacoids: catecholamines, acetylcholine, serotonin and histamine. In: Williams RH (ed) Textbook of endocrinology. Saunders, Philadelphia, p 514

Melmon KL, Rocklin R, Rosenkranz RP (1981) Autacoids as modulators of inflammatory and immune response. Am J Med 71:100–106

Melmon KL, Bourne HR, Weinstein Y, Shearer GM, Krain J, Bauminger S (1974a) Hemolytic plaque formation by leukocytes in vitro. Control by vasoactive hormone. J Clin Invest 53:13–21

Melmon KL, Weinstein Y, Shearer GM, Bourne HR, Bauminger S (1974b) Separation of specific antibody-forming mouse cells by their adherence to insolubilized endogenous hormones. J Clin Invest 53:22–30

Mimh MG, Soter NA, Dvorak HF, Austen KF (1976) Structure of normal skin and the morphology of atopic eczema. J Invest Dermatol 67:305–312

Morley J (1984) Prostaglandins and lymphokines in arthritis. Prostaglandins 8:315–326

Mozes E, Weinstein Y, Bourne HR, Melmon KL, Shearer GM (1974) In vitro correction of antigen-induced immune suppression: effects of histamine, dibutyryl cyclic AMP and cholera enterotoxin. Cell Immunol 11:57–63

Nair MPN, Schwartz SA (1983) Effects of histamine and histamine antagonists on natural and antibody dependent cellular cytotoxicity of human lymphocytes in vitro. Cell Immunol 81:45

Novagrodsky A, Rubin AL, Stenzel KH (1980) A new class of inhibitors of lymphocyte mitogenesis: agents that induce erythroid differentiation in Friend-leukemia cells. J Immunol 124:1892–1897

Payan DG, Goetzl EJ (1983) Specific suppression of human T lymphocyte function by leukotriene B_4. J Immunol 131:551–553

Pepys J (1955) Fixation of tuberculin in skin of tuberculin sensitive human subject. Clin Sci 14:253–265

Rappaport RS, Dodge GR (1983) Effects of prostaglandins on the production of interleukin-2. Adv Exp Med Biol 162:77–82

Razin E, Stevens RL, Austen KL, Caulfield JP, Hein A, Liu FT, Clabby M, Nabel G, Cantor J, Friedman S (1984) Cloned mouse mast cells derived from immunized lymph node cells and from foetal liver cells exhibit characteristics of bone marrow derived mast cells containing chondroitin sulphate E proteoglycan. Immunology 52:563–575

Rocklin RE (1977) Histamine induced suppressor factor (HSF): effect on migration inhibiting factor (MIF) production and proliferation. J Immunol 118:1734–1738

Rocklin RE, Beer DJ (1983) Histamine and immune modulation. Adv Intern Med 28:225

Rocklin RE, Habarek-Davidson A (1984) Pharmacologic modulation in vitro of human histamine-induced suppressor cell activity. Int J Immunopharmacol 6:179–186

Rocklin RE, Greineder DK, Melmon KL (1979) Histamine-induced suppressor factor (HSF): further studies on the nature of the stimulus and the cell which produces it. Cell Immunol 44:404–415

Rocklin RE, Kiselis I, Beer DJ, Rossi P, Maggi F, Bellanti JA (1983) Augmentation of prostaglandin and thromboxane production by human monocytes exposed to histamine-induced suppressor factor (HSF). Cell Immunol 77:92–98

Rola-Pleszczynski M, Lemaire I (1985) Leukotrienes augment interleukin 1 production by human monocytes. J Immunol 135:3958–3961

Rola-Pleszczynski M, Borgeat P, Sirois P (1983a) Leukotriene B_4 induces human suppressor lymphocytes. Biochem Biophys Res Commun 108:15–31

Rola-Pleszczynski M, Borgeat P, Sirois P (1983b) Leukotriene B_4 augments human natural cytotoxic cell activity. Biochem Biophys Res Commun 113:531–537

Roszkowski K, Plaut M, Lichtenstein LM (1977) Selective display of histamine receptors on lymphocytes. Science 195:683–685

Samuelsson B (1983) Leukotrienes: mediators of immediate hypersensitivity reactions and inflammation. Science 220:568–575

Samuelsson B, Paoletti R (eds) (1981) Advances in prostaglandin and thromboxane research, vol 9. Raven, New York

Samuelsson B, Hammerstrom S, Murphy RC, Borgeat P (1980) Leukotrienes and SRS-A. J Allergy 35:375–381

Sanders VM, Munson AE (1984a) Beta adrenoreceptor mediation of the enhancing effect of norepinephrine on the murine primary antibody response in vitro. J Pharmacol Exp Ther 230:183–192

Sanders VM, Munson AE (1984b) Kinetics of the enhancing effect produced by norepinephrine and terbutaline on the murine primary antibody response in vitro. J Pharmacol Exp Ther 231:527–531

Sansoni P, Khan MM, Melmon KL, Engleman EG (1985) Immunoregulatory T cells in man: histamine-induced suppressed T cells are derived from a Leu2$^+$(T8$^+$) subpopulation distinct from that which gives rise to cytotoxic T cells. J Clin Invest 75:650–656

Smith JW, Steiner AL, Parker CW (1971) Human lymphocyte metabolism. Effects of cyclic and noncyclic nucleotides on stimulation by phytohemagglutinin. J Clin Invest 50:442–448

Strober S (1984) Natural suppressor (NS) cells, neonatal tolerance, and total lymphoid irradiation: exploring obscure relationships. Annu Rev Immunol 2:219–237

Targan S (1981) The dual interaction of prostaglandin E_2(PGE$_2$) and interferon (IFN) on NK lytic interaction (recycling) and blockage of pre-NK cell recruitment. J Immunol 127:1424–1428

Webb DR, Nowowiejski I (1981) Control of suppressor cell activation via endogenous prostaglandin synthesis: the role of T cells and macrophages. Cell Immunol 63:321–328

White WB, Ballow M (1985) Modulation of suppressor-cell activity by cimetidine in patients with common variable hypogammaglobulinemia. N Engl J Med 312:198

Wynne-Roberts CR, Anderson CH, Turano AM, Baron M (1978) Light and electron microscopic findings of juvenile rheumatoid arthritis synovium: comparison with normal juvenile synovium. Semin Arthritis Rheum 7:287–302

Yoo D, Lessin LS, Jensen W (1978) Bone marrow mast cells in lymphoproliferative disorders. Ann Intern Med 8:753–757

CHAPTER 15

Lipid Mediators and Lymphocyte Function

M. J. PARNHAM and W. ENGLBERGER

A. Introduction

The recognition that simple lipids are capable of modulating immune responses is a relatively recent development, which has led to an explosive growth in research over the last decade. The lipids involved are all directly or indirectly dependent on the intake of specific polyunsaturated fatty acids, the so-called essential fatty acids (EFAs), in the diet. The essentiality of these fatty acids lies in the fact that they cannot be synthesized by mammalian tissues. The dietary EFA of greatest importance for immunomodulatory lipid mediators is linoleic acid $(18:2)$[1] the precursors of the $\omega 6$ family of EFAs (first double bond at carbon-atom 6), from which γ-linolenic acid $(18:3)$ and arachidonic acid $(20:4)$ are synthesized (Fig. 1). Arachidonic acid is mainly incorporated into the 2 position of membrane phospholipids, from which it is released by hydrolysis (e.g., by phospholipase A_2) on membrane stimulation. This free arachidonic acid is then available for metabolic conversion by a number of enzymatic pathways (Fig. 1).

The major biologically active arachidonic acid metabolic products synthesized by leukocytes are prostaglandin E_2 (PGE_2), prostacyclin (PGI_2), thromboxane A_2 (TxA_2), leukotriene B_4 (LTB_4), and the peptidoleukotrienes LTC_4 and LTD_4, macrophages being the most important white blood cells as a source of these products (GEMSA et al. 1982; BONNEY and HUMES 1984). While eicosanoids, as these products are collectively termed, are generated from macrophages by a variety of stimuli, it is of great relevance to lymphocyte functions and their modulation that lymphocyte-derived lymphokines and antigen-antibody complexes are potent stimulators of PGE_2 release (and presumably other eicosanoids) from macrophages (GORDON et al. 1976; BONNEY et al. 1979). It is now widely accepted that this forms the basis for a feedback control of activated lymphocytes on their own function since it has been confirmed in a number of systems (GOLDYNE and STOBO 1980; GOODWIN and WEBB 1980; CEUPPENS and GOODWIN 1985 a). It was important to show that macrophage-derived PGE_2 is capable of modulating lymphocyte function in order to demonstrate the physiologic relevance of this mechanism; this was first reported by GORDON et al. (1976) and by the group led by WEBB, and has since been confirmed by many authors (GOODWIN and WEBB 1980). For most other eicosanoids generated by macrophages, such a physiologic, as opposed to pharmacologic action on lymphocyte function has yet to be clearly demonstrated. Lymphocytes themselves are a poor source of eicosanoids, except

---

[1] 18 C atoms, 2 double bonds.

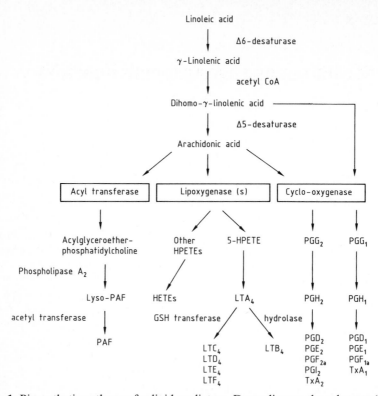

Fig. 1. Biosynthetic pathways for lipid mediators. Depending on the substrate (dihomo-γ-linolenic acid or arachidonic acid), prostaglandins (PGs) and thromboxanes (Txs) containing one or two double bonds, respectively, are formed, each by a separate enzymatic reaction. The products with one double bond are only formed in small amounts. Lipoxygenases insert a peroxide moiety into the fatty acid molecule at any one of the double bonds, forming a variety of hydroperoxy fatty acids (HPETEs). These are converted to the respective hydroxy acids (HETEs), with the exception of 5-HPETE, which is also converted to leukotrienes (LTs). Platelet-activating factor (PAF) is indirectly formed from arachidonic acid in that its precursor molecule is an arachidonyl ether phospholipid from which the fatty acid is hydrolytically removed

perhaps the lipoxygenase product, 15-HETE (GOETZL 1981) although it has been suggested that arachidonic acid from T lymphocytes can be utilized by macrophages to generate its metabolic products (GOLDYNE and STOBO 1982).

Most eicosanoids have an extensive repertoire of biologic activities, PGE_2 having been submitted to the most extensive investigation with regard to the immune system. These latter actions will be considered here, as well as the known activities of other eicosanoids on lymphocyte function. Platelet-activating factor (PAF, acetylglyceroetherphosphatidylcholine, AGEPC) is also generated from membrane phospholipids, an arachidonyl ether phospholipid being a precursor in its synthesis (Fig. 1). It is released on stimulation of a number of cell types, including macrophages, and has potent stimulatory actions on leukocyte functions (O'FLAHERTY and WYLKE 1983). An action of this lipid mediator on lymphocyte function cannot be ruled out and will be discussed.

B. Essential Fatty Acids

I. Role in Lymphocyte Activation

Linoleic and arachidonic acids are major components of the phospholipids of lymphocyte membranes (FERBER and RESCH 1976). Since there is a rapid turnover of the membrane phospholipids as a result of deacylation and reacylation reactions, the lymphocyte membrane can alter its fatty acid composition in response to variations in the lipid milieu (WEYMAN et al. 1977). In most cells, phospholipase A_2 plays an important role in the turnover of membrane phospholipids, but this enzyme has proved difficult to demonstrate in lymphocyte membranes (MERTIN and SMITH 1988). In contrast, TROTTER and FERBER (1981) have demonstrated the existence in thymocytes of an acyl-CoA: lysophosphatide acyltransferase which catalyzes the transfer of arachidonic acid from phosphatidylcholine to phosphatidylethanolamine. This suggests that in lymphocyte membranes, phospholipid turnover involves transfer of the fatty acid between phospholipids, without the participation of phospholipase A_2.

Following stimulation of lymphocytes in vitro with polyclonal mitogens, one of the first most marked changes in lymphocyte membrane phospholipids is an enhanced incorporation of polyunsaturated fatty acids into the 2 position of phosphatidylcholine and phosphatidylethanolamine, associated with activation of acyl-CoA: lysophosphatide acyltransferase (FERBER and RESCH 1976). These authors suggest that the acyltransferase-catalyzed incorporation of unsaturated fatty acids and the resulting increase in membrane fluidity is an essential factor in the coupling of membrane receptor binding and lymphocyte activation. In support of this, the acyl-CoA: lysophosphatide acyltransferase fraction of lymphocyte membranes is closely associated with the concanavalin A-binding fraction on affinity chromatography, and is clearly distinguishable from changes in other membrane-bound enzymes (RESCH 1980). Membrane changes during lymphocyte activation are discussed in detail in Chap. 3.

II. Actions on Lymphocytes In Vitro

On the basis of the foregoing one might expect that addition of arachidonic or linoleic acid to lymphocytes in vitro would stimulate or enhance lymphocyte activation. However, transformation determined by thymidine, uridine, or inositol uptake, plaque formation, immunoglobulin capping, antibody binding, and production of leukocyte migration-inhibiting factor are all inhibited by the addition of either of these two fatty acids to lymphocytes in culture (MEADE and MERTIN 1978; HOOVER et al. 1980; MERTIN 1981; MERTIN and SMITH 1988). MEADE and MERTIN (1978) have drawn attention to the fact that such effects of fatty acids are only detectable in vitro when care is taken over the dissolution of the hydrophobic lipids. Some authors used alcohol to dissolve the compounds before diluting with water, while others first bound the fatty acids to albumin. However, the ratio acid: albumin is crucial and can markedly affect the results obtained (WEYMAN et al. 1977; TONKIN and BROSTOFF 1978). In view of the role of prostaglandins in the regulation of lymphocyte function (discussed in Sect. C), it is highly likely that these inhibitory effects of EFAs in vitro are mediated by conversion of the fatty acids to PGE_2, particularly if appreciable amounts of macrophages are present, as is essential for lymphocyte proliferation. On the other hand, linoleic acid and arachidonic acid have been reported to enhance the number of avid erythrocyte-rosetting T lymphocytes in vitro, a response which may be independent of PGE_2 synthesis (Offner and Clausen 1978). At high concentrations, EFAs are cytotoxic to lymphocytes (Kageyama et al. 1980). Since arachidonic acid can be converted to such a wide variety of products (cf. Fig. 1), it is essential to rule out the mediation of the pharmacologic effects observed by the individual eicosanoids. Cyclooxygenase inhibitors, such as indomethacin, are widely employed to investigate the involvement of PGs, while the advent of dual cyclooxygenase and lipoxygenase inhibitors, such as BW755C, or more selective 5-lipoxygenase inhibitors, such as REV5901 and AA861, means that the possible role of LTs and HETEs/HPETEs can be investigated. In any case, it is important to measure levels of the individual eicosanoids formed in vitro (by radioimmunoassay or high pressure liquid chromatography) to confirm their importance, assaying stable metabolites where the active product is highly unstable (e.g., assay of 6-keto-$PGF_{1\alpha}$ for PGI_2 and TxB_2 for TxA_2).

III. Actions on Lymphocytes In Vivo

Dietary modulation of immune responsiveness and chronic autoimmune diseases has become a subject of particular interest over recent years. Because of the extensive literature on this topic, it is not possible in this brief chapter to deal with all the many facets of the activities of dietary EFAs on the immune response. The reader is referred to a number of review articles for further details (Meade and Mertin 1978; Mertin 1981; Mertin and Stackpoole 1981; Johnston and Marshall 1984; Mertin and Smith 1988).

In assessing data obtained in dietary studies, it is extremely important to define the content of fatty acids and other lipids in the food, so that the effects observed can be related solely to changes in EFAs, rather than being complicated by concomitant changes in other dietary constituents. Furthermore, the levels of arachidonic acid and/or specific eicosanoids in the cells under investigation (e.g., lymphocytes) should also be determined, since the degree of deficiency or enrichment with EFAs can vary according to the cell or organ and the period of dietary treatment. This is of particular importance when EFA-deficient diets are used (Parnham et al. 1979b). Particularly, with studies on EFA-deficient diets but with other treatments as well, it is also important to control the use of fetal calf serum (FCS) for ex vivo studies, since FCS contains EFAs and can thus modify the results obtained (King and Spector 1981; Johnston and Marshall 1984). Other factors which must be borne in mind when carrying out ex vivo studies on lymphocyte function are that the responses to in vivo EFA changes may vary, depending on the organ or tissue from which the cells are removed; the route of antigen administration (i.p. or i.v.) can also affect the intensity of the lymphocyte response, and the concentration of mitogen is crucial in proliferation studies, so that a mitogen concentration-response curve is desirable (Johnston and Marshall 1984).

Bearing these factors in mind, it can be stated that most studies have shown that an EFA-deficient diet leads to an enhancement of lymphocyte responses ex vivo, including T cell proliferation to mitogens or antigens, numbers of plaque-forming cells, and the passive transfer of the delayed-type hypersensitivity (DTH) response in rats (PARNHAM et al. 1979a; MERTIN and STACKPOOLE 1981; JOHNSTON and MARSHALL 1984). Other immune responses which are also enhanced by EFA deficiency include skin allograft rejection in mice and susceptibility to experimental allergic encephalomyelitis in rats (MERTIN 1981; MERTIN and SMITH 1988). These studies would appear to support the in vitro data on the immunosuppressive actions of EFAs on lymphocyte function, possibly through conversion to PGE_2. However, other authors have reported inhibitory effects of EFA deficiency on immune responses in vivo, including DTH in mice, mortality, appearance of dsDNA-specific antibodies and kidney damage in NZB/NZW F_1 mice, and incidence of methylcholanthrene-induced tumors in mice (MERTIN and HUNT 1976; DEWILLE et al. 1981; HURD and GILLIAM 1981). While a selective effect of the reduction of EFA content on a specific lymphocyte subpopulation cannot be ruled out as an explanation for these data, it seems more likely that a reduction in membrane fluidity, resulting from EFA deficiency, probably leads to reduced antigenicity of autoantigens, tumor antigens, and possibly antigen presentation in DTH.

That the pharmacologic response to EFAs in vivo is predominantly immunosuppression has clearly been demonstrated by a number of authors, in particular by MERTIN and his colleagues. Among immune responses inhibited by linoleic and/or arachidonic acid in vivo are skin allograft rejection and graft-versus-host and host-versus-graft reactions in mice and experimental allergic encephalomyelitis in rats and guinea pigs, as well as lymphocyte proliferation to mitogens and antigens and numbers of splenic plaque-forming cells (Ig^+ cells) ex vivo, while thymus weight is reduced (MERTIN 1981; MERTIN and STACKPOOLE 1981; JOHNSTON and MARSHALL 1984; MERTIN et al. 1985; MERTIN and SMITH 1988). It appears that the spleen is an important target for the immunoinhibitory effects of EFAs since splenectomy abrogated the suppression by EFAs of experimental allergic encephalomyelitis, skin allograft survival, and the decrease in thymus weight (MERTIN et al. 1977; MERTIN and STACKPOOLE 1979). Because splenic structural integrity was essential and splenic cells could only reconstitute the inhibitory action of the EFAs on allograft rejection when given on the day of grafting, the authors suggested that EFAs induce splenic suppressor cell activity (MERTIN and STACKPOOLE 1981). A marked increase in splenic PG formation occurs soon after antigen challenge of mice (WEBB and OSHEROFF 1976), while suppression of experimental allergic encephalomyelitis in rats by EFAs is abolished by the cyclooxygenase inhibitor indomethacin and the inhibitory effects of EFAs on graft-versus-host and host-versus-graft response are abrogated by anti-PGE serum (MERTIN and STACKPOOLE 1978; MERTIN et al. 1985). It thus seems likely that EFAs, through conversion to PGE, act, during the induction phase of cell-mediated immune responses, by stimulating T suppressor cells and/or the prostaglandin-induced T cell-derived suppressor factors (PITS), discussed in Sect. C.I.1.f. Data such as these have encouraged clinical trials with diets containing high EFA concentrations with beneficial effects in renal transplantation, multiple sclerosis, and rheumatoid arthritis (McHugh et al. 1977; Mertin 1985; Kremer et al. 1985).

C. Prostaglandin E

PGE_2 is one of the major products of stimulated macrophages (Gemsa et al. 1982; Bonney and Humes 1984) and has been subjected to the most intensive immunologic studies of all the eicosanoids. In many pharmacologic studies, however, PGE_1 has been used, partially because it is somewhat more effective at stimulating adenylate cyclase in vitro than is PGE_2. However, a wide variety of immunoinflammatory data indicate that the effects of PGE_1 and PGE_2 are essentially identical (with the exception of actions on platelets), so that the actions of the two eicosanoids on lymphocyte function can be considered conjointly (Bonta and Parnham 1978).

I. Cell-Mediated Immunity

1. Effects In Vitro

a) Inhibitory Concentrations

One of the most important points to bear in mind in any consideration of the in vitro effects of eicosanoids is the concentration at which they are shown to exert biologic effects. The concentrations of PGE_2 found in inflammatory exudates are in the lower nanogram per milliliter range (i.e., 10^{-8}–10^{-7} mol/l) so that physiologic effects of PGE_2 are expected at these concentrations. In early studies, carried out in the 1970s, PGE_2 was shown to inhibit a number of lymphocyte responses at higher concentration, including T cell proliferation, lymphokine production, cytolysis, and hemolytic plaque formation (Goodwin and Webb 1980). The elegant studies of Gordon et al. (1976), however, clearly demonstrated that PGE_2 and PGE_1 inhibited guinea pig lymphocyte lymphokine (macrophage migration-inhibitory factor, MIF) production in vitro at concentrations which were generated in vitro by macrophages stimulated with guinea pig lymphokines. Commensurate with this, the PG synthesis inhibitor, indomethacin enhanced antigen (tuberculin, PPD)-induced MIF production at concentrations which inhibited PGE_2 formation. Consequently, antigen stimulation of T cells generates lymphokines which stimulate PGE_2 production by macrophages. The concentrations of PGE_2 generated are then able to inhibit T cell lymphokine formation by negative feedback. The authors reported further that PGE_1 and PGE_2 inhibited lymphocyte proliferation, an action not shared by PGA_1 or $PGF_{2\alpha}$. This lack of activity of the A and F series PGs is an important fact to bear in mind, as indomethacin, being a cyclooxygenase inhibitor, could theoretically cause changes in lymphocyte function in vitro by inhibiting the synthesis of a number of eicosanoids. Since these data were reported, a wide variety of T cell responses have been shown to be inhibited by PGE in vitro at physiologic concentrations (10^{-8} mol/l or less). These responses include mitogen responsiveness, antigenic stimulation, erythrocyte rosette formation, and T cell cytotoxicity (Ceuppens and Goodwin

1985a). High affinity binding sites for [³H] PGE$_1$ and [³H] PGE$_2$ have been reported on rat thymocytes and human peripheral blood monocytes, with K_d values in both systems of about 2×10^{-9} mol/l (GOODWIN and WEBB 1980). In human lymphocytes, this rapid binding was associated with a secondary slow binding (over a period of 30–40 min) with a K_d of 6×10^{-9} mol/l (GOODWIN et al. 1979a). The authors suggested, on the basis of temperature dependency, that the secondary process reflected uptake of the labeled PGE. Since the K_d was lower than the IC$_{50}$ of PGE$_2$ against mitogen-induced lymphocyte proliferation ($\sim 10^{-8}$ mol/l), the authors also suggested that binding of the PGE to the 20% FCS present in the incubation medium may have affected the effective concentration measured. As for EFAs, discussed previously, the concentration of FCS and other proteins in the medium must always be carefully controlled and considered in any interpretation of data on the effects of PGE in vitro. It has, in fact, been shown that, in the absence of serum, PGE$_1$ is highly effective in inhibiting phytohemagglutinin (PHA)-induced human lymphocyte proliferation (OKAZAKI et al. 1978).

b) Cyclic AMP Enhancement

As with almost all cell types studied as targets of PGE, cell surface binding and the subsequent inhibition of lymphocyte function by this eicosanoid are associated with an increase in intracellular cyclic AMP levels (BONTA and PARNHAM 1978; GOODWIN and WEBB 1980). GOODWIN et al. (1981) have shown that the concentration-response curve for PGE$_2$ in enhancing human lymphocyte cyclic AMP closely parallels that for its inhibition of mitogenesis. Prolonged incubation of lymphocytes with PGE$_1$ or PGE$_2$ for over 2 h results in desensitization to its stimulatory action on intracellular cyclic AMP (NORDEEN and YOUNG 1978; WEBB 1978). The physiologic relevance of this desensitization is unclear, but the phenomenon must be born in mind when studying effects of PGE in vitro. Differences have been reported in the sensitivity of mouse lymphocytes from the spleen, lymph nodes, thymus, and peripheral blood to the cyclic AMP-enhancing properties of PGE, the mature, cortisone-resistant thymocytes being particularly unresponsive, probably owing to a general insensitivity to cyclic AMP-enhancing agents (BACH 1975; WEBB 1978; ROJO et al. 1982). In human peripheral blood lymphocytes, GOODWIN et al. (1979b) have shown that T$_\gamma$ cells (bearing receptors for the Fc portion of IgG) are approximately sevenfold more sensitive to the cyclic AMP-enhancing properties of PGE$_2$ than the remaining non-T$_\gamma$ cells. They suggested that this finding reflects heterogeneity in the distribution of PGE$_2$ receptors among T cells. This would further suggest that PGE$_2$ acts preferentially on subpopulations of T lymphocytes, a finding supported by results on the inhibitory actions of PGE on lymphocyte functional responses.

c) Differential Sensitivities of Various T Cell Populations

While differential sensitivities of lymphocyte populations to PGE have been reported, it is by no means clear how these differences relate to one another. Both ROJO et al. (1982) and SANCHEZ et al. (1979) reported that T cells from mice and humans, respectively, were more sensitive to PGE than B cells, although in the former study PGE$_2$ inhibited T cell proliferation to concanavalin A, while in the latter, PGE_1 enhanced the number of surface measles virus-binding sites. The sensitivity of human T cell responses to PGE_1 and PGE_2 has been further differentiated into high density cells whose proliferative response to PHA is highly sensitive to inhibition by PGE, and into $OKT4^+$ (helper/inducer T cells) and $OKT8^+$ (suppressor/cytotoxic T cells), proliferation of $OKT4^+$ cells to PHA being inhibited and that of $OKT8^+$ cells being markedly augmented (STOBO et al. 1979; GUALDE and GOODWIN 1982). These data seem to reflect a selectively suppressive action of PGE, augmenting T suppressor cell activity and inhibiting T helper cell activity, as discussed in Sect. C.I.1.f. In any case, the findings highlight an important point in studies on the effects of PGE on lymphocyte function in vitro, namely, that while this eicosanoid is predominantly inhibitory, stimulatory effects may also be observed. These include stimulation of suppressor cells under certain conditions, as described by GUALDE and GOODWIN (1982) and other authors, and induction of theta antigen in splenic cells (CEUPPENS and GOODWIN 1985a). A possible explanation for this apparent paradox of inhibitory and stimulatory actions of PGE may be found in the proposal (MERTIN and SMITH 1986) that the action of PGE on the induction of cell-mediated immune responses can be represented by a bell-shaped concentration-response curve, stimulatory at low concentrations and inhibitory at higher concentrations. One can add to this the effect of the period of treatment with PGE, as exemplified by the finding that overnight preincubation of human lymphocytes enhances their sensitivity to inhibition by PGE_2 (GUALDE and GOODWIN 1982). Thus, not only are T cell responses in vitro differentially sensitive to the concentration of PGE_2 added, but also to the time of addition. Indeed, LEUNG and MIHICH (1982) have proposed that PGE only inhibits T cell proliferation and cytotoxicity during the induction phase of the response, although some contradictory data have been obtained which are as yet unexplained (WARREN et al. 1983).

SIMS et al. (1979) have drawn attention to a further source of possible error in determining the effects of PGE_2 on lymphocyte proliferation in vitro. They found that, while the response of human peripheral blood lymphocytes to PHA exhibited a bell-shaped cell concentration-response curve, the effect of PGE_2 varied between individuals from inhibition to enhancement, being reproducible only at slightly suboptimal cell concentrations (around 10^5 cells/ml). It is therefore worth determining the optimal cell concentration before initiating any studies on eicosanoids and lymphocyte function.

d) Age and Disease

GOODWIN's group has studied a number of factors which may affect the sensitivity of lymphocytes to inhibition by PGE_2. A decreased sensitivity is exhibited by lymphocytes from patients with multiple sclerosis, while an increased sensitivity is exhibited by lymphocytes from healthy subjects over 70 years old, and from subjects who had undergone physical stress, such as surgery or labor (see CEUPPENS and GOODWIN 1985a). In addition, lymphocytes from normal individuals with the $HLA-B_{12}$ haplotype have a decreased sensitivity to PGE_2, which the authors suggested may play a role in genetic predisposition to autoimmune disease (STASZAK et al. 1980). However, lymphocytes from patients with the autoimmune disease rheumatoid arthritis exhibited greater sensitivity than normal to inhibition by PGE$_2$ (see CEUPPENS and GOODWIN 1985 a). The authors suggested that this altered sensitivity is due to prolonged treatment of rheumatoid patients with PG synthesis-inhibiting nonsteroidal anti-inflammatory drugs (NSAIDs), since NSAIDs generally cause enhancement of T lymphocyte responses, including those in elderly subjects (GOODWIN and WEBB 1980).

Lymphocytes from patients with Hodgkin's disease show a depressed proliferative response to PHA which can be markedly enhanced by indomethacin (see GOODWIN and WEBB 1980; CEUPPENS and GOODWIN 1985 a). A glass-adherent PGE$_2$-producing cell was found to be responsible for the suppression, as discussed in Sect. C.I.1.f. These data draw attention to the possible use of NSAIDs as immunostimulants in certain diseases, as confirmed recently by the enhancement by indomethacin in vitro of concanavalin A-induced proliferation of lymphocytes from patients with acquired immune deficiency syndrome (AIDS) (REDDY et al. 1985). In all such studies on the effects of NSAIDs on lymphocyte function, it must be borne in mind that inhibition of cyclooxygenase products other than PGE$_2$ may account for the effects observed, while with NSAIDs such as indomethacin in vitro, proliferative responses to low doses of mitogens are more sensitive to enhancement than responses to higher doses (CEUPPENS and GOODWIN 1985 a).

e) IL-2 Release and Action

The generation of IL-2 (T cell growth factor, TCGF) is essential for the differentiation and proliferation of T cells to mitogenic and antigenic stimulation (Chap. 8). In view of the marked inhibitory effects of PGE on T cell proliferation in vitro, inhibition of IL-2 release would seem a likely mechanism of action. This has been shown to be the case for both mouse splenic and human peripheral blood lymphocytes stimulated with mitogens (BAKER et al. 1981; RAPPAPORT and DODGE 1982). However, in addition to inhibiting IL-2 *release*, PGE has also been shown to inhibit the IL-2-induced proliferation of cytotoxic T cells, indicating inhibition of the *action* of IL-2 (BAKER et al. 1981; TILDEN and BALCH 1982; WOLF and DROEGE 1982). Indomethacin enhanced cytotoxic responses of human T cells only in the absence of added IL-2, indicating that the predominant action of endogenous PGE$_2$ is on IL-2 release and not on IL-2 action, and that NSAIDs may enhance T cell responses by increasing IL-2 production, as shown by RAPPAPORT and DODGE (1982) with indomethacin and fentiazac. More recently, HONDA and STEINBERG (1984) have obtained evidence suggesting that the type of stimulus, whether mitogenic or antigenic (as in mixed lymphocyte cultures) may determine the relative importance of the inhibition by PGE$_2$ of IL-2 release or action. They also suggested that the differential sensitivity of OKT4$^+$ and OKT8$^+$ cells to inhibition by PGE, discussed in Sect. C.I.c, may determine the effects of PGE$_2$ on IL-2 release.

f) T Suppressor Cells and PITS

There is general agreement that, in humans and most animal species, the major PGE$_2$-producing cell is the mononuclear phagocyte. In several human diseases, overproduction of PGE_2 by peripheral blood monocytes has been implicated in the immunosuppression observed. Such conditions include coccidioidomycosis, diffuse cutaneous leishmaniasis, multiple sclerosis, sarcoidosis, and Hodgkin's disease (CEUPPENS and GOODWIN 1985a). The PGE_2-producing cell is glass-adherent, and immunosuppression in the patients can be at least partially abrogated by administration of NSAIDs such as indomethacin. However, in addition to the production of PGE_2 by these glass-adherent monocytes, ROGERS et al. (1980) have shown that glass wool-adherent mouse T cells, when stimulated with PGE_2, generate a soluble peptide which suppresses mitogen-induced lymphocyte proliferation in vitro. On the one hand, this finding draws attention to the importance of defining the cell type involved in suppression of lymphocyte function, ideally with monoclonal antibodies to cell surface receptors, and not simply on the basis of glass wool adherence, as emphasized by GOODWIN and WEBB (1980). On the other hand, the finding offers a possible alternative explanation to inhibition of IL-2 production and/or action for the immunosuppressive activity of PGE_2. ROGERS et al. (1980) characterized two soluble prostaglandin-induced T cell-derived suppressors (PITS) with molecular weights of 35000 ($PITS_\alpha$) and about 5000 ($PITS_\beta$). The PITS were released by PGE_2 rather than synthesized de novo, since cyclophosphamide, at concentrations inhibitory to protein synthesis, did not affect the appearance of PITS. Subsequently, $PITS_\beta$ has been shown to be a mixture of seven different factors, with a variety of suppressive actions on T and B cell functions in vitro (ROGERS 1985). $PITS_{\beta 6}$ appears to be a peptidoleukotriene.

A link may exist between the production of PITS and IL-2 since CHOUAIB et al. (1984) have shown that PGE_2 activates an OKT8$^+$ suppressor cell which in turn inhibits IL-2 production by PHA-stimulated T cells, perhaps through the release of PITS. However, depletion of OKT8$^+$ cells from human peripheral blood monocytes was found by other authors to have no effect on the suppression by PGE_2 of PHA-induced IL-2 release (TILDEN and BALCH 1982), while FISCHER et al. (1985) found that induction of suppression by PGE_2 was mediated by a subpopulation of PGE_2-binding T cells independently of their OKT8$^+$ and OKT4$^+$ phenotype, so that the relationships between PITS and IL-2 have yet to be clearly defined. In any case, other suppressor circuits exist in addition to those mediated by PGE_2 (TING and HARGROVE 1984), emphasizing the fact that in nature there are always a large number of backup processes, T cell suppression being no exception.

g) Natural Killer Cells

In many respects, the regulation of the cytolytic activity of human and mouse natural killer (NK) cells by PGE is similar to its regulation of T cell activity. In most investigations, PGE_2 has been shown to inhibit NK cell activity in vitro, the mechanism involving enhancement of cyclic AMP levels (GOTO et al. 1983; HALL et al. 1983). Interestingly, the suppressive action of PGE_2 is reduced in the absence of T cells, suggesting that a T cell-derived factor, perhaps similar to PITS, may be involved (ZIELINSKI et al. 1984). Another mediator with actions on NK cells is gamma-interferon (IFN-γ) which drives human pre-NK cells to mature

NK cells. In short-term incubations, PGE_2 added within 20 min of IFN-γ inhibits the IFN-γ-driven maturation process, but after 30–40 min, when activation is complete, PGE_2 enhances cytolysis (TARGAN 1981). Longer incubations (18 h) with IFN-α or IFN-β (nonimmune interferons) result in resistance of NK cells to suppression by PGE_2 (LEUNG and KOREN 1982) emphasizing once again the importance of incubation times and timing of PGE_2 addition in the effects of this eicosanoid on lymphocyte function in vitro. Incubation of BCG-augmented mouse NK cells for at least 30 min with indomethacin and aspirin at concentrations which inhibited PGE_2 production in the cell cultures, potentiated NK cell activity and also did so when administered to mice in vivo (TRACEY and ADKINSON 1980), suggesting that the action of endogenous PGE_2 is predominantly inhibitory.

2. Effects In Vivo

Studies on the effects of eicosanoids in vivo are hampered by their rapid breakdown to inactive metabolites. Consequently, there is little point in studying effects of these compounds following oral or intravenous administration. The problem can be at least partially overcome by subcutaneous administration, a procedure frequently used for PGE, whereby the PG is slowly released from a subcutaneous depot. Alternatively, chemically more stable analogs, such as 15-methyl-PGE_1 or 16,16-dimethyl-PGE_2, have been used. When given in this manner, PGE_1 or PGE_2 in daily doses of around 200 μg have been shown in mice to inhibit a number of cell-mediated immune (CMI) responses, including the primary DTH response to sheep red blood cells (SRBC) (PARNHAM et al. 1979a), the DTH response to SRBC in tumor-bearing mice (STYLOS et al. 1979), the rejection of skin allografts (ANDERSON et al. 1977), and the initial (first 30 min) phases of the host-versus-graft and graft-versus-host responses to spleen cells (MERTIN et al. 1984), the latter involving i.p. administration. These data would appear to support the majority of in vitro findings, described in Sect. C.I.1, showing an inhibitory action of PGE on T cell function. Moreover, oral administration of NSAIDs, such as indomethacin, generally results in enhancement of CMI responses in vivo including DTH to *Mycobacterium bovis* or to picric acid-altered albumin in guinea pigs, and allograft rejection and NK cell activity in mice (see CEUPPENS and GOODWIN 1985a). These data suggest that endogenous PGE_2, known to be enhanced in lymphoid organs during a CMI response in mice (LAPP et al. 1980), exerts a negative feedback action on CMI responses in vivo, probably after its release from macrophages. However, stimulatory effects of exogenous PGE administered in vivo have also been reported on DTH to SRBC in normal mice (STYLOS et al. 1979), DTH to tuberculin in rats (PARNHAM et al. 1979a), and the graft-versus-host reaction in mice (LOOSE and DILUZIO 1973). This paradoxical dual action of PGE also corresponds to the findings, discussed earlier, that PGE in vitro may exert either inhibitory or stimulatory effects on T cell responses, depending on the concentration and time of addition, particularly during the early stages of culture. Clarification of the in vivo response to PGE has come from the work of MERTIN et al. (1984). Since NSAIDs are indiscriminate inhibitors of the synthesis of various PGs and may act on lymphocyte function independently of cyclooxygenase inhibition, Mertin and colleagues treated mice with anti-PGE serum as a more selective inhibitory tool. They found that while i.p. PGE administration during the induction phase (first 30 min) inhibits graft-versus-host and host-versus-graft responses in mice, i.p. anti-PGE serum given at a similar time also had an inhibitory action. However, concomitant treatment of mice with anti-PGE serum and PGE_2 (0.1–1 µg) reversed the effect of the serum in a dose-dependent manner. The authors concluded that low, physiologic concentrations of PGE are mediators of the induction of CMI responses – as also proposed by Leung and Mihich (1982) on the basis of in vitro data – an action prevented by anti-PGE serum and restored by exogenous PGE_2. At higher physiologic concentrations of PGE and when exogenous PGE is administered to normal animals (i.e., pharmacologic effect), suppression of CMI responses occurs, also accounting for enhancement by treatment with NSAIDs (Fig. 2).

A role of PGE in the induction of T cell-mediated CMI responses is further supported by the findings that, in autoimmune NZB/NZW and MRL-lpr/lpr mice, which are both associated with T cell defects, prolonged treatment with PGE promotes survival and preserves T cell responses ex vivo (Zurier et al. 1977; Adelman et al. 1980; Kelley et al. 1981; Eastcott and Kelley 1983).

Finally, although space does not allow the topic to be discussed in detail, it should be noted that PGE is a potent selective inhibitor of monocyte progenitor cell expansion (Cline and Golde 1979; Pelus et al. 1982), and also inhibits a variety of macrophage responses (Bonta and Parnham 1982; Parnham et al. 1983a). These actions may well influence the final effect of PGE on CMI responses in vivo and are discussed to some extent in the next section in relation to the humoral immune response. The picture which appears to be emerging from

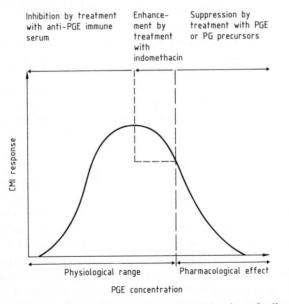

Fig. 2. Hypothetical model of the effect of PGE on the induction of cell-mediated immune responses. (Mertin and Smith 1988)

both in vitro and in vivo studies is that PGE exerts a dual action on T cell function, stimulatory to initial physiologic responses and suppressive when the response threatens to run out of control or when PGE is given pharmacologically. Such a picture is very similar to the dual role proposed for PGE in chronic inflammation (BONTA and PARNHAM 1978).

II. Humoral Immunity

With regard to the action of PGE on the induction of humoral immunity, the literature contains many conflicting data which do not provide a clear-cut mechanism for the PGE-mediated modulation of antibody responses. Initial studies revealed a marked rise in splenic $PGF_{2\alpha}$ levels during the early course of antibody induction. In addition, the induction of an antibody response toward either thymus-dependent or thymus-independent antigens was significantly enhanced by PG synthesis-inhibiting drugs. The authors therefore suggested an intrinsic function of PGs in the regulation of humoral immunity (WEBB and OSHEROFF 1976; ZIMECKI and WEBB 1976). Despite having been the subject of intensive investigation throughout the succeeding decade, the matter remains complex and requires further elucidation.

1. Effects In Vitro

a) Sources of Confusion

Whereas several authors have shown inhibition of in vitro immunoglobulin synthesis by inhibitors of PG synthesis (i.e., NSAIDs) and enhancement of in vitro antibody production or reversal of the NSAID-mediated suppression by addition of exogenous PGE (BURCHIEL and MELMON 1979; WIEDER and WEBB 1981; CEUPPENS and GOODWIN 1982; STAITE and PANAYI 1982), in other studies, opposite effects of PGE or NSAIDs on B cell activity in vitro have been reported (ZIMECKI and WEBB 1976; WEBB and NOWOWIEJSKI 1977; THOMPSON et al. 1984; JELINEK et al. 1985). Slight alterations in experimental procedures may be responsible for these diverging results. For example, the timing of the addition of either PGE or NSAIDs appears to be important for the final response. STAITE and PANAYI (1982) reported that indomethacin added to the culture within the first 8 h inhibited the plaque-forming cell (PFC) response, with little or no effect when added later, although ZIMECKI and WEBB (1976) found enhancement during this period, reaching a peak when NSAIDs were added from 6 h after the time of immunization. A similar time dependence in the response to PGE_2 was observed by EMILIE et al. (1983), PGE_2 causing no effect, enhancement, or inhibition of PGE responses when added from the beginning of the culture, for the first 24 h only, or after a delay of 2 days. While the different effects of NSAIDs may be due to varied effects on arachidonate metabolism, it is clear that the time dependence of the action of PGE_2 requires clarification. B cells from patients with rheumatoid arthritis have been suggested to have progressed beyond PG-mediated immunoregulation, since they show a different sensitivity to indomethacin in comparison with B cells from normal subjects (STAITE et al. 1983). Other reported sources of variation in the response of B cells to PGs include a differential sensitivity to PGE of the primary and secondary antibody response (Wieder and Webb 1981) and a surprising difference in sensitivity of Ig synthesis to effects of PGE_1 and PGE_2. However, while two groups of authors reported this distinction between PGE_1 and PGE_2 over the same dose range, they did not agree on the type of change produced (Morito et al. 1980; Dunne et al. 1981). To explain these confusing data, it has been suggested that either species differences (human, mouse, or rat) or different cell populations (e.g., spleen cells or peripheral blood mononuclear cells) are responsible for diverging results (Staite and Panayi 1984). Although these factors may play some role, it is obvious that a detailed reconsideration of the mechanism of action of PGE on B cells in vitro is necessary.

The induction of an antibody response toward a T-dependent antigen normally involves antigen-processing accessory cells, T cells recognizing antigen in connection with major histocompatibility complex (MHC) class II gene products, T cell-derived growth and differentiation factors, and the clonal expansion and maturation of the B cells themselves. Consequently, every agent like PGE which affects humoral immunity may interfere with one or more steps in the process of B cell activation, quite apart from affecting further regulatory control circuits which suppress an exaggerated immune response. Presumably, even slight changes in these interactions are sufficient to alter the net response to PGE. Only by piecing together the actions of PGE on the individual components, as discussed in Sect. C.II.1.b–d, might it be possible to solve the puzzle posed by the confusing data.

b) Modulation of Ia/HLA-DR Expression and Antigen Presentation

In order to initiate a T-dependent immune response, an antigen must be presented in association with MHC class II coded surface molecules designated HLA-DR in humans and Ia in mice and guinea pigs. Monoclonal Ia-specific antibodies inhibit antigen-induced PFC in mice (Forsgren et al. 1984), indicating a crucial role of Ia molecules in the differentiation of B cells. That PGE is likely to affect the antibody response at this level is suggested by the report that it inhibits lymphokine-induced expression of Ia, but not that of Fc receptors on macrophages (Snyder et al. 1982), while the complement split product C3b generates PGE_2 from guinea pig macrophages and exerts an indomethacin-sensitive inhibition on Ia expression by these cells (Hartung et al. 1983a; Mauer et al. 1984). Similar inhibition by PGE_2 of HLA-DR expression by human monocytes has also been reported (Van Tol et al. 1984). These authors also observed a PGE_2-induced shift to lower concentrations in the optimal antigen (ovalbumin) dose for in vitro PFC responses, suggesting a link between HLA-DR expression, optimal antigen concentration, and PGE_2 action on B cell activation. Since B cells have also been shown to express Ia molecules, an action of PGE_2 on antigen presentation by B cells themselves cannot be ruled out (Chesnut et al. 1982).

c) Effects on Monokines and Lymphokines

A further regulatory action of PGE on humoral immune responses may involve interference with the production or activity of the lymphocyte-activating factor, interleukin 1 (IL-1). The release of IL-1 by murine macrophages has been shown to be inhibited by PGE_2 and PGI_2, and to be enhanced by NSAIDs (KUNKEL et al. 1986). Recently, B cells have also been shown to produce IL-1 (MATSUSHIMA et al. 1985), although the consequences of this for the humoral immune response are not yet clear. It should be noted, however, that IL-1 contamination of different batches of serum added to the incubation medium may be a source of error in studies on in vitro PFC responses (HOFFMANN et al. 1984), in particular when studying PGE-mediated modulation of antibody induction in vitro.

The lymphocyte product IFN-γ probably counteracts the inhibitory action of PGE on the antibody response since it is a B cell-activating factor, possibly acting synergistically with further B cell-activating factors (NAKAGAWA et al. 1985; FRASCA et al. 1985), and suppresses macrophage PGE_2 generation (BORASCHI et al. 1984), although this latter action is dependent on the stimulus to PGE_2 production (BORASCHI et al. 1985). In this way, IFN-γ may initiate a positive feedback reaction, removing the PGE-mediated inhibition of IL-1 release as well as activating T and B cells.

PGE_2 also inhibits T cell generation of IL-2, as discussed in Sct. C.I.1.e and IL-2 has been shown to be essential for the in vitro PFC response (GRANELLI-PIPERNO et al. 1984). Interestingly, B cells have recently been shown to express IL-2 receptors following activation, and high IL-2 concentrations stimulate Ig synthesis by highly purified B cells (MITTLER et al. 1985; MURAGUCHI et al. 1985). Consequently, PGE_2 may inhibit antibody production by inhibiting IL-2 release from T cells, thus preventing IL-2 from acting directly on B cells or inducing the release of further B cell-activating factors from T cells (HOWARD et al. 1983). In this respect, it is important to bear in mind that the requirements of B cell activation for soluble factors vary according to the type of stimulus or antigen used (DEKRUYFF et al. 1985; FALKOFF et al. 1983).

d) Modulation of Regulatory T Cell Circuits

A subpopulation of T cells mediates the suppression of the antibody response by PGE_2 through the generation of the suppressor factor $PITS_{\beta 1}$, which has been shown to suppress the induction of PFC responses in vitro (ROGERS et al. 1985). This factor may play a role in the suppression of B cell activation by PGE_2-binding T suppressor cells reported by other authors (DELFRAISSY et al. 1982; FISCHER et al. 1985). However, a contrasting hypothesis has been put forward by CEUPPENS and GOODWIN (1985b). These authors demonstrated that indomethacin inhibits mitogen-induced Ig synthesis by normal human lymphocytes, an action reversed by the addition of PGE_2, which acts on $OKT8^+$ T suppressor cells (CEUPPENS and GOODWIN 1982). This mechanism is apparently transferable to rheumatoid arthritis since B lymphocytes from rheumatoid arthritis patients who have been treated with indomethacin in vivo exhibit depressed synthesis of rheumatoid factor (RF) (CEUPPENS et al. 1982). CEUPPENS and GOODWIN (1985b) have proposed that PGE_2 formed by RF-triggered monocytes inactivates a T suppressor cell normally regulating T cells, providing help for RF-producing B cells. A vicious circle would ensue in which RF production would proceed uncontrolled and contribute to the arthritis. There is at present no satisfactory explanation for these conflicting data.

2. Effects In Vivo

a) Normal, Healthy Conditions

Little is known about the effects of PGE_2 per se on the humoral immune response in vivo. Most data can only be drawn indirectly from studies with NSAIDs. In these cases, it cannot be concluded with certainty that the effects observed are due to inhibition of PGE_2 production, rather than to effects on the synthesis of other eicosanoids. Studies in mice have often shown that treatment with NSAIDs results in enhancement of the activity of splenic PFC ex vivo (Webb and Osheroff 1976; Webb and Nowowiejski 1977; Schleimer and Benjamini 1981). Webb and Osheroff (1976) reported an enhancement of splenic $PGF_{2\alpha}$ levels during the primary antibody response to SRBC, although at this time PGE_2 radioimmunoassays were not widely used or reliable, so that it is likely that $PGF_{2\alpha}$ was measured out of convenience. In any case, the lower the control antibody response to antigen in vivo, the more pronounced is the enhancement with indomethacin (Webb and Nowowiejski 1977). Enhancement of the antibody response to influenza virus by indomethacin has also been reported in humans, with the primary and secondary antibody responses showing differing sensitivities (Goodwin et al. 1978). Once again, a role of PGE_2 can only be assumed. Should PGE_2 indeed be the target of NSAIDs in enhancing the humoral immune response in vivo, it would appear that its suppressive action, removed by the NSAIDs, is dominant.

b) Autoimmunity and Immune Complex Diseases

During autoimmune diseases (e.g., rheumatoid arthritis, myasthenia gravis) or experimentally induced states of hyperimmunization, the formation of antigen-antibody complexes leads, among other effects, to stimulation of PG production by phagocytes. Modulation of the disease state by PGE and/or NSAIDs may thus be expected. As discussed previously, Ceuppens and Goodwin (1985 b) have proposed that inactivation by PGE_2 of T suppressor cells may contribute to excessive RF production in rheumatoid arthritis. In contrast, PGE administered in vivo, inhibits the mortality and disease symptoms of MRL-lpr/lpr and NZB/NZW mouse strains, both of which have been proposed as models of systemic lupus erythematosus (Zurier et al. 1978; Kelley et al. 1981). In view of B cell hyperactivity in MRL-lpr/lpr mice, it has been proposed that PGE inhibits antibody production in this strain (Kelley et al. 1981), perhaps through an action on the excessive IFN-γ-mediated Ia expression shown to exist on macrophages from these animals (Rosenberg et al. 1984). In a nongenetically determined murine model of glomerulonephritis induced by repeated antigen challenge, the beneficial effect of PGE appears to be due to decreased antibody titres (Kelley and Winkelstein 1980; McLeish et al. 1982).

In summary, while the limited in vivo data on PGE and NSAIDs suggest that PGE may be predominantly inhibitory to the humoral immune response, the findings reported from in vitro studies are contradictory. The amount and type of antigen used, the incubation period employed, and measurement of the primary or secondary antibody response are all contributory factors to these contradictory data.

D. Other Prostaglandins and Thromboxanes

Although injection of mice with SRBC was shown some years ago to cause a marked increase in splenic $PGF_{2\alpha}$ levels (WEBB and OSHEROFF 1976), this cyclooxygenase product and PGs of the A series, formed as chemical breakdown products of PGE, have been shown by several authors to be essentially inactive or only inhibitory at high concentrations against T cell and NK cell responses in vitro (e.g., RAPPAPORT and DODGE 1982; BANKHURST 1982; CEUPPENS and GOODWIN 1985a). LEUNG and MIHICH (1982), however, have described an enhancing effect of $PGF_{2\alpha}$ (10^{-8} mol/l) on the primary cytotoxic response of mouse T cells, when added within 24 h of the antigen. Perhaps $PGF_{2\alpha}$ may play a specific role in lymphocyte toxicity, as supported by a positive correlation between human NK cell cytotoxicity and $PGF_{2\alpha}$ levels in vitro (CHING et al. 1984).

In contrast, PGD_2 and prostacyclin (PGI_2), both of which are as effective as PGE_2 in increasing cyclic AMP levels in human lymphocytes (BURCHIEL and BANKHURST 1979), also inhibit T cell proliferation to mitogens and T cell and NK cell cytotoxicity in vitro (BURCHIEL and BANKHURST 1979; GORDON et al. 1979; LEUNG and MIHICH 1982; LANEFELT et al. 1983). In view of the instability of PGI_2 in solution, it is important to bear in mind the time of administration of this eicosanoid, since the inhibitory effect begins to wane within 20–30 min in culture (BURCHIEL and BANKHURST 1979; GORDON et al. 1979). The breakdown product of PGI_2, $6\text{-keto-}PGF_{1\alpha}$ is, however, inactive (BURCHIEL and BANKHURST 1979; GORDON et al. 1979; LEUNG and MIHICH 1982). Since PGI_2 (usually measured as $6\text{-keto-}PGF_{1\alpha}$) is a major product of stimulated human and mouse macrophages (MORLEY et al. 1979; BONNEY et al. 1980), a role for this PG in endogenous immunosuppression must be considered. Such a role is supported by the finding that the PGI_2 synthesis inhibitor tranylcypromine enhances T cell cytotoxicity when added during the first 24 h of culture (LEUNG et al. 1982), although other actions of the drug cannot be ruled out.

Another major eicosanoid product of stimulated macrophages, particularly in humans, is TxA_2 and its stable metabolite TxB_2 (MORLEY et al. 1979; BONNEY et al. 1980). Several inhibitors of Tx synthesis were shown by KELLY et al. (1979) to inhibit mitogen-induced proliferation of human lymphocytes, but subsequent studies clearly demonstrated that these drug effects were due either to diversion of arachidonic acid metabolism to PGE_2 or to other actions unrelated to effects on eicosanoid synthesis (GORDON et al. 1981; CEUPPENS et al. 1985). Recently, however the TxA_2 receptor antagonist, 13-azaprostanoic acid, has been shown to enhance human NK cell activity in vitro and to reverse the inhibitory effect at 10^{-7} mol/l of the TxA_2 analog, U44069 (ROLA-PLESZCZYNKSI et al. 1985). Since TxA_2 itself has a half-life in aqueous solution of 30 s, studies with this eicosanoid are inevitably difficult, but in view of its possible activity on NK cells, further investigations are warranted.

E. Lipoxygenase Metabolites

Arachidonic acid is metabolized to a variety of oxidized products by different lipoxygenases (as summarized in Fig. 1). Several of these compounds exert proinflammatory activities and are potent modulators of leukocyte function. In particular, the stimulatory effects of LTB_4 on leukocytes (e.g., chemotaxis, adherence, and degranulation) have been the subject of many investigations. A difficulty arising during the study of lipoxygenase metabolites is the fact that they affect one another's synthesis. For instance, it has been reported by VANDERHOEK et al. (1980) that 15-HETE inhibits the 5-lipoxygenase in leukocytes. GOETZL (1981) found that 15-HETE inhibits LTB_4 and 5-HETE synthesis by mitogen-stimulated T lymphocytes, while synthesis of 11-HETE or PGE_2 was not affected. Since immune activation enhances the ability of macrophages to release LTB_4 (HSUEH et al. 1985), inhibition of this release by 15-HETE (if formed in sufficient amounts) may provide a negative feedback on further synthesis of lipoxygenase metabolites.

I. Effects In Vitro

1. Modulation of T Cell Mitogenesis

Early studies pointed toward promotion by lipoxygenase metabolites of mitogen-induced lymphocyte proliferation inasmuch as lipoxygenase inhibitors suppressed this cellular function (KELLY et al. 1979). However, the lipoxygenase inhibitors available at that time lack specificity as they normally inhibit both cyclooxygenase and lipoxygenase (e.g., BW755C, eicosatetraynoic acid) and/or other enzymes (e.g., inhibition of methylation reactions by nordihydroguaretic acid). The development of more selective lipoxygenase inhibitors (e.g., REV5901, AA861), and the use of synthetic lipoxygenase products have partially overcome this problem. In this respect, 15-HETE,5(8, 9, 11, 12, or 15)-HPETE, LTB_4, LTE_4, and LTD_4 are all inhibitory toward lymphocyte proliferation (BAILEY et al. 1982; WEBB et al. 1982; GUALDE et al. 1983, 1985a), inhibition by HETEs depending on the position in the molecule of the hydroxyl group (Low et al. 1984). Consequently, individual lipoxygenase products would appear to be generally inhibitory to T cell mitogenesis. The possible mechanism (or mechanisms) has become apparent from studies on subpopulations of T cells.

Thus, ROLA-PLESZCZYNSKI et al. (1982) reported that LTB_4 *induces* human T suppressor cell activity at concentrations as low as 10^{-14} mol/l. These suppressor cells, which were derived by preincubation with LTB_4, inhibited the mitogen-induced proliferation of cocultivated fresh peripheral blood mononuclear leukocytes, whereas preincubation with LTD_4 or LTE_4 resulted in only weak T suppressor activity. This initial work has been elegantly extended, LTB_4 being shown to enhance the proliferation of purified cytotoxic/suppressor T lymphocytes while inhibiting the helper/inducer T lymphocytes (PAYAN et al. 1984). Similar results were reported for LTB_4 and 15-HPETE by GUALDE et al. (1985a). The net effect of LTB_4 on both T suppressor and T helper populations is inhibition of mitogen-induced T lymphocyte proliferation (PAYAN et al. 1984). Using a fluorescent conjugate of LTB_4 and similarly labeled monoclonal antibodies, the same authors demonstrated that about 8% of T helper/inducer and 14% of T cytotoxic/suppressor cells bind LTB_4. This latter finding may be important in that ROLA-PLESZCZYNSKI (1985) reported that both $T4^+$ and $T8^+$ lymphocyte subsets could be induced by LTB_4 to develop T suppressor activity. With purified $T4^+$ lymphocytes, suppression was mediated by differentiated T lymphocytes bearing the T cytotoxic/suppressor cell marker $T8^+$. The differentiation from $T4^+$ to $T8^+$ lymphocytes was dependent on both the presence of monocytes in the responding cell population and on an intact cyclooxygenase pathway, suggesting that monocyte-derived PGs mediate this particular action of LTB_4.

2. Effects on Monokines and Lymphokines

As discussed in earlier sections, IL-1 released by activated macrophages is essential for the induction in lymphocytes of the release of and sensitivity to IL-2, necessary for lymphocyte activation. Despite the direct inhibitory action of LTB_4 on T cell mitogenesis in vitro, this eicosanoid was reported to enhance IL-1 production by human monocytes and mouse macrophages (ROLA-PLESZCZYNSKI and LEMAIRE 1985; CHENSUE and KUNKEL 1985). The peptido-LTs were weakly stimulatory, depending on the species. As might be expected, lipoxygenase inhibitors inhibited IL-1 production, but only when added prior to the stimulus and depending on the type of stimulus (DINARELLO et al. 1984; KUNKEL and CHENSUE 1985). The relevance of this action of LTB_4 to the final lymphocyte response is as yet unclear. However, a variety of lipoxygenase inhibitors have been shown to suppress IL-1-induced thymocyte proliferation and IL-2 production (by the thymoma cell line EL4) as well as IL-2 production and IL-2-dependent proliferation induced by phorbol myristate acetate and/or concanavalin A (DINARELLO et al. 1983; FARRAR and HUMES 1985; KATO and MUROTA 1985), suggesting that lipoxygenase products may mediate the action of IL-1 and IL-2 on lymphocytes. This suggestion was reinforced by the finding that 5-HETE mitigated the inhibition of IL-1-dependent cell proliferation by 15-HETE (FARRAR and HUMES 1985). 15-HETE, reportedly a major product of activated T cells, also inhibits 5-lipoxygenase (GOETZL 1981), suggesting that 15-HETE and 5-lipoxygenase products, such as 5-HETE, may be physiologic antagonists regulating the action of IL-2.

This also seems to be true for IFN-γ production by lymphocytes, since 15-HETE and lipoxygenase inhibitors suppress, while 5-HETE and LTC_4 partially restore the generation of this lymphokine, LTB_4 and more or less all peptido-LTs actually being able to replace the requirement for IL-2 in this response (FARRAR and HUMES 1985; JOHNSTON and TORRES 1984). The end effect of activation of different lipoxygenases will probably depend on stimulus selectivity and other parameters yet to be defined.

3. Cyclic GMP Enhancement

Cyclic GMP appears to be an important signal in the early phase of lymphocyte activation (HADDEN and COFFEY 1982) and appears to be linked to the lipoxygenase pathway since the inhibition by lipoxygenase inhibitors of lymphocyte mitogenesis is associated with a decrease in cyclic GMP (Coffey et al. 1981). Arachidonic acid itself enhances lymphocyte cyclic GMP (Coffey et al. 1981) as do 15-HETE and LTB$_4$ in T lymphocytes (Mexmain et al. 1985). A possible common target for lipoxygenase products and cyclic GMP is IFN-γ, the diminished production of which can be restored by LTC$_4$ and cyclic GMP (Johnson et al. 1982; Johnson and Torres 1984).

4. NK Cells and T Cell Cytotoxicity

Initial findings that NK cell activity was suppressed by inhibitors of phospholipid methylation and phospholipase A$_2$ pointed toward a possible involvement of eicosanoids (Hoffman et al. 1981). In fact, lipoxygenase inhibitors *did* abrogate human and mouse NK cell activity (Seaman 1984). However, like the regulation of lymphokine activity discussed in Sect. E.I.2, lipoxygenase products appear to exert differing actions on NK cells since 14,15-diHETE has been reported to be inhibitory (Ramstedt et al. 1984) while LTA$_4$, LTB$_4$, and LTD$_4$ enhanced NK cytotoxicity (Rola-Pleszczynski et al. 1984). The enhancing effects of LTs may be secondary to IFN-γ stimulation, since lipoxygenase inhibitors suppressed IFN-γ-induced NK cell activation, but had little effect on NK cells already activated by IFN-γ (Leung et al. 1985).

Although lipoxygenase inhibitors have also been reported to suppress T cell cytotoxicity, Taylor et al. (1985) suggested that this action is independent of arachidonate metabolism because cytotoxic T lymphocytes produce few if any lipoxygenase metabolites. Despite these doubts, lipoxygenase metabolites derived from other cells in close proximity may be regulatory, as Gualde et al. (1983) reported inhibition of T cell cytotoxicity by 15-HPETE.

5. Humoral Immunity

5-HETE, LTB$_4$, and 15-HPETE have been reported to suppress B cell proliferation and immunoglobulin secretion (Goodman and Weigle 1984; Atluru and Goodwin 1984; Gualde et al. 1985b). The inhibitory actions of LTB$_4$ and 15-HPETE may have been due to induction of T suppressor cells present in the cultures (Atluru and Goodwin 1984; Gualde et al. 1985b). 15-HETE, on the other hand, while inhibiting mitogen-induced T cell proliferation, had no effect on lipopolysaccharide-induced mouse B cell proliferation (Bailey et al. 1982). B cells have also been shown to be less sensitive than T cells to inhibition by LTD$_4$ and LTE$_4$ (Webb et al. 1982) so that B cells may be poorly responsive to lipoxygenase products in general. The inhibition of PFC responses in vitro by lipoxygenase inhibition may also be an indirect effect.

II. Effects In Vivo

Little information is available on the immunomodulatory role of lipoxygenase products in vivo. However, in vivo administration of LTB$_4$ or 15-HETE has been reported to inhibit T lymphocyte activity ex vivo (Myers et al. 1984; Aldigier et al. 1984). Enhanced biosynthesis of LTB_4 by immunologically (BCG) activated macrophages or increased 5-lipoxygenase activity in spleen cells of mice with leishmaniasis may thus contribute to decreased immune functions (HSUEH et al. 1985; REINER and MALEMUD 1984). LTB_4 secretion by leukocytes has also been suggested to be responsible for the anergic state of burn-injured patients (BRAQUET et al. 1984).

F. Peroxides

HOFFELD (1981) has shown that a number of agents which inhibit lipid peroxidation enhance the primary antibody response to SRBC and the lipopolysaccharide-induced proliferation of mouse spleen cells in vitro (HOFFELD 1981). The author also found a similar action of 2-mercaptoethanol which raises cellular antioxidant capacity by increasing the availability of intracellular reduced glutathione (GSH). Conversely, by feeding mice a diet deficient in selenium, the activity of the endogenous peroxide-inactivating enzyme glutathione peroxidase (GSH-Px) can be drastically reduced, resulting in an increased endogenous peroxide tone. Mice kept for 7–8 weeks on such a diet exhibit reduced spleen cell proliferation to mitogens and NK cell cytotoxicity, while T cell cytotoxicity is also reduced when the diet is additionally made deficient in the antioxidant, vitamin E (PARNHAM et al. 1983 b; MEEKER et al. 1985). These data indicate that peroxides are inhibitory or possibly damaging to lymphocyte membranes. The advantage of a dietary study over the use of antioxidant compounds (except antioxidant enzymes) is the specificity of action involved, i.e., only GSH-Px is affected, while antioxidants are notoriously nonspecific. However, GSH-Px is only specific to a degree, in that it degrades both lipid peroxides and the H_2O_2 generated by stimulated macrophages and polymorphonuclear leukocytes (PMN). Consequently, the inhibitory effects of selenium deficiency on lymphocyte function can be attributed to either excess lipid peroxide production, excess H_2O_2 production, or both. Indeed, H_2O_2 is generated in sufficient amounts by murine or human macrophages or PMN stimulated in vitro to cause inhibition of mitogen-induced lymphocyte proliferation, NK cell activity, and B cell colony formation (METZGER et al. 1980; SEAMAN et al. 1982; WHISLER and NEWHOUSE 1982). The specificity of the action of H_2O_2 was confirmed in each case by abrogation of the inhibition by catalase, a specific scavenger of H_2O_2. At least when mouse and human macrophages are the sources, the inhibitory action of H_2O_2 appears to be synergistic with that of the concomitantly released PGE_2 (METZGER et al. 1980; WHISLER and NEWHOUSE 1982). From all these studies, it is important to note that when studying the role of peroxides or other reactive oxygen species in the regulation of lymphocyte function, a role of a specific compound can only be confirmed when it can be shown to be generated in concentrations at which it exerts its effects and when a *selective* scavenger is capable of inhibiting the activity. Using these criteria NIWA et al. (1983, 1984) have shown that enhanced PMN H_2O_2 and/or superoxide anion generation may be responsible for the reduced proliferative response to mitogens of T lymphocytes from the venous blood of patients with systemic lupus erythematosus or rheumatoid arthritis.

G. Platelet-Activating Factor

PAF was discovered as a fluid phase mediator of platelet aggregation which was released by antigen challenge of IgE-sensitized rabbit basophilic granulocytes (Henson and Cochrane 1971). The elucidation of the structure of PAF and its biosynthetic pathways revealed that this phospholipid mediator is generated by the cellular pathways giving rise to eicosanoids (see Fig. 1).

Studies on the release of PAF and its effects have been restricted mainly to cells other than lymphocytes, although the existence of PAF precursors in lymphocytes and the release of PAF by human lymphoid cell lines challenged with mitogens have been reported (Sugiura and Waku 1983; Bussolino et al. 1984). However, PAF has also been shown to be a potent stimulator of macrophages, generating, for instance, oxygen radicals (Hartung et al. 1983b). Thus, any effects of PAF and related lysophospholipids on humoral or cell-mediated immunity may be related to alteration of macrophage behavior, rather than that of lymphocytes. Munder et al. (1976) reported that lysolecithin analogs are potentiators of the humoral immune response to SRBC and of the rejection of either genetically different (allograft rejection) or syngeneic implanted tumors in mice. However, such phospholipids may directly alter lymphocyte membrane fluidity and therefore affect both intercellular communication between lymphocytes and their associated functions as suggested by Sellin et al. (1974). It remains to be determined whether PAF itself has any clear effects on lymphocyte responses.

Acknowledgement. We thank Dr. J. Mertin for assistance with our literature search.

Note Added in Proof. Malavasi et al. (1986) have shown that human peripheral blood large granular lymphocytes, depleted of macrophages/monocytes ($<2\%$), when stimulated with a specific anti-Fc receptor monoclonal antibody (AB8.28), generate PAF. Monocyte or granulocyte suspensions did not respond to AB8.28 with PAF generation. G. P. Lewis, at a meeting of the British Inflammation Society, also reported that selected PAF receptor antagonists are capable of inhibiting the IL-2-induced uptake of [^{3}H] thymidine by human peripheral blood lymphocytes (see Parnham and de Brito 1987). Consequently, a role for PAF in lymphocyte function is likely.

References

Adelman N, Ksiazek J, Cohen S, Yoshida T, Zurier RB (1980) Prostaglandin E$_1$ treatment of NZB/WF$_1$ hybrids – Induction of in vitro and in vivo cell-mediated immune responses to DNA. Clin Immunol Immunopathol 17:353–362

Aldigier JC, Gualde N, Mexmain S, Chable-Rabinovitch H, Ratinaud MH, Rigaud M (1984) Immunosuppression induced in vivo by 15 hydroxyeicosatetraenoic acid (15 HETE). Prostaglandins Leukotrienes Med 13:99–107

Anderson CB, Jaffee BM, Graff RJ (1977) Prolongation of murine skin allografts by prostaglandin E. Transplantation 23:444–447

Atluru D, Goodwin JS (1984) Control of polyclonal immunoglobulin production from human lymphocytes by leukotrienes; leukotriene B$_4$ induces an OKT8 (+), radiosensitive suppressor cell from resting, human OKT8 (−) T cells. J Clin Invest 74:1444–1450

Bach M-A (1975) Differences in cyclic AMP changes after stimulation by prostaglandins and isoproterenol in lymphocyte subpopulations. J Clin Invest 55:1074–1081

Bailey JM, Bryant RW, Low CE, Pupillo MB, Vanderhoek JY (1982) Regulation of T-lymphocyte mitogenesis by the leukocyte product 15-hydroxyeicosatetraenoic acid (15-HETE). Cell Immunol 67:112–120

Baker PE, Fahey JV, Munck A (1981) Prostaglandin inhibition of T-cell proliferation is mediated at two levels. Cell Immunol 61:52–61

Bankhurst AD (1982) The modulation of human natural killer cell activity by prostaglandins. J Clin Lab Immunol 7:85–91

Bonney RJ, Humes JL (1984) Physiological and pharmacological regulation of prostaglandin and leukotriene production by macrophages. J Leuk Biol 35:1–10

Bonney RJ, Naruns P, Davies P, Humes JL (1979) Antigen-antibody complexes stimulate the synthesis and release of prostaglandins by mouse peritoneal macrophages. Prostaglandins 18:605–616

Bonney RJ, Davies P, Kuehl FA, Humes JL (1980) Arachidonic acid oxygenation products produced by mouse peritoneal macrophages responding to inflammatory stimuli. J Reticuloendothelial Soc [Suppl] 28:1135–1155

Bonta IL, Parnham MJ (1978) Prostaglandins and chronic inflammation. Biochem Pharmacol 27:1611–1623

Bonta IL, Parnham MJ (1982) Immunomodulatory-antiinflammatory functions of E-type prostaglandins. Minireview with emphasis on macrophage-mediated effects. Int J Immunopharmacol 4:103–109

Boraschi D, Censini S, Tagliabue A (1984) Interferon-γ reduces macrophage-suppressive activity by inhibiting prostaglandin E_2 release and inducing interleukin 1 production. J Immunol 133:764–768

Boraschi D, Censini S, Bartalini M, Tagliabue A (1985) Regulation of arachidonic acid metabolism in macrophages by immune and nonimmune interferons. J Immunol 135:502–505

Braquet M, Ducousso R, Garay R, Guilbaud J, Carsin H, Braquet P (1984) Leukocyte leukotriene B_4 secretion precedes anergy in burn-injured patients. Lancet II:976–977

Burchiel SW, Bankhurst AD (1979) PGI_2 and PGD_2 effects on cyclic AMP and human T-cell mitogenesis. Prostaglandins Med 3:315–320

Burchiel SW, Melmon KL (1979) Augmentation of the in vitro humoral immune response by pharmacologic agents. I. An explanation for the differential enhancement of humoral immunity via agents that elevate cAMP. Immunopharmacology 1:137–150

Bussolino F, Foa R, Malavasi F, Ferrando ML, Camussi G (1984) Release of platelet-activating factor (PAF)-like material from human lymphoid cell lines. Exp Hematol 12:688–693

Ceuppens JL, Goodwin JS (1982) Endogenous prostaglandin E_2 enhances polyclonal immunoglobulin production by tonically inhibiting T suppressor cell activity. Cell Immunol 70:41–54

Ceuppens JL, Goodwin JS (1985a) Immunological responses in treatment with non-steroidal anti-inflammatory drugs, with particular reference to the role of prostaglandins. In: Rainsford KD (ed) Anti-inflammatory and anti-rheumatic drugs, vol 1. CRC, Boca Raton, p 89

Ceuppens JL, Goodwin JS (1985b) Control of antibody and autoantibody production by prostaglandin E. In: Goodwin JS (ed) Prostaglandins and immunity, Nijhoff, Boston, p 99

Ceuppens JL, Rodriguez MA, Goodwin JS (1982) Non-steroid anti-inflammatory agents inhibit the synthesis of IgM rheumatoid factor in vitro. Lancet I:528–530

Ceuppens JL, Vertessen S, Deckmyn H, Vermylen J (1985) Effects of thromboxane A_2 on lymphocyte proliferation. Cell Immunol 90:458–463

Chensue SW, Kunkel SL (1985) Induction of interleukin-1 release by leukotrienes. Fed Prod 44:1270

Chesnut RW, Colon SM, Grey HM (1982) Antigen presentation by normal B cells, B cell tumors, and macrophages: functional and biochemical comparison. J Immunol 128:1764–1768

Ching CY, Ching N, Seto DSY, Hokama Y (1984) Relationships of prostaglandin levels and natural killer (NK) cell cytotoxicity of mononuclear cells in cord blood. J Med 15:233–236

Chouaib S, Chatenoud L, Klatzmann D, Fradelizi D (1984) The mechanisms of inhibition of human IL-2 production II. PGE_2 induction of suppressor T lymphocytes. J Immunol 132:1851–1857

408   M. J. Parnham and W. Englberger

Cline MJ, Golde DW (1979) Cellular interactions in haematopoiesis. Nature 277:177–181
Coffey RG, Hadden EM, Hadden JW (1981) Phytohemagglutinin stimulation of guanylate
    cyclase in human lymphocytes. J Biol Chem 256:4418–4424
DeKruyff R, Clayberger C, Fay R, Cantor H (1985) B cell activation: role of dentritic and
    T cell factors in the response to thymic-independent and -dependent antigens. J Immu-
    nol 134:2860–2866
Delfraissy JF, Galanaud P, Wallon C, Balavoine JF, Dormont J (1982) Abolished in vitro
    antibody response in elderly: exclusive involvement of prostaglandin-induced T sup-
    pressor cells. Clin Immunol Immunopathol 24:377–385
DeWille JW, Fraker PJ, Romsos DR (1981) Effect of dietary fatty acids on delayed-type
    hypersensitivity in mice. J Nutr 111:2039–2041
Dinarello CA, Marnoy SO, Rosenwasser LJ (1983) Role of arachidonate metabolism in the
    immuno-regulatory function of human leukocytic pyrogen/lymphocyte-activating fac-
    tor/interleukin 1. J Immunol 130:890–895
Dinarello CA, Bishai I, Rosenwasser LJ, Coceani F (1984) The influence of lipoxygenase
    inhibitors on the in vitro production of human leukocytic pyrogen and lymphocyte ac-
    tivating factor (interleukin-1). Int J Immunpharmacol 6:43–50
Dunne JV, Foss B, Leung T, McKendry RJR (1981) Effects of prostaglandins E_1 and E_2
    on the vitro production of immunoglobulin by human peripheral blood lymphocytes.
    Prostaglandins Med 6:419–425
Eastcott JW, Kelley VE (1983) Preservation of T-lymphocyte activity in autoimmune
    MRL-*lpr* mice treated with prostaglandin. Clin Immunol Immunopathol 29:78–85
Emilie D, Crevon MC, Galanaud P (1983) Prostaglandin E_2 regulation of human specific
    B cell response: Interaction with a monocyte product. Clin Immunol Immunopathol
    29:415–423
Falkoff RJM, Muraguchi A, Hong JX, Butler JL, Dinarello CA, Fauci AS (1983) The ef-
    fects of interleukin 1 on human B cell activation and proliferation. J Immunol 131:801–
    805
Farrar WL, Humes JL (1985) The role of arachidonic acid metabolism in the activities of
    interleukin 1 and 2. J Immunol 135:1153–1159
Ferber E, Resch K (1976) Phospholipidstoffwechsel stimulierter Lymphozyten. Untersu-
    chungen zum molekularen Mechanismus der Aktivierung. Naturwissenschaften
    63:375–381
Fischer A, LeDeist F, Durandy A, Griscelly C (1985) Separation of a population of human
    T lymphocytes that bind prostaglandin E_2 and exert a suppressor activity. J Immunol
    134:815–819
Forsgren S, Pobor G, Coutinho A, Pierres M (1984) The role of I-A/E molecules in B lym-
    phocyte activation. J Immunol 133:2104–2110
Frasca D, Adorini L, Landolfo S, Doria G (1985) Enhancing effects of IFN-γ on helper
    T cell activity and IL 2 production. J Immunol 134:3907–3911
Gemsa D, Leser H-G, Seitz M, Deimann W, Bärlin E (1982) Membrane perturbation and
    stimulation of arachidonic acid metabolism. Mol Immunol 19:1287–1296
Goetzl EJ (1981) Selective feed-back inhibition of the 5-lipoxygenation of arachidonic acid
    in human T-lymphocytes. Biochem Biophys Res Commun 101:344–350
Goldyne ME, Stobo JD (1980) Prostaglandin E_2 as a modulator of macrophage-T lympho-
    cyte interactions. J Invest Dermatol 74:297–300
Goldyne ME, Stobo JD (1982) Human monocytes synthesize eicosanoids from T lympho-
    cyte-derived arachidonic acid. Prostaglandins 24:623–630
Goodman MG, Weigle WO (1984) Regulation of B-lymphocyte proliferative responses by
    arachidonate metabolites: effect on membrane-directed versus intracellular activators.
    J Allergy Clin Immunol 74:418–425
Goodwin JS, Webb DR (1980) Regulation of the immune response by prostaglandins. Clin
    Immunol Immunopathol 15:106–122
Goodwin JS, Selinger DS, Messner RP, Reed WP (1978) Effect of indomethacin in vivo
    on humoral and cellular immunity in humans. Infect Immun 19:430–433
Goodwin JS, Wiik A, Lewis A, Bankhurst AD, Williams RC (1979 a) High-affinity binding
    sites for prostaglandin E on human lymphocytes. Cell Immunol 43:150–159

Goodwin JS, Kaszubowski PA, Williams RC (1979 b) Cyclic adenosine monophosphate response to prostaglandin E_2 on subpopulations of human lymphocytes. J Exp Med 150:1260–1264

Goodwin JS, Bromberg S, Messner RP (1981) Studies on the cyclic AMP response to prostaglandin in human lymphocytes. Cell Immunol 60:298–307

Gordon D, Bray MA, Morley J (1976) Control of lymphokine secretion by prostaglandins. Nature 262:401–402

Gordon D, Henderson DC, Westwick J (1979) Effects of prostaglandins E_2 and I_2 on human lymphocyte transformation in the presence and absence of inhibitors of prostaglandin biosynthesis. Br J Pharmacol 67:17–22

Gordon D, Nouri AME, Thomas RU (1981) Selective inhibition of thromboxane biosynthesis in human blood mononuclear cells and the effects on mitogen-stimulated lymphocyte proliferation. Br J Pharmacol 74:469–475

Goto T, Herberman RB, Maluish A, Strong DM (1983) Cyclic AMP as a mediator of prostaglandin E-induced suppression of human natural killer cell activity. J Immunol 130:1350–1355

Granelli-Piperno A, Andrus L, Reich E (1984) Antibodies to interleukin 2. Effects on immune responses in vitro and in vivo. J Exp Med 160:738–750

Gualde N, Goodwin JS (1982) Effects of prostaglandin E_2 and preincubation on lectin-stimulated proliferation of human T cell subsets. Cell Immunol 70:373–379

Gualde N, Chable-Rabinovitch H, Motta C, Durand J, Beneytout JL, Rigaud M (1983) Hydroperoxyeicosatetraenoic acids. Potent inhibitors of lymphocyte responses. Biochim Biophys Acta 750:429–433

Gualde N, Atluru D, Goodwin JS (1985 a) Effect of lipoxyenase metabolites of arachidonic acid on proliferation of human T cells and T cell subsets. J Immunol 134:1125–1129

Gualde N, Rigaud M, Goodwin JS (1985 b) Induction of suppressor cells from peripheral blood T cells by 15-hydroperoxyeicosatetraenoic acid (15-HPETE). J Immunol 135:3424–3428

Hadden JW, Coffey RG (1982) Cyclic nucleotides in mitogen-induced lymphocyte proliferation. Immunol Today 3:299–304

Hall TJ, Chen S-H, Brostoff J, Lydyard PM (1983) Modulation of human natural killer cell activity by pharmacological mediators. Clin Exp Immunol 54:493–500

Hartung HP, Hadding U, Bitter-Suermann D, Gemsa D (1983 a) Stimulation of prostaglandin E and thromboxane synthesis in macrophages by purified C3b. J Immunol 130:2861–2865

Hartung HP, Parnham MJ, Winkelmann J, Englberger W, Hadding U (1983 b) Platelet activating factor (PAF) induces the oxidative burst in macrophages. Int J Immunopharmacol 5:115–121

Henson PM, Cochrane CG (1971) Acute immune complex disease in rabbits: the role of complement and of a leukocyte-dependent release of vasoactive amines from platelets. J Exp Med 133:554–571

Hoffeld JT (1981) Agents which block membrane lipid peroxidation enhance mouse spleen cell immune activities in vitro: relationship to the enhancing activity of 2-mercaptoethanol. Eur J Immunol 11:371–376

Hoffman T, Hirata F, Bougnoux P, Fraser BA, Goldfarb RH, Herbermann RB, Axelrod J (1981) Phospholipid methylation and phospholipase A_2 activation in cytotoxicity by human natural killer cells. Proc Natl Acad Sci USA 78:3839–3843

Hoffmann MK, Mizel SB, Hirst JA (1984) IL 1 requirement for B cell activation revealed by use of adult serum. J Immunol 133:2566–2568

Honda M, Steinberg AD (1984) Effects of prostaglandin E_2 on responses of T-cell subsets to mitogen and autologous non-T-Cell stimulation. Clin Immunol Immunopathol 33:111–122

Hoover RL, Bhalla DK, Yanovich S, Inbar M, Karnovsky MJ (1980) Effects of linoleic acid on capping, lectin mediated mitogenesis, surface antigen expression, and fluorescent polarization in lymphocytes and BHK cells. J Cell Physiol 103:399–406

Howard M, Matis L, Malek TR, Shevach E, Kell W, Cohen D, Nakanishi K, Paul WE (1983) Interleukin 2 induces antigen-reactive T cell lines to secrete BC6FI. J Exp Med 158:2024–2039

Hsueh W, Sun FF, Henderson S (1985) the biosynthesis of leukotriene B_4, the predominant lipoxygenase product in rabbit alveolar macrophages, is enhanced during immune activation. Biochim Biophys Acta 835:92–97

Hurd ER, Gilliam JN (1981) Beneficial effect of an essential fatty acid deficient diet in NZB/NZW F_1 mice. J Invest Dermatol 77:381–384

Jelinek DF, Thompson PA, Lipsky PE (1985) Regulation of human B cell activation by prostaglandin E_2. J Clin Invest 75:1339–1349

Johnson HM, Torres BA (1984) Leukotrienes: positive signals for regulation of γ-interferon production. J Immunol 132:413–416

Johnson HM, Areher DL, Torres BA (1982) Cyclic GMP as the second messenger in helper cell requirement for γ-interferon production. J Immunol 129:2570–2572

Johnston DV, Marshall LA (1984) Dietary fat, prostaglandins and the immune response. Prog Food Nutr Sci 8:3–25

Kageyama K, Nagasawa T, Kimura S, Kobayashi T, Kinoshita Y (1980) Cytotoxic activity of unsaturated fatty acids to lymphocytes. Can J Biochem 58:504–508

Kato K, Murota S (1985) Lipoxygenase specific inhibitors inhibit murine lymphocyte reactivity to Con A by reducing IL-2 production and its action. Prostaglandins Leukotrienes Med 18:39–52

Kelley VE, Winkelstein A (1980) Effect of prostaglandin E_1 treatment on murine acute immune complex glomerulonephritis. Clin Immunol Immunopathol 16:316–323

Kelley VE, Winkelstein A, Izui S, Dixon FJ (1981) Prostaglandin E_1 inhibits T-cell proliferation and renal disease in MRL/1 mice. Clin Immunol Immunopathol 21:190–203

Kelly JP, Johnson MC, Parker CW (1979) Effects of inhibitors of arachidonic acid metabolism on mitogenesis in human lymphocytes: possible role of thromboxanes and products of the lipoxygenase pathway. J Immunol 122:1563–1571

King MA, Spector AA (1981) Lipid metabolism in cultured cells. In: Weymouth C, Ham R, Chapple PJ (eds) The growth requirements of vertebrate cells in vitro. Cambridge University Press, New York, p 293

Kremer JM, Bigauoette J, Michalek AV, Timchalk MA, Lininger L, Rynes RI, Huyck C, Zieminski J, Bartholomew LE (1985) Effects of manipulation of dietary fatty acids on clinical manifestations of rheumatoid arthritis. Lancet I:184–187

Kunkel SL, Chensue SW (1985) Arachidonic acid metabolites regulate interleukin-1 production. Biochem Biophys Res Commun 128:892–897

Kunkel SL, Chensue SW, Phan SH (1986) Prostaglandins as endogenous mediators of interleukin 1 production. J Immunol 136:186–192

Lanefelt F, Ullberg M, Jondal M, Fredholm BB (1983) PGE_1 and prostacyclin suppression of NK-cell mediated cytotoxicity and its relation to cyclic AMP. Med Biol 61:324–330

Lapp WS, Mendes M, Kirchner H, Gemsa D (1980) Prostaglandin synthesis by lymphoid tissue of mice experiencing a graft-versus-host reaction: relationship to immunosuppression. Cell Immunol 50:271–281

Leung KH, Koren HS (1982) Regulation of human natural killing. II. Protective effect of interferon on NK cells from suppression by PGE_2. J Immunol 129:1742–1747

Leung KH, Mihich E (1982) Effects of prostaglandins on the development of cell-mediated immunity in culture and on cytolytic activity of in vivo generated effector cells. Int J Immunopharmacol 4:205–217

Leung KH, Ehrke MJ, Mihich E (1982) Modulation of the development of cell-mediated immunity: possible role of the products of the cyclo-oxygenase and the lipoxygenase pathways of arachidonic acid metabolism. Int J Immunopharmacol 4:195–204

Leung KH, Ip MM, Koren HS (1985) The role of the lipoxygenase in regulation of NK activity. In: Herbermann RB (ed) Mechanisms of cytotoxicity by NK cells. Academic, New York, p 253

Loose LD, DiLuzio NR (1973) Effect of prostaglandin E_1 on cellular and humoral immune responses. J Reticuloendothel Soc 13:70–77

Low EE, Pupillo MB, Bryant RW, Bailey JM (1984) Inhibition of phytohemagglutinin-induced lymphocyte mitogenesis by lipoxygenase metabolites of arachidonic acid: structure activity relationships. J Lipid Res 25:1090–1095

Malavasi F, Tetta C, Funaro A, Bellone G, Ferrero E, Colli Franzone A, Dellabona P, Rusci R, Matera L, Camussi G, Caligaris-Cappio F (1986) Fc receptor triggering induces expression of surface activation antigens and release of platelet-activating factor in large granular lymphocytes. Proc Natl Acad Sci USA 83:2443–2447

Matsushima K, Procopio A, Abe H, Scala G, Ortaldo JR, Oppenheim JJ (1985) Production of interleukin 1 activity by normal human peripheral blood B lymphocytes. J Immunol 135:1132–1136

Mauer U, Burger R, von Steldern D, Bitter-Suermann D, Hadding U (1984) Expression of Ia antigens on macrophages is reduced after stimulation with homologous C3b. J Immunol 132:2802–2806

McHugh MI, Wilkinson R, Elliott RW, Field EJ, Dewar P, Hall RR, Taylor RMR, Uldall PR (1977) Immunosuppression with polyunsaturated fatty acids in renal transplantation. Transplantation 24:263–267

McLeish KR, Gohara AF, Gunning WT (1982) Suppression of antibody synthesis by prostaglandin E as a mechanism for preventing murine immune complex glomerulonephritis. Lab Invest 47:147–152

Meade CJ, Mertin J (1978) Fatty acids and immunity. Adv Lipid Res 16:127–165

Meeker HC, Eskew ML, Scheuchenzuber W, Scholz RW, Zarkower A (1985) Antioxidant effects on cell-mediated immunity. J Leuk Biol 38:451–458

Mertin J (1981) Essential fatty acids and cell-mediated immunity. Prog Lipid Res 20:851–856

Mertin J (1985) Drug treatment of patients with multiple sclerosis. In: Koetsier JC (ed) Demyelinating diseases. Elsevier, Amsterdam, p 187 (Handbook of clinical neurology, vol 3)

Mertin J, Hunt R (1976) Influence of polyunsaturated fatty acids on survival of skin allografts and tumor incidence in mice. Proc Natl Acad Sci USA 73:928–931

Mertin J, Smith AD (1988) Immune modulation by prostaglandins and their precursors. In: Willis AL (ed) Handbook of prostaglandins and related lipids, vol 4. CRC, Boca Raton, (in press)

Mertin J, Stackpoole A (1978) Suppression by essential fatty acids of experimental allergic encephalomyelitis enhanced by indomethacin. Prostaglandins Med 1:283–291

Mertin J, Stackpoole A (1979) The spleen is required for the suppression of experimental allergic encephalomyelitis by prostaglandin precursors. Clin Exp Immunol 36:449–455

Mertin J, Stackpoole A (1981) Prostaglandin precursors and the cell-mediated immune response. Cell Immunol 62:293–300

Mertin J, Meade CJ, Hunt R, Sheena J (1977) Importance of the spleen for the immunoinhibitory action of linoleic acid in mice. Int Arch Allergy Appl Immunol 53:469–473

Mertin J, Stackpoole A, Shumway SJ (1984) Prostaglandins and cell-mediated immunity. The role of prostaglandin E_1 in the induction of host-versus-graft and graft-versus-host reactions in mice. Transplantation 37:396–402

Mertin J, Stackpoole A, Shumway S (1985) Nutrition and immunity: the immunoregulatory effect of n-6 essential fatty acids is mediated through prostaglandin E. Int Arch Allergy Appl Immunol 77:390–395

Metzger Z, Hoffeld T, Oppenheim JJ (1980) Macrophage-mediated suppression. I. Evidence for participation of both hydrogen peroxide and prostaglandins in suppression of murine lymphocyte proliferation. J Immunol 124:983–988

Mexmain S, Cook J, Aldigier JC, Gualde N, Rigaud M (1985) Thymocyte cyclic GMP response to treatment with metabolites issued from the lipoxygenase pathway. J Immunol 135:1361–1365

Mittler R, Rao P, Olini G, Westberg E, Newman W, Hoffman W, Hoffmann M, Goldstein G (1985) Activated human B cells display a functional IL 2 receptor. J Immunol 134:2393–2399

Morito T, Bankhurst AD, Williams RC (1980) Studies on the modulation of immunoglobulin production by prostaglandins. Prostaglandins 20:383–390

Morley J, Bray MA, Jones RW, Nugteren DH, van Dorp DA (1979) Prostaglandin and thromboxane production by human and guinea-pig macrophages and leucocytes. Prostaglandins 17:730–736

Munder PG, Weltzien HU, Modolell M (1976) Lysolecithin analogs: a new class of immuno-potentiators. In: Miescher PA (ed) Immunopathology. Schwabe, Basel, p 411

Muraguchi A, Kehrl JH, Longo DL, Volkman DJ, Smith KA, Fauci AS (1985) Interleukin 2 receptors on human B cells – Implications for the role of interleukin 2 in human B cell function. J Exp Med 161:181–197

Myers MJ, Ades EW, Jackson WT, Petersen BH (1984) Possible in vivo modulation of the immune system by the leukotriene, LTB$_4$. I. Delayed suppression of cellular immunity. J Clin Lab Immunol 15:205–209

Nakagawa T, Hirano T, Nakagawa N, Yoshizaki K, Kishimoto T (1985) Effect of recombinant IL 2 and γ-IFN on proliferation and differentiation of human B cells. J Immunol 134:959–966

Niwa Y, Sakane T, Shingu M, Yokoyama MM (1983) Effect of stimulated neutrophils from the synovial fluid of patients with rheumatoid arthritis on lymphocytes. A possible role of increased oxygen radicals generated by the neutrophils. J Clin Immunol 3:228–240

Niwa Y, Sakane T, Shingu M, Yokoyama MM (1984) Role of stimulated neutrophils from patients with systemic lupus erythematosus in disturbed immunoreactivity, with special reference to increased oxygen intermediates generated by the neutrophils. J Clin Lab Immunol 14:35–43

Nordeen SK, Young DA (1978) Refractoriness of the cyclic AMP response to adenosine and prostaglandin E$_1$ in thymic lymphocytes. Dependence on protein synthesis and energy-providing substrates. J Biol Chem 253:1234–1239

Offner H, Clausen J (1978) The enhancing effect of unsaturated fatty acids on E rosette formation. Int Arch Allergy Appl Immunol 56:376–379

O'Flaherty JT, Wykle RL (1983) Biology and biochemistry of platelet-activating factor. Clin Rev Allergy 1:353–367

Okazaki T, Shimizu M, Arbesman CE, Middleton E (1978) Prostaglandin E and mitogenic stimulation of human lymphocytes in serum-free medium. Prostaglandins 15:423–427

Parnham MJ, de Brito F (1987) Meeting report: modern aspects of inflammation. Agents Actions 22:248–250

Parnham MJ, Schoester G-AP, van der Kwast TH (1979a) Enhancement by prostaglandin E$_1$ and essential fatty acid deficiency of the passive transfer of delayed hypersensitivity to PPD in rats. Comparison with effects on delayed hypersensitivity to SRBC in mice. Int J Immunopharmacol 1:119–126

Parnham MJ, Vincent JE, Zijlstra FJ, Bonta IL (1979b) The use of essential fatty acid deficient rats to study pathophysiological roles of prostaglandins. Comparison of prostaglandin production with some parameters of deficiency. Lipids 14:407–412

Parnham MJ, Bittner C, Winkelmann J (1983a) Chemiluminescence from mouse resident macrophages: characterization and modulation by arachidonate metabolites. Immunopharmacol 5:277–291

Parnham MJ, Winkelmann J, Leyck S (1983b) Macrophage, lymphocyte and chronic inflammatory responses in selenium deficient rodents. Association with decreased glutathione peroxidase activity. Int J Immunopharmacol 5:455–461

Payan DG, Missirian-Bastian A, Goetzl EJ (1984) Human T-lymphocyte subset specificity of the regulatory effects of leukotriene B$_4$. Proc Natl Acad Sci USA 81:3501–3505

Pelus LM, Saletan S, Silver RT, Moore MAS (1982) Expression of Ia-antigens on normal and chronic myeloid leukemic human granulocyte-macrophage colony-forming cells (CFU-GM) is associated with the regulation of cell proliferation by prostaglandin E. Blood 59:284–292

Ramstedt U, Serhan CN, Lundberg U, Wigzell H, Samuelsson (1984) Inhibition of human natural killer cell activity by (14R, 15S)-14,15-dihydroxy-5Z, 8Z, 10E, 12E-icosatetraenoic acid. Proc Natl Acad Sci USA 81:6914–6918

Rappaport RS, Dodge GR (1982)) Prostaglandin E inhibits the production of human interleukin 2. J Exp Med 155:943–948

Reddy MM, Manvar D, Ahuja KK, Moriarty ML, Grieco MH (1985) Augmentation of mitogen-induced proliferative responses by in vitro indomethacin in patients with acquired immune deficiency syndrome and AIDS-related complex. Int J Immunopharmacol 7:917–921

Reiner NE, Malemud CJ (1984) Arachidonic acid metabolism in murine leishmaniasis (donovani): ex-vivo evidence for increased cyclooxygenase and 5-lipoxygenase activity in spleen cells. Cell Immunol 88:501–510

Resch K (1980) The role of the plasma membrane in the initiation of lymphocyte activation. In: Kaplan JG (ed) The molecular basis of immune cell function. Elsevier/North-Holland, Amsterdam, p 109

Rogers TJ (1985) The role of arachidonic acid metabolites in the function of murine suppressor cells. In: Goodwin JS (ed) Prostaglandins and immunity. Nijhoff, Boston, p 79

Rogers TJ, Nowowiejski I, Webb DR (1980) Partial characterization of a prostaglandin-induced suppressor factor. Cell Immunol 50:82–93

Rogers TJ, deHaven JI, Donnelly RP (1985) Suppression of B-cell and T-cell responses by the prostaglandin-induced T-cell derived suppressors (PITS)-III. Production of PITS$_\beta$ factors from T-cell hybridomas. Int J Immunopharmacol 7:153–156

Rojo JM, Pilar PM, Barasoain I, Portoles A (1982) Exogenous additions of prostaglandins variably after the blastogenic response of B and T lymphocytes from different mice lymphoid organs. Immunopharmacology 4:95–104

Rola-Pleszczynski M (1985) Differential effects of leukotriene B_4 on T4$^+$ and T8$^+$ lymphocyte phenotype and immunoregulatory functions. J Immunol 135:1357–1360

Rola-Pleszczynski M, Lemaire I (1985) Leukotrienes augment interleukin 1 production by human monocytes. J Immunol 135:3958–3961

Rola-Pleszczynski M, Borgeat P, Sirois P (1982) Leukotriene B_4 induces human suppressor lymphocytes. Biochem Biophys Res Commune 108:1531–1537

Rola-Pleszczynski M, Gagnon L, Rudzinska M, Borgeat P, Sirois P (1984) Human natural cytotoxic cell activity: enhancement by leukotrienes (LT)A$_4$, B$_4$ and D$_4$ but not by stereoisomers of LTB$_4$ or HETEs. Prostaglandins Leukotrienes Med 13:113–117

Rola-Pleszczynski M, Gagnon L, Bolduc D, LeBreton G (1985) Evidence for the involvement of the thromboxane synthase pathway in human natural cytotoxic cell activity. J Immunol 135:4114–4119

Rosenberg YJ, Steinberg AD, Santoro TJ (1984) The basis of autoimmunity in MRL-lpr/lpr mice: a role for self Ia-reactive T cells. Immunol Today 5:64–67

Sanchez ME, Maki DVJ, McLaren LC, Bankhurst AD (1979) Modulation of the adherence of human lymphocytes to measles-infected cells by prostaglandin E$_1$: a differential effect on lymphocyte subpopulations. Prostaglandins 18:35–41

Schleimer RP, Benjamini E (1981) Effects of prostaglandin synthesis inhibition on the immune response. Immunopharmacology 3:205–219

Seaman WE (1984) Human and murine natural killer cell activity may require lipoxygenation of arachidonic acid. J Allergy Clin Immunol 74:407–411

Seaman WE, Gindhart TD, Blackman MA, Dalal B, Talal N, Werb Z (1982) Suppression of natural killing in vitro by monocytes and polymorphonuclear leukocytes. Requirement for reactive metabolites of oxygen. J Clin Invest 69:876–888

Sellin D, Wallach DFH, Weltzien HU, Resch K, Sprenger E, Fischer H (1974) Intercellular communication between lymphocytes in vitro. Eur J Immunol 4:189–193

Sims T, Clagett JA, Page RC (1979) Effects of cell concentration and exogenous prostaglandin on the interaction and responsiveness of human peripheral blood leukocytes. Clin Immunol Immunopathol 12:150–161

Snyders DS, Beller DI, Unanue ER (1982) Prostaglandins modulate macrophage Ia expression. Nature 299:163–165

Staite ND, Panayi GS (1982) Regulation of human immunoglobulin production in vitro by prostaglandin E$_2$. Clin Exp Immunol 49:115–122

Staite ND, Panayi GS (1984) Prostaglandin regulation of B-lymphocyte function. Immunol Today 5:175–178

Staite ND, Ganczakowski M, Panayi GS, Unger A (1983) Prostaglandin-mediated immunoregulation: reduced sensitivity of in vitro immunoglobulin production to indomethacin in rheumatoid arthritis. Clin Exp Immunol 52:535–542

Staszak C, Goodwin JS, Troup GM, Pathak DR, Williams RC (1980) Decreased sensitivity to prostaglandin and histamine in lymphocytes from normal HLA-B12 individuals: a possible role in autoimmunity. J Immunol 125:181–185

Stobo JD, Kennedy MS, Goldyne ME (1979) Prostaglandin E modulation of the mitogenic response of human T cells. Differential response of T-cell subpopulations. J Clin Invest 64:1188–1195

Stylos WA, Chirigos MA, Papademetriou V (1979) The modulatory effect of exogenously added prostaglandin E$_1$ or E$_2$ on the delayed-type hypersensitivity reaction of normal or tumored mice. J Immunopharmacol 1:521–533

Sugiura T, Waku K (1983) Ether phospholipids in macrophages, polymorphonuclear leukocytes, lymphocytes and platelets: high levels of 1-O-alkyl-2-acyl-sn-glycero-3-phosphorylcholine. In: Benveniste J, Arnoux B (eds) Platelet-activating factor and structurally related ether-lipids. Elsevier, Amsterdam, p 291

Targan SR (1981) The dual interaction of prostaglandin E_2 (PGE$_2$) and interferon (IFN) on NK lytic activation: enhanced capacity of effector-target lytic interactions (recycling) and blockage of pre-NK cell recruitment. J Immunol 127:1424–1428

Taylor AS, Howe RC, Morrison AR, Sprecher H, Russell JH (1985) Inhibition of cytotoxic T lymphocyte-mediated lysis by ETYA: effect independent of arachidonic acid metabolism. J Immunol 134:1130–1135

Thompson PA, Jelinek DF, Lipsky PE (1984) Regulation of human B cell proliferation by prostaglandin E_2. J Immunol 133:2446–2453

Tilden AB, Balch CM (1982) A comparison of PGE$_2$ effects on human suppressor cell function and on interleukin 2 function. J Immunol 129:2469–2473

Ting CC, Hargrove ME (1984) Regulation of the activation of cytotoxic T lymphocytes by prostaglandins and antigens. J Immunol 133:660–666

Tonkin CH, Brostoff J (1978) Do fatty acids exert a specific effect on human lymphocyte transformation in vitro? Int Arch Allergy Appl Immunol 57:171–176

Tracey DE, Adkinson NF (1980) Prostaglandin synthesis inhibitors potentiate the BCG-induced augmentation of natural killer cell activity. J Immunol 125:136–141

Trotter J, Ferber E (1981) CoA-dependent cleavage of arachidonic acid from phosphatidylcholine and transfer to phosphatidylethanolamine in homogenates of murine thymocytes. FEBS Lett 128:237–241

Vanderhoek JY, Bryant RW, Bailey JM (1980) Inhibition of leukotriene biosynthesis by the leukocyte product 15-hydroxyeicosatetraenoic acid. J Biol Chem 255:10064–10066

Van Tol MJD, Zijlstra J, Thomas CMG, Zegers BJM, Ballieux RE (1984) Distinct role of neonatal and adult monocytes in the regulation of the in vitro antigen-induced plaque-forming cell response in man. J Immunol 133:1902–1908

Warren RQ, Thomas FT, Thomas JM (1983) Immunoregulatory effects of prostaglandin on human MLR and CML responses. Transplant Proc 15:1866–1867

Webb DR (1978) The effects of prostaglandins on cAMP levels in subpopulations of mouse lymphocytes. Prostaglandins Med 1:441–453

Webb DR, Osheroff PL (1976) Antigen stimulation of prostaglandin synthesis and control of immune responses. Proc Natl Acad Sci USA 73:1300–1304

Webb DR, Nowowiejski I (1977) The role of prostaglandins in the control of the primary 19S immune response to sRBC. Cell Immunol 33:1–10

Webb DR, Nowowiejski I, Healy C, Rogers TJ (1982) Immunosuppressive properties of leukotriene D_4 and E_4 in vitro. Biochem Biophys Res Commun 104:1617–1622

Weyman C, Morgan SJ, Belin J, Smith AD (1977) Phytohemagglutinin stimulation of human lymphocytes. Effect of fatty acids on uridine uptake and phosphoglyceride fatty acid profile. Biochim Biophys Acta 496:155–166

Whisler RL, Newhouse Y (1982) Inhibition of human B lymphocyte colony responses by endogenous hydrogen peroxide and prostaglandins. Cell Immunol 69:34–45

Wieder KJ, Webb DR (1981) The effect of prostaglandin metabolism on immunoglobulin and antibody production in naive and educated whole spleen cells. Prostaglandins Med 7:79–90

Wolf M, Droege W (1982) Inhibition of cytotoxic responses by prostaglandin E_2 in the presence of interleukin 2. Cell Immunol 72:286–293

Zielinski CC, Gisinger C, Binder C, Mannhalter JW, Eibl MM (1984) Regulation of NK cell activity by prostaglandin E_2: the role of T cells. Cell Immunol 87:65–72

Zimecki M, Webb DR (1976) The regulation of the immune response to T-independent antigens by prostaglandins and B cells. J Immunol 117:2158–2164

Zurier RB, Damjanov J, Sayadoff DM, Rothfield NF (1977) Prostaglandin E_1 treatment of NZB/NZW F$_1$ hybrid mice. II. Prevention of glomerulonephritis. Arthritis Rheum 20:1449–1456

Zurier RB, Damjanov I, Miller PL, Biewer BF (1978) Prostaglandin E_1 treatment prevents progression of nephritis in murine lupus erythematosus. J Clin Lab Immunol 1:95–98

CHAPTER 16

Thymic Hormones and Lymphocyte Functions

J.-F. Bach and M. Dardenne

A. Introduction

The differentiation of lymphocytes from precursor cells involves a complex series of events, and several factors control this sequential transformation of T cells. The thymic epithelium plays a central and apparently unique role in the first phases. It is during its direct contact with the thymic epithelium that the prothymocyte (whether or not it is already committed to the T cell lineage) is transformed into the immature cortical thymocyte, and eventually into the "postthymic thymocyte." This transformation is associated with the acquisition of antigenic markers, and the formation of the repertoire of anti-self receptors necessary for the cognitive functions of T cells (see Chap. 1).

It is not known whether thymic hormones intervene in these first phases of differentiation in addition of the inducing effect on differentiation alloantigens which comprise functionally important molecules (e.g., Thy-1 and Lyt-2 antigens). Later stages of maturation, which lead the T cell to the post-thymic stage (the still immunologically incompetent cell which leaves the thymus) and to the mature T cell, are under thymic hormone control. Other factors may participate in the very last stages, for example, antigen stimulation, in particular through the production of interleukin 2 (IL-2). It should be noted, however, that IL-2 may only operate as an amplification circuit since it is exclusively produced by mature T cells which must, by definiton, have differentiated under thymic control.

Several thymic hormones have been described, and it has not yet been determined how many molecules intervene physiologically as mediators of thymic humoral function. As far as chemically well-defined peptides are concerned, one is confronted with a series of molecular entities with no apparent relationship. So far, from this series, four distinct peptides have been identified: thymopoietin, thymosin α1, thymic humoral factor (THF), and thymulin (formerly called FTS), with molecular weights ranging from 800 to 5500. To date, only three of them have been chemically synthesized: thymopoietin, thymosin α1, and thymulin. Before discussing the main biologic effects of these peptides on T lymphocytes, we shall give a brief review of their main characteristics.

B. Chemistry of the Four Available Thymic Peptides

I. Thymosin α 1

Thymosin α1 was the first peptide to be isolated from thymosin fraction 5 and sequenced. It consists of 28 amino acid residues and has a molecular weight of 3108 (GOLDSTEIN et al. 1977). Both natural and synthetic peptides show several (and indentical) biologic activities. Thymosin α1 increases mitogenic responses of murine lymphocytes, stimulates antibody production, enhances production of the macrophage migration-inhibitory factor, and augments the number of Thy-1$^+$ Lyt-1,2,3$^+$ cells (AHMED et al. 1979; GOLDSTEIN et al. 1983). It also increases the expression of terminal deoxynucleotidyltransferase (TdT). Although in some of these assay systems thymosin α1 seems to have a higher specific activity than thymosin fraction 5, it is difficult to distinguish the role of thymosin α1 from other biologically produced thymosin fraction 5 peptides.

II. Thymopoietin

Thymopoietin was characterized by its neuromuscular effects rather than by its action on the immune system. The development of experimental models of myasthenia gravis led to the detection of a thymic hormone influence on neuromuscular transmission, and electromyographic assays were used to monitor the fractionation of thymic extracts (GOLDSTEIN and LAU 1980). By this means, thymopoietin was isolated and the biochemically homogeneous polypeptide was shown to be potent (>4 ng per mouse) in the neuromuscular assays. Thymopoietin was ultimately shown to induce various T cell-specific alloantigens in vitro in the Komuro-Boyse assay.

Thymopoietin is a 49 amino acid polypeptide isolated to chemical homogeneity from thymic extracts. Its complete amino acid sequence has been determined. There are two forms (termed thymopoietin I and II) which differ by only two amino acid substitutions. A synthetic pentapeptide has the complete activity of thymopoietin and is selective for T cell differentiation in vitro (GOLDSTEIN et al. 1979). Thymopoietin (or its pentapeptide fragment TP5) has been shown to enhance several T cell functions in vivo (rejection of the 3LL carcinoma, prevention of autoimmunity in mice, and generation of cytotoxic T cells). Recently, a peptide related to thymopoietin has been isolated from the spleen. This peptide, named splenin, has an amino acid sequence very close to that of thymopoietin I and II, but shows two minor differences, particularly on residue 34 which is included in the TP5 sequence.

III. Thymulin

Thymulin, formerly called FTS, is a nonapeptide initially prepared from porcine serum, but also isolated to purity from human serum and calf thymus (BACH 1983). Thymulin binds zinc (DARDENNE et al. 1982) with a dissociation constant of 10^{-7} M (as evaluated by equilibrium chromatography), and the presence of zinc is necessary for its biologic activity. More than 40 analogs of thymulin have been synthesized and immunologically evaluated (in bioassays and receptor assays) permitting the localization of the molecule's activity to the seven terminal amino acids. Some analogs have been shown to bind to the receptor and to inhibit thymulin activity, behaving like antihormones (PLÉAU et al. 1979). Thymulin is exclusively produced by the thymic epithelium. It circulates in the blood, and a portion of it is bound to a 40–60 kdalton carrier molecule. It is subject to the action of several inhibitors (BACH 1983).

Thymulin apparently acts exclusively on T cells. It binds to T cell membrane receptors with high affinity: there are two sites with $K_d = 10^{-9}$ and 10^{-7} M, without negative cooperativity (PLÉAU et al. 1980). Thymulin has been shown to enhance the functions of the various T cell subsets (BACH 1983). Interestingly, thymulin shows a preferential action on suppressor T cells at high doses, particularly in normal recipients. At low doses, or in immunodeficient patients, it is more difficult to predict which T cell subset will be preferentially stimulated.

IV. Thymic Humoral Factor

Using an in vitro graft-versus-host assay, TRAININ and SMALL (1970) characterized a low molecular weight peptide called thymic humoral factor (THF). Using a crude thymic extract dialysate as the source of THF, TRAININ et al. (1979) showed that THF was capable of restoring the competence of lymphoid cells from neonatally thymectomized mice, enabling them to participate in mixed lymphocyte reactions, to kill tumor cells, and to respond to T lectins. The administration of THF to humans suffering from either primary or secondary immunodeficiencies resulted in the restoration of cellular immunocompetence. Immune maturation of thymus-derived lymphoid cells after exposure to THF in vitro or in vivo occurs via an obligatory rise in cellular cAMP levels (KOOK and TRAININ 1974). THF was isolated by stepwise gel filtration through Sephadex columns. When fractions were tested in a graft-versus-host assay in vitro, the pure THF material was found to be a polypeptide with a molecular weight of 3000. Its amino acid sequence has not yet been elucidated.

C. Effect of Thymic Hormones on Lymphocyte Markers and Functions

Thymic factors do not act identically on different lymphocyte subsets. The analysis and discussion of the functions that are the most readily affected by the various available thymic factors should prove useful for the understanding of the role of thymic factors in T cell differentiation. Indirect evidence, essentially based on the work of STUTMAN (1978), indicates that thymic factors probably act at the level of a so-called post-thymic precursor cell, as found in neonatal spleen. Such a post-thymic cell has already encountered the thymic influence, probably by direct contact with the epithelium, where, in addition to receiving the antigen-nonspecific maturation signal, it has gained its anti-H-2 (or Ia) receptors that will be needed for the various T cell cognitive functions.

Data obtained with purified or synthetic thymic factors are generally compatible with this hypothesis. There are some reports that thymic factors might act in nude mice or totally T cell-deprived mice (thymectomized, irradiated, reconstituted with anti-theta serum-treated bone marrow cells) but these publications either concern cell markers (Bach et al. 1975; Scheid et al. 1975) and provide no direct information on functional T cell differentiation, or relate to T cell functions (Ikhehara et al. 1975), but these have not been confirmed. Most data obtained either in vitro or in vivo, derive from studies in normal adult thymectomized, partially T cell-deprived, NZB or aged mice, that may show some degree of T cell deficiency, but that share the property of possessing post-thymic cells.

I. Marker Studies

Marker studies indicate that the various types of T cell differentiation antigens may be induced in precursor cells that are devoid of such markers. This was initially shown by us for the theta antigen, with various thymic extracts (Bach et al. 1971), and has now been confirmed and extended for Lyt-1,2, and 3 antigens, TL antigens, and xenogeneic antigens (Scheid et al. 1975). Most available thymic factors appear to induce such differentiation antigens. In particular, thymulin induces the theta and Lyt antigens in the mouse, and xenogeneic T cell antigens in the human (Bach 1983; Incefy et al. 1980).

Other T cell markers are induced by thymic factors. In particular, TdT expression is modified by incubation of immature lymphoid cells with thymic factors. Interestingly, the effects differ according to the cell type considered. TdT is increased by thymosin in nude mouse spleen cells (Pazmino et al. 1978), and decreased in normal bone marrow cells by snythetic thymulin in bovine serum albumin gradient-separated human bone marrow cells (Incefy et al. 1980). Human E-rosettes are seemingly increased in vitro and in vivo by all available factors (Wara et al. 1975; Zaizov et al. 1979; Incefy et al. 1975, 1980).

II. Effect on T Cell Functions

Most T cell functions have been reported to be induced or enhanced by thymic factors (provided the appropriate recipient is selected). Thymic hormones enhance T cell mediated *cytotoxicity* in thymectomized mice. This effect is particularly clear in adult thymectomized mice with the Brunner assay (Bach 1977). Similarly, thymulin also acts on T cells involved in delayed-type hypersensitivity induced by dinitrofluorobenzene (DNFB) (Erard et al. 1979). It restores a normal response in adult thymectomized mice. The effect of thymic hormones on *Helper* T cells as studied on sheep red blood cell-specific antibody production is much less clear, perhaps owing to a simultaneous action on suppressor T cells.

In fact, thymic hormones have recently proven to be remarkably active on *suppressor* T cells in various in vitro and in vivo systems (Bach 1983; Erard et al. 1979). Given in vivo to normal mice, thymulin suppresses the generation of alloantigen-reactive T cells or DNFB-sensitive T cells.Given at 10–100 ng, it may prolong skin allograft survival. Lastly, in vitro, thymulin and thymosin fraction 5 (Calabrese et al. 1980; Horowitz et al. 1977) markedly reconstitute the depressed capacity of most lupus patients to generate suppressor T cells after Con A activation, assessed on pokeweed mitogen-driven immunoglobulin synthesis.

This new effect of thymic factors complicates the interpretation of the functional biologic data observed previously, but widens the potential therapeutic applications. It appears, as far as thymulin is concerned, that the suppressor effect is essentially observed at high "pharmacologic" thymulin doses, while other effects are seen at lower, presumably physiologic doses. Whether this difference in dose is related to a difference in cellular receptors of suppressor T cells compared with helper T cells or other T cells, is not known. Whether it is related to a pharmacologic stimulation of mature suppressor cells or to an induction of maturation of suppressor T cell precursors has not been determined. Note, however, that a nonspecific inhibitory effect on immune responses is unlikely, as the effect can be prevented by pretreatment of recipient mice with low doses of cyclophosphamide, known to inhibit suppressor T cells selectively in various systems.

It is interesting to note that this effect of thymulin on suppressor cells probably explains most of its preventive effects observed in NZB autoimmune mice (decrease in polyvinylpyrrolidone-specific antibody production, prevention of the Sjögren syndrome; BACH et al. 1980). A simultaneous effect on helper T cells probably explains the accelerated production of IgG DNA-specific antibodies also observed in these mice.

III. Mode of Action at the Cellular Level

As with any hormone, the action of thymic hormones should be discussed at two levels: receptor and second messenger. The hormone receptor has only been studied in detail for thymulin for which high affinity receptors have been identified on lymphoblastoid T cell lines (not on B or null cell lines; PLÉAU et al. 1980) and thymopoietin (ANDHYA et al. 1984). However, receptors for neither thymulin nor thymopoietin have yet been characterized on normal lymphoid cells, and it is still impossible to define the distribution of receptor-bearing cells.

There has been an intensive search for a second messenger. Data indicate that only THF readily stimulates cyclic AMP (KOOK and TRAININ 1974). Thymulin factor 5 and thymopoietin stimulate cyclic GMP (BACH et al. 1979). The recent reports that thymulin (GUALDE et al. 1982; RINALDI-GARACI et al. 1985) and thymosin α1 (RINALDI-GARACI et al. 1983) stimulate prostaglandin synthesis might suggest that prostaglandins could represent a putative second messenger which in turn could stimulate cyclic AMP synthesis. This hypothesis was proposed several years ago when we showed that indomethacin, which inhibits prostaglandin synthesis, also inhibits thymulin action, while prostaglandins and cyclic AMP mimic the effects of thymic hormone on the differentiation of alloantigens (BACH and BACH 1973).

D. Conclusions

The fact that the thymus is a lymphocyte-differentiating gland has been extensively documented (Chap. 1). Thymic epithelial cells play a central role by influencing the different steps of intrathymic maturation. They present the different products of the major histocompatibility complex to lymphocytes. They secrete chemotactic factors, enabling the colonization of the gland by pre-T cells, and produce thymic hormones whose biologic activities have been demonstrated in vivo and in vitro at the different stages of T cell differentiation. These hormones can provide some of the signals necessary for T lymphocyte maturation and should, therefore, have therapeutic applications in the future.

References

Ahmed A, Wong DM, Thurman GB, Low TLK, Goldstein AI (1979) T lymphocyte maturation cell surface markers and immune function, induced by T lymphocyte cell free products and thymosin polypeptides. Ann NY Acad Sci 332:81–94

Andhya T, Talle MA, Goldstein G (1984) Thymopoietin radioreceptor assay utilizing lectin-purified glycoprotein from a biologically responsive T-cell line. Arch Biochem Biophys 234:167–177

Bach JF (1983) Thymulin (FTS-Zn). Clin Immunol Allergy 3:133–157

Bach JF, Dardenne M, Goldstein AL, Guha A, White A (1971) Appearance of T cell markers in bone marrow rosette-forming cells after incubation with purified thymosin, a thymic hormone. Proc Natl Acad Sci USA 68:2734–2738

Bach JF, Bach MA, Charreire J, Dardenne M, Pleau JM (1979) The mode of action of thymic hormones. Ann NY Acad Sci 332:23–32

Bach MA (1977) Lymphocyte mediated cytotoxicity: effect on ageing of adult thymectomy and thymic factor. J Immunol 119:641–648

Bach MA, Bach JF (1973) Studies on thymic products. IV: The effects of cyclic nucleotides and prostaglandins on rosette forming cells. Interaction with thymic factor. Eur J Immunol 3:778

Bach JF, Dardenne M, Pleau JM, Bach MA (1975) Isolation, biochemical characteristics and biologic activity of a circulating thymic hormone in the mouse and in the human. Ann NY Acad Sci 249:186–210

Bach MA, Droz D, Noel LH, Blanchard D, Dardenne M, Peking A (1980) Effect on long-term treatment with circulating thymic factor on murine lupus. Arthritis Rheum 23:1351–1358

Calabrese LH, Bach JF, Currie T, Vitt D, Clough J, Krakauer RS (1981) Development of systemic lupus erythematosus following thymectomy for myasthenia gravis. Studies of suppressor cell functions. Arch Intern Med 141:253–255

Dardenne M, Pleau JM, Nabarra B, Lefrancier P, Derrien M, Choay J, Bach JF (1982) Contribution of zinc and other metals to the biological activity of the serum thymic factor. Proc Natl Acad Sci USA 79:5370–5373

Erard D, Charreire J, Auffredou MT, Galanaud P (1979) Regulation of contact sensitivity to DNFB in the mouse: effects of ageing on adult thymectomy and thymic factor. J Immunol 123:1573–1576

Goldstein AL, Low TLKL, McAdoo M, McLure J, Thurman GB, Rossio JJ, Lay CY et al. (1977) Thymosin α1: isolation and sequence analysis of an immunologically active thymic polypeptide. Proc Natl Acad Sci USA 74:725–729

Goldstein AL, Low TLH, Latz MM, Hall NR, Naylor PH (1983) Thymosins. Clin Immunol Allergy 3:119–132

Goldstein G, Lau C (1980) Thymopoietin and immunoregulation. In: Beer RF, Bassett EG (eds) Polypeptide hormones. Raven, New York, pp 459–465

Goldstein G, Scheid MP, Boyse EA, Schlesinger DH, van Vauwe J (1979) A synthetic pentapeptide with biological activity characteristic of the thymic hormone thymopoietin. Science 204:1309–1310

Gualde N, Rigaud M, Bach JF (1982) Stimulation of prostaglandin synthesis by the serum factor (FTS). Cell Immunol 70:363–366

Horowitz S, Borcheling W, Moorthy AV, Chesney R, Schulte-Wissermann H, Hong R (1977) Induction of suppressor T cells in systemic lupus erythematosus by thymosin and cultured thymic epithelium. Science 197:999–1001

Ikhehara S, Hamashima Y, Masuda T (1975) Immunological restoration of both thymec-tomized and athymic nude mice by a thymus factor. Nature 258:335–337

Incefy GS, L'Esperance P, Good RA (1975) In vitro differentiation of human marrow cells into T lymphocytes by thymic extracts using the rosette technique. Clin Exp Immunol 19:475–483

Incefy GS, Mertelsmann R, Dardenne M, Bach JF, Good RA (1980) Induction of differ-entiation in human marrow T cell precursors by the synthetic serum thymic factor (FTS). Clin Exp Immunol 40:396–400

Kook AI, Trainin N (1974) Hormone like activity of a thymus hurmoral factor on the in-duction of immune competence in lymphoid cells. J Exp Med 139:193–207

Pazmino NH, Ihle JM, Goldstein AL (1978) Induction in vivo and in vitro of terminal deoxynucleotidyl transferase by thymosin in bone marrow cells from athymic mice. J Exp Med 147:708–718

Pléau JM, Dardenne M, Blanot D, Bricas I, Bach JF (1979) Antagonistic analogue of serum thymic factor (FTS) interacting with the FTS cellular receptor. Immunol Lett 1:179–182

Pléau JM, Fuentes V, Morgat JL, Bach JF (1980) Specific receptors for the serum thymic factor (FTS) in lymphoblastoid cultured cell lines. Proc Natl Acad Sci 77:2861–2865

Rinaldi-Garaci C, Garaci E, DelGobbo V, Favalli C, Jezzi R, Goldstein AL (1983) Modu-lation of endogenous prostaglandins by thymosin $\alpha 1$ in lymphocytes. Cell Immunol 80:57–65

Rinaldi-Garaci C, Jezzi T, Baldassarre AM, Dardenne M, Bach JF, Garaci E (1985) Effect of thymulin on intracellular cyclic nucleotides and prostaglandin E_2 in peanut agglu-tinin fractionated thymocytes. Eur J Immunol 15:548–552

Scheid MP, Goldstein G, Boyse EA (1975) Differentiation of T cells in nude mice. Science 190:1211–1222

Stutman O (1978) Intrathymic and extrathymic T cell maturation. Immunol Rev 42:138–184

Trainin N, Small M (1970) Studies on some physicochemical properties of a thymus hu-moral factor conferring immunocompetence on lymphoid cells. J Exp Med 132:885–889

Trainin N, Rotter V, Yakir Y, Leve R, Handzel Z, Shahat B, Zaizov R (1979) Biochemical and biological properties of THF in animal and human models. Ann NY Acad Sci 332:9–22

Wara DW, Goldstein AL, Doyle W, Amman AJ (1975) Thymosin activity in patients with cellular immunodeficiency. N Engl J Med 292:70–74

Zaizov RR, Vogel I, Wolack B, Cohen IJ, Varsano I, Shohat B, Handzel Z et al. (1979) The effect of THF in lymphoproliferative and myeloproliferative diseases in children. Ann NY Acad Sci 332:172–183

Part 4

CHAPTER 17

Glucocorticosteroids

T. W. Behrens and J. S. Goodwin

A. Introduction

Over the last four decades, glucocorticosteroids have assumed a major role in the treatment of allograft rejection and a number of allergic, autoimmune, and malignant diseases in humans. Pharmacologic doses of corticosteroids profoundly suppress a wide variety of nonspecific inflammatory responses and specific immunologic processes. Despite the progress of recent years, the precise mechanisms whereby corticosteroids exert their powerful effects remain uncertain. However, it is increasingly clear that lymphocytes, as primary effectors of cellular and humoral immune responses, mediate many of the clinically useful properties of glucocorticosteroids. Following a brief historical persepective, this chapter will review the effects of corticosteroids on T and B lymphocyte function, and summarize what is known about the mechanism of action of steroids.

It is important to note the striking differences in susceptibility to corticosteroids between species (CLAMAN 1972). Steroid-sensitive species, including the mouse, rat, and rabbit, experience dramatic lymphoid depletion following steroid treatment, characterized by shrinkage of the thymus, spleen, and peripheral lymph nodes, and lysis of peripheral blood lymphocytes. In contrast, human and guinea pig lymphoid cells are resistant to the lytic effects of steroid administration. This fundamental difference in steroid sensitivity should lead to cautious interpretation of the literature, especially in applying data from steroid-sensitive animals to humans. Another potential problem in the interpretation of early studies is that suprapharmacologic doses of steroids, clearly unobtainable in vivo, were often added to in vitro cultures (CUPPS and FAUCI 1982). Unless otherwise stated, this chapter will focus on human experimental data and studies investigating the effects of physiologic or pharmacologic concentrations of corticosteroids.

B. History

The early studies of ADDISON (1855) and BROWN-SEQUARD (1856) established for the first time that the adrenal glands are essential for life. By 1930, the profound effects of adrenocortical extracts on sodium balance and carbohydrate metabolism were recognized, and in 1932 Harvey CUSHING described the syndrome of hypercortisolism. A decade of fruitful basic research ensued and, by 1943, organic chemists has isolated and identified the structures of 28 adrenal cortex steroids

(Reichstein and Shoppee 1943). Several of these were found to be biologically active, including cortisol, cortisone, and corticosterone. Dougherty and White (1944) discovered that glucocorticosteroids caused lysis of lymphoid tissue in mice, and in 1948 Forsham and his co-workers reported a transient lymphocytopenia in humans following ACTH administration (Hills et al. 1948). Following the synthesis of cortisone by Kendall et al. (1934) in sufficient quantities for clinical use, Hench et al. (1949) reported the dramatic reversal of the inflammatory manifestations of rheumatoid arthritis with cortisone administration. Interestingly, Hench had noted as early as 1929 that arthritis patients sometimes experienced a remission when pregnant or jaundiced, and he suspected a steroid metabolite. His discovery brought widespread attention, and in 1950 Hench, Kendall and Reichstein were jointly awarded the Nobel Prize in Medicine and Physiology.

As corticosteroids became available to investigators in the 1950s, the immunosuppressive and anti-inflammatory properties of these agents were recognized. In 1951, Billingham et al. reported that cortisone prolonged the life of skin homografts in rabbits. Early animal studies focused on the effects of steroids on antibody production, allergic hypersensitivity, tumor and transplantation immunity, and delayed cell-mediated reactions (for review see Gabrielsen and Good 1967). Therapeutic trials of corticosteroids for a wide variety of human diseases were initiated, and initial research examined the gross clinical and metabolic effects of steroids. Initial enthusiasm for the clinical use of steroids was tempered by the profound side effects of high dose therapy. Subsequently, the explosion of knowledge regarding basic cell and molecular biology during the ensuing 35 years have provided many insights into the mechanisms of the diverse actions of steroids. Several excellent reviews summarize this exciting period (Gabrielsen and Good 1967; David et al. 1970; Baxter and Forsham 1972; Claman 1972).

C. Effects of Steroids on Lymphocyte Function In Vivo

In general, T lymphocytes are more sensitive to the in vivo immunosuppressive effects of corticosteroids than are B lymphocytes. Fauci et al. (1976) emphasized the importance of the redistribution of lymphocytes and monocytes in mediating corticosteroid action in humans. A single dose of corticosteroids in humans results in a 70% decline in circulating lymphocytes and a 90% decline in circulating monocytes. T lymphocytes, especially helper T cells, are depleted from the circulation to a greater extent than B lymphocytes in response to corticosteroids. This occurs within 4–6 h and reverts to normal by 24 h (Fauci and Dale 1974). A similar phenomenon occurs daily during chronic steroid administration. The lymphocytopenia appears to be due to redistribution of circulating lymphocytes to other lymphoid compartments, particularly the bone marrow, and not to cell lysis or death. The normal migration of lymphocytes from the peripheral circulation to secondary lymphoid tissues and back occurs rapidly (approximately 12 times per day) and is not random. Specific molecules present on the surface of circulating lymphocytes and the cells lining postcapillary high endothelial venules direct the lymphocyte traffic in a precise, though poorly understood, manner. Presumably, corticosteroids alter the specific recognition molecules or surface charge on the cell membranes, and either enhance exit of lymphocytes from the circulation or block reentry.

B lymphocytes are relatively resistant to the in vivo immunosuppressive effects of corticosteroids in humans. Early studies, using low doses of steroids, reported no effects on serum immunoglobulin levels in humans (SCHWARTZ 1968). Specific antibody synthesis following inoculation with pneumococcal capsular polysaccharide, pertussis vaccine, diphtheria toxoid, and streptococcal O-antigens are not affected by glucocorticoid therapy (for review see DAVID et al. 1970). However, serum IgG, IgA, and IgM levels are suppressed following a brief course of daily high dose methylprednisolone with maximal suppression 2–4 weeks after treatment. This reflects an initial increase in immunoglobulin catabolism, and subsequent decreased production (BUTLER and ROSSEN 1973). Alternate day prednisone therapy was found to enhance the primary antibody response to keyhole limpet hemocyanin immunization in a group of asthmatic children, but had no effect on the secondary immunization (TUCHINDA et al. 1972). An increase in both total and specific IgE levels was noted in a group of asthmatic patients following steroid treatment (POSEY et al. 1978). In vivo prednisolone was shown to enhance the serum IgM and IgG concentrations in a patient with common variable hypogammaglobulinemia, and immunoglobulin levels fell to their baseline 3 months after steroid therapy was completed (WALDMANN et al. 1978). In vivo steroids may augment immunoglobulin levels in certain clinical situations by inhibiting suppressor cell function (WALDMANN et al. 1978).

Cell-mediated immune reactions are generally inhibited by in vivo corticosteroids. Patients on steroids are often anergic, reflecting an inability to express cutaneous delayed hypersensitivity despite previous sensitization. LONG and FAVOUR (1950) were the first to demonstrate suppression of the tuberculin reaction in humans after systemic cortisone therapy, and VOLLMER (1951) showed suppression after local injection of cortisone into the skin test site. BOVORNKITTI et al. (1960), using repeated purified protein derivative (PPD) tests, showed that 68 of 70 patients treated with prednisone 40 mg/day converted from a positive to a negative tuberculin test within 2 weeks. The skin test reaction reconverted to a positive test 6 days after prednisone therapy was stopped. Steroid-induced anergy may result as much from impaired recruitment of macrophages to the skin test site as from suppression of T lymphocyte function (WESTON et al. 1973). The role of corticosteroid inhibition of macrophage function in cell-mediated immunity is reviewed elsewhere (CUPPS and FAUCI 1982). Glucocorticoids, generally in combination with other immunosuppressive agents, are routinely administered following kidney, heart, and liver allograft transplantation. Steroids are believed to suppress graft rejection by inhibiting the proliferation of alloreactive T lymphocytes and the generation of cytotoxic T lymphocytes (KEOWN and STILLER 1986). Intravenous corticosteroids alone can reverse acute graft rejection (OST et al. 1983).

D. Effects of Steroids on Lymphocyte Function In Vitro

Lacking adequate in vivo models, investigators have focused on in vitro lymphocyte function to characterize the immunomodulatory effects of corticosteroids. In many systems, glucocorticoids must be present early in the culture period for the maximal in vitro effect. This suggests that in vitro steroids primarily affect early immunoregulatory events, and are less effective in modulating an established response (CRUPPS and FAUCI 1982).

I. Humoral Immunity

B lymphocytes are central in the induction of humoral immunity. B cells in the G_0 (resting) stage are stimulated to enter the G_1 phase of the cell cycle by crosslinkage of their surface immunoglobulin molecules with such multivalent ligands as antigen, immunoglobulin-specific antibodies, or protein A of *Staphylococcus aureus* (Fig. 1; Chap. 1). Other signals essential to B cell activation and maturation are provided by activated T helper cells. Interaction of T helper cells with HLA-DR molecules on the surface of resting B cells is necessary for the transition from G_0 to G_1. Activated B cells in the G_1 cell cycle proliferate after binding T cell-derived B cell growth factors to specific membrane receptors. The B cell then be-

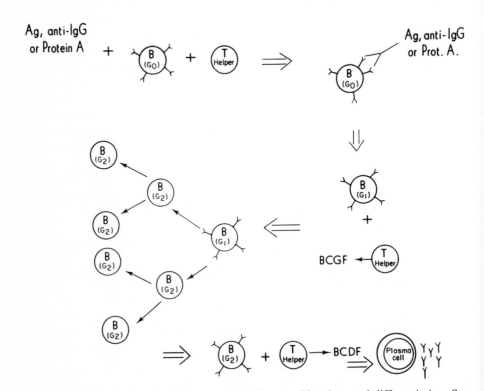

Fig. 1. Normal events in B lymphocyte activation, proliferation, and differentiation. See text for details

gins DNA synthesis, and divides. The daughter B cells of this activation pathway express receptors for another soluble T cell product called B cell differentiation factor, which promotes terminal plasma cell differentiation (Chaps. 1 and 2).

Studies investigating in vitro B cell function following in vivo corticosteroid therapy have shown variable results, usually demonstrating either no change or decreased responsiveness to pokeweed mitogen stimulation (SAXON et al. 1978). Most studies investigating the effects of steroids on B cell function have used systems where B cell function was dependent on the accessory cell functions of monocytes and T cells. More recent studies have clarified the specific actions of corticosteroids on B lymphocyte function (BOWEN and FAUCI 1984; CUPPS et al. 1985). Using a system studying purified human peripheral blood and tonsillar B cells, in the absence of accessory cells, CUPPS et al. (1985) have demonstrated a complex graded effect of in vitro corticosteroids on B lymphocyte activation, proliferation, and differentiation. Early events in B cell activation and proliferation induced by *Staphylococcus aureus* Cowan I (SAC) or high dose anti-IgM are profoundly inhibited by in vitro corticosteroids. Hydrocortisone blocks resting (G_0) purified B cells from enlarging, acquiring activation antigens, and progressing to the G_1 cell cycle phase. Furthermore, all RNA and DNA synthesis is inhibited. Corticosteroids must be present in culture during the first 24 h to be effective. SAC-stimulated cultures were found to require accessory cells for the steroid in-

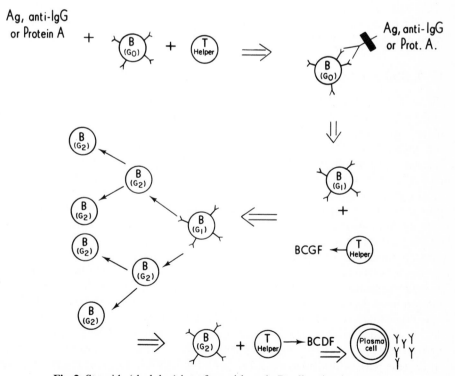

Fig. 2. Steroids (*dark bar*) interfere with early B cell activation events

hibition, whereas monocyte depletion of anti-IgM-stimulated B cells had no effect. Intermediate steps in B cell proliferation, as measured by responsiveness to B cell growth factor, are less sensitive to the suppressive effects of in vitro corticosteroids. Late events in the B cell cycle, specifically differentiation to an immunoglobulin-secreting state, are resistant to in vitro corticosteroid suppression. In summary, once the resting B cell has received a sufficient signal to become activated, steroids have only minimal effects on proliferative events (Cupps et al. 1985). The effects of steroids on B cell function are summarized in Fig. 2.

In several systems where B cell function is dependent on T lymphocytes or T cell-derived factors, in vitro corticosteroids actually augment immunoglobulin production. In 1981, Grayson et al. reported that steroids induced polyclonal immunoglobulin production in cultures of human lymphocytes in the absence of mitogen. The response to steroids was comparable in magnitude to that produced by pokeweed mitogen, although it was delayed, peaking at 8–10 days of culture. Our laboratory has recently determined that fetal calf serum or other minor antigenic stimuli are necessary for the observed corticosteroid stimulation of immunoglobulin production in the absence of mitogen (Sierakowski and Goodwin 1986). These profound effects of physiologic concentrations of corticosteroids undoubtably play an important role in the in vivo humoral immune response to antigenic stimuli. There is considerable evidence in several systems that suppressor cells are inhibited by corticosteroids (Piccolella et al. 1985; Haynes and Fauci 1979), and loss of tonic suppressor influences may explain the increase in immunoglobulin production seen. A recent study supports this concept. Paavonen (1985) found that glucocorticoids enhanced immunoglobulin synthesis in a pokeweed mitogen-driven system by selectively inhibiting a T8$^+$ T suppressor cell.

II. Cellular Immunity

The initial event in T cell activation is recognition by the T cell of both specific antigen and major histocompatibility complex molecules on an antigen-presenting, or accessory, cell. Following recognition, a soluble product of the accessory cell, interleukin 1 (IL-1), is secreted and serves as an additional signal (Chap. 7). T cell activation is followed by proliferation and expansion of antigen-specific activated T cells. Interleukin 2 (IL-2) is a glycoprotein of molecular weight 17000 produced by activated T lymphocytes (Chap. 8). All subsets of peripheral T lymphocytes can develop specific IL-2 receptors and proliferate in the presence of IL-2. Once stimulated by IL-2, T lymphocytes produce a variety of lymphokines, including gamma interferon, lymphotoxin, and B cell growth and differentiation factors, and are activated for their various effector functions (Fig. 3).

Corticosteroids suppress most in vitro T lymphocyte proliferative responses, and they appear to interfere with early activation events. T lymphocyte blast formation in response to concanavalin A (Con A) is markedly suppressed by pharmacologic doses of corticosteroids both in vivo and in vitro. Phytohemagglutinin (PHA)-induced blast formation is also generally suppressed by corticosteroids. Steroid sensitivity in PHA-induced proliferation increases as the mitogen concentration decreases (Goodwin et al. 1979), and this shift in the dose-response curve likely accounts for the varying susceptibility to corticosteroid inhibition reported

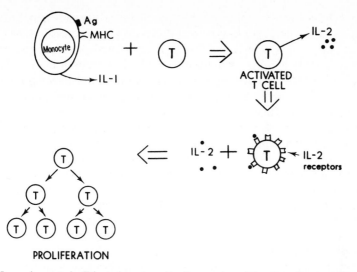

Fig. 3. Normal events in T lymphocyte activation and proliferation. See text for details

in the literature. Depletion of macrophages in an in vitro system also increased the steroid sensitivity to PHA (BLOMGREN and ANDERSSON 1976), suggesting that macrophage interactions or soluble products are important in determining steroid sensitivity. Pokeweed mitogen-induced blast transformation of T lymphocytes is less steroid sensitive than the PHA response in vitro. As with PHA, suboptimal doses of pokeweed mitogen increase the steroid sensitivity of lymphocyte cultures (GORDON and NOURI 1981), and likely account for differences in steroid sensitivity reported (BLOMGREN and ANDERSSON 1976).

T lymphocyte responses to antigen stimulation are also suppressed by corticosteroids. In vivo, corticosteroids suppressed proliferation induced by the antigens tetanus toxoid and streptokinase-streptodornase, and the inhibitory steroid dose is less than that needed in mitogen-driven systems (FAUCI and DALE 1974).

Both autologous and allogeneic mixed lymphocyte reactions are inhibited by corticosteroids. The allogeneic response is partially inhibited by pretreatment of the lymphocyte donor in vivo with pharmacologic doses of hydrocortisone or prednisone (KATZ and FAUCI 1979), or by pharmacologic concentrations of hydrocortisone in the in vitro cultures. The autologous reaction is much more sensitive to steroid inhibition. Low dose prednisone (10 mg orally) inhibits the autologous mixed lymphocyte reaction, but not the allogeneic, 2 h after drug administration (HAHN et al. 1980). Physiologic concentrations of hydrocortisone (10^{-8} M) suppressed the autologous mixed lymphocyte reaction without effect on the allogeneic reaction in vitro (ILFELD et al. 1977). This interesting finding suggests an in vivo role for corticosteroids in suppressing autoreactive T lymphocyte clones.

Natural killer (NK) cells and antibody-dependent cell-mediated cytotoxicity (ADCC) effector cells are important in vivo in tumor surveillance, acute graft rejection, and lysis of virally infected cells. In vitro, corticosteroids have varying effects on NK activity, ranging from suppression (PARRILLO and FAUCI 1979; PEDERSEN and BEYER 1986) to no effect (ONSRUD and THORNSBY 1981). In vivo, PARRILLO and FAUCI (1979) found that 12 mg dexamethasone suppressed NK activity at 24 and 48 h, with normalization by 96 h. PEDERSEN et al. (1986) documented a fall in NK cell activity following high dose pulse methylprednisolone therapy in patients with rheumatoid arthritis. ONSRUD and THORNSBY (1981) found increased NK cell activity 4 h after a 300 mg dose of hycrocortisone to normal subjects, whereas KATZ et al. (1984) found no significant effect 4 h after a 400 mg dose. ADCC appears to be relatively resistant to in vivo corticosteroids (PARRILLO and FAUCI 1979; KATZ et al. 1984), while inhibition has been noted in vitro (NAIR and SCHWARTZ 1984). Suppressor cells and their soluble products regulate NK and ADCC activities, and the discrepancies noted in the literature may be due to varying degrees of suppressor cell inhibition.

Suppressor cells in a variety of systems are inhibited by corticosteroids. In a *Candida* antigen-driven in vitro system, PICCOLELLA et al. (1985) found that dexamethasone inhibits the differentiation of T suppressor cells. Dexamethasone added at the beginning of cultures inhibited proliferation of mononuclear cells and IL-1 and IL-2 production. Delaying the addition of dexamethasone 1–4 days actually enhanced proliferation, owing to inhibition of T suppressor activity. The in vitro addition of hydrocortisone before the generation of Con A-induced suppressor cells blocks the development of suppressor cell activity in a pokeweed mitogen-driven system (HAYNES and FAUCI 1979). In most in vitro systems studied, suppressor cells, once generated, are resistant to the inhibitory effects of steroids. The naturally occurring suppressor cells seen in certain patients with common variable hypogammaglobulinemia (WALDMANN et al. 1978), and subjects who are "nonresponders" to pokeweed mitogen lymphocyte stimulation (HAYNES and FAUCI 1979), are sensitive to in vivo and in vitro steroids.

E. Effects of Steroids on Monokines and Lymphokines In Vitro

Many of the suppressive effects of glucocorticoids would appear to be secondary to inhibition of the production and action of a variety of lymphokines and monokines. These substances are proteins or peptides that communicate between cells of the immune system, carrying messages that stimulate cells to proliferate, differentiate, or perform specific functions. These proteins act through high affinity receptors on the surface membrane of their target cells, and are involved in the amplification of immune responses.

IL-1 is a polypeptide of molecular weight 17 500, produced by monocytes and macrophages following antigen presentation and interaction with T cells (Chap. 7). This monokine enhances T lymphocyte functions by promoting production of IL-2, colony-stimulating factor, gamma interferon, and other lymphokines. IL-1 also enhances specific cytotoxic and natural killer functions, and modulates suppressor cell activity. IL-1 directly increases B cell expression of surface immunoglobulin receptors and the production and secretion of antibody (Chap. 5). B cell proliferation is also enhanced, through direct effects and via T

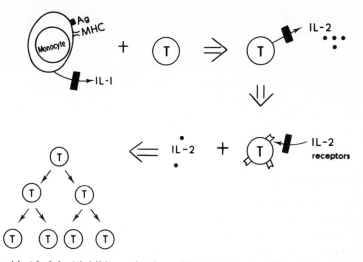

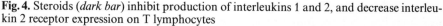

Fig. 4. Steroids (*dark bar*) inhibit production of interleukins 1 and 2, and decrease interleukin 2 receptor expression on T lymphocytes

helper cell production of B cell growth factor. Corticosteroids are one of the few classes of agents capable of inhibiting the production of IL-1. Pharmacologic doses of steroids inhibit not only the production of IL-1, but the expression of Ia molecules on macrophages (SNYDER and UNANUE 1982). Given the key role of IL-1 in enhancing lymphocyte function, steroid inhibition of IL-1 is likely to be an important immunosuppressive effect of these drugs in vivo (Fig. 4).

Corticosteroids profoundly inhibit IL-2 production and subsequent proliferation of mitogen-stimulated T lymphocytes, and the cytolytic capability of T lymphocytes in the mixed lymphocyte reaction (GILLIS et al. 1979 a,b). Addition of exogenous IL-2 restores normal levels of proliferation and cytolysis. The observation that exogenous IL-2 restores proliferation suggests that corticosteroids do not affect the initial activation events of lymphocytes, rather they block the passage of the cell through an early cell cycle phase (LARSSON 1980). The study by BETTENS et al. (1984) supports this hypothesis. The authors found that the initial events in T cell activation by PHA were unaltered by corticosteroids, but these cells remained in the early G_1 phase of the cell cycle, owing to insufficient RNA synthesis for proliferation. Addition of IL-2 overcame this blockade and allowed progression through the cell cycle. At the level of DNA transcription, corticosteroids inhibit the synthesis of IL-2 mRNA (ARYA et al. 1984), and partially inhibit the synthesis of IL-2 receptor mRNA and subsequent IL-2 receptor expression (Fig. 4; REED et al. 1986). Steroid-treated cells are able to upregulate their IL-2 receptors and proliferate in response to exogenous IL-2, similar to untreated lymphocytes.

Gamma-interferon is a glycosylated peptide of molecular weight 20–25000, produced by mitogen- or antigen-activated T lymphocytes. In addition to a number of complex actions on cellular and humoral immunity, gamma interferon activates macrophages to increase bactericidal and tumoricidal actions and to enhance expression of Fc receptors for IgG (Chap. 9). Glucocorticoids block the production of gamma interferon by T lymphocytes (Guyre et al. 1981), and this inhibition occurs at the level of DNA transcription (Arya et al. 1984). By inhibiting gamma interferon production, steroids diminish Fc receptor expression on accessory cells, and likely subsequent Fc receptor-mediated clearance by the reticuloendothelial system. This phenomenon may account for the beneficial effect of glucocorticoids in autoimmune hemolytic anemia and immune complex disease.

F. Mechanisms of Action

Like other steroid hormones, corticosteroids are generally believed to act by influencing gene transcription. Earlier theories of steroid action, including stabilization of cellular and lysosomal membranes, and alterations of protein, glucose, and lipid metabolism and transport, have been replaced by explanations at the molecular level. Specific intracytoplasmic receptors for the hormone ($2-6 \times 10^4$ receptors per cell) are found in all glucocorticoid-responsive tissues, including lymphocytes. In human lymphocytes, there does not appear to be a correlation between numbers of specific glucocorticoid receptors and sensitivity to steroids (Lippman and Barr 1977). Following penetration of the cell membrane, glucocorticoids bind to a specific receptor protein, and the hormone-receptor complex undergoes a poorly understood activation step. The complex accumulates in the nucleus, binds to chromosomal DNA, initiates DNA transcription, and new messenger RNA appears. The messenger RNA relocates to the cytoplasm, attaches to ribosomes, and serves as a template for new protein synthesis (O'Malley 1984).

One of the best described actions of glucocorticoids is inhibition of arachidonic acid release. Vane (1971) demonstrated the nonsteroidal anti-inflammatory drugs, such as aspirin inhibit the synthesis of prostaglandins. In 1975, Gryglewski et al. and several other groups showed that corticosteroids inhibit the release of arachidonic acid from membrane phospholipids, and proposed that their anti-inflammatory activity is due to this action. This hypothesis was difficult for many investigators to accept because it was already generally accepted that nonsteroidal anti-inflammatory drugs (NSAID) work via inhibition of arachidonic acid metabolism, and that the anti-inflammatory effects of corticosteroids are clearly different and more powerful than those of NSAID. The understanding of arachidonic acid metabolism at that time was essentially as a straight line synthetic pathway from membrane phospholipid to arachidonic acid to the prostaglandins (Fig. 5). Thus, if corticosteroids and NSAID inhibit at different points on the same pathway, they should have very similar actions. This problem was clarified when Samuelsson (1983) and others identified the lipoxygenase metabolic pathways for arachidonic acid (Fig. 6).

This more complex schema of arachidonic acid metabolism allows us to give serious consideration to the possibility that many of the pharmacologic and perhaps physiologic actions of corticosteroids are indeed via inhibition of arachidonic acid release from membrane phospholipid, because corticosteroids inhibit

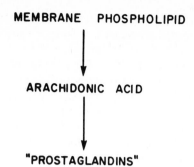

Fig. 5. Arachidonic acid metabolism as understood in the 1970s

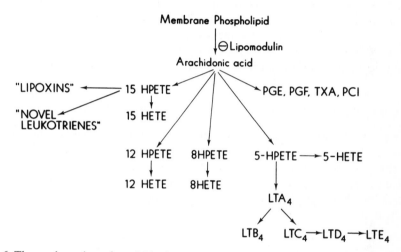

Fig. 6. The modern view of arachidonic acid metabolism. Lipomodulin inhibits the release of arachidonic acid from membrane phospholipids

both cyclooxygenase and lipoxygenase products. Clearly, the evidence supporting this concept has grown considerably over the past few years. Inhibitors of RNA and protein synthesis block the steroid effect, suggesting that steroids induce the synthesis of an inhibitor of arachidonic acid release (DANON and ASSOULINE 1978). FLOWER and BLACKWELL (1978) in England, and HIRATA et al. (1980) at the National Institutes of Health, identified a phospholipase A_2-inhibitory glyco-protein, termed macrocortin or lipomodulin, that is synthesized and released by cells on exposure to corticosteroids. Lipomodulin has been shown to inhibit ra-diolabeled arachidonic acid release from phospholipids directly. By inhibiting phospholipase A_2, glucocorticoids prevent the biosynthesis of the proinflamma-tory eicosanoids, including the prostaglandins, hydroxy acids, and leukotrienes. Because arachidonic acid metabolites are known to induce vasodilation, chemo-taxis of neutrophils, and mast cell activation, many of the nonspecific anti-inflam-matory properties of glucocorticoids may be explained by regulation of lipomo-dulin synthesis.

Several lines of evidence suggest that steroid-induced lipomodulin synthesis is important for the immunosuppressive actions of steroids. Lipomodulin inhibits NK cell activity and ADCC in vitro in a dose-dependent manner via phospholipase inhibition (HATTORI et al. 1983). The antiphospholipase activity of lipomodulin may mediate the inhibition of early activation events in human B cells by steroids (BOWEN and FAUCI 1984). Several recent studies have investigated the role of arachidonic acid metabolites as second messengers for cellular events. Lipoxygenase products mediate the proliferative response of mouse thymocytes to IL-1 (DINARELLO et al. 1983), and arachidonic acid and several of its lipoxygenase products are second messengers for gamma interferon production in a murine splenocyte model (JOHNSON et al. 1986). It would be interesting to investigate the effects of corticosteroids in these models. Finally, HIRATA et al. (1981) found autoantibodies against lipomodulin in the sera of patients with rheumatoid arthritis and systemic lupus eryhtematosus. These authors suggest that lipomodulin-specific antibody increases the metabolism of arachidonic acid to its inflammatory metabolites, and may, in part, account for the efficacy of glucocorticoids in the treatment of these disorders.

G. Conclusion

Corticosteroids have powerful effects on the humoral and cellular immune response in humans. Clinical use of these agents is limited by the equally powerful side effects of prolonged or high dose therapy. A better understanding of the mechanism of action of steroids should allow the development of new therapeutic agents which have similar immunosuppressive properties to corticosteroids, without the limiting side effects.

References

Addison T (1855) On the constitutional and local effects of disease of the suprarenal capsules. Highley, London
Arya SK, Wong-Staal F, Gallo RC (1984) Dexamethasone-mediated inhibition of human T cell growth factor and gamma-interferon messenger RNA. J Immunol 133:273–276
Baxter JD, Forsham PH (1972) Tissue effects of glucocorticoids. Am J Med 53:573–589
Bettens F, Kristensen F, Walker C, Schwulera U, Bonnard GD, deWeck AL (1984) Lymphokine regulation of activated (G$_1$) lymphocytes. II. Glucocorticoid and anti-Tac-induced inhibition of human T lymphocyte proliferation. J Immunol 132:261–265
Billingham RE, Krohn RL, Medawan PB (1951) Effect of cortisone on survival of skin homografts in rabbits. Br Med J 4716:1157–1163
Blomgren H, Andersson B (1976) Steroid sensitivity of the PHA and PWM responses of fractionated human lymphocytes in vitro. Exp Cell Res 97:233–240
Bovornkitti S, Kangsadal P, Sathirapat P (1960) Reversion and reconversion rate of tuberculin skin reactions in correlation with the use of prednisone. Dis Chest 38:51–55
Bowen DL, Fauci AS (1984) Selective suppressive effects of glucocorticoids on the early events in the human B cell activation process. J Immunol 133:1885–1890
Brown-Sequard CE (1856) Recherches experimentales sur al physiologie et la pathologie des capsules surrenales. C R Seances Acad Sci [D] (Paris) 43:422–425
Butler WT, Rossen RD (1973) Effects of corticosteroids on immunity in man. Decreased serum IgG concentration caused by 3 or 5 days of high doses of methylprednisolone. J Clin Invest 52:2629–2640

Claman HN (1972) Corticosteroids and lymphoid cells. N Engl J Med 287:388–397

Cupps TR, Fauci AS (1982) Corticosteroid-mediated immunoregulation in man. Immunol Rev 65:133–155

Cupps TR, Gerrard TL, Falkoff RJM, Whalen G, Fauci AS (1985) Effects of in vitro corticosteroids on B cell activation, proliferation and differentiation. J Clin Invest 75:754–761

Cushing H (1932) The basophil adenomas of pituitary body and their clinical manifestations. Bull Johns Hopkins Hosp 50:137–195

Danon A, Assouline G (1978) Inhibition of prostaglandin biosynthesis by corticosteroids requires RNA and protein synthesis. Nature 273:552–553

David DS, Grieco MH, Cushman P (1970) Adrenal glucocorticoids after twenty years. A review of their clinically relevant consequences. J Chronic Dis 22:637–711

Dinarello CA, Marnoy SO, Rosenwasser LJ (1983) Role of arachidonate metabolism in the immunoregulatory function of human leukocytic pyrogen/lymphocyte-activating factor/interleukin-1. J Immunol 130:890–895

Dougherty TF, White A (1944) Influence of hormones on lymphoid tissue structure and function. The role of the pituitary adrenotrophic hormone in the regulation of the lymphocytes and other cellular elements of the blood. Endocrinology 35:1–15

Fauci AS, Dale DC (1974) The effect of in vivo hydrocortisone on subpopulations of human lymphocytes. J Clin Invest 53:240–246

Fauci AS, Dale DC, Balow JE (1976) Glucocorticosteroid therapy: mechanisms of action and clinical considerations. Ann Intern Med 84:304–315

Flower RJ, Blackwell GJ (1978) Anti-inflammatory steroids induce biosynthesis of a phospholipase A_2 inhibitor which prevents prostaglandin generation. Nature 278:456–458

Gabrielsen AE, Good RA (1967) Chemical suppression of adaptive immunity. Adv Immunol 6:91–230

Gillis S, Crabtree GR, Smith KA (1979a) Glucocorticoid-induced inhibition of T cell growth factor production. I. The effect on mitogen-induced lymphocyte proliferation. J Immunol 123:1624–1631

Gillis S, Crabtree GR, Smith KA (1979b) Glucocorticoid-induced inhibition of T cell growth factor production. II. The effect on the in vitro generation of cytolytic T cells. J Immunol 123:1632–1638

Goodwin JS, Messner RP, Williams RC (1979) Inhibitors of T-cell mitogenesis: effect of mitogen dose. Cell Immunol 45:303–308

Gordon D, Nouri AME (1981) Comparison of the inhibition by glucocorticosteroids and cyclosporin A of mitogen-stimulated human lymphocyte proliferation. Clin Exp Immunol 44:287–294

Grayson J, Dooley NJ, Koski IR, Blaese RM (1981) Immunoglobulin production induced in vitro by glucocorticoid hormones. J Clin Invest 68:1539–1547

Gryglewski RJ, Panczenko B, Korbut R, Grodzinsky L, Ocetkiewicz A (1975) Corticosteroids inhibit prostaglandin release from perfused mesenteric blood vessels of rabbit and from perfused lungs of sensitized guinea pigs. Prostaglandins 10:343–355

Guyre PM, Bodwell JE, Munck A (1981) Glucocorticoid actions on the immune system: Inhibition of production of an Fc-receptor-augmenting factor. J Steroid Biochem 15:35–39

Hahn BH, MacDermott RP, Jacobs SB, Pletscher LS, Beale MG (1980) Immunosuppressive effects of low doses of glucocorticoids: effects on autologous and allogeneic mixed leukocyte reactions. J Immunol 124:2812–2817

Hattori T, Hirata F, Hoffman T, Hizuta A, Herberman RB (1983) Inhibition of human natural killer activity and antibody dependent cellular cytotoxicity by lipomodulin, a phospholipase inhibitory protein. J Immunol 131:662–665

Haynes BF, Fauci AS (1979) Mechanisms of corticosteroid action on lymphocyte subpopulations. IV. Effects of in vitro hydrocortisone on naturally occurring and mitogen-induced suppressor cells in man. Cell Immunol 44:157–168

Hench PS, Kendall EC, Slocumb CH, Polley HF (1949) The effect of a hormone of the adrenal cortex (17-hydroxy-11-dehydrocorticosterone: compound E) and of pituitary adrenocorticotropic hormone on rheumatoid arthritis: preliminary report. Proc Staff Meet Mayo Clin 24:181–197

Hills AG, Forsham PH, Finch CA (1948) Changes in circulating leukocytes induced by administration of pituitary adrenocorticotrophic hormone (ACTH) in man. Blood 3:755–768

Hirata F, Schiffman E, Yenkatasubramanian K, Salomen D, Axelrod J (1980) A phospholipase A$_2$ inhibitory protein in rabbit neutrophils induced by glucocorticoids. Proc Natl Acad Sci USA 77:2533–2538

Hirata F, del Carmine R, Nelson CA, Axelrod J et al. (1981) Presence of autoantibody for phospholipase inhibitory protein, lipomodulin, in patients with rheumatic diseases. Proc Natl Acad Sci USA 78:3190–3194

Ilfield DN, Krakauer RS, Blaese RM (1977) Suppression of the human mixed lymphocyte reaction by physiologic concentrations of hydrocortisone. J Immunol 119:428–434

Johnson HM, Russell JK, Torres BA (1986) Second messenger role of arachidonic acid and its metabolites in interferon-gamma production. J Immunol 137:3053–3056

Katz P, Fauci AS (1979) Autologous and allogeneic intercellular interactions: modulation by adherent cells, irradiation, and in vitro and in vivo corticosteroids. J Immunol 123:2270–2277

Katz P, Zaytoun AM, Lee JH (1984) The effects of in vivo hydrocortisone on lymphocyte-mediated cytotoxicity. Arthritis Rheum 27:72–78

Kendall EC, Mason HL, McKenzie BF, Myers CS, Koelsche GA (1934) Isolation in crystalline form of hormone essential to life from suppressed cortex. Its chemical nature and physiologic properties. Trans Assoc Am Physicians 49:147–152

Keown PA, Stiller CR (1986) Control of rejection of transplanted organs. Adv Intern Med 31:17–46

Larsson E-L (1980) Cyclosporing A and dexamethasone suppress T cell responses by selectively acting at distinct sites of the triggering process. J Immunol 124:2828–2833

Lippman ME, Barr R (1977) Glucocorticoid receptors on purified subpopulations of human peripheral blood lymphocytes. J Immunol 118:1977–1981

Long JB, Favour CB (1950) The ability of ACTH and cortisone to alter delayed type bactericidal hypersensitivity. Bull Johns Hopkins Hosp 87:186–202

Nair MPN, Schwartz SA (1984) Immunomodulatory effects of corticosteroids on natural killer and antibody-dependent cellular cytotoxic activities of human lymphocytes. J Immunol 132:2876–2882

O'Malley BW (1984) Steroid hormone action in eucaryotic cells. J Clin Invest 74:307–312

Onsrud M, Thornsby E (1981) Influence of in vivo hydrocortisone on some human blood lymphocyte subpopulations. I. Effect on natural killer cell activity. Scand J Immunol 13:573–579

Ost L, Tillegard A, Lundgren G et al. (1983) Treatment of renal allograft rejection with reduced IV steroid doses. Transplant Proc 15:563–565

Paavonen T (1985) Glucocorticoids enhance the in vitro Ig synthesis of pokeweed mitogen-stimulated human B cells by inhibiting the suppressive effect of T8$^+$ T cells. Scand J Immunol 21:63–71

Parrillo JE, Fauci AS (1979) Comparison of the effector cells in human spontaneous cellular cytotoxicity and antibody-dependent cellular cytotoxicity: differential sensitivity of effector cells to in vivo and in vitro corticosteroids. Scand J Immunol 8:99–107

Pedersen BK, Beyer JM (1986) Characterization of the in vitro effects of glucocorticosteroids on NK cell activity. Allergy 41:220–224

Piccolella E, Vismara D, Lombardi G et al. (1985) Effect of glucocorticoids on the development of suppressive activity in human lymphocyte response to a polysaccharide purified from Candida albicans. J Immunol 134:1166–1171

Posey WC, Nelson HS, Branch B, Pearlman DS (1978) The effects of acute corticosteroid therapy for asthma on serum immunoglobulin levels. J Allergy Clin Immunol 62:340–348

Reed JC, Abidi AH, Alpers JD, Hoover RG, Robb RJ, Nowell PL (1986) Effect of cyclosporin A and dexamethasone on interleukin-2 receptor gene expression. J Immunol 137:150–154

Reichstein, Shoppee CW (1943) The hormones of the adrenal cortex. Vitamin Horm 1:346–413

Samuelsson B (1983) Leukotrienes: mediators of immediate hypersensitivity reactions and inflammation. Science 220:568–578

Saxon A, Stevens RH, Ramer SJ, Clements PJ, Yu DTY (1978) Glucocorticoids administered in vivo inhibit human suppressor T lymphocyte function and diminish B lymphocyte responsiveness in in vitro immunoglobulin synthesis. J Clin Invest 61:922–930

Schwartz RS (1968) Immunosuppressive drug therapy. In: Rapaport FH, Dausett J (eds) Human transplantation, vol 28. Grune and Stratton, New York, pp 440–471

Sierakowski S, Goodwin JS (1986) Glucocorticoid-induced immunoglobulin production. Requirement for fetal calf serum. Clin. Exp. Immunol. in press, 1988

Snýder DS, Unanue ER (1982) Corticosteroids inhibit murine macrophage Ia expression and interleukin-1 production. J Immunol 129:1803–1805

Tuchinda M, Newcomb RW, DeVald BL (1972) Effect of prednisone treatment on the human immune response to keyhole limpet hemocyanin. Int Arch Allergy 42:533–544

Vane JR (1971) Inhibition of prostaglandin synthesis as a mechanism of action for aspirin-like drugs. Nature [New Biol] 231:232–235

Vollmer H (1951) The local effects of cortisone on the tuberculin reaction. J Pediatr 39:22–32

Waldmann TA, Blaese RM, Broder S, Krakauer RS (1978) Disorders of suppressor immunoregulatory cells in the pathogenesis of immunodeficiency and autoimmunity. Ann Intern Med 88:226–238

Weston WL, Mandel MJ, Yeckley JA et al. (1973) Mechanism of cortisol inhibition of adoptive transfer of tuberculin sensitivity. J Lab Clin Med 82:366–371

CHAPTER 18

Slow Acting Antirheumatics

P. E. LIPSKY

A. Introduction

Rheumatoid arthritis (RA) is a chronic disease that produces systemic symptoms and a variety of extra-articular manifestations as well as inflammation of the joints with the capacity to cause damage to articular cartilage and erosion of periarticular bone. Since the etiology of the disease is unknown, therapy is not directed toward cure, but rather toward suppression of one or other aspects of the inflammatory process, in the hope of ameliorating local and systemic symptoms, and also preventing joint destruction.

A number of therapeutic agents have been utilized in the medical management of RA. Clinical experience has suggested that these drugs fall into three general classes. The first class includes aspirin and the other nonsteroidal anti-inflammatory drugs (NSAIDs; see Chap. 26). These agents are able to inhibit cyclooxygenase activity and, thus, the production of various arachidonic acid metabolites, including prostaglandins, prostacyclin, and thromboxane. Although these drugs exert anti-inflammatory, analgesic, and antipyretic effects, and thus offer symptomatic relief, they have not been shown to alter the course of the disease nor to prevent the development of damage to bone or cartilage.

A second group of drugs includes the systemic immunosuppressive drugs such as azathioprine and cyclophosphamide. These agents appear to be active by virtue of their capacity to suppress systemic immune responsiveness and thereby the immunologic reactivity that lies at the basis of the chronic inflammatory process in the joint. These agents have been shown to slow the rate of articular damage in some patients.

A third group of drugs that includes gold compounds, antimalarials, D-penicillamine and, perhaps, levamisole and sulfasalazine have also been shown to suppress rheumatoid inflammation. These drugs differ from the NSAIDs in that they have minimal nonspecific anti-inflammatory activities. Moreover, they differ from the immunosuppressive agents by having minimal capacity to inhibit systemic immune responsiveness. Despite this, therapy with these antirheumatic agents appears to modify the course of the disease, ameliorating signs, symptoms, and serologic correlates of inflammation in many patients, slowing the pace of articular damage in some, and inducing remissions in a few (LIPSKY 1983). This activity has suggested that these compounds exert a unique therapeutic effect on rheumatoid inflammation that has been used to characterize them as disease-modifying antirheumatic drugs (DMARDs).

B. Characteristics of Therapy

DMARDs exert a number of activities in patients with RA that suggest that they belong to a functionally defined class of pharmacologic agents (LIPSKY 1983). The concept that these drugs are specific antirheumatoid agents derives from the observation that they are active in treating RA, but have minimal demonstrable nonspecific anti-inflammatory effects. With few exceptions, their effectiveness at suppressing inflammation appears to be largely limited to the treatment of RA. Therapy with these drugs is characterized by a delayed onset of clinical effect and, thus, they have been called "slow acting." The gradual suppression of the signs and symptoms of inflammation may not be apparent until weeks or months after the initiation of therapy, and can take 6 months or longer to reach a maximum. Once suppression of disease activity has been achieved, it may last for months or even years with continued administration of the drug. In addition, active inflammation may remain quiescent for weeks or even months after the drug has been discontinued. This is to be contrasted with the clinical response to NSAIDs which, when observed, is prompt and persists only as long as the drug is continued.

The terms "remission-inducing" and "disease-modifying" have been used because of the potential of these agents to alter the course of the disease and retard its progress. Thus, suppression of disease activity achieved with these agents results not only in amelioration of local and systemic symptoms, but also frequently leads to normalization of serologic correlates of disease activity, including acute phase reactants and the immunoglobulin-specific autoantibody, rheumatoid factor. In addition, therapy with these agents may suppress the development of new erosive changes in periarticular bones. It should be pointed out, however, that while these drugs may cause clinical and serologic improvement in many patients, induction of a complete remission of disease activity remains a relatively uncommon event. Moreover, slowing of the progression of bone erosions has not been convincingly demonstrated to occur as a result of therapy with most of these agents (IANNUZZI et al. 1983).

None of these agents was initially developed specifically to treat RA. Rather, these drugs were tested in an attempt to suppress a suspected, but usually hypothetical, etiologic process, or because a chance clinical observation suggested possible efficacy. While clinical experience has shown these agents to be effective in the treatment of RA, the original rationales for their use have, in general, not been substantiated. The striking similarity of the clinical effect of these agents in the treatment of RA has suggested that the DMARDs may share a common property that explains their activity in this disease. Whereas each of these agents has been shown to exert a variety of pharmacologic actions, the putative common activity that defines them as effective in the treatment of RA has not been clearly elucidated.

C. The Immunologic Basis of Rheumatoid Arthritis

Although the initiating stimulus has not been identified, established rheumatoid synovitis is characterized by persistent immunologic activity (ZVAIFLER 1973).

The synovial tissue is infiltrated with mononuclear cells, often collected into aggregates or follicles around small blood vessels. The T lymphocyte is the most frequent infiltrating cell, although macrophages, mast cells, B cells, and antibody-secreting plasma cells may also be seen. Polymorphonuclear leukocytes are uncommon. T4 helper/inducer cells are found in greater numbers than T8 suppressor/cytotoxic cells, and are frequently found in close proximity to Ia-expressing antigen-presenting cells (DUKE et al. 1982; KLARESKOG et al. 1982). It has been suggested that the inflammatory process in the synovial tissue is driven by the T4 helper/inducer cells infiltrating the synovium. Evidence for this includes: (a) the predominance of T4 cells in the synovium (DUKE et al. 1982; KLARESKOG et al. 1982); (b) the local production of lymphokines such as interleukin 2, gamma interferon, monocyte chemotactic factor, and leukocyte migration-inhibition factor (DEGRE et al. 1983; HUSBY and WILLIAMS 1985) by these infiltrating T cells; and (c) amelioration of the disease by removal of T cells with thoracic duct drainage (PAULUS et al. 1977) or suppression of their function by total lymphoid irradiation (KOTZIN et al. 1981; TRENTHAM et al. 1981). Since T lymphocytes produce a variety of cytokines that promote B cell proliferation and differentiation into antibody-secreting cells, T cell activation may also promote local B cell stimulation and antibody formation. The resultant production of immunoglobulin and rheumatoid factor can lead to immune complex formation, with consequent complement activation and exacerbation of the inflammatory process by the production of anaphylotoxins such as C3a and C5a, and chemotactic factors such as C5a. The tissue inflammation is reminiscent of delayed-type hypersensitivity reactions occurring in response to soluble antigens or microorganisms.

The response is likely to be triggered by a T4 cell recognizing relevant antigenic fragments in the context of Ia molecules encoded by genes of the major histocompatibility complex displayed by an antigen-presenting cell. In RA, it is unclear whether this represents a response to an exogenous antigen or to altered autoantigens such as collagen or immunoglobulin. Alternatively, it could represent responsiveness to activated Ia-positive autologous cells such as might occur as a result of Epstein-Barr virus infection. After initial activation, T4 cells produce interleukin 2 (IL-2) that serves to amplify the response by facilitating T and B cell proliferation and differentiation. In addition, the activated T cells produce gamma interferon that serves as a potent activator of macrophages, amplifying their capacity to cause tissue damage. Gamma interferon can also stimulate cells that are normally Ia-negative, such as fibroblasts and endothelial cells, to express class II products of the major histocompatibility gene complex. As a result, these cells may become antigen-presenting cells and further amplify the local immune response in the synovial tissue.

Overriding the chronic inflammation in the synovial tissue is an acute inflammatory process in the synovial fluid. The exudative synovial fluid contains a large number of polymorphonuclear leukocytes and relatively few mononuclear cells. A number of mechanisms may play a role in stimulating the exudation of synovial fluid (ZVAIFLER 1973; BEUTLER and CERAMI 1986; DINARELLO 1984). Locally produced immune complexes can activate complement and generate anaphylotoxins and chemotactic factors. Local production of macrophage factors such as interleukin 1 (IL-1), tumor necrosis factor (TNF), and the lipoxygenase pathway metabolite of arachidonic acid, leukotriene B_4 (LTB$_4$) may also play a role in the emigration of polymorphonuclear leukocytes. Thus, TNF and LTB$_4$ are powerful chemoattractants for polymorphonuclear leukocytes, whereas all three macrophage products can enhance interactions between circulating neutrophils and postcapillary venules. Once in the synovial fluid, the polymorphonuclear leukocytes can ingest immune complexes, with the resultant production of reactive oxygen metabolites and other mediators of inflammation, further adding to the inflammatory milieu.

The immunologic reactivity in the synovial tissue also leads to the damage of bone and cartilage. Much of this damage occurs in juxtaposition to the inflamed synovium or pannus that spreads to cover the articular cartilage. This vascular granulation tissue is composed of proliferating fibroblasts, small blood vessels, and a variable number of mononuclear cells. The macrophage-derived cytokines IL-1 and TNF may play an important role by stimulating the cells of the pannus to release prostaglandin E_2, collagenase, and other neutral proteases. Cytokines such as IL-1 or catabolin and TNF may also activate chondrocytes in situ, stimulating them to produce proteolytic enzymes that can degrade cartilage locally. IL-1 may also stimulate local bone demineralization by directly activating osteoclasts. Finally, cytokines such as lymphotoxin and TNF may contribute to local tissue damage by interfering with the metabolic activity of the cellular elements.

The immunologic activity in the synovial tissue may also explain a number of the systemic manifestations of RA. Cytokines produced in the inflamed synovium, such as IL-1 and TNF, may produce a number of systemic symptoms and also the increase in circulating levels of acute phase reactants associated with RA. In addition, immune complexes formed between rheumatoid factor and immunoglobulin molecules may account for some of the extra-articular manifestations.

Figure 1 is a schematic representation of some of the cellular interactions occurring in the rheumatoid synovium, and indicates how this ongoing immunologic reactivity may account for the superimposed acute inflammatory response in the synovial fluid, the damage to bone and cartilage, and the systemic features of RA. This model of rheumatoid inflammation suggests that therapeutic agents which share the capacity to suppress the local signs and symptoms of RA, and correct systemic manifestations of the disease as well as retard damage to bone and cartilage, are likely to exert their effect on the inflammation in the synovial tissue, which acts as the driving force behind the disease process. As depicted in Fig. 1, the nature of rheumatoid inflammation suggests that immunologic processes play a role in its initiation and perpetuation. Whether the ongoing reactivity represents specific or polyclonal responses to exogenous or self-antigens, or is the consequence of defective immunoregulatory mechanisms, the net result is chronic immunologically mediated inflammation with the capacity to promote both the local and systemic manifestations of the disease. One of the initial events in the induction of an immune response is the interaction of antigen-presenting cells with antigen-specific T lymphocytes (see Chap. 2). The pharmacologic inhibition of this interaction could explain the therapeutic benefit of DMARDs in RA. The nature of rheumatoid inflammation therefore suggests the hypothesis that DMARDs may be effective because of their capacity to function as immu-

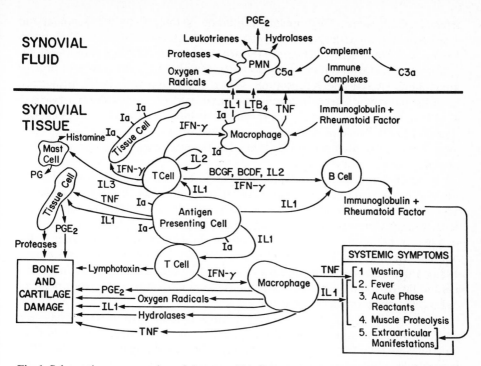

Fig. 1. Schematic representation of rheumatoid inflammation. Abbreviations: BCDF B cell differentiation factor; BCGF B cell growth factor; IFNγ gamma interferon; IL-1 interleukin 1; IL-2 interleukin 2; IL-3 interleukin 3; LTB_4 leukotriene B_4; PG prostaglandin; PMN polymorphonuclear cells; TNF tumor necrosis factor

nosuppressive agents, and thereby limit the ongoing immune responsiveness that perpetuates the inflammation. Support for this idea comes from the finding that other procedures known to suppress systemic immune responsiveness have been shown to ameliorate rheumatoid inflammation. Thus, thoracic duct drainage (PAULUS et al. 1977), peripheral lymphapheresis and lymphoplasmapheresis (WALLACE et al. 1979; KARSH et al. 1981), total lymphoid irradiation (KOTZIN et al. 1981; TRENTHAM et al. 1981), and treatment with immunosuppressive agents such as azathioprine or cyclophosphamide (COOPERATING CLINIC OF THE AMERICAN RHEUMATISM ASSOCIATION 1970; CURREY et al. 1974) have all been shown to be effective in the treatment of RA (see also Chaps. 19 and 23).

D. Disease-Modifying Antirheumatic Drugs

Gold compounds were the first of DMARDs to be described. Despite the documentation of clinical efficacy (RESEARCH SUBCOMMITTEE OF THE EMPIRE RHEUMATISM COUNCIL 1960a,b), an adequate explanation for the action of gold compounds in RA has remained elusive. A number of mechanisms have been proposed based on various effects of gold compounds observed in a number of different model systems. These include inhibition of the activity of lysosomal and other cellular and extracellular enzymes (ENNIS et al. 1968; NECHAY 1980), interference with complement activation (SCHULTZ et al. 1974; BURGE et al. 1978), inhibition of prostaglandin biosynthesis (STONE et al. 1975), alterations in protein interactions (ADAM and KUHN 1968; WALZ and DIMARTINO 1972), protection from the damaging effects of locally produced oxidizing molecules (CUPERUS et al. 1985), as well as various nonspecific anti-inflammatory effects (VERNON-ROBERTS 1979). While each of these may explain some of the actions of gold compounds, none has been generally accepted as the mechanism by which gold compounds alter the course of RA.

The possibility that gold compounds may suppress immune responsiveness was suggested by the clinical observation that immunoglobulin levels (LORBER et al. 1978) and rheumatoid factor titers (RESEARCH SUBCOMMITTEE OF THE EMPIRE RHEUMATISM COUNCIL 1960a) often decrease in patients treated with gold compounds. In addition, gold therapy has been shown to cause a reduction in the number of circulating lymphocytes in patients with RA (HANLY and BRESNIHAN 1985), and a decrease in the number of circulating cells capable of making rheumatoid factor spontaneously or in response to in vitro stimulation with polyclonal B cell activators (OLSEN et al. 1984).

The capacity of gold compounds to suppress immune responsiveness has been confirmed with in vitro studies. Initially, gold sodium thiomalate and gold thioglucose were found to inhibit proliferative responses of human peripheral blood mononuclear cells stimulated with either antigens or mitogenic lectins (LIPSKY and ZIFF 1977). Inhibition of responsiveness was noted with concentrations of gold comparable to those achieved in the synovial tissue as a result of therapeutic administration. Inhibition of responsiveness did not require the continuous presence of the gold compound. Rather, human peripheral blood mononuclear cells could be preincubated with gold sodium thiomalate, after which their capacity to respond to antigens or mitogens in vitro was markedly inhibited. A prolonged exposure of more than 72 h to pharmacologically achievable concentrations of gold sodium thiomalate was necessary before loss of responsiveness was noted on subsequent culture.

Striking morphological changes were noted in the monocytes concomitant with the loss of antigen and mitogen responsiveness (UGAI et al. 1979; GHADIALLY et al. 1982). The monocytes developed large intracytoplasmic vacuoles that contained deposits of gold-containing material, whereas lymphocyte morphology was unchanged. Since initiation of antigen- and mitogen-induced human T lymphocyte proliferation requires the active participation of monocytes, it was possible that the preincubation with gold had interfered with lymphocyte activation not by altering T cell function, but rather by inhibiting the capacity of monocytes to function as requisite accessory cells. Experiments carried out to examine this possibility indicated that gold inhibited the accessory function of the monocytes, but had no inhibitory effect on the potential responsiveness of the lymphocytes (LIPSKY and ZIFF 1977). These data suggested the conclusion that the action of gold compounds in RA might result from the capacity of these drugs to inhibit the functional capability of mononuclear phagocytes involved in the initiation of the chronic, immunologically mediated inflammatory synovitis.

Mononuclear phagocytes are involved not only in the initiation of immune responses, but also in the expression of immunologically mediated inflammatory responses by virtue of their phagocytic, degradative, and secretory capabilities. Gold compounds have been found to interfere with a number of other functional activities of mononuclear phagocytes that allow them to function as effector cells at sites of chronic inflammation, such as pinocytosis and phagocytosis (UGAI et al. 1979). In addition, gold compounds have been found to inhibit a number of other functions of monocytes, including their response to chemotactic stimuli (Ho et al. 1978) and their capacity to produce complement components (LITTMAN and SCHWARTZ 1982).

Auranofin (*S*-triethylphosphine gold 2,3,4,6-tetra-*O*-acetyl-1-thio-β-D-glu-copyranoside) is an orally absorbable gold containing DMARD (CHAFFMAN et al. 1984). Because of the phosphine group, auranofin exerts a number of effects not shared with injectable gold compounds, including the capacity to suppress various immune responses in vivo in laboratory animals. Auranofin also exerts a number of anti-inflammatory and immunosuppressive activities. However, at concentrations of gold equivalent to those attained in the synovial fluid of treated patients (~ 0.3 µg/ml; GOTTLIEB 1982), auranofin appears to suppress the accessory cell function of mononuclear phagocytes, while having minimal effects on other cell types (SALMERON and LIPSKY 1982). A number of other functions of monocytes are also inhibited by auranofin (SCHEINBERG et al. 1982). Unlike injectable gold compounds, auranofin inhibits monocyte function rapidly and at low concentrations, presumably because of the lipophilicity conveyed by the triethylphosphine group.

The results of the in vitro experiments support the idea that a major action of gold compounds involves inhibition of various functions of mononuclear phagocytes. This conclusion is consistent with a number of in vivo observations made in both human subjects and experimental animals. Thus, gold is sequestered in organs rich in mononuclear phagocytes. Within rheumatoid synovial tissue, gold accumulates in the lysosomes of type A synovial cells and other macrophages (VERNON-ROBERTS et al. 1976). The function of mononuclear phagocytes in vivo is also altered in experimental animals and patients with rheumatoid arthritis as a result of gold treatment (VERNON-ROBERTS et al. 1973; JESSOP et al. 1973). In view of the critical role of mononuclear phagocytes in both the induction and expression of immunologically mediated inflammatory responses, interference with their function by gold compounds may well explain the efficacy of chrysotherapy in reducing rheumatoid inflammation.

The mechanism by which gold compounds inhibit mononuclear phagocyte function involves the binding of the gold moiety to surface suflhydryl-containing compounds, followed by uptake into the cell (LIPSKY and ZIFF 1977; UGAI et al. 1979). As a result, all of the functional consequences of mononuclear phagocyte exposure to gold can be prevented by sulfhydryl-containing reducing agents, including thiol compounds which themselves are disease-modifying drugs, such as D-penicillamine (LIPSKY and ZIFF 1977). This may be important in understanding the effectiveness of gold compounds in patients with RA, as active disease is associated with markedly depressed levels of serum sulfhydryl-containing reducing compounds (LORBER et al. 1964). The decreased levels of these inhibitors of the action of gold on mononuclear phagocytes may facilitate the efficacy of these disease-modifying drugs in patients with RA.

The mechanism of action of antimalarials in RA has also not been clearly delineated. A number of observations have indicated that these disease-modifying drugs may alter monocyte function. For example, chloroquine inhibits human monocyte chemotaxis and phagocytosis in vitro (NORRIS et al. 1977). In addition, chloroquine has been shown to inhibit the capacity of human monocytes to function as antigen-presenting cells and as accessory cells required for mitogen-induced T cell activation (SALMERON and LIPSKY 1983). These findings indicate that antimalarials may be similar to gold compounds in that their action as DMARDs may result from their capacity to inhibit monocyte function. One particular action of chloroquine on monocyte function may be especially important in understanding the action of this agent in RA. At pharmacologically attainable concentrations (< 1 μg/ml), chloroquine appears to inhibit the release of IL-1 by monocytes (SALMERON and LIPSKY 1983). In view of the wide spectrum of activities of IL-1 on cells of the immune system, and in promoting various aspects of the inflammatory response (DINARELLO 1984; Chap. 7), modulation of the release of this cytokine could well explain some of the activities of the antimalarials in RA.

D-Penicillamine was first used to treat RA because of the belief that it could directly dissociate IgM rheumatoid factor in vivo, with a consequent loss of its agglutinating capacity and a resultant amelioration of the symptoms of RA. Clinical trials have confirmed that D-penicillamine is effective in the treatment of RA (MULTICENTRE TRIAL GROUP 1973). Despite its well-described clinical efficacy, the mechanism of action of D-penicillamine in RA remains unclear at the present time. D-Penicillamine has been shown to decrease rheumatoid factor titers in treated patients (MULTICENTRE TRIAL GROUP 1973). However, it is unlikely that this effect results from D-penicillamine-induced dissociation of serum or synovial fluid IgM rheumatoid factor since the concentration of D-penicillamine attained in vivo is several hundred fold less than that needed to dissociate macroglobulins. In addition, rheumatoid factor titers remain depressed for prolonged periods after the cessation of drug therapy. It would thus appear that the reduction in rheumatoid factor titers is a secondary phenomenon that reflects an amelioration of the underlying inflammatory process.

A number of observations in treated patients have suggested that D-penicillamine might exert an immunosuppressive action and, thus, act by suppressing the ongoing immune response that underlies the chronic inflammation. In this regard, therapy with penicillamine often results in decreased rheumatoid factor titers (MULTICENTRE TRIAL GROUP 1973) and immunoglobulin levels (BLUESTONE and GOLDBERG 1973).

The possibility that the effectiveness of D-penicillamine in RA might result from its capacity to function as an immunosuppressive agent is supported by the in vitro observation that D-penicillamine inhibits mitogen- and antigen-induced human T cell activation (LIPSKY and ZIFF 1978, 1980; LIPSKY 1984). Penicillamine-mediated inhibition of lymphocyte responsiveness specifically requires the presence of copper ions. A number of other metal ions such as zinc, iron, mercury, and gold were found to be unable to augment the inhibitory capacity of penicillamine. However, penicillamine is not unique in its ability to inhibit lymphocyte responsiveness in the presence of copper ions. A variety of other thiol-containing compounds, in the reduced, but not oxidized form, are also inhibitory in the presence of copper. Significantly, compounds which have been shown in preliminary trials to be effective in the treatment of RA, such as 2-mercaptopropionylglycine (AMOR et al. 1980), 5-thiopyridoxine (HUSKISSON et al. 1980), and captopril (MARTIN et al. 1984) were found to be comparable to D-penicillamine in suppressing mitogen responsiveness in the presence of copper ions (LIPSKY 1981).

In contrast to the action of gold and antimalarials that inhibited the accessory cell function of mononuclear phagocytes, D-penicillamine and other thiol-containing DMARDs were found to inhibit T lymphocyte function directly, while causing no alteration of mononuclear phagocyte function (LIPSKY and ZIFF 1978). Helper T cells were particularly sensitive to the inhibitory action of D-penicillamine (LIPSKY and ZIFF 1980). Recent studies of the function of lymphocytes in treated patients have confirmed that administration of D-penicillamine can inhibit helper T cell function (OLSEN et al. 1984).

Inhibition of lymphocyte function is dependent on the presence of copper ions and results from the copper-mediated oxidation of the thiol group of penicillamine, leading to the generation of hydrogen peroxide (LIPSKY 1984; STARKEBAUM and ROOT 1985; STAITE et al. 1985). Of interest, monocytes, but not other cells found in the rheumatoid synovium, were able to protect T cells from inhibition by virtue of their abundant content of catalase (LIPSKY 1984). These results suggest that the functional competence of mononuclear phagocytes within the inflamed synovium may play a critical role in determining the therapeutic effectiveness of D-penicillamine and other thiol-containing disease-modifying drugs. Other features of the rheumatoid synovium may also be important in determining the effectiveness of therapy with D-penicillamine. For example, the immunosuppressive activity of D-penicillamine requires the drug to be in the reduced form; the oxidized disulfide is inactive (LIPSKY and ZIFF 1978). The rheumatoid synovium is characterized by diminished perfusion and intense inflammation, with resultant local acidosis (WALLIS et al. 1985). Since maintenance of D-penicillamine in the reduced thiol form is favored when the pH is lowered, the local environment of the rheumatoid synovium may facilitate the immunosuppressive capacity of D-penicillamine.

E. Summary

The evidence suggests that immunosuppression is an action that is shared by DMARDs, and thus supports the view that disease modification may result from suppression of the immunologic activity that underlies rheumatoid inflammation. The possibility that other DMARDs such as sulfasalazine may suppress immune responses remains to be determined. Gold compounds and antimalarials appear to be active by virtue of their capacity to depress various functions of mononuclear phagocytes, while D-penicillamine and other thiol-containing agents act by inhibiting a number of the activities of T lymphocytes. The conclusion that DMARDs have different sites of immunosuppressive action in RA may explain the observation that the success rate of treatment with one is comparable, regardless of antecedent therapy with another (STEVEN et al. 1982). It is important that unique features of the rheumatoid synovium such as sulfhydryl reactivity, pH, and the integrity of mononuclear phagocyte function may influence the activities of these agents within the affected tissue. DMARDs may therefore function as regionally active immunosuppressive agents whose inhibitory capacity is predicated on the nature of rheumatoid inflammation.

References

Adam M, Kuhn K (1968) Investigations on the reaction of metals with collagen in vivo. I. Comparison of the reaction of gold thiosulfate with collagen in vivo and in vitro. Eur J Biochem 3:407–410

Amor B, Mery C, Degery A (1980) Tiopronine. New antirheumatic slow acting drug in rheumatoid arthritis. Rev Rheum 47:157–162

Beutler B, Cerami A (1986) Cachectin and tumour necrosis factor as two sides of the same biological coin. Nature 320:584–588

Bluestone R, Goldberg LS (1973) Effect of D-penicillamine on serum immunoglobulins and rheumatoid factor. Ann Rheum Dis 32:50–52

Burge JJ, Fearon DT, Austen KF (1978) Inhibition of the alternative pathway of complement by gold sodium thiomalate in vitro. J Immunol 120:1626–1630

Chaffman M, Brodgen RN, Heel RC, Speight TM, Avery GS (1984) Auranofin. A preliminary review of its pharmacological properties and therapeutic use in rheumatoid arthritis. Drugs 27:378–424

Cooperating Clinics of the American Rheumatism Association (1970) A controlled trial of cyclophosphamide in rheumatoid arthritis. N Engl J Med 283:883–889

Cuperus RA, Muijsers AO, Wever R (1985) Antiarthritis drugs containing thiol groups scavenge hypochloride and inhibit its formation by myeloperoxidase from human leukocytes. Arthritis Rheum 28:1228–1233

Currey HLF, Harris J, Masin RM, Woodland J, Beveridge T, Roberts CJ, Vere DW, Dixon AStJ, Owen Smith B (1974) Comparison of azathioprine, cyclophosphamide and gold in treatment of rheumatoid arthritis. Br Med J 3:763–766

Degre M, Mellbye OJ, Clarke-Jenssen O (1983) Immune interferon in serum and synovial fluid in rheumatoid arthritis and related disorders. Ann Rheum Dis 42:672–676

Dinarello CA (1984) Interleukin 1. Rev Infect Dis 1:51–95

Duke O, Panayi GS, Janossy G, Poulter LW (1982) An immunohistological analysis of lymphocyte subpopulations and their microenvironment in the synovial membranes of patients with rheumatoid arthritis using monoclonal antibodies. Clin Exp Immunol 49:22–30

Ennis RS, Granda JL, Posner AS (1968) Effect of gold salts and other drugs on the release and activity of lysosomal hydrolases. Arthritis Rheum 11:756–764

Ghadially FN, Lipsky PE, Yang-Stepphuhn SE, Lalonde J-MA (1982) The morphology and atomic composition of aurosomes produced by sodium aurothiomalate in human monocytes. Ann Pathol 2:117–125

Gottlieb NL (1982) Comparative pharmacokinetics of parenteral and oral gold compounds. J Rheum [Suppl] 8:99–109

Hanly JG, Bresnihan B (1985) Reduction of peripheral blood lymphocytes in patients receiving gold therapy for rheumatoid arthritis. Ann Rheum Dis 44:299–301

Ho PPK, Young AL, Southland GL (1978) Methyl ester of N-formyl-methionyl-leucyl-phenylalanine: chemotactic responses of human blood monocytes and inhibition of gold compounds. Arthritis Rheum 21:133–136

Husby G, Williams RC Jr (1985) Immunohistochemical studies of interleukin-2 and γ-interferon in rheumatoid arthritis. Arthritis Rheum 28:174–181

Huskisson EC, Jaffe IA, Scott J, Dieppe PA (1980) 5-Thiopyridoxine in rheumatoid arthritis: clinical and experimental studies. Arthritis Rheum 23:106–110

Iannuzzi L, Dawson N, Zein N, Kushner I (1983) Does drug therapy slow radiographic deterioration in rheumatoid arthritis? N Engl J Med 309:1023–1028

Jessop JD, Vernon-Roberts B, Harris J (1973) Effects of gold salts and prednisolone on inflammatory cells. I. Phagocytic activity of macrophages and polymorphs in inflammatory exudates studied by a "skin-window" technique in rheumatoid and control patients. Ann Rheum Dis 32:294–300

Karsh J, Klippel JH, Plotz PH, Decker JL, Wright DG, Flye MW (1981) Lymphapheresis in rheumatoid arthritis. A randomized trial. Arthritis Rheum 24:867–873

Klareskog L, Forsum U, Wigren A, Wigzell H (1982) Relationship between HLA-DR expression cells and T lymphocytes of different subsets in rheumatoid synovial tissue. Scand J Immunol 15:501–507

Kotzin BL, Strober S, Engelman EG, Calin A, Hoppe RT, Kansas GS, Terrell CP, Kaplan HS (1981) Treatment of intractable rheumatoid arthritis with total lymphoid irradiation. N Engl J Med 305:969–976

Lipsky PE (1981) Modulation of lymphocyte function by copper and thiols. Agents Actions [Suppl] 8:95–102

Lipsky PE (1983) Remission-inducing therapy in rheumatoid arthritis. Am J Med 74(4b):40–49

Lipsky PE (1984) Immunosuppression by D-penicillamine in vitro: inhibition of human T lymphocyte proliferation by copper or ceruloplasmin-dependent generation of hydrogen peroxide and protection by monocytes. J Clin Invest 73:56–65

Lipsky PE, Ziff M (1977) Inhibition of antigen and mitogen-induced human lymphocyte proliferation by gold compounds. J Clin Invest 59:455–466

Lipsky PE, Ziff M (1978) The effect of D-penicillamine on mitogen-induced human lymphocyte proliferation: synergistic inhibition by D-penicillamine and copper salts. J Immunol 120:1006–1013

Lipsky PE, Ziff M (1980) Inhibition of human helper T cell function in vitro by D-penicillamine and $CuSO_4$. J Clin Invest 65:1069–1976

Littman BH, Schwartz P (1982) Gold inhibition of the production of the second complement component by lymphokine-stimulated human monocytes. Arthritis Rheum 25:288–296

Lorber A, Pearson CM, Meredith WL, Gantz-Mandell LE (1964) Serum sulfhydryl determinations and significance in connective tissue diseases. Ann Intern Med 61:423–434

Lorber A, Simon T, Leeb J, Peter A, Wilcox S (1978) Chrysotherapy. Suppression of immunoglobulin synthesis. Arthritis Rheum 21:785–791

Martin MFR, McKenna F, Bird HA, Surrall KE, Dixon J, Wright V (1984) Captopril: a new treatment for rheumatoid arthritis. Lancet 1:1325–1327

Multicentre Trial Group (1973) Controlled trial of D(−)-penicillamine in severe rheumatoid arthritis. Lancet 1:275–280

Nechay BR (1980) Inhibition of adenosine thriphosphatases by gold. Arthritis Rheum 23:464–470

Norris DA, Weston DL, Smas WM (1977) The effect of immunosuppressive and anti-inflammatory drugs on monocyte function in vitro. J Lab Clin Med 90:569–580

Olsen N, Ziff M, Jasin HE (1984) Spontaneous synthesis of IgM rheumatoid factor by blood mononuclear cells from patients with rheumatoid arthritis: effect of treatment with gold salts or D-penicillamine. J Rheumatol 11:17–21

Paulus HE, Machleder HI, Levine S, Yu DTY, MacDonald NS (1977) Lymphocyte involvement in rheumatoid arthritis. Studies during thoracic duct drainage. Arthritis Rheum 20:1249–1262

Research Subcommittee of the Empire Rheumatism Council (1960a) Gold therapy in rheumatoid arthritis. Report of a multi-centre controlled trial. Ann Rheum Dis 19:95–119

Research Subcommittee of the Empire Rheumatism Council (1960b) Gold therapy in rheumatoid arthritis. Final report of a multi-centre controlled trial. Ann Rheum Dis 20:315–334

Salmeron G, Lipsky PE (1982) Modulation of human immune responsiveness in vitro by auranofin. J Rheum [Suppl 8] 9:25–32

Salmeron G, Lipsky PE (1983) Immunosuppressive potential of antimalarials. Am J Med 75(1A):19–24

Scheinberg MA, Santos LMB, Finkelstein AE (1982) The effect of auranofin and sodium aurothiomalate on peripheral blood monocytes. J Rheum 9:366–369

Schultz DR, Volanakis JE, Arnold PJ, Gottlieb NL, Sakai K, Stroud RM (1974) Inactivation of C1 in rheumatoid synovial fluid, purified C1 and C1 esterase by gold compounds. Clin Exp Immunol 17:395–406

Staite ND, Messner RP, Zoschke DC (1985) In vitro production and scavenging of hydrogen peroxide by D-penicillamine: relationship to copper availability. Arthritis Rheum 28:914–921

Starkebaum G, Root RK (1985) D-Penicillamine: analysis of the mechanism of copper-catalyzed hydrogen peroxide generation. J Immunol 134:3371–3378

Steven MM, Hunter JA, Murdoch RM, Cappell HA (1982) Does the order of second-line treatment of rheumatoid arthritis matter? Br Med J 284:79–81

Stone KJ, Mather SJ, Gibson PP (1975) Selective inhibition of prostaglandin biosynthesis by gold and phenylbutazone. Prostaglandins 10:241–251

Trentham DE, Belli JA, Anderson RJ, Buckley JA, Goetzl EJ, David JR, Austin KF (1981) Clinical and immunologic effects of fractionated total lymphoid irradiation in refractory rheumatoid arthritis. N Eng J Med 305:976–982

Ugai K, Ziff M, Lipsky PE (1979) Gold-induced changes in the morphology and functional capabilities of human monocytes. Arthritis Rheum 22:1352–1360

Vernon-Roberts B (1979) Action of gold salts on the inflammatory response and inflammatory cell function. J Rheum [Suppl] 5:120–129

Vernon-Roberts B, Jessop JD, Dore J (1973) Effects of gold salts and prednisone on inflammatory cells. II. Suppression of inflammation and phagocytosis in the rat. Ann Rheum Dis 32:301–307

Vernon-Roberts B, Dore JL, Jessop JD, Henderson WJ (1976) Selective concentration and localization of gold in macrophages of synovial and other tissue during and after chrysotherapy in rheumatoid patients. Ann Rheum Dis 35:477–486

Wallace DJ, Goldfinger D, Gatti R, Lowe C, Fan P, Bluestone R, Klinenberg JR (1979) Plasmapheresis and lymphoplasmapheresis in the management of rheumatoid arthritis. Arthritis Rheum 22:703–710

Wallis WJ, Simkin PA, Nelp WB (1985) Low synovial clearance of iodide provides evidence of hypoperfusion in chronic rheumatoid synovitis. Arthritis Rheum 28:1096–1104

Walz DT, Dimartino JJ (1972) Effect of anti-arthritic drugs on sulfhydryl reactivity of rat serum. Proc Soc Exp Biol Med 140:263–268

Zvaifler NJ (1973) The immunopathology of joint inflammation in rheumatoid arthritis. Adv Immunol 16:265–236

CHAPTER 19

Cyclophosphamide

R. R. BARTLETT

A. Introduction

The alkylating agent cyclophosphamide (CY) was first described in 1958 by AR-
NOLD et al. and has been subjected to extensive study as a chemotherapeutic agent
in the tumor field. Interest in the immunosuppressive activity of this agent has expanded gradually, following the initial observation that the substance possessed
an inherent selectivity for lymphoid cells (BERENBAUM and BROWN 1963, 1964;
SANTOS and OWENS 1966; MANNY and SCHWARTZ 1971; MARBROOK and BAGU-
LEY 1971).

Historically, CY was one of a large number of nitrogen mustard derivatives
designed to release nornitrogen mustard after selective activation by enzymes
within tumor cells (ARNOLD et al. 1958). Soon it became apparent that the toxicity
of CY was dependent on an earlier activation event which took place in the microsomes of the liver (FOLEY et al. 1961). It was later found that its greater cytotoxic
effects on tumor cells could be attributed to much less efficient enzymatic detoxi-
fication of primary oxidation products in malignant cells than in normal cells, owing to the absence or lower concentrations of the appropriate enzymes (CONNORS
1975). Clinically, CY has proved to be a relatively safe and effective drug for
cancer chemotherapy.

In this chapter, I will limit my review of the activity of CY to its effects on
lymphocytes. The immunosuppressive potential of this agent has been extensively
studied, especially ragarding its apparent selectivity for certain T lymphocytes
(TURK et al. 1972; ASKENASE et al. 1975) and B cells (LERMAN and WEIDANZ 1970;
TURK and POULTER 1972). Further, the use of this drug to promote tolerance has
also undergone extensive analysis (AISENBERG and DAVIS 1968; MANNY and
SCHWARTZ 1970; HOWARD and COURTENAY 1974).

Alkylating agents are compounds that transfer alkyl groups to other substances. According to the number of groups that a single molecule can donate,
alkylating agents can be monofunctional, bifunctional, or trifunctional. They
often require chemical activation or enzymatic conversion before they can donate
alkyl groups. Generally, it is considered that alkylating agents exert their immunosuppressive activity by inhibiting nuclear DNA replication (WHITEHOUSE 1975;
see also Chap. 4). DNA contains several sites vulnerable to attack by alkylating
agents, of which the primary ones are shown in Fig. 1. Of these sites, the most vulnerable is the nitrogen atom at position 7 in guanine, usually accounting for about
90% of the total alkylation (LUDLUM 1975). The alkylation of DNA can have one
of the following consequences. First of all, the addition of methyl or ethyl groups

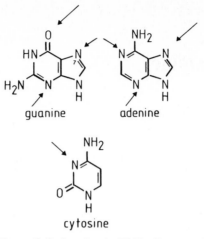

Fig. 1. Base alkylation sites in DNA. (Ludlum 1975)

to guanine can cause it to behave as a base analog of adenine and thereby produce pairing errors. Second, alkylated guanine may loosen its bonds with the sugar-phosphate backbone and leach out, resulting in the production of depurinated gaps in the DNA chain. These gaps, in turn, may interfere with DNA replication or cause shortening of the nucleotide chain. A third possibility is that bifunctional agents may bind simultaneously to both strands, and cross-link them, thus blocking the replication of DNA.

Rapidly proliferating cell populations are considerably more sensitive to alkylating substances than those that are not undergoing division. This is exemplified clearly by the characteristic side effects of prolonged CY administration on such tissues as hair follicles, testes, ovaries, bone marrow, and lymphoid cells (Shand 1979).

B. Effects of Cyclophosphamide on Cells of the Immune System

In rodents, single doses in the LD_{10} range (300 mg/kg in mice) induce, in 2–3 days, marked thymus cortex shrinking and a profound loss of cells in the B lymphocyte zones of lymph nodes and spleen, whereas T cell areas are, histologically, relatively spared (Turk and Poulter 1972). After such treatment, profound lymphopenia, involving both T and B cells, is observable without marked changes in the hematocrit, an indication of the relative selectivity of CY for lymphoid tissue.

Natural killer (NK) cells are also affected by treatment with CY. A marked decrease in NK cell activity per unit number of splenocytes was observed in mice 2 days after a single 150 mg/kg injection (Mantovani et al. 1978), complete recovery occurring, however, within 7–8 days.

Treatment of various animal species with CY results in a decrease in the amount of circulating monocytes (Evans et al. 1980), and, since at least large doses rapidly reduce the number of long-lived resident peritoneal macrophages, it seems possible that this agent not only interferes with monocyte precursors, but can be directly cytotoxic to mature mononuclear phagocytes. Further, impaired degradation of antigen-antibody complexes and phagocytosis of bacteria by peritoneal macrophages has been reported (GADEBERG et al. 1975), although others have observed an increase in phagocytosis by murine macrophages after long-term treatment with this drug (BUHLES and SHIFRINE 1977).

C. Immunomodulation by Cyclophosphamide

I. Immunosuppression and Immunostimulation In Vivo

CY can be immunosuppressive or immunostimulatory with respect to T and B cell responses. The effects of this agent depend on the dose employed as well as on the relationship of the time of drug administration to the time of antigen challenge. Early experiments performed with CY indicated that it was a potent immunosuppressive agent for T-dependent antigens (STENDER et al. 1963; BERENBAUM and BROWN 1964; SANTOS and OWENS 1966). The suppression of humoral immune responses by CY is dose dependent, and, if mice are administered 150 mg/kg at the same time as antigen, i.e., sheep red blood cells (SRBC), the subsequent plaque-forming cell responses (see Chap. 5) is abrogated (SHAND 1979). Owing to the fact that the efficacy of the drug is expressed most potently on rapidly dividing cell populations, the greatest immunosuppression is observed when it is administered at the time of, or shortly after, antigen exposure. Lymphocytes treated with CY prior to stimulation with antigen show progressively less inhibition as the time interval between drug and antigen presentation increases. In mice, complete functional recovery from the activity of CY has been found to be established within 6–7 days after its application (SHAND 1979).

Not only is T-dependent antibody production inhibited by treating mice with CY, but the response to T-independent antigens is also suppressed (HOWARD and COURTENAY 1974; SHAND and HOWARD 1978; BARTLETT 1986). We have found that in mice the proliferative response of lymphocytes to lipopolysaccharide (LPS) or dextran sulfate, two T-independent B cell mitogens, is almost completely eliminated when CY is given for 5 days at an oral dosage of 10 mg kg^{-1} day^{-1} (BARTLETT 1986). Lymphocytes from healthy Lewis rats, treated for 12 days with 7 mg kg^{-1} day^{-1} CY, displayed a greatly reduced response to mitogens 10 days after treatment was discontinued (BARTLETT and SCHLEYERBACH 1985).

That CY may have effects on the immune response other than suppression has been shown in several studies. MAQUIRE and ETTORE (1967) observed that guinea pigs treated with 10 mg/kg CY for 5 days before sensitization with dinitrochlorobenzene (DNCB) showed an enhanced contact skin response to DNCB 14 days later. These initial observations were expanded by TURK and POULTER (1972), who found that pretreatment with 300 mg/kg CY, a dose that deplete B cell-dependent areas of peripheral lymphoid tissue, augments the response to DNCB and inhibits antibody production. Further studies examining delayed-type hypersensitivity (DTH) demonstrated that augmentation of the T cell response and the suppression of antibody production, both of which follow pretreatment with CY, could be dissociated (ASKENASE et al. 1975). Furthermore, DUCLOS et al. (1977) reported that CY pretreatment decreased antibody production by splenocytes of athymic nude mice (without T cells), but increased antibody production by spleen cells from normal mice. These results indicate that low doses of CY do affect B cells, but a subpopulation of regulating T cells in normal mice is predominantly affected. The enhancement of DTH (RAMSHAW et al. 1976) and mediation of cytotoxic T cells (RÖLLINGHOFF et al. 1972) is secondary to the inactivation of a subpopulation of T lymphocytes, most likely suppressor T cells. Along this line, HARDT et al. (1981) reported on a Lyt-23$^+$ CY-sensitive T cell that regulates the activity of an IL-2 inhibitor in vivo. This inhibitor effectively counteracts the nonspecific activity of the Lyt-1$^+$ helper T cell-derived IL-2. Treatment with CY eliminates this inhibitor, thus allowing an increased immune response to occur.

The evidence for augmentation of the immune response by CY has lead to investigations of its use as a means of enhancing the immune reponse against tumors (reviewed by EHRKE and MIHICH 1984). A pitfall in many of these experiments has been the variability with which the enzymatic activation of CY occurs within various mouse strains (HURME et al. 1980). The availability of the active metabolites at the target cell depends on the level of enzymatic activity which, being under genetic control, might show considerable interspecies or even interindividual differences.

When comparing the efficacy of immunosuppressive agents for potentiating the immune response, TURK and PARKER (1973) found that CY was the most effective, followed by melphalan, azathioprine, and methothrexate. GOTO et al. (1981) described similar effects using anticancer drugs on the DTH response to methylated serum albumin in mice; these included carbazylaquinone, thio-TEPA (N,N',N''-triethylenethiophosphoramide), nitrogen mustard-N-oxide, mitomycin C, adriamycin, 5-fluorouracil, vincristine, cyclocytidine, and methotrexate. The first six of these substances were shown to be significantly more effective than CY.

II. Tolerance Induction and Termination

Any manipulation that depresses the immune response nonspecifically will favor tolerance induction (see Chap. 1). Generally, large doses of immunosuppressive agents, which produce relatively profound nonspecific immunodepression, are necessary if one is to induce long-lasting tolerance. Concerning CY, the most effective procedure to induce tolerance in mice is to treat the animals 1 day before antigen exposure with approximately 300 mg/kg (SISKIND 1984).

The mechanism by which nonspecific immunodeppression facilitates tolerance induction has not been definitively determined (Chap. 1). Possibilities suggested by SISKIND (1984) are: (a) prevention of concomitant immunization when the antigen is administered; (b) destruction of mature peripheral lymphoid cells, leading to a shift toward an immature cell population known to be more susceptible to tolerance induction; (c) a shift in the helper/suppressor T cell ratio such that suppression becomes dominant; and (d) preferential killing of cells stimulated to proliferate by the antigen. It is very likely that different immunosuppressive agents influence different tolerance mechanisms. In the case of CY-induced tolerance to SRBC, based on cell transfer studies and the ability of thymectomy to slow down recovery, it appears that this substance causes T cell nonresponsiveness (SISKIND 1984). This despite the fact, already mentioned, that when CY is administered purely for its nonspecific immunosuppressive effect, this agent preferentially depletes the animal of B cells. Further, it has been found that CY is very effective in potentiating tolerance to relatively T-independent polysaccharide antigens (HOWARD and COURTENAY 1974). This implies a direct effect on B lymphocytes, and certainly demonstrates that simple inhibition of the immune response by killing rapidly dividing cells cannot account for the facilitation of tolerance induced by this agent (SISKIND 1984). In addition, it could be shown that the tolerance induced by CY was dependent on the inherent tolerogenicity rather than the immunogenicity of the antigen (DESAYMARD and HOWARD 1975; HOWARD and HALE 1978; HOWARD and SHAND 1979). It is interesting to note that, although CY-treated murine lymphoid cells cap normally on exposure to rabbit anti-mouse immunoglobulin antiserum, they behave like immature B cells in that they are deficient in the capacity to reexpress surface immunoglobulins (SHAND and HOWARD 1978).

Procedures that facilitate the induction of tolerance: the use of CY, X-irradiation, thoracic duct drainage, etc., tend to deplete the animal of mature peripheral lymphoid cells. Subsequent repopulation of the peripheral lymphoid system with newly arising cells from the bone marrow would tend to transiently yield a "less mature" lymphocyte population that might be more susceptible to tolerance induction (SISKIND 1984; Chap. 1).

CY not only induces immunological tolerance, but it can also terminate the tolerant state. Guinea pigs that have been rendered tolerant to DNCB contact sensitivity by intravenous injection of a large dose of dinitrobenzene sulfonate (DNBSO$_3$), lose this tolerance after treatment with 250 mg/kg CY 3 days before attempted sensitization (TURK and PARKER 1982). Once the tolerant state had been broken, the animals remained responsive after subsequent challenge with specific antigen. It appears likely that this tolerant state is mediated by suppressor T cell activity, and that its termination by CY is the result of eliminating, or inhibiting, this cell type (TURK et al. 1972). However, in this model, if one allowed a 14-day gap between the CY pretreatment and attempted sensitization, the animals were subsequently found to remain nonresponsive. In this case, the effect of the CY was only temporary, and delay of sensitization allowed the regeneration of the suppressor cell population (TURK and PARKER 1982).

III. In Vitro Activities

CY, in its native form, is toxic neither to tumor cells nor to lymphocytes when they are incubated together with the agent in culture (CONNORS et al. 1974; SHAND 1978). However, if instead of native CY, serum from animals injected a short time previously with the drug is added to the cultures, then toxicity is observed (BERENBAUM et al. 1973), thus demonstrating the presence of active metabolites in the circulation. Further, it is possible to activate CY in vitro by employing liver homogenates or isolated liver microsomes in conjunction with a nicotinamide adenine

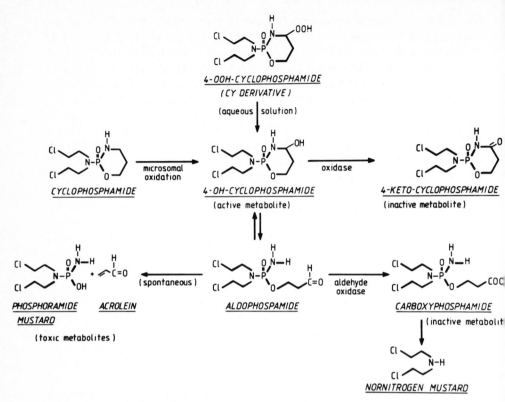

Fig. 2. The metabolic pathway of cyclophosphamide. (Modified from Connors 1975, Cowens et al. 1984)

dinucleotide phosphate-glucose-6-dehydrogenase-generating system. The active metabolites formed by this procedure show antitumor as well as immunosuppressive activity (Brock and Hohorst 1963; Connors et al. 1970, 1974; Shand 1978).

The metabolic activation of CY results in several compounds, depicted in Fig. 2, which have also been chemically synthesized. It has been shown that the metabolites that are effective in suppressing B cell function in vitro are only those species with alkylating activity (Shand and Howard 1979). These include 4-hydroxycylophosphamide (4-OH-CY), and phosphoramide mustard (PM) (Fig. 2). 4-Hydroperoxycyclophosphamide (4-OOH-CY) is a derivative of CY that in aqueous solution is spontaneously converted to 4-OH-CY, the first metabolite to be formed in the mammalian organism during the natural degradation process. Tables 1 and 2 show the results of studies on the activity of CY, 4-OOH-CY, and carboxyphosphamide (CP) on cultured lymphocytes. Only 4-OOH-CY has immunosuppressive activity on both mitogen-induced lymphocyte proliferation and the development of plaque-forming cells (PFC) to SRBC. We do observe, however, that at very high concentrations of CP (10^{-5} M), the formation of PFC to SRBC is significantly reduced (Table 1), whereas the effects on T and B cell mitogen-induced proliferation are unaffected (Table 2). Thus, according to our data

Table 1. In vitro effects of agents on the development of plaque-forming cells (PFC) to sheep red blood cells (SRBC)[a]

Compound	Dose (M)	Change (%)
Cyclophosphamide (CY)	10^{-5}	+ 8
	10^{-6}	− 8
	10^{-7}	+ 18
4-Hydroperoxy cyclophosphamide (4-OOH-CY)	10^{-5}	−100
	10^{-6}	−100
	10^{-7}	− 34
Carboxyphosphamide (CP)	10^{-5}	− 69
	10^{-6}	− 15
	10^{-7}	− 5

[a] Murine splenocytes (6×10^6 cells) were incubated together with 3×10^6 SRBC and various concentrations of drugs or solvent. After 5 days of incubation (37° C, 5% CO_2), the Jerne PFC assay was performed as described by CUNNINGHAM and SZENBERG (1968)

Table 2. In vitro effects of agents on the mitogen induced lymphocyte proliferation[a]

Substance	Concentration (M)	Mitogen (cpm $\times 10^3 \pm$ SD)				
		Con A	PHA	DXS	LPS	PWM
None	0	54 ±14	10 ±2	22 ±2	20 ±1.6	8 ±0.4
Cyclophosphamide (CY)	10^{-5}	61 ± 2.0	8.6±0.5	23 ±3.0	20 ±3	9 ±1.2
	10^{-6}	46 ± 9.0	11 ±2.0	22 ±3.0	22 ±2	8 ±1.0
	10^{-7}	44 ±13.0	13 ±4.0	21 ±3.4	19 ±1	6 ±1.1
4-Hydroperoxycyclophosphamide (4-OOH-CY)	10^{-5}	1.2± 0.1	0.1±0.02	0.2±0.01	0.1±0.1	0.1±0.1
	10^{-6}	1.4± 0.2	4.1±0.2	4 ±0.1	3.7±1.0	3.0±0.02
	10^{-7}	53 ± 5.0	9.5±0.4	27 ±4.0	18 ±3.0	9.2±1.4
Carboxyphosphamide (CP)	10^{-5}	47 ± 5	9.5±1.4	18 ±4	16 ±0.6	7 ±1.0
	10^{-6}	49 ± 9	10.4±1.2	18 ±3	20 ±4.0	9 ±1.5
	10^{-7}	54 ±14	14 ±3.3	17 ±1	18 ±4.0	7 ±1.3

[a] Murine splenocytes were incubated together with the agents and mitogens indicated. For each group, six replicates were set up. After 48 h incubation (37° C, 5% CO_2), the cultures were given 0.25 µCi/ml [^{3}H]thymidine, 24 h later the cells were harvested and the amount of radioactivity incorporated in the DNA determined. Con A concanavalin A; PHA phytohemagglutinin A; DXS dextran sulfate; LPS lipopolysaccharide; PWM pokeweed mitogen. 4-OOH-CY and CP were generous gifts of Asta-Werke, Degussa Pharma Gruppe, Federal Republic of Germany.

and the results of others (SHAND and HOWARD 1979; DIAMANTSTEIN et al. 1979; KAUFMANN et al. 1980), it can be said that 4-OOH-CY and microsomally activated CY in vitro mimic the effects of CY in vivo.

Experiments conducted in vivo have indicated that pretreatment with a low dose of CY may have selective effects on T suppressor lymphocytes (MAGUIRE and ETTORE 1967; ASKENASE et al. 1975; RAMSHAW & 1976; RÖLLINGHOFF et al. 1972). To further clarify this point investigations were conducted in several laboratories to test the effects of the primary metabolite of CY on lymphocyte cultures. Not only does the CY derivative 4-OOH-CY decompose in aqueous solution to the naturally occurring metabolite 4-OH-CY, but both molecules are equivalent in their cytotoxicity and their ability to cross-link DNA (COWENS et al. 1984), and so this molecule has been chosen most often to conduct such studies. DIAMANTSTEIN et al. (1979), reported that treatment of splenocytes with 4-OOH-CY, at a concentration that does not affect the ability of B lymphocytes to respond to mitogens, augments the response to a T-dependent antigen, but not to a T-independent antigen. This group further demonstrated that various T lymphocyte subpopulations involved in mediation and regulation of DTH responses to SRBC differ in their susceptibilities to the in vitro action of 4-OOH-CY (KAUFMANN et al. 1980), thus providing direct evidence for the validity of the notion that the enhancement of DTH to SRBC by CY in vivo is due to selective elimination of precursors of T suppressor cells. These findings parallel those reported by COWENS et al. (1981, 1984), demonstrating that 1 h incubation of murine splenocytes with 15 μM 4-OOH-CY abrogated the development of T suppressor cells, but did not affect the development of the allogen-specific cytotoxic T cell response. The elimination of suppression was found to be dose dependent, with an ED_{50} value of about 7.9 μM 4-OOH-CY (COWENS et al. 1984). The same group has also found parallel effects in the human cytotoxic T-lymphocyte response to a lymphoblastoid cell line (SMITH et al. 1982).

Extending these observations, DIAMANTSTEIN et al. (1981) reported that suppressor T cells of humoral immune responses and effector T cells mediating DTH are resistant to doses of 4-OOH-CY that abolish the activities of suppressor T cells of DTH and helper T cells of the humoral immune response. Further, this group used this compound to define the relative suceptibilities of T cells involved in the immune response of mice to an intracellular pathogen, *Listeria monocytogenes*. The specific T cell proliferation and interleukin production in vitro, as well as adoptive protection and DTH reactions in vivo, all proved to be markedly resistant to the action of 4-OOH-CY, indicating a considerable homogeneity within the cellular immune response to intracellular pathogens (KAUFMANN et al. 1984).

If one accepts that 4-OOH-CY in vitro reflects the action of CY in vivo, then these results suggest that not only B cells, but also T cell subsets are affected by CY, and that certain subpopulations of T cells involved in cellular and/or humoral immunity may also differ in their sensitivities to the action of the drug. Concerning tolerance termination with CY, it has been shown that in vitro treatment with 4-OOH-CY of spleen cells from mice that are not responsive to heterologous erythrocytes terminates this tolerance, thus allowing the successful transfer of the DTH reaction to recipient animals (KAUFMANN et al. 1980).

D. Effects of Cyclophosphamide on Autoimmune Animal Models

The immunosuppressive aspects of CY have allowed this agent to be used to slow down the progression of autoimmune diseases in animal models of various human autoimmune disorders. In the following, data will be presented concerning the effects of CY on disease development and lymphocyte modulation in a selection of animals with varying self-reactive "rheumatic" diseases.

I. Adjuvant Arthritis Disease of Lewis Rats

The adjuvant disease is perhaps the most widely used animal model to study the reaction of antirheumatic agents. A single injection of a dispersion of certain dried, heat-killed mycobacteria, or their cell wall components, in a suitable oily vehicle, into the hindpaw, induces the disease in certain rat strains (PEARSON 1956; KOHASHI et al. 1976; CHANG et al. 1981). It has been shown that the adjuvant disease can be transferred from a sick to a healthy animal with lymphoid cells (MACKENZIE et al. 1978), but not with serum (CURREY and ZIFF 1968).

Altered lymphocyte responses in humans with rheumatoid arthritis have been assessed by many investigators, and found to be commonly depressed (RAWSON and HUANG 1974; LANCE and KNIGHT 1974; SANY and CLOT 1976). In rats with the experimentally induced disease, a decreased spleen cell responsiveness to mitogens has been described (KOUROUNAKIS and KAPUSTA 1976; BINDERUP et al. 1980; BARTLETT and SCHLEYERBACH 1985). In our laboratory, we use CY as a standard substance for pharmacologic screening in this animal model of arthritic disease. Our experience is that doses of CY that inhibit the development of the disease are also immunosuppressive (BARTLETT and SCHLEYERBACH 1985). Considering that suppressor T cells are very sensitive to CY, and treatment with low doses of this agent leads to an increased cellular response, we have attempted, unsuccessfully, to restore the proliferative response of lymphocytes in these animals by administering doses of CY that only slightly suppress the disease (BARTLETT and SCHLEYERBACH 1985). This lack of success may be due to the presence of adherent suppressor macrophages in the spleens of animals with adjuvant disease (KOUROUNAKIS and KAPUSTA 1976; BINDERUP et al. 1980), that are not so sensitive to the effects of this drug. Activated macrophages produce large amounts of prostaglandins (PG) of the E series (PGE_1 and PGE_2), which are known to depress the immune response (GOODWIN et al. 1977; Chap. 15). Although CY does have anti-inflammatory activity (WALZ et al. 1971), there is no evidence that it inhibits the production of PG.

II. Murine Models for Systemic Lupus Erythematosus

Systemic lupus erythematosus (SLE) is an autoimmune disease that can affect virtually any organ in the body, and is characterized by the development of antibodies against certain types of self-antigens, the most prevalent of which are the antibodies to double-stranded DNA (dsDNA) (DECKER et al. 1979). Primarily, the antibodies formed against dsDNA complex together, and, with complement, deposit in the small blood vessels, leading to widespread vasculitis (Arthus lesions). The deposits are especially threatening if they are formed in the renal glomeruli, as this leads to glomerulonephritis and renal failure.

The impressive list of autoantibodies in SLE suggests the existence of a fundamental disturbance of the immune system, in which a B cell hyperactivity is reflected. The nature of this disease has been studied for a number of years in animal models. The New Zealand black (NZB) mouse was the first animal to be described as developing a spontaneous SLE-disease, characterized principally by the development of autoimmune hemolytic anemia (THEOFILOPOULOPOS et al. 1979). Several other strains of mice have been described more recently that also develop SLE spontaneously. These include MRL lpr/lpr (MRL/l), BXSB, and a cross between NZB and New Zealand white (NZW) mice (B/W).

1. Disease of New Zealand Mice

The effects of CY on the development of disease in New Zealand mice has been studied by several groups (e.g., RUSSEL and HICKS 1968; CASEY 1968; MORRIS et al. 1976). How this drug affects progress of the disease, or the survival of these animals depends greatly on the therapeutic regimens employed. It has been found that regular administration of CY effectively reduces DNA antibodies, as well as other antinuclear antibodies, markedly reduces glomerular immune complex deposition, and prolongs the life of the autoimmune New Zealand mice (MORRIS et al. 1976). However, it has been observed that pneumonia is more common in mice that have been treated with CY (HOROWITZ et al. 1969). Prolonged and frequent administration on CY is not necessary for protection against the autoimmune disease of these mice (MORRIS et al. 1976). The effects of CY on the immune responses seem to be much longer lasting than its effects on the hematopoietic system (MANNY and SCHWARTZ 1970; MORTON et al. 1972), which may account for the finding that widely spaced doses of CY reduce the harmful production of autoantibodies (MORRIS et al. 1976) without continous suppression of the hematopoietic system.

2. MRL/l Mice: A Model for SLE and Rheumatoid Arthritis

This relatively new animal model for autoimmune diseases has features distinguishing it from New Zealand and other mouse strains with SLE-like disease, i.e., articular involvement such as swelling of the hindpaws, pannus formation, proliferation of synovial tissue, degradation of articular cartilage, and the presence of circulating rheumatoid factor (for review see BARTLETT et al. 1986). These features indicate that this murine strain may serve well as a model for rheumatoid arthritis.

MRL/l mice are homozygous for the lpr gene, and characteristically develop a profound lymphoproliferation in which an expansion of a T cell subset bearing an inactive Lyt-1^+2^- phenotype (helper T cell) dominates (LEWIS et al. 1981). Paradoxically, in the face of massive T cell expansion, splenocytes and lymph node cells from these mice display greatly impaired interleukin 2 (IL-2) production, and proliferate poorly in response to T and B cell mitogens (ALTMAN et al. 1981; BARTLETT et al. 1986).

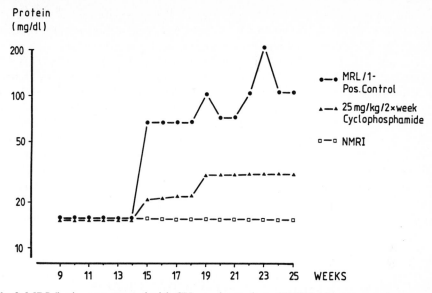

Fig. 3. MRL/l mice were treated with CY or solvent alone. NMRI mice were used as a non-autoimmune control. The amount of protein in the urine was determined weekly for each group, using Alustix (Ames Division, Miles Laboratories, Elkhard)

Table 3. Effect of CY treatment on disease development in autoimmune MRL/l mice[a]

Mice strain		MRL/l	MRL/l	NMRI
Treatment		None	25 mg/kg (twice weekly)	None
Spleen	Weight (mg)	668	330	226
	Cells ($\times 10^6$)	120	36	30
DNA-specific antibodies (titer)		4000	400	< 40
Anti-SRBC (IgM)	PFC/spleen	162	52	5247
	Antibody (titer)	4	16	2078
Mitogen-induced lymphocyte proliferation (cpm $\times 10^3$)	Con A (0.5 µg/ml)	3 ± 0.2	19 ± 1.6	89 ± 3
	PHA (0.5%)	3 ± 0.5	6 ± 0.3	35 ± 1
	DXS (30 µg/ml)	8 ± 0.4	17 ± 0.9	29 ± 1
	LPS (10 µg/ml)	8 ± 0.9	14 ± 1.6	15 ± 0.7

[a] Female MRL/l mice were treated with CY twice weekly with an oral dose of 25 mg/kg for 24 weeks, starting when the animals were 8 weeks old. At 1 week before termination of treatment, the mice were injected (i.p.) with 5×10^8 SRBC. On the 5th day after immunization, the animals were bled, and the spleens removed (8–10 mice per group). The splenocytes of each group were pooled, and tested for their response to mitogens and the formation of PFC to SRBC. The antibody titer to SRBC and DNA was determined individually for each mouse. For abbreviations see Tables 1 and 2.

Our experience with CY is that this agent's effects on the MRL/l disease are dependent on the dose regime used. CY given daily (7 mg/kg) reduces the production of antibodies to DNA and the development of glomerulonephritis (S. POPOVIĆ and R. BARTLETT 1986, unpublished work). On the other hand, we have observed that 25 mg/kg CY, given twice weekly, reduced not only the development of proteinuria (Fig. 3) and the antibodies to DNA (Table 3), but improved the response of lymphocytes to mitogens (Table 3) and restored the phorbol myristate acetate (PMA)-induced oxidative burst of macrophages (POPOVIĆ and BARTLETT 1986). Because the weight of the spleens of these animals was closer to normal than that of diseased mice (Table 3), it seems reasonable to speculate that the rapidly proliferating, nonfunctional helper T cells are more sensitive to the alkylating character of this drug than "normal" lymphocytes, thus enabling the immune response to be partially restored. This hypothesis should, of course, be confirmed by further studies, such as flow cytometric analysis of lymphocyte subpopulations.

E. Clinical Aspects of Cyclophosphamide Therapy

CY has been used clinically to modulate several diseases. Usually, the immunosuppressive aspects of this compound have been employed to inhibit autoimmune processes associated with SLE (STEINBURG et al. 1971), rheumatoid arthritis (STEINBERG 1973), multiple sclerosis (HOMMES 1978; BRINKMAN et al. 1983; TEN BERGE et al. 1982), etc. The use of CY to induce tolerance has become common practice, and, along with the introduction of other immunosuppressive drugs, has ushered in the era of human allogeneic organ transplantation.

Toxicity has been a major limiting factor in the use of CY. Leukopenia is frequent, but usually controllable when low doses are employed, and is usually reversed after drug withdrawal (FAUCI et al. 1983). Severe bacterial infections can occur (DECKER 1973), but their incidence can be minimized by maintaining the white blood cell count above 3000 (polymorphonuclear cell count >1500) (FREUNDLICH and ZURIER 1984). Thrombocytopenia is fairly common, but less frequent than with other alkylating agents (FREUNDLICH and ZURIER 1984). Hemorrhagic cytopenia occurs in 5%–10% of the patients treated with CY, and often requires drug discontinuation (PLOTZ et al. 1979). Like most alkylating agents, CY is a weak carcinogen, and secondary malignancies have been observed in cancer patients who have received this drug for long periods of time (HARRIS 1979).

F. Summary

CY is an alkylating agent that displays immunomodulating characteristics that can be, depending on the dosage and therapy schedule employed, either immunosuppressing or immunostimulatory. The apparently contradictory effects of CY result from the differing sensitivity of various lymphocyte subpopulations to its cytotoxic activity.

CY must be processed by liver microsomes before active metabolites can be formed. Because CY must be enzymatically activated, and because of the variability with which this activation occurs within different mouse strains, the availability of the active metabolites at the target cell depends on the level of enzyme activity. This, being under genetic control, might show considerable interspecies or even interindividual differences. Experiments in which the activity of the primary metabolite of CY, 4-OH-CY, was investigated have shown that the responses of both T and B cells in vitro are influenced. This probably reflects the in vivo activity of CY after liver metabolization.

The immunosuppressive effects of CY become apparent if this drug is administered after antigen stimulation has occurred. These aspects of immunosuppression have made CY very useful for curtailing the detrimental aspects of various autoimmune diseases, as well as for the induction of tolerance. One of the drawbacks of chronic immunosuppression by cytotoxic drugs are the side effects, e.g., increased risk of infection, hemorrhagic cystitis, malignancy.

The immunostimulatory effects of CY are considered to be related to the elimination of B and/or T suppressor cells which are highly sensitive to the cytotoxic effects of this drug. Although the experimental interest in CY as an immunopotentiating substance dates back to the late 1960s, adequate clinical trials have not been conducted. Thus, it is premature to speculate on the potential usefulness of CY in augmenting immunity to clinically important antigens in patients with cancer or other diseases associated with immunosuppression. However, the realization that CY, and other cytotoxic agents, can potentiate the immune response has given reseachers a new perspective on immunoregulation, and, thus, novel possibilities for immunopharmacologic intervention.

Acknowledgments. The author thanks Ms. S. Popović for allowing her unpublished data on the effects of cyclophosphamide on MRL/l mice to be used for this chapter, and Dr. P. Hilgard, Asta-Werke, Degussa Pharma Gruppe, for providing cyclophosphamide derivatives and helpful information on the literature relating to these derivatives. Further, the skilled technical assistance of Ms. D. Tessmann and Ms. D. Heck is acknowledged.

References

Aisenberg AC, Davis C (1968) The thymus and recovery from cyclophosphamide-induced tolerance to sheep erythrocytes. J Exp Med 128:35–46

Altman A, Theofilopoulos AN, Weiner R, Katz DH, Dixon FJ (1981) Analysis of T-cell function in autoimmune murine strains. Defects in production of and responsiveness to interleukin-2. J Exp Med 154:791–808

Arnold H, Bourseaux F, Brock N (1958) Chemotherapeutic action of a cyclic nitrogen mustard phosphamide ester (B-518-ASTA) in experimental tumours of the rat. Nature 181:931

Askenase PW, Hayslen BJ, Gershon RK (1975) Augmentation of delayed type hypersensitivity by doses of cyclophosphamide which do not affect antibody responses. J Exp Med 141:697–702

Bartlett RR (1986) Immunopharmacological profile of HWA 486, a novel isoxazol derivative. II. In vivo immunomodulating effects differ from those of cyclophosphamide, prednisolone, or cyclosporin A. Int J Immunopharmacol 8:199–204

Bartlett RR, Schleyerbach R (1985) Immunopharmacological profile of a novel isoxazol derivative, HWA 486, with potential antirheumatic activity. I. Disease modifying action on adjuvant arthritis of the rat. Int J Immunopharmacol 7:7–18

Bartlett RR, Raiss RX, Popović S, Schleyerbach R (1986) Immunological, histological, and ultrastructural studies in autoimmune MRL/l-Mice. In: Kuettner K, Schleyerbach R (eds) Articular cartilage biochemistry. Raven, New York, pp 391–412

Berenbaum MC, Brown IN (1963) Prolongation of homograft survival in mice with single doses of cyclophosphamide. Nature 200:84

Berenbaum MC, Brown IN (1964) Dose-response relationship for agents inhibiting the immune response. Immunology 7:65–71

Berenbaum MC, Cope WA, Double JA (1973) The effect of microsomal enzyme inhibition on the immunosuppressive and toxic effects of cyclophosphamide. Clin Exp Immunol 14:257–270

Binderup L, Bramm E, Arrigoni-Martelli E (1980) Splenic suppressor cells in adjuvant arthritic rats: effect of D-penicillamine. Agents Actions [Suppl] 7:199–203

Brinkman CJJ, Nillesen WM, Hommes OR (1983) T-cell subpopulations in blood and cerebrospinal fluid of multiple sclerosis patients: effect of cyclophosphamide. Clin Immunol Immunopathol 29:341–348

Brock N, Hohorst HJ (1963) Über die Aktivierung von Cyclophosphamide in vivo und in vitro. Arzneimittelforsch 13:1021–1031

Buhles WC, Shifrine M (1977) Effects of cyclophosphamide on macrophage numbers, functions and progenitor cells. J Reticuloendothel Soc 21:285–297

Casey TP (1968) Immunosuppression by cyclophosphamide in NZB × NZW mice with lupus nephritis. Blood 32:436–444

Chang Y-H, Pearson CM, Chedid L (1981) Adjuvant polyarthritis. V. Induction by N-acetyl-muramyl-L-alanyl-D-isoglutamine, the smallest peptide subunit of bacterial peptidoclycan. J Exp Med 153:1021–1026

Connors TA (1975) Bioactivation and cytotoxicity. In: Bridges JW, Chasseaud LF (eds) Progress in drug metabolism. Wiley, London, pp 41–75

Connors TA, Grover PL, McLoughlin AM (1970) Mircosomal activation of cyclophosphamide in vivo. Biochem Pharmacol 19:1533–1535

Connors TA, Cox PJ, Farmer PB, Foster AB, Jarman M (1974) Some studies of the active intermediates formed in the microsomal metabolism of cyclophosphamide and isophosphamide. Biochem Pharmacol 23:115–129

Cowens JW, Ozer H, Ehrke J, Colvin M, Mihich E (1981) Inhibition of the development of suppressor cells in culture by 4-hydroperoxycyclophosphamide. Fed Proc 40:1096

Cowens JW, Ozer H, Ehrke MJ, Greco WR, Colvin M, Mihich E (1984) Inhibition of the development of suppressor cells in culture by 4-hydroperoxycyclophosphamide. J Immunol 132:95–100

Cunningham AJ, Szenberg A (1968) Further improvements in the plaque technique for detecting single antibody forming cells. Immunology 14:599–608

Currey HLS, Ziff M (1968) Suppression of adjuvant disease in the rat by heterologous antilymphocyte globulin. J Exp Med 127:185–193

Decker JL (1973) Toxicity of immunosuppressive drugs in man. Arthritis Rheum 16:89–91

Decker JL, Steinberg AD, Reinertsen JL, Platz PH, Balow JE, Klippel JH (1979) Systemic lupus erythematosus: evolving concepts. Ann Intern Med 91:587–591

Desaymard C, Howard JG (1975) Role of epitope density in the induction of immunity and tolerance with thymus-independent antigens. II. Studies with 2,4-dinitrophenyl conjugates in vivo. Eur J Immunol 5:541–545

Diamantstein T, Willinger W, Reiman J (1979) T-suppressor cells sensitive to cyclophosphamide and to its in vitro active derivative 4-hydroperoxycyclophosphamide control the mitogenic response of murine splenic B cells to dextran sulfate. J Exp Med 150:1571–1576

Diamantstein T, Klos M, Hahn H, Kaufmann SHE (1981) Direct in vitro evidence for different susceptibilities to 4-hydroperoxycyclophosphamide of antigen-primed T cells regulating humoral and cell-mediated immune responses to sheep erythrocytes. J Immunol 126:1717–1719

Duclos H, Galamand P, Devinsky O, Maillot M-C, Dormout J (1977) Enhancing effect of low dose cyclophosphamide treatment on the in vitro antibody response. Eur J Immunol 7:679–684

Ehrke MJ, Mihich E (1984) Immunologic effects of anticancer drugs. In: Kuemmerle MP (ed) Clinical chemotherapy, vol 3. Thieme, Stuttgart, pp 475–499

Evans R, Madison LD, Eidlen DM (1980) Cyclophosphamide-induced changes in the cellular composition of a methylcholanthrene-induced tumor and their relation to bone marrow and blood leukocyte levels. Cancer Res 40:395–402

Fauci AS, Maynes BF, Katz P, Wolff SM (1983) Wegener's granulomatosis: prospective clinical and therapeutic experience with 85 patients 21 years. Ann Intern Med 98:76–85

Foley GE, Friedman OM, Drolet BP (1961) Studies on the mechanism of action of cytoxan. Evidence of activation in vivo and in vitro. Cancer Res 21:57–63

Freundlich B, Zurier RB (1984) Immunomodulators in the treatment of selected autoimmune diseases. In: Fenichel RL, Chirigos MA (eds) Immune modulation agents and their mechanisms. Dekker, New York, pp 289–321

Gadeberg OV, Rhodes JM, Larsen SO (1975) The effect of various immunosuppressive agents on mouse peritoneal macrophages and on the in vitro phagocytosis of *Escherichia coli* 04:K3:H5 and degradation of ^{125}I-labelled HSA-antibody complexes by these cells. Immunology 28:59–70

Goodwin JS, Messner RP, Bankhurst AD (1977) Suppression of human T-cell mitogenesis by prostaglandin. J Exp Med 146:1719–1734

Goto M, Mitsuoka A, Sugiyama M, Kitane M (1981) Enhancement of delayed hypersensitivity reaction with varieties of anticaner drugs. J Exp Med 154:204–209

Hardt C, Röllinghoff M, Pfizenmaier K, Mosmann H, Wagner H (1981) Lyt-23[+] cyclophosphamide-sensitive T cells regulate the activity of an interleukin 2 inhibitor in vivo. J Exp Med 154:262–274

Harris CC (1979) A delayed complication of cancer therapy – cancer. JNCI 63:275–277

Hommes OR (1978) Intensive immuno-suppressive treatment of chronic progressive multiple sclerosis. Ned Tijdschr Geneeskd 122:1545–1551

Horowitz RE, Dubois EK, Weiner J et al. (1969) Cyclophosphamide treatment of mouse systemic lupus erythematosus. J Lab Invest 21:199–206

Howard JG, Courtenay BM (1974) Induction of tolerance to polysaccharide in B lymphocytes by exhaustive immunization and during immunosuppression with cyclophosphamide. Eur J Immunol 4:603–608

Howard JG, Hale C (1978) Drug-promoted B-cell tolerance induction: a selective activity of cyclophosphamide dependent on the tolerogenicity of thymus-independent antigens. Eur J Immunol 8:492–496

Howard JG, Shand FL (1979) The nature of drug-induced B-cell tolerance. Immunol Rev 43:43–68

Hurme M, Bang BE, Sihvola M (1980) Genetic differences in the cyclophosphamide-induced immune suppression: Weaker suppression of T-cell cytotoxicity by cyclophosphamide activated by CBA mice. Clin Immunol Immunopathol 17:38–42

Kaufmann SHE, Hahn H, Diamantstein T (1980) Relative susceptibilities of T-cell subsets involved in delayed-type hypersensitivity to sheep red blood cells to the in vitro action of 4-hydroperoxycyclophosphamide. J Immunol 125:1104–1108

Kaufmann SHE, Metelmann C, Diamantstein T, Hahn H (1984) Short communication: resistance to 4-hydroperoxycyclophosphamide of T-cells involved in cell mediated antibacterial immunity. Int J Immunopharmacol 6:81–85

Kohashi O, Pearson CM, Shimono T, Kotani B (1976) Preparation of various fractions from *Mycobacterium smegmatis*, their arthritogenicity, and their preventive effect on adjuvant disease. Int Arch Allergy Appl Immunol 51:451–460

Kourounakis L, Kapusta MA (1976) Restoration of diminished T-cell function in adjuvant induced disease by methotrexate. J Rheumatol 3:346–354

Lance EM, Knight SC (1974) Immunologic reactivity in rheumatoid arthritis, response to mitogens. Arthritis Rheum 17:513–520

Lerman SP, Weidanz WP (1970) The effect of cyclophosphamide on the ontogeny of the humoral immune response in chickens. J Immunol 105:614–619

Lewis DE, Giorgi JV, Warner NL (1981) Flow cytometry analysis of T-cells and continuous T-cell lines from autoimmune MRL/l-mice. Nature 289:298–300

Ludlum DB (1975) Molecular biology of alkylation: an overview. In: Sartorelli AC, Johns DG (eds) Antineoplastic and immunosuppressive agents. Springer, Berlin Heidelberg New York, pp 6–17 (Handbook of experimental pharmacology; vol 38/2)

MacKenzie AR, Pick CR, Sibley PR, White BP (1978) Suppression of rat adjuvant disease by cyclophosphamide pretreatment; evidence for an antibody mediated component in the pathogenesis of the disease. Clin Exp Immunol 32:86–96

Maguire C, Ettore VL (1967) Enhancement of dinitrochlorobenzene (DNCB) contact sensitization by cyclophosphamide in guinea pigs. J Invest Dermatol 48:39–43

Manny A, Schwartz RS (1970) On the mechanism of immunological tolerance in cyclophosphamide-treated mice. Clin Exp Immunol 6:87–99

Manny A, Schwartz RS (1971) Periodicity during recovery of immune response after cyclophosphamide treatment. Blood 37:692–695

Mantovani A, Luini W, Peri G, Vecchi A, Spreafico F (1978) Effect of chemotherapeutic agents on natural cell-mediated cytotoxicity in mice. J Natl Cancer Inst 61:1255–1261

Marbrook J, Baguley BC (1971) The recovery of immune responsiveness after treatment with cyclophosphamide. Int Arch Allergy Appl Immunol 41:802–812

Morris AD, Esterly J, Chase G, Sharp GC (1976) Cyclophosphamide protection in NZB/NZW disease. Arthritis Rheum 19:49–55

Morton JT, Brown M, Siegel BW (1972) Influence of cytoxan and poly I-C on early antinuclear responses in New Zealand Black mice. Proc Soc Exp Biol Med 139:1417–1419

Pearson CM (1956) Development of arthritis, periarthritis and periostitis in rats given adjuvants. Proc Soc Exp Biol Med 91:95–101

Plotz PH, Klippel JH, Decker JL, Grauman D, Wolff B, Brown BC, Rutt G (1979) Bladder complications in patients receiving cyclophosphamide for systemic lupus erythematosus or rheumatoid arthritis. Ann Intern Med 91:221–223

Popović S, Bartlett R (1986) Disease modifying activity of HWA 486 on the development of SLE in MRL/l mice. Agents Actions 19:313–314

Ramshaw IA, Bretscher PA, Parish CR (1976) Regulation of immune response. I. Suppression of delayed-type hypersensitivity by T-cells from mice expressing humoral immunity. Eur J Immunol 6:674–679

Rawson AJ, Huang TC (1974) Lymphocytes in rheumatoid arthritis. I. Response to allegeneic cells and to phytomitogens. Clin Exp Immunol 16:41–46

Röllinghoff M, Starzinski-Powitz A, Pfizenmaier K, Wagner H (1972) Cyclophosphamide-sensitive T-lymphocytes suppress the in vivo generation of antigen-specific cytotoxic T-lymphocytes. J Exp Med 145:455–461

Russell PF, Hicks JD (1968) Cyclophosphamide treatment of renal disease in (NZB × NZW) F1 hybrid mice. Lancet I:440:446

Santos GW, Owens AH (1966) 19s and 7s antibdoy production in cyclophosphamide- or methotrexate-treated rats. Nature 209:622–624

Sany J, Clot J (1976) Stimulation of lymphocytes from rheumatoid arthritis patients by mitogens and IgG. Allergy Immunol 22:147–159

Shand FL (1978) The capacity of microsomally-activated cyclophosphamide to induce immunosuppression in vitro. Immunology 35:1017–1025

Shand FL (1979) The immunopharmacology of cyclophosphamide. Int J Immunopharmacol 1:165–171

Shand FL, Howard JG (1978) Cyclophosphamide inhibited B-cell receptor regeneration as a basis for drug-induced tolerance. Nature 271:255–257

Shand FL, Howard JG (1979) Induction in vitro of reversible immunosuppression and inhibition of B-cell receptor regeneration by defined metabolites of cyclophosphamide. Eur J Immunol 9:17–21

Siskind GW (1984) Immunologic tolerance. In: Paul WE (ed) Fundamental immunology. Raven, New York, pp 537–558

Smith J, Cowens W, Nussbaum-Blumenson A, Sheedy D, Mihich E, Ozer H (1982) Functional separation of human suppressor and cytotoxic T subsets defined in vitro by 4-hydroperoxy-cyclophosphamide (4-HC). Fed Proc 41:797–801

Steinberg AD (1973) Efficacy of immunosuppressive drugs in rheumatic diseases. Arthritis Rheum 16:92–96

Steinburg AD, Kaltreider HB, Staples PS et al. (1971) Cyclophosphamide in lupus nephritis: a controlled trial. Ann Intern Med 75:165–171

Stender HS, Strauch D, Winter H, Textor W (1963) The effect of cyclophosphamide on antibody formation with fractional and massive dosage. Arzneimittelforsch 13:1031–1034

Ten Berge RJM, van Walbeek HK, Schellekens PTA (1982) Evaluation of the immunosuppressive effects of cyclophosphamide in patients with multiple sclerosis. Clin Exp Immunol 50:495–502

Theofilopoulos AN, Eisenberg RA, Bourdon M, Crowell JS, Dixon FJ (1979) Distribution of lymphocytes identified by surface markers in murine strains with systemic lupus erythematosus-like syndromes. J Exp Med 149:516–534

Turk JL, Parker D (1973) Further studies on B-lymphocyte suppression in delayed hypersensitivity indicating a possible mechanism for Jones-Mote hypersensitivity. Immunology 24:751–757

Turk JL, Parker D (1982) Effect of cyclophosphamide on immunological control mechanisms. Immunol Rev 65:99–113

Turk JL, Poulter LW (1972) Selective depletion of lymphoid tissue by cyclophosphamide. Clin Exp Immunol 10:285–296

Turk JL, Parker T, Poulter LW (1972) Functional aspects of the selective depletion of lymphoid tissue by cyclophosphamide. Immunology 23:493–501

Walz DT, DiMarino MJ, Misher A (1971) Adjuvant-induced arthritis in rats. II. Drug effects on physiologic, biochemical, and immunologic parameters. J Pharmacol Exp Ther 178:223–231

Whitehouse MW (1975) Timely appraisal: ectopic (exocellular) nucleic acid as a drug target especially in rheumatoid arthritis and certain cancers (?). Agents Actions 5:508–511

CHAPTER 20

Lobenzarit (CCA)

Y. Shiokawa

A. Introduction

Lobenzarit (CCA) is an antiarthritic agent synthesized by Chugai Pharmaceutical Co., Ltd, Tokyo, Japan. It was selected for investigation as a result of immuno-pharmacologic screening tests of various immunologic responses induced by the interactions of immunocompetent cells. Extensive studies of lobenzarit have revealed significant effects on the immune system. In animals the compound has proven to be effective in preventing and reducing the severity of glomerulonephritis in NZB/NZW F_1 hybrid mice, which are immunologically predisposed to the disease. It also inhibits the development of spontaneous arthritis and nephritis in MRL/Mp-lpr/lpr (MRL/l) mice.

Rheumatoid arthritis (RA) is generally recognized as an autoimmune disease and in recent years, attempts have been made to treat RA patients by normalizing the underlying immune disorders. Levamisole and D-penicillamine, which may be regarded as pioneer drugs in this approach, frequently cause serious adverse reactions, and their clinical application may produce a number of problems (Chap. 18).

Clinical evaluation of lobenzarit in multicenter cooperative trials in patients with RA began in Japan in 1977. Subsequently, controlled double-blind trials of lobenzarit versus placebo in RA patients have demonstrated the significant effectiveness and usefulness of lobenzarit. No serious adverse reactions such as those reported with levamisole and D-penicillamine have been encountered in patients receiving lobenzarit.

B. Chemistry

Lobenzarit is a diphenylamine derivative. It forms pale yellowish crystals, and is soluble in water, insoluble in ether and acetone, and stable under both acidic and alkaline conditions.

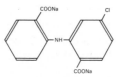

Lobenzarit disodium (CCA, disodium 4-chloro-2, 2′-iminodibenzoate) $C_{14}H_8ClNO_4Na_2$, molecular weight 335.65

C. Toxicology

No abnormalities have been observed at a daily dose of 12.5 mg/kg in a chronic toxicity study in dogs. At higher doses, slight decreases occurred in kidney and liver weights. Histopathologic changes observed in rats after chronic administration of lobenzarit in daily doses of 100 mg/kg or more are slight dilatation of the renal tubules and minor edematous changes in the epithelium of the gastric mucosa. Lobenzarit is neither teratogenic nor mutagenic.

D. Pharmacokinetics

Approximately 60% of orally administered lobenzarit is absorbed in rats. The maximum plasma level is observed 1 h after oral administration in dogs. The major route of excretion is the urine, and more than 80% is excreted unchanged within 48 h. The biologic half-life is 8 h.

E. Immunopharmacologic Studies

I. Prevention of Autoimmune Disease and Immunomodulation in MRL/Mp-lpr/lpr (MRL/l) Mice

In a study by ABE et al. (1981), male MRL/l mice were given 25 mg/kg lobenzarit p.o. three times a week, beginning at 8 weeks of age, and animals were killed for histologic examination of the joints and kidneys when they were 20 weeks old. There was a significant reduction in the degree of subsynovial soft tissue edema and of synovial cell proliferation in the treated group. Also, destruction of cartilage and replacement by granulomatous tissue tended to be suppressed in the treated group, but not significantly compared with a control group.

Untreated animals eventually developed lupus-like nephritis (proliferative glomerulonephritis) with subsequent progression of the lesions (membranous, membranoproliferative changes), whereas in the lobenzarit-treated animals, thickening of the basement membrane and immune deposits were only mild. Electron microscopic examinations also provided evidence of suppression of the development of the characteristic lesions in the kidneys of treated mice.

OHSUGI et al. (1985 b) investigated the serologic features and improvement of immunologic abnormalities during the period of prominent clinical manifestations (17–19 weeks of age) in male MRL/l mice that had been given daily oral lobenzarit since the age of 6–8 weeks. Animals were examined for the effects of lobenzarit on polyclonal B cell activation. Adult mice had increased numbers of immunoglobulin-secreting cells, elevation of trinitrophenyl-specific antibody, and higher levels of circulating immunoglobulins compared with the young (8-week-old) mice.

The elevation of serum IgG was significantly suppressed following treatment with lobenzarit, but the serum IgM concentration was not appreciably affected.

Table 1. Prophylactic effect of lobenzarit on developing arthritis and immunologic abnormality in MRL/Mp-lpr/lpr mice

Items	Control group	Lobenzarit-treated group	
Development of autoimmune diseases			
Arthritis		Prophylactic effect[a]	
Nephritis		Decrease in IC deposit[a]	
Lymphadenopathy[b]	1.31 ±0.13[c]	0.79 ±0.11	$P<0.01$
Serum autoantibodies[d]			
Rheumatoid factor (IgG)	0.446±0.068	0.257±0.038	$P<0.02$
(IgM)	0.479±0.048	0.493±0.048	
Anti-ssDNA (IgG)	0.733±0.060	0.601±0.053	
(IgM)	0.300±0.051	0.372±0.044	
Polyclonal B cell activation			
Serum anti-TNP (IgG)	0.510±0.040	0.310±0.050	$P<0.01$
(IgM)	0.200±0.027	0.210±0.030	
Serum immunoglobulins[e]			
(IgG$_1$)	1559±193	842±146	$P<0.01$
(IgG$_2$)	316± 59	169± 25	$P<0.05$
(IgM)	44± 7	60± 15	
Immunoglobulin-secreting cells per 10^5 spleen cells			
(IgG)	285± 45	147± 34	$P<0.05$
(IgM)	64± 16	48± 8	
LPS-induced immunoglobulin-secreting cells per 10^6 spleen cells			
(IgG)	166± 44	67± 24	$P<0.1$
(IgM)	415± 80	309± 61	

[a] ABE et al. (1981a).
[b] Weight of mesenteric lymph node (g).
[c] Mean±SE.
[d] Measured by ELISA method ($OD_{500 nm} - OD_{550 nm}$).
[e] mg/dl.

In the lobenzarit-treated animals, there was a significant decrease of circulating IgG autoantibodies although their serum levels were still not as low as the levels in young mice. These results suggest that lobenzarit inhibits the development of autoimmune diseases in MRL/l mice by altering their inherited immunologic abnormalities (Table 1).

II. Prevention of Autoimmune Disease and Immunomodulation in NZB/NZW F$_1$ Hybrid Mice

NZB/NZW F$_1$ mice receiving lobenzarit daily, p.o., beginning at 9 weeks of age, were compared with untreated controls with regard to the incidence and severity of proteinuria and survival rate (OHSUGI et al. 1978). Controls began developing proteinuria as they reached 28 weeks of age, and a marked increase of proteinuria ensued, leading to a mortality rate as high as 70% at 45 weeks. Severe proteinuria was also evident in the survivors. Lobenzarit-treated animals had a greatly reduced incidence and severity of proteinuria compared with the age-matched controls, and the mortality rate was less than 20%. The medium duration of survival was markedly prolonged in the lobenzarit-treated groups, i.e., 60 weeks at 5 mg/kg and 62 weeks at 50 mg/kg, compared with 38 weeks in the control group.

NZB/NZW F_1 mice were given oral doses of lobenzarit during weeks 13–28, and then killed for histopathologic study of the kidneys. Characteristic renal lesions were noted in untreated controls, including swollen glomeruli, conspicuous fibrinoid and hyaline degeneration of the glomerular capillary vessels, and emergence of a periodic acid–Schiff (PAS)-positive substance. In mice receiving 50 mg kg^{-1} day^{-1} lobenzarit, the development of these glomerular changes was significantly suppressed. Similar suppression, but of a lesser degree, was noted in mice given lobenzarit in doses of 5 mg kg^{-1} day^{-1}. An immunofluorescence study also demonstrated significantly reduced immunoglobulin deposits in the glomeruli of mice treated with lobenzarit (Ohsugi et al. 1985a).

Treatment with lobenzarit significantly suppressed the progressive elevation of serum nuclear-specific and DNA-specific antibodies, which occurred with advancing age in the untreated controls. Furthermore, the treated mice produced significantly less natural thymocytotoxic autoantibody (NTA) which is fairly selectively cytotoxic to suppressor T lymphocytes (Nakano et al. 1983).

Table 2. Enhancement of Con A-induced suppressor T cell activity toward anti-SRBC PFC responses by treatment with lobenzarit (CCA)[a] in NZB/NZW F_1 hybrid mice

Suppressor activation	Treatment	PFC per culture	Suppression (%)
Experiment 1			
None	None	115 ± 43[b]	
Con A in vitro (5 µg/ml)	H₂O	93 ± 31	19[c]
Con A in vitro (5 µg/ml)	CCA (5 mg/kg)	82 ± 49	29
Con A in vitro (5 µg/ml)	CCA (50 mg/kg)	18 ± 7	84
Con A in vitro (5 µg/ml)	Young mice	34 ± 3	71
Experiment 2			
None	None	120 ± 10	
Con A in vitro (5 µg/ml)	H₂O	70 ± 26	42
Con A in vitro (5 µg/ml)	CCA (10 mg/kg)	24 ± 19	80
Con A in vitro (5 µg/ml)	CCA (50 mg/kg)	8 ± 2	93
Con A in vitro (5 µg/ml)	Young mice	4 ± 1	97

[a] Administration of CCA was started at 9 weeks of age, and 26 weeks later the suppressor T cell activity was assayed by the suppression of splenic anti-SRBC PFC responses.
[b] Mean ± SE.
[c] The percentage suppression was determined by the following formula:

$$100 - \frac{\text{number of PFC of culture with suppressor cells}}{\text{number of PFC of culture without suppressor cells}} \times 100.$$

Table 3. Responsiveness of thymocytes to Con A in NZB/NZW F_1 mice treated with lobenzarit (CCA) daily from 9 to 28 weeks of age

Concentration of Con A (µg/ml)	[³H]Thymidine incorporation					
	Control		CCA 5 mg/kg		CCA 50 mg/kg	
	cpm	S.I.[a]	cpm	S.I.	cpm	S.I.
0	516	1.0	238	1.0	281	1.0
2.5	3937	7.6	3528	14.8	7110	25.3
5	5720	11.1	7232	34.0	20221	72.0
10	3077	6.0	5955	25.0	8755	31.2

[a] The stimulation index (S.I.) was expressed as the ratio of counts per minute of Con A-containing culture to that of nonstimulated culture.

NZB/NZW F_1 mice were treated with lobenzarit, 10 or 50 mg/kg p.o., daily from the 9th to the 35th week of life, and then their spleen cells were tested for concanavalin A (Con A)-induced suppressor T cell activity. The mitogen-induced suppressor T cells of lobenzarit-treated mice markedly inhibited the hemolytic plaque-forming cell response, compared with the T cells in untreated controls. The suppressor T cells of the treated animals, aged 35 weeks, were virtually as active as those of young (10-week-old) mice in this respect (Table 2). The data indicate that lobenzarit effectively prevented the decline of suppressor T cell function with advancing age in NZB/NZW F_1 mice.

To examine the effect of lobenzarit on the decline of thymus function associated with aging, NZB/NZW F_1 mice were given daily oral doses of lobenzarit at 9–28 weeks, and subsequently their thymic cells were tested for blastoid transformation by Con A. The lobenzarit-treated groups displayed thymocyte responses to stimulation by the mitogen 2–7 times as great as that of cells from untreated controls (Table 3). The results show a preventive effect of lobenzarit against the decline of thymocyte reponses associated with aging.

Thus, lobenzarit has been shown to suppress the production of NTA and nuclear-specific and DNA-specific antibodies, and to prevent the development of lupus-like nephritis, with a consequent marked prolongation of survival, in NZB/NZW F_1 mice. The data seem to indicate that these effects are attributable to the immunoregulatory activity of the compound, e.g. preventing the depression of suppressor T cell function with aging.

III. Therapeutic Effect on Adjuvant Arthritis in Rats

Rats were dosed p.o. daily with lobenzarit from days 16 to 22 after an injection of adjuvant into the hindpaw, and their hindleg volumes were measured to assess the therapeutic effect of the treatment on swelling. The treatment with lobenzarit in doses of 50 mg kg^{-1} day^{-1} produced a significant reduction of hindleg swelling (OHSUGI et al. 1977b). The therapeutic effect of lobenzarit against adjuvant arthritis was abolished by treating rats with anti-thymocyte serum (ATS).

In rats with adjuvant arthritis induced after they had been deprived of short-lived T lymphocytes by thymectomy at the age of 1 month, treatment with lobenzarit had no appreciable effect on hindleg swelling (Ohsugi et al. 1983).

Involution of the thymus was significantly inhibited by administration of lobenzarit in rats with adjuvant arthritis.

It is thus clear that lobenzarit prevents the progression of adjuvant arthritis in rats. These studies show that suppressor T cells, which are short-lived, can be eliminated by thymectomy, and are highly susceptible to ATS, probably play an important role in the antiarthritic effect of the compound.

IV. No Inhibitory Effect on Acute Inflammation

Lobenzarit was tested for anti-inflammatory activity against carrageenan-induced hindpaw edema and against cotton pellet-induced granuloma formation in rats. Neither experimental model of local acute inflammatory reactions was affected by lobenzarit. Furthermore, the compound caused no significant inhibition of prostaglandin biosynthesis (Tanemura et al. 1984). These findings indicate that lobenzarit has pharmacologic actions distinct from those of the structurally similar mefenamic acid and other nonsteroidal anti-inflammatory agents (Chap. 26).

V. Immunoregulatory Effects

Lobenzarit enhances immune responses by activation of helper T cells in cases of depressed helper T cell function (Nakazawa et al. 1984; Watanabe et al. 1983; Tanemura et al. 1984); conversely, lobenzarit lowers immune responses by stimulating suppressor T cells in circumstances where excessive immune reactions occur owing to depressed T cell function, thereby restoring the immune reactions to a normal level (Yamamoto et al. 1982). The compound is thus considered to have the properties of an immunomodulator. It has also been shown that lobenzarit exerts little or no effect on normal immune responses, but augments immune reactions only when they are depressed by insufficient antigenic stimulation (Ohsugi et al. 1977a).

VI. Effects on Immunocompetent Cells

The effects of lobenzarit on lymphocytes are summarized in Table 4.

1. Activation of Helper T Lymphocytes

A study of the effect of lobenzarit on helper T lymphocytes with BALB/c mouse spleen cells was reported by Yamamoto et al. (1983). Lobenzarit enhanced the induction of human γ-globulin (HGG)-specific helper T cells in vitro when the dose of antigen was suboptimal, but it had no appreciable effect on reactions evoked with an optimal dose of antigen. Similar findings were also noted in vivo as augmentation of keyhole limpet hemocyanin (KLH)-specific helper T cell activity was observed only in animals immunized with suboptimal doses of antigen.

Table 4. Effects on immunocompetent cells

1. Activation of helper T lymphocytes
2. Activation of suppressor T lymphocytes
     i) Con A-induced suppressor T cell activity in aged NZB/NZW F_1 hybrid mice
    ii) KLH-specific suppressor cells
   iii) Con A-induced suppressor T cell in vitro
    iv) Adjuvant arthritis in rats
     v) Delayed-type hypersensitivity
3. Activation of killer T cells
4. Augmentation of proliferative response of mouse spleen cells to T cell mitogens
5. Augmentation of natural killer cell activity in the spleen
6. Increase in Lyt-2^+, and decrease in Lyt-1^+ spleen cells
7. Production of IFN
8. Induction of IL-2

2. Activation of Suppressor T Lymphocytes

The effects of lobenzarit on suppressor T cells have also been investigated with BALB/c mouse spleen cells. The induction of KLH-specific suppressor T cells was enhanced by lobenzarit in vitro only when suboptimal doses of antigen were used for induction. Similar results were obtained with lobenzarit in vivo (YAMAMOTO et al. 1983). In a study conducted to explore the effect of lobenzarit on suppressor T cell induction with Con A, OGAWA and TSUNEMATSU (1982) observed that lobenzarit enhanced the induction only in cultures with submaximal doses of the mitogen.

OHSUGI et al. (1985a) measured the Con A-induced suppressor T cell activity in spleen cell populations form NZB/NZW F_1 mice after 4 weeks of treatment with daily oral doses of lobenzarit. This treatment began at 9 months of age, by which time the suppressor T cell activity (i.e., suppression of sheep red blood cell-specific antibody production) had presumably already been lowered. Untreated controls had markedly depressed suppressor T cell activity compared with young mice, but in the lobenzarit-treated mice there was a significant recovery from the depression.

The enhancement of suppressor T cell activity by lobenzarit has been implicated in the mechanism that underlies the previously described inhibitory effect of the compound on adjuvant arthritis in rats (OHSUGI et al. 1983). This is also true of the effect on delayed-type hypersensitivity in mice (ITOH et al. 1983).

3. Activation of Killer T Cells (HSV-specific)

Enhanced induction of HSV-specific killer T cells was demonstrated with lobenzarit in cultures of C3H/He mouse spleen cells (ITOH et al. 1983).

4. Proliferation of Mouse Spleen Cells

Lobenzarit has been shown to enhance the proliferation of BALB/c mouse spleen cells stimulated in vitro with such T cell mitogens as Con A and phytohemagglutinin (PHA), whereas the compound exerted no detectable influence on the spleen

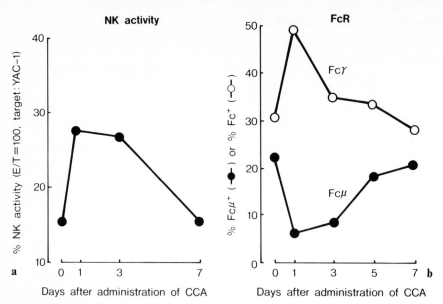

Fig. 1 a, b. Enhancement of NK activity and Fc receptor modification by lobenzarit in mice: time course of changes after dosing. Spleen cells from C3H/He mice were assayed for NK activity (**a**), measured with YAC-1 cells as target cells at an effector: target cell ratio of 100:1, and for FcμR- or FcγR-positive cells (**b**) on days 0, 1, 3, 5, and 7 after an oral dose of 100 mg/kg lobenzarit

cells proliferation with lipopolysaccharide (LPS), a B cell mitogen (Hata et al. 1980).

5. Augmentation of NK Activity

The NK activity in the spleen cell population of C3H/He mice increased following an oral dose of lobenzarit, and returned to the initial level 7 days after dosing (Fig. 1a; Itoh et al. 1983).

6. Splenic Lymphocyte Surface Markers

It has been demonstrated that lobenzarit influences certain lymphocyte surface markers (see also Chap. 6). As seen in Table 5, the proportion of Lyt-1$^+$ (helper/inducer T) cells decreased and that of Lyt-2$^+$ (suppressor/killer T) cells increased in the spleen of C3H/He mice 1 day after administration of lobenzarit (in vivo). This also occurred in cultures of C3H/He mouse spleen cells after 3 h incubation with lobenzarit (in vitro). In the same test system, Fcγ receptor-positive cells increased and Fcμ receptor-positive cells decreased following administration of lobenzarit, as shown in Fig. 1b (Itoh et al. 1983).

7. IFN-γ Production

Lobenzarit, given to mice orally at 10–100 mg/kg, induced interferon production (IFN-γ) at 40–80 units/ml in the circulating blood (Itoh et al. 1983).

Table 5. Changes in Lyt antigen-positive cell population following treatment with lobenzarit (CCA)

Experiment	Reagents	Dose	Lyt-1 (%)	Lyt-2 (%)
1[a] In vitro	None		30	11
	CCA	10 ng/ml	22	20
	IFN	100 units/ml	21	20
2[b] In vivo	None		37	16
	CCA	100 mg/kg per mouse p.o.	16	28
	IFN	10^4 units per mouse i.p.	19	32

[a] Spleen cells from C3H/He mice were incubated with CCA or interferon for 3 h, and subsequently assayed for Lyt-positive cells. Data are given as mean of two separate tests.
[b] Groups of C3H/He mice received a single dose of CCA or interferon, and their spleen cells 24 h after dosing were tested for Lyt antigen. Data are given as mean of two separate tests.

8. Induction of Interleukin 2

Y. SHIOKAWA and C. ABE (1985) studied the effects of lobenzarit on induction of interleukin 2 (IL-2) in vivo and in vitro. They found that lobenzarit was a poor inducer of IL-2.

F. Clinical Studies

I. Multicenter Double-Blind Controlled Study

SHIOKAWA et al. (1984) conducted multicenter double-blind controlled trials to investigate the efficacy of lobenzarit in the treatment of RA. The study at 46 medical institutions compared treatment with lobenzarit and an inert placebo. Both groups of patients received 25 mg t.i.d. indomethacin as a basal regimen during the study period of 16 weeks. Group 1 (115 patients) received lobenzarit 80 mg t.i.d., and Group 2 (115 patients) received placebo, t.i.d. orally. A significant improvement was noted in grip strength, the number of swollen joints, 1-h erythrocyte sedimentation rate, and the Lansbury activity index both in the patients receiving lobenzarit and those receiving placebo. The degree of improvement was greater in the patients who received lobenzarit. The most notable clinical improvement was the change in the number of swollen joints and the changes in the Lansbury activity index. The mean change in the Lansbury activity index at each examination period is shown in Fig. 2 for lobenzarit- and placebo-treated patients. The improvement in the Lansbury activity index was significantly greater in the patients receiving lobenzarit than in the patients receiving placebo at weeks 12 or 16 ($P < 0.05$). At week 16, overall clinical effectiveness was also significantly higher in Group 1 (63%) than in Group 2 (43%) ($P < 0.05$). The investigators concluded that lobenzarit is a safe and effective agent against RA when used in conjunction with indomethacin.

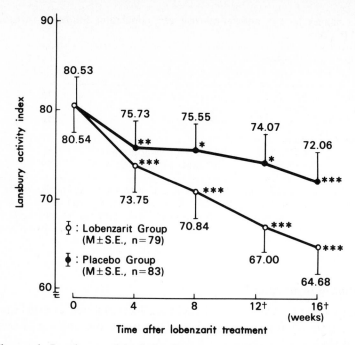

Fig. 2. Changes in Lansbury activity index. Intragroup and intergroup statistical analyses were carried out with the Student's *t*-test at 4, 8, 12, and 16 weeks after the beginning of treatment. *Asterisks* represent significant differences from the prestudy value: * $P<0.05$; ** $P<0.01$; ***$P<0.001$. Prestudy values: lobenzarit group 80.54 ± 3.04; placebo group 80.53 ± 3.19. *Daggers* indicate a significant difference between groups at the times specified, $P<0.05$. The Lansbury activity index was calculated from the duration of morning stiffness, the grip strength, the number of active joints, and the 1-h erythrocyte sedimentation rate

II. Long-Term Study

In order to study the effect of long-term treatment with lobenzarit, a clinical study was performed by Maeda (1985) to assess the effectiveness of the drug taken over extended periods by RA patients. A group of 95 patients with classical or definite RA according to the diagnostic criteria of the American Rheumatism Association received lobenzarit daily in doses of 80 mg t.i.d., with defined doses of nonsteroidal anti-inflammatory agents as basal therapy regimens. Analysis of data for the degree of improvement using the Lansbury activity index, with stratification of patients according to duration of illness after onset, disclosed a greater efficacy of lobenzarit therapy in patients whose duration of illness was less than 3 years as compared with those having suffered from the disease for longer periods. As a result, it was shown by the investigators that lobenzarit does indeed have favorable characteristics as a second-line drug, but usually affords greater clinical benefit when used as a first-line drug (Fig. 3).

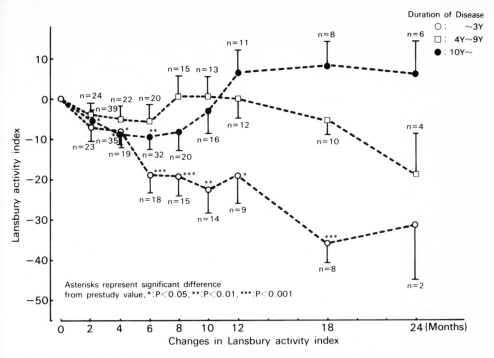

Fig. 3. Changes in Lansbury activity index. Statistics were analyzed with the Student's *t*-test at 2–24 months after the beginning of treatment. *Asterisks* represent significant differences from the prestudy value: * $P < 0.05$; ** $P < 0.01$; *** $P < 0.001$. The Lansbury activity index was calculated from the duration of morning stiffness, the grip strength, the number of active joints, and the 1-h erythrocyte sedimentation rate

III. Global Assessment of Radiologic Changes in the Hand

A comparative clinical trial of lobenzarit (CCA) versus gold salts thiomalate (GST) and D-penicillamine (D-Pc) conducted to assess the effect of lobenzarit on joint destruction in RA was reported by ARITOMI (1985). At the start, 6 months, and 1, 2, 3, and 4 years, radiographic features of the hands were evaluated by the method of LARSEN et al. (1977) as to the degree of erosion of the wrist, carpometacarpal, metacarpophalangeal, and proximal interphalangeal joints. The erosion was evaluated in categories of: (1) no change; (2) questionable; (3) mild erosion; (4) moderate erosion; or (5) marked erosion. Each patient was rated on a seven-point scale according to the degree of improvement of erosion compared with the pretreatment status: (1) markedly improved; (2) moderately improved; (3) slightly improved; (4) unchanged; (5) slightly worsened; (6) worsened; or (7) markedly worsened.

No significant difference was observed among the three treatment groups at any of the five periods of assessment regarding the degree of progress of the disease (Table 6). Analysis of the data with stratification of patients according to stage of RA at the start of medication revealed a significant delay in deterioration in the joints of patients receiving lobenzarit whose initial condition was stage IV

Table 6. Total global assessment of radiographic scores of both hands (as proposed by the Drug Efficacy Evaluation Committee of the Japan Rheumatism Association)[a]

Time (years)	Drug	Sum of overall improvement scores of both hands[a]												Total	H test
		<4	4	5	6	7	8	9	10	11	12	13	14		
0.5	CCA						2	1	2					5	
	d-Pc						3							3	
	GST						5	2	1					8	
	Total						10	3	3					16	N.S.
1	CCA					1	5	6	5	1	1			19	
	d-Pc						7	2	7	1				17	
	GST						13		6	4	1	1		25	
	Total					1	25	8	18	6	2	1		61	N.S.
2	CCA					1			5		3		1	10	
	d-Pc						2		1	3	3	2		11	
	GST						2	2	4	1	3		1	13	
	Total					1	4	2	10	4	9	2	2	34	N.S.
3	CCA						1		2	1	2			6	
	d-Pc						2		1	1	5	1		10	
	GST						2		1	1		1	3	8	
	Total						5		4	3	7	2	3	24	N.S.
4	CCA										2		1	3	
	d-Pc										1	1	2	4	
	GST						1		1				2	4	
	Total						1		1		3	1	5	11	N.S.
Total	CCA					2	8	7	14	2	8		2	43	
	d-Pc						14	2	9	5	9	4	2	45	
	GST						23	4	13	6	4	2	6	58	
	Total					2	45	13	36	13	21	6	10	146	N.S.

[a] Each joint of either hand was rated for degree of improvement on a seven-point scale, assigning 1 point for "markedly improved" and 7 points for "markedly worsened". The sum of scores for both hands was recorded as degree of improvement in both hands. Therefore, it was 8 points in the case of "unchanged" in both hands, or 14 points in the case of bilaterally "markedly improved".

(CCA, 10; D-Pc, 16; GST, 10), compared with patients receiving gold salts ($P<0.05$) (data not shown). The investigators concluded that lobenzarit is a re-mission-inducing drug with efficacy comparable to that of GST and D-Pc, which are known to retard the progress of radiographic deterioration in joints (see Chap. 18).

IV. Immunopharmacologic Data in Humans

1. Interrelation of OKT8$^+$ T Cells and Lansbury Activity Index

The interrelation of changes in the percentage of OKT8$^+$ T cells in peripheral blood and in the RA activity in patients receiving lobenzarit (80 mg, t.i.d.) was investigated by SONOZAKI and MITSUI (1984). The degree of improvement in the Lansbury rheumatoid activity index was related to changes in precentage of cir-culating OKT8$^+$ T lymphocytes in each RA patient. There was a greater degree of improvement in the index in patients who recovered normal OKT8$^+$ T cell per-centages (group A), compared with the groups showing no change (B and C), or a decline (D). The difference in Lansbury index improvement was statistically sig-nificant between groups A and B ($P<0.01$) and also between group A and the groups showing no change (B and C) ($P<0.01$). The investigator concluded that the changes in percentage OKT8$^+$ T cells may reflect the clinical status of RA (Fig. 4).

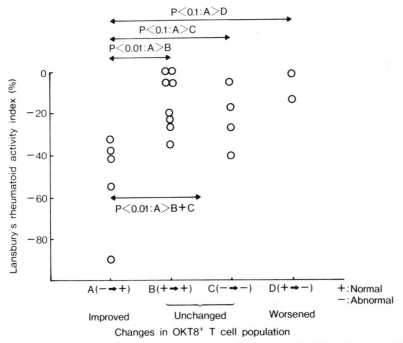

Fig. 4. Distribution of patients by degree of improvement in the Lansbury rheumatoid ac-tivity index in four groups classified according to type of OKT8$^+$ T cell population changes

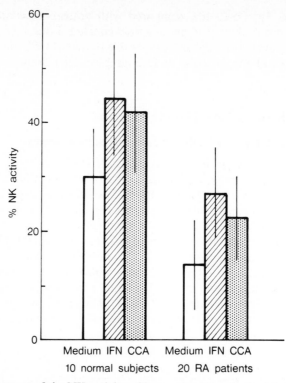

Fig. 5. Enhancement of the NK activity of human lymphocytes by lobenzarit. Peripheral blood lymphocytes from normal subjects and RA patients were used as effector cells. The NK activity of the cells against K562 target cells was assayed at an effector: target cell ratio of 10:1 in the presence of medium alone (*open*), 500 units/ml human IFN (*hatched*), or 10 ng/ml lobenzarit (*stippled bars*), and expressed as the mean ±SD

2. Enhancement of NK Activity

Depressed natural killer (NK) activity in RA and its augmentation with lobenzarit in vitro was investigated by Iтон et al. (1983). The specimens studied were from 20 patients with classical or definite RA and 10 age- and sex-matched normal controls. The NK activity of the patients' cells was significantly lower than that of the control group. However, the NK activity in RA was increased following incubation with 500 units/ml human IFN-β, and was restored almost to normal levels. The NK activity of mononuclear cells from both RA and normal subjects was also significantly increased following incubation with 10 ng/ml lobenzarit (Fig. 5).

3. Suppression of Ia Antigen Expression and Interleukin 1 Production

The effect of lobenzarit on lentinan-induced Ia expression and IL-1 production by normal human monocytes as activated macrophages was investigated by Iтон (1983). The Ia expression and IL-1 production induced by 10 μg/ml lentinan (see Chap. 25) were markedly suppressed in the presence of lobenzarit, 10 μg/ml. The investigators have thus postulated that lobenzarit may exert its antirheumatic ef-

Table 7. Effect of lobenzarit on suppressing Ia expression and IL-1 production by activated human macrophages

Agents added	Dose (µg/ml)	Cells[a] (%)		IL-1[b] (units/ml)
		OKIa1	OKM1	
Control		19.3	90	8.4
Activated macrophages	10	31.2	89	205
Lobenzarit	10	10.4	89	8.5
Activated macrophages + lobenzarit	10 + 10	11.4	93	12.8

[a] Adherent cells from peripheral blood were incubated for 2 days with RPMI 1640 medium containing lentinan and/or lobenzarit. The percentages of OKIa1[+] (human DR antigen) and OKM1[+] (human monocyte-directed antigen) cells were determined by indirect immunofluorescence.
[b] Culture supernatants were collected, dialyzed, concentrated, and tested for their IL-1 activities with non-peanut agglutinin-agglutinated mouse (PNA[−]) thymocytes.

fect by suppressing Ia expression and IL-1 production by activated macrophages (Table 7).

V. Side Effects

Of 115 cases studied in a double-blind trial by SHIOKAWA et al. (1984), 44 (38.3%) had adverse reactions to lobenzarit. The commonest adverse reactions to lobenzarit were related to gastrointestinal disorders in 26 cases (23%), skin disorders in 10 cases (9%), renal dysfunction in 5 cases (4%), disorders of the nervous system, etc. Long-term study revealed that the incidence and type of adverse reactions were almost the same as those encountered in the double-blind trial. All side effects were mild in nature and reversible. None of the side effects necessitated discontinuation of the drug.

G. Conclusions

Lobenzarit exerts various kinds of enhancing effects on lymphocytes and is significantly therapeutic in RA. However, it is not known whether lobenzarit affects some particular mechanism in the pathogenesis of RA by correcting specific abnormalities. Further studies are needed to determine the drug's mechanism of action. Lobenzarit was launched in 1986 in Japan as a remission-inducing, immunomodulating drug for RA.

References

Abe C, Shiokawa Y, Ohishi T, Hata S, Takagaki Y (1981) The effect of N-(2-carboxyphenyl)-4-chloroanthranilic acid disodium salt (CCA) on spontaneous autoimmune disorders in MRL/l mice. Ryumachi [Suppl] 21:165
Aritomi H (1985) Radiographic evaluation of the effect of remission inducing drugs in rheumatoid arthritis. In: Nobunaga T (ed) 3rd symposium on clinical trial of drugs – assessments of efficacy for immunomodulators. Nagai-shoten, Osaka, p 103–104

Hata S, Nakano T, Niki R, Takagaki Y, Sakai S (1980) Effect of CCA on the experimental amyloidosis induced by lipopolysaccharide in C3H/He mice. Jpn J Inflammation 1:145

Itoh K (1983) Mechanism of suppression of chronic inflammation by CCA. I. Effect of CCA on activated macrophage. 4th Conference of the Japanese Society of Inflammation, Tokyo

Itoh K, Kurane I, Saito F, Kawakami K, Kosaka S, Kumagai K (1983) The IFN-inducing ability and immunoregulatory action of CCA. Clin Immunol 15:242

Larsen A, Dale K, Eek M (1977) Radiographic evaluation of rheumatoid arthritis and related conditions by standard reference films. Acta Radiol [Diagn] (Stockh) 18:481

Maeda A (1985) A long-term clinical trial of CCA. In: Nobunaga T (ed) 3rd symposium on clinical trials of drugs – assessments of efficacy for immunomodulators. Nagai-shoten, Osaka, p 78–79

Nakano T, Yamashita Y, Ohsugi Y, Sugawara Y, Hata S, Takagaki Y (1983) The effect of CCA (lobenzarit disodium) on the suppressor T cell function and the production of autoantibodies in NZB × NZW F_1 mice. Immunopharmacology 5:293

Nakazawa T, Abe C, Shiokawa Y, Kamijo K (1984) Carboxyphenyl chloroanthranilic acid (CCA) in the modulation of immune response in mice. Int J Tissue React 6:23

Ogawa H, Tsunematsu T (1982) Effects of immunomodulating agents on human suppressor T lymphocytes. Allergy 31:207

Ohsugi Y, Nakano T, Hata S, Matsuno T, Nishii Y, Takagaki Y (1977a) Disodium N-(2-carboxyphenyl)-4-chloroanthranilate: enhancement of immune response in mice. Chem Pharm Bull (Tokyo) 25:2143

Ohsugi Y, Hata S, Tanemura M, Nakano T, Matsuno T, Takagaki Y, Nishii Y, Shindo M (1977b) N-(2-carboxyphenyl)-4-chloroanthranilic acid disodium salt: a novel anti-arthritic agents without anti-inflammatory and immunosuppressive activities. J Pharm Pharmacol 29:636

Ohsugi Y, Nakano T, Hata S, Niki R, Matsuno T, Nishii Y, Takagaki Y (1978) N-(2-carboxyphenyl)-4-chloroanthranilic acid disodium salt: prevention of autoimmune kidney disease in NZB/NZW F_1 hybrid mice. J Pharm Pharmacol 30:126

Ohsugi Y, Nakano T, Hata S (1983) A novel anti-arthritic agent, CCA (lobenzarit sodium); and the role of thymus-derived lymphocytes in the inhibition of rat adjuvant arthritis. Immunopharmacology 6:15

Ohsugi Y, Nakano T, Ueno K, Fukui H, Niki R, Sugawara Y, Hata S (1985a) An immunopharmacological profile of lobenzarit disodium (CCA), a new immunomodulating anti-rheumatic drug. Int J Immunother 1:85

Ohsugi Y, Nakano T, Ueno K, Sugawara Y (1985b) CCA pharmacology: preclinical evaluation for effects on experimental arthritis and immunomodulative effects. In: Nobunaga T (ed) 3rd symposium on clinical trials of drugs – assessments of efficacy for immunomodulators. Nagai-shoten, Osaka, p 67–69

Shiokawa Y, Abe C (1985) Immunotherapy of connective tissue disease. Proceedings of the 3rd international conference on immunopharmacology, Florence, Italy, 6–9 May 1985. In: Chedid L (ed) Advances in immunopharmacology, p 75–81

Shiokawa Y, Horiuchi Y, Mizushima Y, Kageyama T, Shichikawa K, Ofuji T, Honma M et al. (1984) A multicenter double-blind controlled study of lobenzarit, a novel immunomodulator, on rheumatoid arthritis. J Rheumatol 11:615

Sonozaki T, Mitsui H (1984) T cell abnormality in rheumatoid arthritis and effect of immunopotentiator. Ryumachi 24:3

Tanemura M, Kaiho S, Mizuno K, Nogaki K, Hata S, Takagaki Y (1984) Effect of an immunomodulator agent CCA on inflammatory response in various animal models. Jpn J Inflammation 4:239

Watanabe H, Yanagawa A, Shoji Y, Mizushima Y (1983) A study of the immunomodulating effect of CCA. Jpn J Inflammation 3:156

Yamamoto I, Ohmori Y, Sasano M (1982) CCA: an immunopharmacological profile in vivo and in vitro. Drug Exp Clin Res 8:5

Yamamoto I, Ohmori H, Sasano M (1983) Effect of N-(2-carboxyphenyl)-4-chloroanthranilic acid disodium salt (CCA) on the induction of helper and suppressor T cells in vitro and in vivo. Jpn J Pharmacol 33:859

CHAPTER 21

Cyclosporins: Immunopharmacologic Properties of Natural Cyclosporins

P. C. HIESTAND and H. U. GUBLER

A. Introduction

The fungi *Tolypocladium inflatum* Gams and *Cylindrocarpon lucidum* Booth are the producers of a series of cyclic oligopeptides called cyclosporins. To date, about 30 of these natural peptides have been isolated and characterized with respect to their chemical composition and immunopharmacologic properties. All these peptides are structurally related to cyclosporin A, and are composed of 11 amino acids. Usually these peptides differ from cyclosporin A by not more than one amino acid.

Many review articles have appeared describing the in vivo and in vitro pharmacologic properties of cyclosporin A (see SHEVACH 1985). Cyclosporin A is a fairly selective inhibitor of effector functions and proliferation of T lymphocytes in vitro (BOREL and WIESINGER 1977; WIESINGER and BOREL 1979), effects that are due to a selective interference with interleukin 2 (IL-2) transcription (KROENKE et al. 1984). Unlike other immunosuppressive agents, cyclosporin A does not alter the proliferation of IL-2-independent lymphocytic cell lines, nor for that matter, cell lines of nonlymphocytic origin. Thus cyclosporin A is not merely a cytotoxic or cytostatic agent which affects lymphocytes. Cyclosporin A inhibits primary and secondary immune responses in vivo (BOREL et al. 1976, 1977), suppresses delayed-type hypersensitivity reactions (BOREL et al. 1977), inhibits the localized (HIESTAND et al. 1985) and systemic (BOREL et al. 1976) graft-versus-host reaction, and is a powerful suppressant of graft rejection (BOREL et al. 1976). In models of autoimmunity, it has been shown to suppress autoantibody formation in a murine lupus erythematosus model (NZB/NZW F$_1$) (ISRAEL-BIET et al. 1983; JONES and HARRIS 1985; GUNN 1985) and in a rat model of experimental allergic myasthenia gravis (DRACHMANN et al. 1985). Beside inhibiting the production of autoantibodies, cyclosporin A also reduces or inhibits the development of clinical symptoms in lupus erythematosus (ISRAEL-BIET et al. 1983; JONES and HARRIS 1985; GUNN and RYFFEL 1985), experimental allergic encephalomyelitis (BOREL et al. 1976), adjuvant-induced polyarthritis (BOREL et al. 1976), insulin-dependent diabetes (STILLER et al. 1983), experimental autoimmune uveitis (NUSSENBLATT et al. 1981), and experimental autoimmune thyroiditis (VLADUTIU 1983; HASSMAN et al. 1985).

To investigate the possible utility of other cyclosporins produced by *T. inflatum* as immunosuppressive agents we have characterized their immunopharmacologic effects in a variety of in vitro test systems, known to be affected by cyclosporin A. A few natural cyclosporins with considerable in vitro activity as well

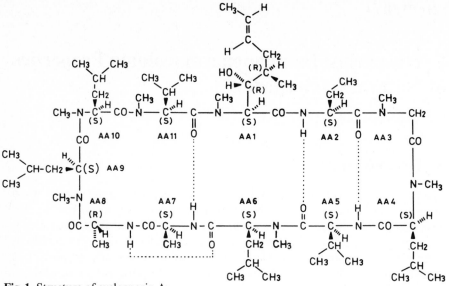

Fig. 1. Structure of cyclosporin A

as some inactive analogs were chosen for further investigation in vivo, using models that were considered analogous to their in vitro counterparts. The data presented in this chapter also illustrate the range of immunopharmacologic activities of cyclosporin A which have been used to characterize the properties of this molecule with respect to its immunomodulatory profile.

C. *lucidum* and T. *inflatum* were identified in 1970 as the producers of a number of neutral peptides. This peptide mixture proved to be weakly antifungal in vivo and did not cause acute toxicity. The discovery of immunosuppressive activity induced by this peptide mixture in vivo led to the purification (DREYFUSS et al. 1976) and chemical (RUEGGER et al. 1976) and biologic characterization (BOREL et al. 1976, 1977) of the first natural cyclosporin: cyclosporin A (Fig. 1).

Further natural cyclosporins have subsequently been isolated and characterized: cyclosporin C (DREYFUSS et al. 1976; TRABER et al. 1977a), cyclosporins B, D, and E (TRABER et al. 1977b). So far, 28 natural cyclosporin have been identified and characterized as neutral, highly lipophilic, cyclic peptides composed of 11 amino acids. The majority of these amino acids are in the *N*-methylated form (Table 1; VON WARTBURG and TRABER 1986). The following section provides a brief description of the in vitro and in vivo models we have used to profile the activity of various cyclosporins. The results are shown in the accompanying tables.

B. In Vitro Methods

All cyclosporins were dissolved in ethanol/Tween-80 (10:1 v/v) at a concentration of 20 mg/ml, and diluted with medium to the required final concentration. Compounds were added to all in vitro systems at the time of addition of the antigen or mitogen.

Table 1. Structures of natural cyclosporins (Cs)

Metabolite	1	2	3	4	5	6	7	8	9	10	11
Cs-A	C₉-AS	Abu	Sar	MeLeu	Val	MeLeu	Ala	D-Ala	MeLeu	MeLeu	MeVal
Cs-B	C₉-AS	Ala	Sar	MeLeu	Val	MeLeu	Ala	D-Ala	MeLeu	MeLeu	MeVal
Cs-C	C₉-AS	Thr	Sar	MeLeu	Val	MeLeu	Ala	D-Ala	MeLeu	MeLeu	MeVal
Cs-D	C₉-AS	Val	Sar	MeLeu	Val	MeLeu	Ala	D-Ala	MeLeu	MeLeu	MeVal
Dihydro-Cs-D	Dihydro-C₉-AS	Val	Sar	MeLeu	Val	MeLeu	Ala	D-Ala	MeLeu	MeLeu	MeVal
Cs-E	C₉-AS	Abu	Sar	MeLeu	Val	MeLeu	Ala	D-Ala	MeLeu	MeLeu	Val
Cs-F	Desoxy-C₉-AS	Abu	Sar	MeLeu	Val	MeLeu	Ala	D-Ala	MeLeu	MeLeu	MeVal
Cs-G	C₉-As	Nva	Sar	MeLeu	Val	MeLeu	Ala	D-Ala	MeLeu	MeLeu	MeVal
Cs-H	C₉-AS	Abu	Sar	MeLeu	Val	MeLeu	Ala	D-Ala	MeLeu	MeLeu	D-MeVal
Cs-I	C₉-AS	Val	Sar	MeLeu	Val	MeLeu	Ala	D-Ala	MeLeu	Leu	MeVal
Cs-K	Desoxy-C₉-AS	Val	Sar	MeLeu	Val	MeLeu	Ala	D-Ala	MeLeu	MeLeu	MeVal
Cs-L	N-Desmethyl-C₉-AS	Abu	Sar	MeLeu	Val	MeLeu	Ala	D-Ala	MeLeu	MeLeu	MeVal
Cs-M	C₉-AS	Nva	Sar	MeLeu	Nva	MeLeu	Ala	D-Ala	MeLeu	MeLeu	MeVal
Cs-N	C₉-AS	Nva	Sar	MeLeu	Val	MeLeu	Ala	D-Ala	MeLeu	Leu	MeVal
Cs-O	MeLeu	Nva	Sar	MeLeu	Val	MeLeu	Ala	D-Ala	MeLeu	MeLeu	MeVal
Cs-P	N-Desmethyl-C₉-AS	Thr	Sar	MeLeu	Val	MeLeu	Ala	D-Ala	MeLeu	MeLeu	MeVal
Cs-Q	C₉-AS	Abu	Sar	Val	Val	MeLeu	Ala	D-Ala	MeLeu	MeLeu	MeVal
Cs-R	C₉-AS	Abu	Sar	MeLeu	Val	Leu	Ala	D-Ala	MeLeu	Leu	MeVal
Cs-S	C₉-AS	Thr	Sar	Val	Val	MeLeu	Ala	D-Ala	MeLeu	MeLeu	MeVal
Cs-T	C₉-AS	Abu	Sar	MeLeu	Val	MeLeu	Ala	D-Ala	MeLeu	Leu	MeVal
Cs-U	C₉-AS	Abu	Sar	MeLeu	Val	Leu	Ala	D-Ala	MeLeu	MeLeu	MeVal
Cs-V	C₉-AS	Abu	Sar	MeLeu	Val	MeLeu	Abu	D-Ala	MeLeu	MeLeu	MeVal
Cs-W	C₉-AS	Thr	Sar	MeLeu	Val	MeLeu	Ala	D-Ala	MeLeu	MeLeu	Val
Cs-X	C₉-AS	Nva	Sar	MeLeu	Val	Leu	Ala	D-Ala	Leu	MeLeu	MeVal
Cs-Y	C₉-AS	Nva	Sar	MeLeu	Val	Leu	Ala	D-Ala	MeLeu	MeLeu	MeVal
Cs-Z	Methylamino-octanoic acid	Abu	Sar	MeLeu	Val	MeLeu	Ala	D-Ala	MeLeu	MeLeu	MeVal

C₉-AS = [2S, 3R, 4R, 6E]-3-hydroxy-4-methyl-2-methylamino-6-octenoic acid
Abu = L-α-aminobutyric acid; Nva = L-norvaline; MeVal = N-methyl-L-valine; MeLeu = N-methyl-L-leucine; Sar = sarcosine.

Table 2. Effect of cyclosporins A–Z on proliferative responses of mouse lymphocytes to mitogenic stimulation in vitro

Cyclosporin	IC_{50} (μg/ml)		
	Con A[a]	IL-2[b]	LPS[c]
Cs-A	0.0016	0.0016	0.0033
Cs-B	<0.04	<0.04	<0.04
Cs-C	<0.04	<0.04	<0.04
Cs-D	1.15	0.58	0.5
Dihydro-Cs-D	1.0	0.52	0.75
Cs-E	ND	ND	ND
Cs-F	0.117	0.23	0.086
Cs-G	0.06	0.095	0.027
Cs-H	>1	>1.0	0.22
Cs-I	>5	ND	1.8
Cs-K	0.14	0.38	0.101
Cs-L	0.37	2.2	0.26
Cs-M	<0.04	<0.04	<0.04
Cs-N	0.072	0.52	0.56
Cs-O	0.49	0.72	0.25
Cs-P	0.048	0.103	0.052
Cs-Q	0.95	2.9	0.48
Cs-R	1.0	0.65	0.2
Cs-S	ND	ND	ND
Cs-T	0.025	0.075	0.024
Cs-U	ND	ND	ND
Cs-V	0.56	0.5	0.24
Cs-W	0.38	0.48	0.85
Cs-X	0.25	0.51	0.2
Cs-Y	0.442	4.1	0.177
Cs-Z	0.551	2.0	0.29

[a] Proliferative response to stimulation with the lectin concanavalin A.
[b] Interleukin 2 generated in spleen cell cultures by use of concanavalin A and assayed by use of an IL-2-dependent cytotoxic T cell line.
[c] Proliferative response to stimulation with lipopolysaccharide (from *Salmonella typhimurium*).

I. Proliferative Response of Lymphocytes to Mitogenic Stimulation
(Janossy and Greaves 1971, 1973; Greaves and Janossy 1972)

Spleen cells ($0.5–1 \times 10^6$ cells) from mice (BALB/c, C57/BL, and other strains) were incubated for 3 days with either Con A (1–5 μg/ml) or LPS (25–75 μg/ml). Proliferation of lymphocytes was assessed by labeled thymidine incorporation into DNA (Table 2).

II. Generation of Soluble Factors Affecting the Immune Response

1. Interleukin 2 (Mosmann 1983)

Interleukin 2 (IL-2) was induced by mitogen stimulation of mouse spleen cells. After 48 h, supernatants were collected and assayed for their IL-2 content by use of an IL-2-dependent cell line. The growth of these cells was assayed after a further 48 h by an enzymatic assay which measures mitochondrial activity (Table 2).

III. Proliferative Response of Lymphocytes to Allogeneic Stimulation: Murine Mixed Lymphocyte Reaction (MEO 1979)

Spleen cells (0.5×10^6) from BALB/c mice (female 8–10 weeks) were coincubated for 5 days with 0.5×10^6 irradiated (2000 rad) or mitomycin C-treated spleen cells from CBA mice (female, 8–10 weeks). The irradiated allogeneic cells induce a proliferative response in the BALB/c spleen cells which can be measured by incorporation of [³H] thymidine into DNA. Since the stimulator cells were irradiated (or mitomycin C treated) they do not respond to the BALB/c cells with proliferation, but retain the ability to provide an antigenic stimulus (Table 3).

Table 3. Effect of cyclosporins A–Z on growth and function of mouse lymphocytes stimulated by allogeneic cells in vitro

Cyclosporin	IC_{50} (µg/ml)	
	MLR[a]	CML[b]
Cs-A	0.0036	0.0067
Cs-B	0.099	<0.04
Cs-C	< 0.04	<0.04
Cs-D	0.13	0.09
Dihydro-Cs-D	0.24	0.34
Cs-E	0.15	ND
Cs-F	1.043	ND
Cs-G	0.0085	0.083
Cs-H	12.5	ND
Cs-I	2.0	ND
Cs-K	> 1	0.67
Cs-L	0.074	0.047
Cs-M	0.04	<0.04
Cs-N	0.09	<0.04
Cs-O	> 1.0	0.23
Cs-P	0.095	0.063
Cs-Q	> 1	>5
Cs-R	0.378	0.48
Cs-S	> 5	ND
Cs-T	0.0348	0.04
Cs-U	0.401	ND
Cs-V	0.031	0.069
Cs-W	> 1	0.37
Cs-X	0.61	0.17
Cs-Y	> 1	0.29
Cs-Z	> 1	2.45

[a] Mixed lymphocyte reaction.
[b] Cell-mediated lympholysis (generation of cytotoxic lymphocytes).

IV. Induction of Cytotoxic T Cells
in a One-Way Mixed Lymphocyte Reaction
(Brunner et al. 1968)

Spleen cells 10^6 from BALB/c mice (female, 8–10 weeks) were incubated in the presence of 10^6 irradiated (2000 rad) spleen cells from CBA mice (female, 8–10 weeks). In this one-way MLR, the irradiated allogeneic lymphocytes provide the antigenic stimulus and induce the proliferation of cytotoxic T lymphocytes derived from the BALB/c spleen cell mixture. After 5 days incubation, 10^5 spleen cells from CBA mice, previously stimulated in vitro with LPS and labeled with Cr^{51}, were added for a further 3 h incubation. During this time, cytotoxic T cells lyse the CBA target cells, thereby releasing their incorporated isotope into the supernatant of the culture. Aliquots of the cell-free culture supernatants were counted in a gamma counter (Table 3).

V. Primary Humoral Immune Response to Sheep Red Blood Cells
(Mishell and Dutton 1966, 1967)

Mouse spleen cells (OF1, female, 8–10 weeks, 10^7) were cocultured with sheep erythrocytes (SRBC, 3×10^7) for 3 days in 1 ml medium in 24-well plates. Lymphocytes were harvested, washed, and plated at a density of 10^6 cells onto soft agar with fresh antigen (SRBC). Complement (guinea pig serum) was added 60–90 min later and the incubation continued for a further 60 min after which the number of hemolytic plaques was counted under a microscope. During the 3-day incubation period, the lymphocytes were sensitized to the antigen (SRBC). On subsequent incubation with antigen, B lymphocytes secrete specific antibody which binds to the antigen in the vicinity of the secretory lymphocyte. Addition of complement causes lysis of the antibody-coated erythrocytes, yielding a plaque. Each plaque represents a single antibody-producing cell (Table 4).

VI. Secondary Humoral Immune Response
Against a T Cell-Specific Antigen (DNP-KLH) In Vitro
(Hiestand et al. 1985)

BALB/c mice (female, 8–10 weeks) were sensitized by i.p. injection of 10 μg DNP-KLH (specific activity 6–8 mol DNP per mol KLH) mixed with 0.5 ml alum. After 3 weeks, animals were boosted with 10 μg DNP-KLH i.p. Spleen cell suspensions were prepared 2 weeks after the final injection of antigen and incubated (cell density 0.5×10^6 cells in 0.2 ml final incubation volume) with 2 ng DNP-KLH for 7 days. Lymphocytes which were sensitized in vivo (memory cells) recognize the antigen during the in vitro incubation, and respond with the secretion of specific antibody. Antibodies were detected in the supernatants by use of an ELISA technique. Substances to be tested were added at the time of antigen challenge to determine their ability to stimulate or inhibit antibody formation (Table 4).

Table 4. Effect of cyclosporins A–Z on the formation of plaque-forming cells and on antibody formation in vitro

Cyclosporin	IC$_{50}$ (µg/ml)	
	Primary humoral response to SRBC	Secondary humoral response to DNP-KLH
Cs-A	0.036	0.026
Cs-B	0.21	0.155
Cs-C	0.038	ND
Cs-D	0.44	1.25
Dihydro-Cs-D	0.33	>1.0
Cs-E	0.2	0.0982
Cs-F	0.55	>1.0
Cs-G	0.014	0.01
Cs-H	>1.0	>1.0
Cs-I	3.6	1.85
Cs-K	>1.0	2.1
Cs-L	0.39	>1.0
Cs-M	0.25	0.59
Cs-N	0.15	0.5
Cs-O	>1.0	>1.0
Cs-P	0.27	0.62
Cs-Q	>1.0	>1.0
Cs-R	>1.0	>1.0
Cs-S	>1.0	>1.0
Cs-T	0.034	0.092
Cs-U	0.34	0.22
Cs-V	0.04	>1.0
Cs-W	0.55	>1.0
Cs-X	0.69	0.2
Cs-Y	>1.0	0.285
Cs-Z	>1.0	>1.0

VII. Cytotoxic and Cytostatic Activity in Vitro with the P-815 Mastocytoma Cell Line (STAEHELIN 1962)

A Costar 96-well plate was filled with medium (100 µl per well), compounds to be tested were added to the top row in a 25-µl aliquot, mixed then 25 µl was removed and added to the next lower row until the end of the plate was reached. The last 25 µl was discarded. Then, 100 µl cell suspension (P-815 mastocytoma cells, 30 000 cells per well) was added to each well, and the plates were incubated for 48 h at 37 °C in a humidified atmosphere of air $+5\%–7\%$ CO$_2$.

Cell proliferation was assessed by use of a cell counter or by an enzymatic-colorimetric assay: plates were centrifuged for 10 min at 3000 rpm (IEC Centra-7R). Supernatant was discarded, the cells were washed once with PBS (Dulbecco without calcium and magnesium) and 50 µl per well 0.5% Triton X-100 solution (0.5 ml Triton X-100 in 99.5 ml water) was added and the plates shaken vigorously for 5–10 min at room temperature. Substrate (p-nitrophenyl-N-acetyl-β-

D-glucosaminide, 50 µl per well) was added before incubation for 60 min at 37 °C. Then 150 µl 2N NaOH was added, and the plates were read at 405 nm.

All natural cyclosporins behave like cyclosporin A in this test system in that they do not inhibit IL-2-independent proliferating cell lines. Therefore, they do not possess cytostatic or cytotoxic potential up to a concentration of more than 1 µg/ml. Above this concentration, around 2–10 µg/ml, they are cytotoxic to cells in vitro.

C. In Vivo Methods

All cyclosporins were dissolved in a minimal amount of ethanol and diluted to the final concentration with olive oil. The final concentration of ethanol in this mixture was less than 5%.

I. Formation of Plaque-Forming Cells (Humoral Immune Response)
(JERNE and NORDIN 1963; JERNE et al. 1963)

Mice were immunized by the i.v. injection of 10^8 sheep erythrocytes (SRBC) and treated on three consecutive days with the drugs under investigation. Spleen cell suspensions were prepared 4 days after immunization and 10^6 lymphocytes were plated onto soft agar in the presence of indicator cells (SRBC) and complement. Lysis of the indicator cells due to secretion of specific antibody and the presence of complement yielded plaques. The number of plaques per plate were counted and corrected for the number of plaques per spleen (Table 5).

Table 5. Effect of orally administered natural cyclosporins on humoral and cell-mediated immune responses in vivo

Cyclosporin	ED_{50} (mg/kg)			ED_{30} (mg/kg)
	GvH[a]	PFC (IgM)[b]		DTH (oxazolone)[c]
	Rat	Mouse	Rat	Mouse
Cs-A	≦36	55	3–6	70
Cs-B	>50	>100	ND	70
Cs-C	25	50	ND	ND
Cs-D	25	25	ND	>70
Dihydro-Cs-D	44	150	>20	35
Cs-F	>50	ND	ND	>70
Cs-G	38	45	3–6	35
Cs-H	ND	>100	ND	ND
Cs-M	≦50	52	ND	ND

[a] Localized graft-versus-host reaction in female rats.
[b] IgM-secreting plaque-forming cells assayed either on day 4 (mice) or on day 6 (rat).
[c] Delayed-type hypersensitivity reaction (oxazolone skin test in the mouse).

II. Delayed-Type Hypersensitivity Reaction in Mice

1. Oxazolone Skin Test (DIETRICH and HESS 1970)

OFl mice (female, 8–12 weeks) were sensitized by painting their shaved abdomens with a solution of an antigen (oxazolone) in ethanol. After 9 days, they were challenged with the same antigen applied to the left ear. The right ear remained untreated and served as the individual's negative control. After 24 h, the thickness of both ears was measured by means of an automated microcaliper. The difference in thickness between the treated left and the untreated right ear provided a parameter to evaluate the reaction. When sensitized lymphocytes recognize the antigen during the challenging phase, they move to the site of challenge and initiate a local inflammatory response, resulting in edema and hence an increased ear thickness. The delayed-type hypersensitivity (DTH) reaction is mediated by the release of soluble factors effecting the immune response (lymphokines, e.g., chemotactic factors, differentiation-inducing factors, maturation factors, growth factors; Table 5).

III. Localized Graft-Versus-Host Reaction (FORD et al. 1980)

Spleen cells (10^7) from 6-week-old female Wistar/Furth (WF) rats were injected subcutaneously on day 0 into the left hindpaw of female (F344 × WF)F$_1$ rats weighing about 100 g. Animals were treated with the test compound for 4 consecutive days and the popliteal lymph nodes were removed and weighed on day 7. The difference in weight between the two lymph nodes was taken as the parameter for evaluating the reaction (Table 5).

D. Autoimmune Disease Models

I. Freund's Adjuvant-Induced Arthritis (BILLINGHAM and DAVIES 1979)

OFA and Wistar rats (male or female, 150 g body weight) were injected intracutaneously at the base of the tail or in the hindpaw with 0.1 ml mineral oil containing 0.6 mg lyophilized heat-killed *Mycobacterium smegmatis*. In the developing arthritis model, treatment was started immediately after the injection of the adjuvant (days 1–18); in the established arthritis model, treatment was started on day 14, when the secondary inflammation was well developed (days 14–20). At the end of the experiment, the swelling of the joints was measured by means of a microcaliper. ED$_{50}$ is the oral dose in mg/kg which reduces the swelling (primary or secondary) to half that of the controls.

Cyclosporins that were inactive in the developing arthritis model were, with a few exceptions, not tested in the established disease (Table 6).

Table 6. Effect of orally administered cyclosporins A–Z on adjuvant-induced arthritis in rats

Cyclosporin	ED_{50} (mg/kg)	
	Developing	Established
Cs-A	6	12
Cs-B	20	28
Cs-C	3	14
Cs-D	4	>10
Dihydro-Cs-D	8	27
Cs-E	>30	ND
Cs-F	>30	ND
Cs-G	5	14
Cs-H	>60	>60
Cs-I	ND	ND
Cs-K	ND	>20
Cs-L	>15	ND
Cs-M	5	15
Cs-N	>10	ND
Cs-O	>10	ND
Cs-P	>10	ND
Cs-Q	>13	ND
Cs-R	ND	ND
Cs-S	>10	ND
Cs-T	>10	ND
Cs-U	>10	ND
Cs-V	>14	ND
Cs-W	ND	ND
Cs-X	ND	ND
Cs-Y	>10	ND
Cs-Z	ND	ND

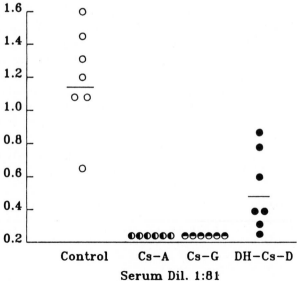

II. Formation of Autoantibodies in Experimental Allergic Myasthenia Gravis (LENNON et al. 1975)

The formation of autoantibodies against the acetylcholine receptor was induced in the rat by intracutaneous injection of purified acetylcholine receptor suspended in Freund's complete adjuvant. The receptor was isolated by affinity chromatography of extracts from the electric organs of *Torpedo californica* on immobilized *Naja naja siamensis* neurotoxin (Fig. 2; FULPIUS et al. 1981).

E. Transplantation Models

I. Skin Allograft Reaction in Mice (HIESTAND et al. 1985 a,b)

Fitted pinchgrafts of skin from female C57/BL donors were transplanted to female BALB/*c* mice. The survival time of the transplant was recorded (Table 7).

II. Kidney Allograft Reaction in Rats (HIESTAND et al. 1985 a,b)

One kidney from a female F344 rat was transplanted to a unilaterally (left side) nephrectomized WF recipient rat. Treatment commenced on the day of transplantation, and was continued for 14 days. The recipient's original right kidney was removed 7 days after transplantation, leaving the recipient relying on the performance of the donor kidney. Survival of the animal was taken as the parameter for a functional graft (Table 7).

III. Heterotopic Heart Transplantation in Rats (HIESTAND et al. 1985 a,b)

Heterotopic heart allografts (F344 rats) were transplanted into WF rats by the donor aorta and right pulmonary artery, anastomosed end-to-side to the recipient's abdominal aorta and inferior vena cava. Heart muscle was fully perfused and beating; left atrium and ventricle remained empty. Coronary venous blood returned via the right atrium, the right ventricle, and the pulmonary artery of the transplant to the recipient's inferior vena cava (Table 7).

Fig. 2. Experimentally induced allergic myasthenia gravis in rats. Acetylcholine receptor isolated from *Torpedo californica* was injected subcutaneously on day 0 in combination with Freund's complete adjuvant into the backs of 8-week-old female Lewis rats. Additional adjuvant (*Bordetella pertussis*) was administered into the hindfootpads. Animals were treated orally with cyclosporins at a dose of 25 mg/kg, starting on the day of immunization for 14 days. Autoantibody titers were determined at weekly intervals by use of an ELISA technique. Results show the individual autoantibody titers of 6–7 rats per group after a 1-week treatment period.

Table 7. Prevention of graft rejection in rats by orally administered natural cyclosporins[a]

Cyclosporin	Dose (mg/kg)	Graft survival (days ± SD)		Heterotopic heart	Skin allograft
		Kidney allograft			
		Dead/total	Survival (days)		
Controls	–	5/5	9.6±0.5	6.8±0.8	8.3±0.5
Cs-A	14×20	ND	ND	112.5±43.3	16.9±1.8
	14×10	0/5	>245	>150	ND
	14×7.5	0/5	>365	ND	ND
	14×5	5/5	11.7±2.08	ND	ND
Cs-B	14×7.5	4/5	26.5±18.1 (11, 12, 35, 48, >80)[c]	ND	ND
Cs-C	14×7.5	0/5	>120	ND	ND
Dihydro-Cs-D	14×10	4/6	17±10.7[b]	18.4±5.8	16.6±1.8
	14×20	ND	ND	17.3±7.8[b]	20.3±1.9
Cs-G	14×20	ND	ND	>112	ND
	14×10	0/5	>60	>300	ND
	14×7.5	0/5	>365	ND	ND
	14×5	4/5	10.5±0.58	ND	ND

[a] Treatment commenced on the day of transplantation and continued for 14 consecutive days.

[b] Three of five heart grafts and four of six kidney grafts were acutely rejected. Two animals in each group kept the graft for more than 60 days, after which rejection occurred.

[c] Graft survival time in days. One graft was not rejected.

F. Discussion

The fungus *Tolypocladium inflatum* produces a number of cyclic peptides, one of which (cyclosporin A) has been shown to possess powerful immunosuppressive properties in vitro and in vivo (BOREL and WIESINGER 1977; WIESINGER and BOREL 1979; BOREL et al. 1976, 1977; HIESTAND et al. 1985; ISRAEL-BIET et al. 1983; GUNN 1985; DRACHMAN et al. 1985; GUNN and RYFFEL 1985; VLADUTIU 1983; JONES and HARRIS 1985; STILLER et al. 1983; NUSSENBLATT 1981; HASSMAN et al. 1986). The primary interaction of cyclosporin A with events leading to cell activation is still unknown. However, it has been demonstrated that cyclosporin A selectively inhibits the transcription of factors involved in the activation of T lymphocytes (KROENKE et al. 1984). This makes cyclosporin A the first selective, low molecular weight, immunosuppressive agent to be used extensively in organ transplantation in humans. Although cyclosporin A inhibits lymphocyte activation, primary defense mechanisms against bacterial or viral infections are not apparently compromised by the fairly low dose of cyclosporin A used clinically in transplantation. Thus, antibody formation can still be observed in patients given cyclosporin A (SCHWARTZ et al. 1986).

One major drawback associated with the clinical use of cyclosporin A, however, is an adverse effect on renal function. Therefore, a cyclosporin derivative devoid of this action would be desirable. With this in mind, a large number of natural, synthetic, and semisynthetic cyclosporin derivatives have been investigated in models which were affected by cyclosporin A.

No general rule can be drawn from the in vitro data regarding structure-activity relationships. However, it seems clear that amino acids, 2, 5, and 10 can be manipulated without loss of immunosuppressant activity. Slight modifications are also permitted on amino acid 1. Changes of the residue in position 2 from γ-aminobutyric acid (cyclosporin A) to valine leads to a decrease of overall activity. However, activity is largely retained if threonine or norvaline is substituted at this position. Hydrogenation of the double bond in the C_9 amino acid (position 1) does lead to a change in the activity profile with a generalized decreased potency in various transplant models, in humoral immune responses, and in the adjuvant-induced arthritis model. Surprisingly, activity in the delayed-type hypersensitivity model is retained.

Structural changes at amino acid residues 4, 6, and 11 usually lead to complete loss of activity. To gain further information on structure-activity relationships, most of the in vitro active, as well as some of the inactive cyclosporins have been assayed with in vivo systems to confirm their in vitro activity under conditions that take pharmacokinetics and the metabolism of the various derivatives into account.

One fact that became apparent from these investigations is that activity in the Freund's adjuvant-induced polyarthritis model in the rat seems to be a good indicator of effectiveness in transplantation models. A similar correlation exists with activity in the graft-versus-host model, with only one exception (a synthetic derivative) in about 600 analogs tested. Nevertheless, these findings should be treated with caution since only a minority of the available cyclosporins have been investigated in the time-consuming transplant models.

Inhibition of antibody formation only partially correlates with other activities. The only correlation with activity in humoral immune responses is found in autoimmune disease models which depend primarily on autoantibody formation (e.g., systemic lupus erythematosus and myasthenia gravis). Compounds such as dihydrocyclosporin D, which do not affect primary humoral immune responses (plaque-forming cell assay) are without therapeutic effect in the NZB/NZW F1 mouse lupus model and in experimental allergic myasthenia gravis (see Fig. 2).

One other point became clear during the investigation of these natural cyclosporins. None of analogs possessed greater potency than cyclosporin A in either in vitro or in vivo tests.

In conclusion, it can be stated that only a few natural cyclosporin analogs (cyclosporin A, C, D, G, and M) have been found to be active in vivo, even though several derivatives did show appreciable in vitro activity. The lack of correlation between in vitro and in vivo potency may reflect differences in the bioavailability and pharmacokinetic behavior of these different cyclosporins.

References

Billingham MEJ, Davies GE (1979) Experimental models of arthritis in animals as screening tests for drugs to treat arthritis in man. In: Vane JR, Ferreira SH (eds) Handbook of experimental pharmacology, vol 50/II. Springer, Berlin Heidelberg New York, p 108

Borel JF, Wiesinger D (1977) Effect of cyclosporin A on murine lymphoid cells. In: Lucas DO (ed) Regulatory mechanisms in lymphocyte activation. Academic NY, p 716

Borel JF, Feurer C, Gubler HU, Staehelin H (1976) Biological effects of cyclosporin A: a new antilymphocytic agent. Agents Actions 6:468

Borel JF, Feurer C, Magnee C, Staehelin H (1977) Effects of the new antilymphocytic peptide cyclosporin A in animals. Immunology 32:1017

Brunner KT, Mauel J, Cerottini JC, Chapuis B (1968) Quantitative assay of the lytic action of immune lymphoid cells on ^{51}Cr-labelled allogeneic target cells in vitro; inhibition by isoantibody and by drugs. Immunology 14:181

Dietrich FM, Hess R (1970) Hypersensitivity in mice. I. Induction of contact sensitivity to oxazolone and inhibition by various chemical compounds. Int Arch Allergy 38:246

Drachman DB, Adams RN, McIntosh K, Pestronk A (1985) Treatment of experimental myasthenia gravis with cyclosporin A. Clin Immunol Immunopathol 34:174

Dreyfuss M, Haerri E, Hofmann H, Kobel H, Pache W, Tscherter H (1976) Cyclosporin A and C. New metabolites from *Trichoderma polysporum* (link ex Pers.) Rifai. Eur J Appl Microbiol 3:125

Ford WL, Burr W, Simonsen M (1970) A lymph node weight assay for the graft-versus-host activity of rat lymphoid cells. Transplantation 10:258

Fulpius BW, Bersinger NA, James RW, Schwendimann B (1981) Isolation and purification of the nicotinic acetylcholine receptor from *Torpedo* electric organ. In: Azzi A, Brodbeck U, Zahler P (eds) Membrane proteins. Springer, Berlin Heidelberg New York, p 70

Greaves M, Janossy G (1972) Elicitation of selective T and B lymphocyte responses by cell surface binding ligands. Transplant Rev 11:87

Gunn HC (1985) Successful treatment of autoimmunity in (NZB/NZW)F1 mice with cyclosporine and (Nva^2)-cyclosporin. I. Reduction of autoantibodies. Clin Exp Immunol 64:225

Gunn HC, Ryffel B (1985) Successful treatment of autoimmunity in (NZB/NZW)F1 mice with cyclosporin and (Nva^2)-cyclosporine. II. Reduction of kidney pathology. Clin Exp Immunol 64:234

Hassman RA, Dieguez C, Rennie P, Weetman AP, Hall R, McGregor AM (1985) The influence of cyclosporin A on the induction of experimental autoimmune thyroid disease in the PVG/c rat. Clin Exp Immunol 59:10

Hiestand PC, Gunn HC, Gale JM, Ryffel B, Borel JF (1985a) Comparison of the pharmacological profiles of cyclosporine, (Nva^2)-cyclosporine and (Val^2)dihydrocyclosporine. Immunology 55:249

Hiestand PC, Gunn H, Gale J, Siegl H, Ryffel B, Donatsch P, Borel JF (1985b) The immunosuppressive profile of a new natural cyclosporine analogue: Nva^2-cyclosporine. Transplant Proc 17:1362

Israel-Biet D, Noel LH, Bach M-A, Dardenne M, Bach JF (1983) Marked reduction of DNA antibody production and glomerulopathy in thymulin (FTS-Zn) or cyclosporin A treated (NZB × NZW)F1 mice. Clin Exp Immunol 54:359

Janossy G, Greaves MF (1971) Lymphocyte activation. I. Response of T and B lymphocytes to phytomitogens. Clin Exp Immunol 9:483

Janossy G, Greaves MF, Doenhoff MJ, Snajdr S (1973) Lymphocyte activation. V. Quantitation of the proliferative responses to mitogens using defined T and B cell population. Clin Exp Immunol 14:581

Jerne NK, Nordin AA (1963) Plaque formation in agar by single antibody-producing cells. Science 140:405

Jerne NK, Nordin AA, Henry C (1963) The agar plaque technique for recognizing antibody-producing cells. In: Amos B, Koprowski H (eds) Cell bound antibodies. Wistar Institute, Philadelphia, pp 109

Jones MG, Harris G (1985) Prolongation of life in female NZB/NZW (f1) hybrid mice by cyclosporin A. Clin Exp Immunol 59:1

Kroenke M, Leonard WJ, Depper JM, Arya SK, Wong-Staal F, Gallo RC, Waldmann TA, Greene WC (1984) Cyclosporin A inhibits T-cell growth factor gene expression at the level of mRNA transcription. Proc Natl Acad Sci USA 81:5214

Lennon VA, Lindstrom JM, Seybold ME (1975) Experimental autoimmune myasthenia: a model of myasthenia gravis in rats and guinea pigs. J Exp Med 141:1365

Meo T (1979) The MLR in the mouse. In: Lefkovits J, Pernis B (eds) Immunological Methods. Academic NY, p 227

Mishell RI, Dutton RW (1966) Immunization of normal mouse spleen cell suspensions in vitro. Science 153:1004

Mishell RL, Dutton RW (1967) Immunization of dissociated spleen cell cultures from normal mice. J Exp Med 126:423

Mosmann T (1983) Rapid colorimetric assay for cellular growth and survival: application to proliferation and cytotoxicity assays. J Immunol Methods 65:55

Nussenblatt RB, Rodrigues MM, Wacker WB, Cevario SJ, Salinas-Carmona MC, Gery I (1981) Cyclosporin A. Inhibiton of experimental autoimmune uveitis in Lewis rats. J Clin Invest 67:1228

Ruegger A, Kuhn M, Lichti H, Loosli HR, Huguenin R, Quiquerez C, Von Wartburg A (1976) Cyclosporin A, ein immunosuppressiv wirksamer Pilzmetabolit aus *Trichoderma polysporum* (LINK ex PERS.) Rifai. Helv Chim Acta 59:1075

Schwartz A, L'age Stehr J, Offermann G (1986) The transfer of LAV/HTLV III infection by renal transplantation. Clinical course in four cases. Klin Wochenschr 64:200

Shevach EM (1985) The effects of cyclosporin A on the immune system. Ann Rev Immunol 3:397

Staehelin H (1962) A simple quantitative test for cytostatic agents using nonadhering cells in vitro. Med Exp 7:92

Stiller CR, Laupacis PA, Keown PA, Gardell C, Dupre J, Thibert P, Wall W (1983) Cyclosporine. Action, pharmacokinetics, and effect in the BB rat model. Metabolism 32:69

Traber R, Kuhn M, Loosli HR, Pache W, Von Wartburg A (1977a) Neue Cyclopeptide aus *Trichoderma polysporum* (LINK ex PERS)RIFAI: die Cyclosporine B, D and E. Helv Chim Acta 60:1568

Traber R, Kuhn M, Ruegger A, Lichti H, Loosli HR, Von Wartburg A (1977 b) Die Struktur von Cyclosporin C. Helv Chim Acta 60:1247

Vladutiu AO (1983) Effect of cyclosporine on experimental autoimmune thyroiditis in mice. Transplantation 35:518

Von Wartburg A, Traber R (1986) Chemistry of the natural cyclosporin metabolites. Prog Allergy 38:28

Wiesinger D, Borel JF (1979) Studies on the mechanism of action of cyclosporin A. Immunobiology 156:454

CHAPTER 22

Muramyl Dipeptides

M. PARANT and L. CHEDID

A. Introduction

Synthetic muramyl dipeptide or MDP (AcMur-L-Ala-D-iGln) is able to replace killed mycobacteria in complete Freund's adjuvant (CFA) for the induction of both humoral and cellular immunity (ELLOUZ et al. 1974). The structural requirements for the adjuvant activity were investigated by comparing a large series of analogs, and found to be rather narrow. Initially, the adjuvant effect of MDP was demonstrated in a water-in-oil emulsion. However, its clinical use became a reasonable goal when it was shown to possess immunoadjuvant properties, even when administered in saline (CHEDID et al. 1976; AUDIBERT et al. 1976), and when synthetic analogs lacking untoward effects were prepared (CHEDID et al. 1982; ALLISON et al. 1986). Some of the steps in the research into the biologic adjuvant effects of MDPs have been reported in reviews articles (ADAM 1985; AUDIBERT et al. 1985; TAKADA and KOTANI 1985).

Hydrophilic muramyl peptides that display an adjuvant effect in vivo and in vitro when used in saline solution represent valuable tools to analyze the detailed cellular mechanisms underlying the enhancement of immune responses. In addition, MDP and many of its derivatives are nonimmunogenic when given alone or in CFA, in contrast to more complex adjuvants of bacterial origin, e.g., *Bordetella pertussis*, BCG, peptidoglycan, or lipopolysaccharide (LPS). Antibodies to MDP can only be elicited by immunization with MDP covalently linked to particular carriers (REICHERT et al. 1980), allowing the production of hybridomas, secreting antibodies that bind to MDP determinants (BAHR et al. 1983).

An immunoadjuvant may interact with the host immune system by increasing the number of cells participating in the response and/or by improving the function of individual cells. The cells on which MDPs act have not been unequivocally identified. There are only a few studies concerned with direct measurements of the in vivo effects of MDP on changes in compartments of the immune system, and on subsequent function in vitro. To define the possible mode of action of MDPs, many investigations have been conducted in various tissue culture systems, in the presence or in the absence of additional immunogenic determinants. The purpose of this chapter is to describe the influence of MDPs on host responses in which most of the relationships between lymphocytes and accessory cells are known (ALLISON 1984). Direct or indirect effects of MDPs on lymphocyte cultures will then be examined in an attempt to establish a clear correlation between in vivo and in vitro responses.

B. In Vivo Quantitative and Qualitative Changes in Specific Immune Responses Produced by MDPs

The initial effect of MDPs seems to be, in most cases, on nonimmunocompetent cells. In the literature, numerous data have been reported on macrophage activation by MDPs (for review see Leclerc and Chedid 1983). Since antibdoy is produced by cells of the B lymphocyte lineage, accessory cells could interact with B cells or could augment the helper effect of T lymphocytes (Allison 1984).

I. Characteristics of Antibody Responses After MDP Treatment

MDPs have been shown to enhance humoral immunity to a variety of natural and synthetic vaccines (Audibert et al. 1985), and also to numerous laboratory antigens (for review see Adam 1985). Immune responses to thymus-dependent antigens are increased to a much greater extent than those to thymus-independent antigens, indicating the importance of T lymphocytes (see Chap. 1).

Both humoral and cellular immunity are increased by MDPs in IFA (incomplete Freund's adjuvant). However, the potentiation of antibody synthesis does not depend on the use of a lipid vehicle. Hydrophilic MDPs may specifically stimulate humoral immunity when administered in saline simultaneously with an antigen, even when given by separate routes (Chedid et al. 1976; Audibert et al. 1976).

Modifications induced by MDP in the class of antibody to a given antigen have been minimally evaluated. The available data indicate that muramyl peptides possess the capacity to influence isotype selection by B lymphocytes. In guinea pigs that receive either MDP in IFA or CFA with ovalbumin (Ova), IgG2 antibody levels are increased (Kotani et al. 1975). After immunization, either in saline or in water-in-oil emulsion, specific antibodies obtained in mice against bovine serum albumin (BSA) or against dinitrophenyl (DNP)-Ova are predominantly of the IgG1 isotype (Leclerc et al. 1978; Heymer et al. 1978), although MDP can increase the anti-BSA response within all isotypes (Strauch and Wood 1982). A predominance of the IgG1 response was also observed in mice immunized against DNP-poly (Glu-Ala-Tyr) (DNP-GAT) or DNP-Ova (Löwy et al. 1980), and a significant increase in both IgM and IgG anti-hapten plaque-forming cells after immunization with trinitrophenyl (TNP)-Ova and MDP (Sugimoto et al. 1978). IgE antibodies against Ova were obtained in mice given large doses of both MDP and antigen by the intraperitoneal route (Ohkuni et al. 1979), whereas an MDP conjugated to the same antigen could inhibit the induction of IgE responses (Kishimoto et al. 1979). In saliva and in serum, IgA immune responses were elicited in rats or rabbits after immunization by the oral route or through the respiratory system (Morisaki et al. 1983; Taubman et al. 1983; Butler et al. 1983). It is obvious that the nature of the antigen may also influence isotypes of the antibody response.

Mice were used to evaluate the genetic influence on the adjuvant effect of MDP since several immunomodulators (BCG, LPS) are known to be under genetic control. Differences in responsiveness to the adjuvant effect have been noted, whereas nonspecific stimulation of resistance to infections did not show similar strain variations (PARANT 1979). The adjuvant effect of MDP was comparatively determined on the immune response of mice to BSA, bacterial α-amylase, and GAT. An analysis of inbred and congeneic strains has indicated that responses to MDP are influenced by at least two genes. Strong responses to MDP were obtained only in strains that carried neither the H-2^b locus nor the C57B1 background. Because of the various levels of possible adjuvant action in hosts, it is not surprising to find multigenic control in their responses (STARUCH and WOOD 1982).

II. T Cell-Mediated Responses

The induction of cell-mediated reactions by MDPs critically depends on the immunization scheme and on the vehicle in which antigen and adjuvant are injected. MDP can augment T cell-mediated immunity, provided that it is either used together with antigens that do not induce humoral antibody formation (GISLER et al. 1979) or administered in suitable vehicles, water-in-oil emulsions, liposomes, or polymers (for review see ALLISON 1984). Substitution with appropriate side chains, which may also alter MDP localization in strategic tissue compartments, provides another means of inducing T cell-mediated responses (YAMAMURA et al. 1976; PARANT et al. 1980). Induction of delayed-type hypersensitivity (DTH), autoimmune diseases, and generation of cytotoxic T cells have been used in these studies. However, most, if not all, cell-mediated systems are macrophage dependent, and the role of macrophage activation cannot always be determined.

Transfer experiments of syngeneic thymocytes and bone marrow cells into irradiated recipients have shown that exposure of T-derived lymphocytes to MDP is essential for the manifestation of its effect on the response to SRBC (LÖWY et al. 1977). Clearly, stimulation of the helper T cell function was demonstrated in mice immunized with hapten-carrier conjugates. MDP was given in saline 1 h before TNP-Ova or TNP-keyhole limpet hemocyanin (KLH) and the increased anti-hapten response was linked to the generation of helper cells directed to the carrier portion (SUGIMOTO et al. 1978; LÖWY et al. 1980). These results confirm the previous observation on the T cell dependency of the adjuvant effect of MDP on anti-sheep red blood cell (SRBC) responses, although in some cases an additional proliferation of pluripotential B cell precursors brought about by MDP was suggested (PRUNET et al. 1978).

In vivo, the local proliferative T cell response in a graft-versus-host-reaction was significantly enhanced by MDP (MATTER 1979). The generation of cytotoxic T cells has been extensively studied after administration of hydrophilic and lipophilic MDP derivatives. Thus, MDP increases the lytic activity of peritoneal cells in mice immunized with P-815 cells, but the enhanced T cell activity does not confer protection for nonimmunocompetent hosts (MATTER 1979). Moreover, the highly lipophilic 6-O-mycoloyl-MDP markedly stimulates the cytotoxic response to allogeneic tumor cells in mice (YAMAMURA et al. 1976), and can suppress fibrosarcoma growth in syngeneic mice when inoculated in small droplets with tumor cells (AZUMA et al. 1978). In mice immunized with syngeneic methylcholanthrene tumors coupled covalently with a spacer and MDP, the antitumor cytotoxicity is T cell-mediated and non-H-2 restricted (EGGERS and TARMIN 1984).

The cross-reactivity between an MDP derivative and BCG was used to increase tumor-specific immunity. In BCG-primed mice, haptenic compound enhanced helper T cell activity, specific T cell proliferative responses, and DTH reactions. When such mice were immunized with syngeneic tumor cells modified by binding with the cross-reactive MDP derivative, a specific protective immunity was generated as well as in vitro cytotoxic T cell responses (Hamaoka et al. 1985).

III. Immunosuppression

The stimulatory effect of MDP can be inhibited by a single injection of the same compound before adjuvant-promoted immunization, and this effect is adjuvant type specific (Gisler et al. 1979). Pretreatment of mice with high doses of MDP suppresses the SRBC-specific antibody response, and this effect is dependent on the route of antigen administration (Leclerc et al. 1979a; Souvannavong and Adam 1980). The inhibition thus induced by MDP is mediated by suppressor T cells and by an inhibition of interleukin 2 (IL-2) production (Leclerc and Chedid 1983). Antigen-specific suppression with a purified fragment of BSA can be strongly enhance by MDP. Results of cell transfer imply that specific suppressor T cells are generated by this treatment, but do not rule out the possible role of splenic suppressor/inducer B lymphocytes (Ferguson et al. 1983). A selective suppression of the IgE response has been reported after preadministration of antigen-conjugated MDP. These conjugates abrogate the IgE antibody responses to the relevant allergens by activating IgE class-specific suppressor T cells without affecting the IgG response (Kishimoto et al. 1979).

DTH reactions to BCG and to *Listeria* cell walls are suppressed by pretreatment with MDP in an oily emulsion. In this system, MDP-induced nonspecific T suppressor cells inhibit the ability of DTH effector T cells to elicit DTH reactions (Kato et al. 1984). In this study, it seems that the generation of splenic suppressor T-cells requires an intravenous injection of MDP in the emulsion, whereas by another route or in saline MDP was inactive 2 weeks later. According to other reports concerned with the suppression of antibody formation, MDP can be administered in saline a few days before the antigen, and the inhibitory effect is transient (Leclerc et al. 1979a; Brumer and Stevens 1985).

C. In Vivo Changes in Cell Compartments of the Immune System Following MDP Administration

The studies that were performed to evaluate the influence of MDP on lymphoid organs were conducted in animals given the glycopeptide alone, and may therefore be different from responses occurring after immunization. LPS which is often used with MDP in comparative assays is a potent immunogen, and differences in the properties may reflect their distinct capacity for eliciting a specific immune response by themselves rather than differences in adjuvant effect.

The retention of circulating lymphocytes in the draining lymph node, known as lymphocyte trapping, has been proposed as an important mechanism for the adjuvant effect. Following subcutaneous inoculation of MDP in a water-in-oil emulsion, a dose-related increase in lymphocyte traffic into the rat regional lymph node and early changes in blood flow were found and were similar to those produced by CFA injection (ANDERSON 1985).

Intraperitoneal treatment of mice with MDP in saline, without addition of antigen, induces lymph node hyperplasia (BRUMER and STEVENS 1981), whereas no change is shown in spleen and liver weight (TANAKA et al. 1977; BRUMER and STEVENS 1981). The lymph node hyperplasia is associated with a hyperresponsiveness of cells to T mitogens. On the other hand, a transient depression in the response of spleen cells to T and B cell mitogens is simultaneously observed, and the data suggest that splenic suppressor T cells may be responsible. The deficient production of IL-2 is also consistent with reports indicating that large doses of MDP may induce immunosuppression (BRUMER and STEVENS 1981, 1985).

After a single injection of a large dose of MDP to mice, WUEST and WACHSMUTH (1982) found that the relative leukopenia occurring within 8 h was due to low lymphocyte counts. With daily injections, low doses of MDP provoked lymphocytosis, whereas larges doses still resulted in leukopenia. In the same study, it was also reported that three daily injections of MDP induce an increase in the number of macrophage progenitor cells in the marrow.

Adjuvant MDPs stimulate the phagocytic activity of the reticuloendothelial system (RES) when injected in saline, with or without addition of a protein antigen (TANAKA et al. 1977). However, effective doses are higher than those inducing an adjuvant effect, and MDP which is an active adjuvant in guinea pigs does not stimulate RES function in these animals (TANAKA et al. 1977; WATERS and FERRARESI 1980).

Surprisingly, it has been reported that the expression of peritoneal macrophage Ia was unaffected by MDP administration, in contrast to the effect of LPS. Furthermore, MDP did not enhance or depress the induction of Ia-positive macrophages by T cell stimuli (BEHBEHANI et al. 1985). Other accessory cell populations deserve to be examined in this respect.

NK (natural killer) cell activity may be enhanced in the spleen of mice several days after MDP administration, but is not correlated with the stimulation of peritoneal cells (SHARMA et al. 1981). After an intravenous injection of a lipophilic MDP derivative N-acetylmuramyl-L-alanyl-D-isoglutaminyl-L-alanylphosphatidylethanolamine (MTP-PE) incorporated into liposomes, an enhancement of NK cell activity was found in the lung and the liver, but not in the spleen. The results indicate a potential role of interstitial NK activity in the increased host resistance to the formation of experimental metastases (TALMADGE et al. 1985). These data also emphasize the need to consider the effect of immunomodulators on organ-associated NK cell activity.

D. Role of Lymphocyte Populations in Antibody Responses of Cell Cultures Stimulated with MDPs

In vitro methods for immunizing lymphocytes are well established and may provide information as to whether or not an immunoadjuvant has a direct action on lymphoid cells. The central problem is first to determine the formation of helper T cells since, for most antigens, the inductive process requires the interaction of antigen and T cells with B cell precursors, and second to evaluate the importance of accessory cells.

In vitro MDP has been shown to potentiate the immune responses of normal mouse spleen cells to SRBC (Specter et al. 1977) and to a T-independent antigen TNP-PAA (trinitrophenyl polyacrylamide) (Leclerc et al. 1979b). The ability of MDPs to allow for a plaque response against SRBC in cultures of spleen cells from T cell-deficient nude mice was investigated since polyclonal B cell activators such as LPS have been found to replace T cells in the induction of immune responses. MDP can stimulate primary immune responses to SRBC in spleen cell cultures from nude mice (Watson and Whitlock 1978; Leclerc et al. 1979b; Février et al. 1979). There are several possible ways of exerting a T cell-replacing activity. Depending on the experimental system, the authors found some differences in the mode of action. The results suggest that MDP either functions as a polyclonal stimulator, like LPS (Specter et al. 1978), and induces the maturation of T cell precursors to helper T cells (Février et al. 1979), or interacts directly with B cells to mimic the helper T signal (Watson and Whitlock 1978).

A stimulation of accessory cells cannot be excluded in all these experiments (Watson and Whitlock 1978). However, in assays conducted with various populations of mouse spleen cells, Sugimura et al. (1979) have demonstrated that MDP can increase the PFC (plaque-forming cell) reponse if added after antigenic stimulation, i.e., after antigen presentation by macrophages. The results indicate that MDP interacts with T and B lymphocytes, and that it does not replace the T cell function. Further studies have provided indications of a proliferation in pluripotential B cell precursors (Prunet et al. 1978), or a stimulating effect of MDP on a late stage of the differentiation of B cells into antibody-producing cells (Souvannavong and Adam 1984). The role of a cooperating cell population and of soluble factors released from a few cells could be reevaluated, particularly with mediators obtained by recombinant DNA technology.

Peyer's patch cell preparations from various mouse strains contain approximately equal number of T and B cells, but less than 1% macrophages. MDP was shown to promote higher responses to SRBC in such cell cultures. After addition of splenic macrophages from a responsive strain, MDP promoted good immune responses in C3H/HeJ cell preparations which are not reactive to MDP. Therefore, whereas in this model Con A (concanavalin A) enhances T helper cell activity, MDP and also LPS require the presence of responsive macrophages for augmentation of immune responses (Kiyono et al. 1982).

The generation of cytotoxic T cells has been measured in vitro in the presence of MDPs. Enhanced cytotoxic responses were obtained in an allogeneic system at optimal or suboptimal antigen concentrations (Azuma et al. 1976; Matter 1979), and also in a syngeneic system (Igarashi et al. 1977). With higher doses of antigen, MDP significantly reduces cytotoxic responses. It has been suggested that activation of macrophages by MDP may elicit both amplifying and suppressive responses (Matter 1979). Pretreatment of mice with MDP also inhibits the in vitro generation of cytotoxic T lymphocytes (Leclerc et al. 1979a).

E. In Vitro Direct Responses of Lymphocytes to MDP in the Absence of Antigenic Stimulation

I. Mitogenic Effect of MDPs

For some time, the B cell mitogenicity of MDP had been controversial (AZUMA et al. 1976; SPECTER et al. 1977). As compared with LPS, the stimulation induced by MDP is weak, and requires more sensitive culture conditions to be demonstrated. Nevertheless, the mitogenic response to MDP is consistent. Thymidine incorporation and blast cell formation are increased in spleen cells from normal or nude mice incubated with MDP (DAMAIS et al. 1977; TAKADA et al. 1979b; WATSON and WHITLOCK 1978; GISLER et al. 1979). In contrast, MDP fails to trigger the division of T cells by itself, as shown with cortisone-resistant thymus cells (GISLER et al. 1979). T cells contribute minimally, if at all, to the DNA synthesis in murine B cells. However, MDP-induced mitogenic responses require prolonged incubation. A component of the cell culture other than the number of dividing B cells limits the magnitude of the response. This is likely to be the macrophages (WOOD and STARUCH 1981). When estimated by clonal expansion analysis with limiting dilution (see Chap. 12), synthetic MDP and some derivatives do not directly stimulate splenic or bone marrow B cells, in contrast to lipid A, confirming the participation of other cell populations in the effect of MDP on B cells (SAIKO-TAKI et al. 1985).

There are considerable differences in the susceptibility of spleen cells from various mouse strains to the mitogenic effect of MDP (DAMAIS et al. 1978). A comparative study in hybrids and backcross progeny has shown that the mitogenic effects of MDP and LPS are linked to different genes. There was apparently no genetic correlation between the in vitro adjuvant and mitogenic effects of MDP. Thus, C3H/He strains, which respond poorly to MDP as a mitogen, respond well to it as an adjuvant (CHEDID et al. 1976; DAMAIS et al. 1978; WOOD and STARUCH 1981). Nevertheless, by testing several MDP analogs in a high responder strain, a correlation between the structural requirements for adjuvant activity and mitogenicity has been tentatively established (DAMAIS et al. 1978).

II. Polyclonal Activation

Polyclonal B cell activation is usually related to a mitogenic stimulus. A marked increase in the number of antibody-forming cells to SRBC has been reported in cultures incubated with MDP in the absence of antigen (SPECTER et al. 1977). A similar increase in background responses to a T-dependent and a T-independent antigen has been obtained in cell cultures from nude mice (LECLERC et al. 1979b; SAIKO-TAKI et al. 1980). These observations are compatible with the notion that MDP acts as a polyclonal activator, but alternatively it might reflect an MDP-induced potentiation of responsiveness to culture constituents such as fetal calf serum known to cross-react with SRBC (GISLER et al. 1979). Further, TPA (12-O-tetradecanoylphorbol 13-acetate) was shown to inhibit the MDP-induced polyclonal response of cultured murine spleen cells, whereas it enhanced MDP mitogenicity, indicating a dissociation between proliferative and polyclonal re-

sponses to MDP as well as to LPS. The dual effects may result from the stimulation by TPA of accessory cells, and thereafter the activation of suppressor cells
(Ferguson et al. 1982). In another model with only a few B cells maintained in
the culture, MDP and its derivatives were unable to stimulate clonal expansion,
indicating that immunologic activities of MDPs may be mediated by the activated
T cells and/or macrophages via cell-cell interaction or soluble factors (Saiko-Taki
et al. 1985). In human peripheral blood mononuclear cell cultures, MDP and
some adjuvant-active analogs failed to induce in vitro proliferation and/or polyclonal activation. However, MDPs enhanced pokeweed mitogen-induced immunoglobulin synthesis, at least in terms of IgA and IgM levels, while no enhancement of IgG was seen (Bahr et al. 1984).

III. Influence of MDPs on Mitogenic Responses

MDP and hydrophilic analogs do not possess direct mitogenic activity on T lymphocytes (Gisler et al. 1979; Hadden et al. 1979). The addition of MDP to peripheral blood cells has been reported to have enhancing and suppressive effects
on the Con A response, depending on the donor and on the dose of mitogen.
Again, this effect could be operating through positive and negative regulation by
monocytes (Bahr et al. 1984).

In mouse mixed lymphocyte cultures, a potentiation of T cell proliferation is
induced by MDP. The enhancement of thymidine uptake was seen with suboptimal doses of irradiated histoincompatible lymphocytes (Gisler et al. 1979;
Matter 1979). A lack of effect has been reported with human cells in two-way
mixed lymphocyte cultures incubated with MDP (Bahr et al. 1984).

IV. Effect of MDP on Thymoma Cell Lines

Thymoma cell lines (see Chap. 12) represent a good opportunity for determining
the effect of MDPs on cellular models of the T lymphocyte system. The growth
of murine cell lines is not modified by MDP unless macrophages are present in
the culture. A macrophage-mediated inhibition is induced by MDP on the growth
of cell lines possessing phenotypic markers characteristic of T helper (Lyt-1^+2^+),
T cytotoxic/suppressor (Lyt-1^-2^+), and T precursor lymphocytes (Lyt-1^+2^+). In
the case of thymomas having the Lyt-1^-2^+ phenotype, the inhibition is prostaglandin synthetase dependent (Phillips et al. 1984).

V. In Vitro NK Cell Induction

Administration of MDP to CBA/J mice induces an enhancement of the splenic
NK activity. In the same study, mouse spleen cells were incubated for 18 h with
various doses of MDP. NK cell activity against YAC-1 target cells was significantly increased at higher effector: target cell ratios (Sharma et al. 1981). Liposomes incorporating the lipophilic MTP-PE increase NK cell activity in the lung
and the liver, but not in the spleen. In vitro these liposomes do not augment
splenic NK cell activity, although they strongly increase the tumoricidal effect of
macrophages (Talmadge et al. 1985).

F. In Vitro Indirect Responses of Lymphocytes to MDPs

Many data suggest that the regulation of the numbers and the activity of macrophages play a major role in the stimulation of immune responses by MDPs (for review see LECLERC and CHEDID 1982; ALLISON 1984; TAKADA and KOTANI 1985). Moreover, evidence has accumulated suggesting that the principal mediator released by adjuvants is interleukin-1 (IL-1) (STARUCH and WOOD 1983; ALLISON 1984). It is accepted that the accessory cell function of macrophages, or other cells, not only involves the presentation of antigen in the context of the Ia glycoproteins, but also the release of IL-1 or the expression of membrane IL-1 (OPPENHEIM et al. 1986; KURT-JONES et al. 1985; Chap. 7). A prominent role of IL-1 is apparent in regulation of the growth of mature T cells activated by lectins and antigens, which proliferate and then produce IL-2. IL-1 can also act directly on a subpopulation of activated B cells to stimulate proliferation and differentiation to immune globulin secretion, a synergistic effect being observed with T cell-derived lymphokines (ALLISON 1985; OPPENHEIM et al. 1986).

The production of IL-1 (originally described as lymphocyte-activating factor or LAF) by human mononuclear cells incubated with MDP was first reported by OPPENHEIM et al. (1980). In the same study, cell line macrophages, which are completely devoid of lymphocytes, could be stimulated by MDP to produce LAF after prolonged incubation. It has repeatedly been demonstrated in other assays that macrophages can be activated by MDP without the aid of lymphocytes (PABST and JOHNSTON 1980; NAGAO et al. 1981). Peritoneal macrophages from mice (OPPENHEIM et al. 1980), guinea pigs (IRIBE et al. 1982), or rabbits (DAMAIS et al. 1982) incubated with MDP also produced IL-1. The first observation leading anyone to question whether IL-1 might be a family of molecules was made during the course of investigations with MDP derivatives. Incubation of human monocytes or rabbit macrophages with MDP produces supernatant fluids containing both LAF and EP (endogenous pyrogen) activities among other monokines such as CSF (colony-stimulating factor), D factor, and TNF (tumor necrosis factor). In contrast, cells incubated with a nonpyrogenic adjuvant analog such as murabutide (DAMAIS et al. 1982) or MDP(threonyl) (ALLISON 1985) did not release EP by producing comparable levels of LAF. There are already indications that IL-1-α and IL-1-β, now obtained by DNA transfer technology, differ in at least some important biologic activities (ALLISON 1985; Chap. 7).

MDP-induced IL-1 production by mouse macrophages was also found to be under genetic control (ABEHSIRA-AMAR et al. 1985) as has already been shown for B cell mitogenic responses (DAMAIS et al. 1978). It has been reported, for example, that resident or elicited peritoneal macrophages from C3H/HeJ mice were not stimulated by MDP to produce IL-1 although these mice are known to respond to the adjuvant effect of MDP (CHEDID et al. 1976; STARUCH and WOOD 1983). The results indicate that this mouse strain is very susceptible to the adjuvant effect of IL-1, and that smaller amounts can be sufficient (STARUCH and WOOD 1982). This work, demonstrating the in vivo adjuvant effect of IL-1, has strengthened the hypothesis proposed by ALLISON and colleagues in 1970 that macrophages are the primary cell targets for adjuvants (ALLISON 1984). The role of IL-1 in the stimulation of immune responses is likely to be established by the use of various forms of IL-1 now produced by recombinant DNA technology.

G. Conclusions

Nonimmunogenic hydrophilic MDPs have been used for analyzing immunoregulatory mechanisms in various cell culture systems. Studies have confirmed that interaction between macrophages and lymphocytes is involved in the activation of helper T cells and/or B cells by the adjuvant glycopeptides. Moreover, most of the results indicate that the primary target cells for MDP action are accessory cells which release IL-1 on stimulation. This is likely to be a common mechanism by which adjuvants exert their effects, although other mediators may also be elicited. Some of the undesirable side effects that are induced by MDPs may be related to macrophage activation. However, nontoxic MDPs such as murabutide or MDP (threonyl) are still able to induce IL-1 release, thus indicating a selective stimulation of macrophages. Although in vivo more than 90% of parenterally administered MDP is cleared from the body within 2 h (Parant 1979), the correlation of in vivo and in vitro models appears to be excellent in many cases.

In the future, adjuvant formulation or manipulation of synthetic compounds should allow one to select the desired properties. Studies are being pursued to determine the effects on lymphocytes of lipophilic MDPs and of polymerized or conjugated derivatives. After incorporation into a synthetic vaccine (Audibert et al. 1985), the effects of an MDP analog on cells are likely to be altered.

References

Abehsira-Amar O, Damais C, Parant M, Chedid L (1985) Strain dependence of muramyl dipeptide-induced LAF (IL-1) release by murine-adherent peritoneal cells. J Immunol 134:365–368

Adam A (1985) Synthetic adjuvants. Wiley, New York

Allison AC (1984) Immunological adjuvants and their mode of action. In: Bell R, Torrigiani G (eds) New approaches to vaccine development. Schwabe, Basel, p 133

Allison AC (1985) The interleukin-1 family of molecules. Bioessays 3:260–263

Allison AC, Byars NE, Waters RV (1986) Immunologic adjuvants: efficacy and safety considerations. In: Nerbig RM, Gough PM, Kaeberle ML, Whetstone CA (eds) Advances in carriers and adjuvants for veterinary biologics. The Iowa State University Press, Ames, p 91

Anderson AO (1985) Multiple effects of immunological adjuvants on lymphatic microenvironments. I. Role of immunologically-relevant angiogenesis in the mechanisms of action of CFA, MDP and avridine. Int J Immunother 1:185–195

Audibert F, Chedid L, Lefrancier P, Choay J (1976) Distinctive adjuvanticity of synthetic analogs of mycobacterial water-soluble components. Cell Immunol 21:243–249

Audibert F, Leclerc C, Chedid L (1985) Muramyl peptides as immunopharmacological responses modifiers. In: Torrence PF (ed) Biological response modifiers. Academic, New York, p 307

Azuma I, Sugimura K, Taniyama T, Yamawaki M, Yamamura Y, Kusumoto S, Okada S, Shiba T (1976) Adjuvant activity of mycobacterial fractions: immunological properties of synthetic N-acetylmuramyl dipeptide and related compounds. Infect Immun 14:18–27

Azuma I, Sugimura K, Yamawaki M, Uemiya M, Kusumoto S, Okada S, Shiba T, Yamamura Y (1978) Adjuvant activity of synthetic 6-O-"mycoloyl"-N-acetylmuramyl-L-alanyl-D-isoglutamine and related compounds. Infect Immun 20:600–607

Bahr GM, Eshhar Z, Ben-Yitzhak R, Modabber FZ, Arnon R, Sela M, Chedid L (1983) Monoclonal antibodies to the synthetic adjuvant muramyl dipeptide: characterization of the specificity. Molec Immunol 20:745–752

Bahr GM, Modabber FZ, Morin A, Terrier M, Eyquem A, Chedid L (1984) Regulation by muramyl dipeptide (MDP) of the lymphoproliferative responses and polyclonal activation of human peripheral blood mononuclear cells. Clin Exp Immunol 57:178–186

Behbehani K, Beller DI, Unanue ER (1985) The effects of beryllium and other adjuvants on Ia expression by macrophages. J Immunol 134:2047–2049

Brumer E, Stevens DA (1981) Opposite modulation of lymph node cell and spleen cell responses to mitogens by muramyl dipeptide and its desmethyl analog. Cell Immunol 59:195–204

Brumer E, Stevens DA (1985) Mechanisms in opposite modulation of spleen cell and lymph node cells responses to mitogens following muramyl dipeptide treatment in vivo. Cell Immunol 91:505–514

Butler JE, Richerson HB, Swanson PA, Kopp WC, Suelzer MT (1983) The influence of muramyl dipeptide on the secretory immune response. In: McGhee JR, Mestecky J (eds) Secretory immune system. Ann Acad Sci 409:669–687

Chedid L, Audibert F, Lefrancier P, Choay J, Lederer E (1976) Modulation of the immune response by a synthetic adjuvant and analogs. Proc Natl Acad Sci USA 73:2472–2475

Chedid LA, Parant MA, Audibert FM, Riveau GJ, Parant FJ, Lederer E, Choay JP, Lefrancier PL (1982) Biological activity of a new synthetic muramyl peptide adjuvant devoid of pyrogenicity. Infect Immun 35:417–424

Damais C, Parant M, Chedid L (1977) Nonspecific activation of murine spleen cells in vitro by a synthetic immunoadjuvant (N-acetylmuramyl-L-analyl-D-isoglutamine). Cell Immunol 34:49–56

Damais C, Parant M, Chedid L, Lefrancier P, Choay J (1978) In vitro spleen cell responsiveness to various analogs of MDP (N-acetylmuramyl-L-alanyl-D-isoglutamine), a synthetic immunoadjuvant, in MDP high-responder mice. Cell Immunol 35:173–179

Damais C, Riveau G, Parant M, Gerota J, Chedid L (1982) Production of lymphocyte activating factor in the absence of endogenous pyrogen by rabbit or human leukocytes stimulated by a muramyl dipeptide derivative. Int J Immunopharmacol 4:451–462

Eggers AE, Tarmin L (1984) T-cell nature of adjuvant peptide-induced antitumor cell-mediated cytotoxicity. J Biol Response Mod 3:387–390

Ellouz F, Adam A, Ciorbaru R, Lederer E (1974) Minimal structural requirements for adjuvant activity of bacterial peptidoglycan derivatives. Biochem Biophys Res Commun 59:1317–1325

Ferguson TA, Fish LA, Baxter CS, Michael JG (1982) Concomitant enhancement of B-cell mitogenesis and inhibition of antibody synthesis by a phorbol ester (41481). Proc Soc Exp Biol Med 171:83–87

Ferguson TA, Krieger NJ, Pesce A, Michael JG (1983) Enhancement of antigen-specific suppression by muramyl dipeptide. Infect Immun 39:800–806

Février M, Duquenne C, Birrien JL, Liacooulos P (1979) Maturation of nu/nu mouse spleen pre-T cells induced in vitro by muramyl dipeptide. In: Kaplan JG (ed) Molecular basis of immune cell function. Elsevier, Amsterdam, p 499

Gisler RH, Dietrich FM, Baschang C, Brownbill A, Schumann G, Staber FG, Tarcsay L, Wachsmuth ED, Dukor P (1979) New developments in drugs enhancing the immune response: activation of lymphocytes and accessory cells by muramyl dipeptides. In: Turk JL, Parker D (eds) Drugs and immune responsiveness. McMillan, London, p 133

Hadden J, Englard A, Sadlik JR, Hadden EM (1979) The comparative effects of isoprinosine, levamisole, muramyl dipeptide and SM 1213 on lymphocyte and macrophage proliferation and activation in vitro. Int J Immunopharmacol 1:17–27

Hamaoka T, Takai Y, Kosugi A, Mizushima Y, Shima J, Kusama T, Fujiwara H (1985) The augmentation of tumor-specific immunity using haptenic muramyl dipeptide (MDP) derivatives. I. Synthesis of a novel haptenic MDP derivative cross-reactive with Bacillus Calmette-Guérin and its application to enhanced induction of tumor immunity. Cancer Immunol Immunother 20:183–188

Heymer B, Finger H, Wirsing CH (1978) Immunoadjuvant effects of the synthetic muramyl dipeptide (MDP) N-acetylmuramyl-Lalanyl-D-isoglutamine. Z Immunitätsforsch 155:87–92

Igarashi T, Okada M, Azuma I, Yamamura Y (1977) Adjuvant activity of synthetic N-ace-tylmuramyl-L-alanyl-D-isoglutamine and related compounds on cell-mediated cytotox-icity in syngeneic mice. Cell Immunol 34:270–278

Iribe H, Koga T, Onoue K, Kotani S, Kusumoto S, Shiba T (1982) Enhanced production of T-cell activating factors by macrophages exposed in vitro to MDP and its adjuvant-active analogs. In: Yamamura Y, Kotani S, Azuma I, Koda A, Shiba T (eds) Immu-nomodulation by microbial products and related synthetic compounds. Excerpta Medica, Amsterdam, p 213 (International congress series, vol 563)

Kato K, Yamamoto KI, Kimura T, Azuma I, Askenase PW (1984) Suppression of BCG cell wall induced delayed type hypersensitivity by pretreatment with killed BCG: induc-tion of nonspecific suppressor T-cells by the adjuvant portion (MDP) and of specific suppressor T-cells by the antigen portion (TAP). J Immunol 132:2790–2795

Kishimoto T, Hirai Y, Nakanishi K, Azuma I, Nagamatsu A, Yamamura Y (1979) Reg-ulation of antibody response in different immunoglobulin classes. VI. Selective sup-pression of IgE response by administration of antigen-conjugated muramyl peptides. J Immunol 123:2709–2715

Kiyono H, McGhee JR, Kearney JF, Michalek SM (1982) Enhancement of in vitro im-mune responses of murine Peyer's patch cultures by concanavalin A, muramyl dipep-tide and lipopolysaccharide. Scand J Immunol 15:329–339

Kotani S, Watanabe Y, Kinoshita F, Shimono T, Morisaki I, Shiba T, Kusumoto S, Tarumi Y, Ikenaka K (1975) Immunoadjuvant activities of synthetic N-acetylmuramyl peptides or -amino acids. Biken J 18:105–111

Kurt-Jones EA, Virgin HW, Unanue ER (1985) Relationship of macrophage Ia and mem-brane IL-1 expression to antigen presentation. J Immunol 135:3652–3654

Leclerc C, Chedid L (1982) Macrophage activation by synthetic muramyl peptides. In: Pick E (ed) Lymphokines, vol 7. Academic, New York, pp 1–21

Leclerc C, Chedid L (1983) Suppression of IL-2 production by muramyl dipeptide and de-rivatives. In: Oppenheim JJ, Cohen S (eds) Interleukins, lymphokines and cytokines. Academic, New York, p 699

Leclerc C, Audibert F, Chedid L (1978) Influence of a synthetic adjuvant (MDP) on qual-itative and quantitative changes of serum globulins. Immunology 35:963–970

Leclerc C, Juy D, Bourgeois E, Chedid L (1979a) In vivo regulation of humoral and cellular immune responses of mice by a synthetic adjuvant, N-acetylmuramyl-L-alanyl-D-iso-glutamine, muramyl dipeptide or MDP. Cell Immunol 45:199–206

Leclerc C, Bourgeois E, Chedid L (1979b) Enhancement by MDP of in vitro nude mice responses to a T-dependent antigen. Immunol Commun 8:55–64

Löwy I, Bona C, Chedid L (1977) Target cells for the activity of a synthetic adjuvant: mura-myl dipeptide. Cell Immunol 29:195–199

Löwy I, Leclerc C, Bourgeois E, Chedid L (1980) Inhibition of mitogen induced polyclonal activation by a synthetic adjuvant, muramyl dipeptide (MDP). J Immunol 124:320–325

Matter A (1979) The effects of muramyl dipeptide (MDP) in cell-mediated immunity. A comparison between in vitro and in vivo systems. Cancer Immunol Immunother 6:201–210

Morisaki I, Michalek SM, Harmon CC, Torii M, Hamada S, McGhee JR (1983) Effective immunity to dental caries: enhancement of salivary anti-*Streptococcus mutans* antibody responses with oral adjuvants. Infect Immun 40:577–591

Nagao S, Miki T, Tanaka A (1981) Macrophage activation by muramyl dipeptide (MDP) without lymphocyte participation. Microbiol Immunol 25:41–50

Ohkuni H, Norose Y, Ohta M, Hayama M, Kimura Y, Tsujimoto M, Kotani S, Shiba T, Kusumoto S, Yokogawa K, Kawata S (1979) Adjuvant activities in production of rea-ginic antibody by bacterial cell wall peptidoglycan or synthetic N-acetylmuramyl di-peptides in mice. Infect Immun 24:313–318

Oppenheim JJ, Togawa A, Chedid L, Mizel S (1980) Components of mycobacteria and muramyl dipeptide with adjuvant activity induce lymphocyte activating factor. Cell Immunol 50:71–81

Oppenheim JJ, Kovacs EJ, Matsushima K, Durum SK (1986) There is more than one in-terleukin-1. Immunol Today 7:45–56

Pabst MJ, Johnston RB (1980) Increased production of superoxide anion by macrophages exposed in vitro to muramyl dipeptide or lipopolysaccharide. J Exp Med 151:101–114

Parant M (1979) Biologic properties of a new synthetic adjuvant muramyl dipeptide (MDP). Springer Semin Immunopathol 2:101–118

Parant MA, Audibert FM, Chedid LA, Level MR, Lefrancier PL, Choay JP, Lederer E (1980) Immunostimulant activities of a lipophilic muramyl dipeptide derivative and of desmuramyl peptidolipid analogs. Infect Immun 27:825–831

Phillips NC, Bahr GM, Modabber RZ, Chedid L (1984) Modulation of the growth of murine thymoma cell lines having different Lyt-phenotypes by MDP and MDP(D-D): macrophage-mediated inhibition of in vitro cell growth. Int J Immunopharmacol 6:577–585

Prunet J, Birrien JL, Panijel J, Liacopoulos P (1978) On the mechanisms of early recovery of specifically depleted lymphoid cell populations by nonspecific activation of T-cells. Cell Immunol 37:151–161

Reichert C, Carelli C, Jolivet M, Audibert F, Lefrancier P, Chedid L (1980) Synthesis of conjugate containing N-acetylmuramyl-L-analyl-D-isoglutamine (MDP). Their use as hapten-carrier systems. Mol Immunol 17:357–363

Saito-Taki T, Tanabe MJ, Mochizuki H, Matsumoto T, Nakano M, Takada H, Tsujimoto M, Kotani S, Kusumoto S, Shiba T, Yokogawa K, Kawata S (1980) Polyclonal B-cell activation by cell wall preparations of gram-positive bacteria. Microbiol Immunol 24:209–218

Saito-Taki T, Nakano M, Kiso M, Hasegawa A (1985) Comparison of murine B-cell clonal expansions by synthetic lipid A and muramyl dipeptide analogs. Microbiol Immunol 29:1111–1120

Sharma SD, Tsai V, Krahenbuhl JL, Remington JS (1981) Augmentation of mouse natural killer cell activity by muramyl dipeptide and its analogs. Cell Immunol 62:101–109

Souvannavong V, Adam A (1980) Opposite effects of the synthetic adjuvant N-acetylmuramyl-L-alanyl-D-isoglutamine on the immune response in mice depending on experimental conditions. Eur J Immunol 10:654–656

Souvannavong V, Adam A (1984) Restoration and stimulation of the in vitro immune response of B-cells to sheep erythrocytes by interleukines and muramyl dipeptide (MDP). Biochem Biophys Res Commun 125:431–439

Specter S, Friedman H, Chedid L (1977) Dissociation between the adjuvant vs mitogenic activity of a synthetic muramyl dipeptide for murine splenocytes. Proc Soc Exp Biol Med 155:349–352

Specter S, Cimprich R, Friedman H, Chedid L (1978) Stimulation of enhanced in vitro immune response by the synthetic adjuvant, muramyl dipeptide. J Immunol 120:487–491

Staruch MJ, Wood DD (1982) Genetic influence on the adjuvanticity of muramyl dipeptide in vivo. J Immunol 128:155–181

Staruch MJ, Wood DD (1983) The adjuvanticity of interleukin-1 in vivo. J Immunol 130:2191–2194

Sugimoto M, Germain RN, Chedid L, Benacerraf B (1978) Enhancement of carrier-specific helper T-cell function by the synthetic adjuvant. N-acetylmuramyl-L-alanyl-D-isoglutamine (MDP). J Immunol 120:980–981

Sugimura K, Uemiya M, Saiki I, Azuma I, Yamamura Y (1979) The adjuvant activity of synthetic N-acetyl muramyl dipeptide: evidence of initial target cells for the adjuvant activity. Cell Immunol 43:137–149

Takada H, Kotani S (1985) Immunopharmacological activities of synthetic muramyl peptides. In: Stewart-Tull DES, Davies M (eds) Immunology of the bacterial cell envelope. Wiley, Chichester, p 119

Takada H, Tsujimoto M, Kato K, Kotani S, Kusumoto S, Inage M, Shiba T, Yano I, Kawata S, Yokogawa K (1979 a) Macrophage activation by bacterial cell walls and related synthetic compounds. Infect Immun 25:48–53

Takada H, Tsujimoto M, Kotani S, Kusumoto S, Inage M, Shiba T, Nagao S, Yano I, Kawata S, Yokogawa K (1979 b) Mitogenic effects of bacterial cell walls, their fragments, and related synthetic compounds on thymocytes and splenocytes of guinea pigs. Infect Immun 25:645–652

Talmadge JE, Schneider M, Collins M, Phillips H, Herberman RB, Wiltrout RH (1985) Augmentation of NK cell activity in tissue specific sites by liposomes incorporating MTP-PE. J Immunol 135:1477–1483

Tanaka A, Nagao S, Saito R, Kotani S, Kusumoto S, Shiba T (1977) Correlation of stereo-chemically specific structure in muramyl dipeptide between macrophage activation and adjuvant activity. Biochem Biophys Res Commun 77:621–627

Taubman MA, Ebersole JL, Smith DJ, Stack W (1983) Adjuvants for secretory immune responses. Ann NY Acad Sci 409:637–649

Waters RV, Ferraresi RW (1980) Muramyl dipeptide stimulation of particle clearance in several animal species. J Reticuloendothel Soc 28:457–471

Watson J, Whitlock C (1978) Effect of a synthetic adjuvant on the induction of primary immune responses in T-cell-depleted spleen cultures. J Immunol 121:383–389

Wood DD, Staruch MJ (1981) Control of the mitogenicity of muramyl dipeptide. Int J Immunopharmacol 3:31–44

Wuest B, Wachsmuth E (1982) Stimulatory effect of N-acetylmuramyl dipeptide in vivo: proliferation of bone marrow progenitor cells in mice. Infect Immun 37:452–462

Yamamura Y, Azuma I, Sugimura K, Yamawaki M, Kusumoto S, Okada S, Shiba T (1976) Adjuvant activity of 6-O-mycoloyl-N-acetylmuramyl-L-alanyl-D-isoglutamine. Gann 67:867–877

CHAPTER 23

Antipurines and Purine Metabolism

G. WOLBERG

A. General Introduction

The study of the involvement of purines in lymphocyte function has been highlighted by two dramatic and unrelated discoveries. The first, the discovery in 1958 that 6-mercaptopurine (6-MP) had marked immunosuppressive properties (SCHWARTZ et al. 1958), was followed by the wide use of its S-substituted analog, azathioprine (Aza), to prevent rejection of kidney transplants (MURRAY et al. 1967). The second, the discovery by GIBLETT that deficiencies in either of two enzymes of the purine catabolic pathway, adenosine deaminase (ADA) (GIBLETT et al. 1972) or purine nucleoside phosphorylase (PNP) (GIBLETT et al. 1975), were associated with immunodeficiency disease, led to many studies involving purine metabolism in lymphocytes as well as the modulation of lymphocyte function by purines.

B. Antipurines: 6-Mercaptopurine and Azathioprine

I. Historical Perspective/Background

Studies concerning the effects of the thiopurines, including Aza and 6-MP, on the immune response in general, and on lymphocytes in particular, have spanned an era of enormous growth in our knowledge of the cells involved in the immune response. The structures of Aza and 6-MP are as follows:

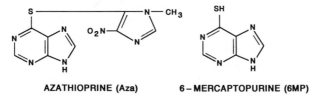

AZATHIOPRINE (Aza)   6 – MERCAPTOPURINE (6MP)

6-MP was synthesized at the Wellcome Research Laboratories in 1951 and within 1.5 years was used in the clinic to treat leukemia. Aza was synthesized in 1957 as a masked form of 6-MP and, within 6 years, was found to be superior to 6-MP in dog renal allografts (CALNE et al. 1962) and to be effective in human renal transplantation (MURRAY et al. 1963). The role of the lymphocyte in the immune response was only beginning to be studied, and lymphocyte subsets were some years from discovery. Textbooks on immunology made almost no references to lymphocytes. The work of many investigators, including GLICK et al. (1956),

GOOD et al. (1962), MILLER (1961), CLAMAN et al. (1966), and DAVIES et al. (1967) led to the establishment of the role of thymus-dependent or T lymphocytes and bone marrow-derived or B lymphocytes in the immune response (see Chap. 1). It was not until 1970 that GERSHON and KONDO reported suppressor cell activity, 1975 that natural killer cells were described (HERBERMAN et al. 1975; KIESSLING et al. 1975), and 1979 that monoclonal antibodies defining inducer/helper T lymphocytes (OKT4) and human suppressor/cytotoxic T lymphocytes (OKT8) became available (REINHERZ et al. 1979). Thus, our present understanding of the effects of 6-MP and Aza on lymphocytes has emerged slowly and the total picture may have to wait for further discoveries of lymphocyte subsets.

II. Metabolism

Much is known concerning the metabolism of 6-MP and Aza, and a comprehensive review is available in a previous volume of this series (ELION and HITCHINGS 1975). However, it may be useful to discuss this topic briefly in order to illustrate the complexity involved in the precise mechanism of action of these agents or their active metabolites. Since Aza is a methylnitroimidazole-substituted derivative of 6-MP, and was originally synthesized as a slow-release or less toxic form of 6-MP, it has generally been assumed that the biologic effects of Aza were attributable solely to its cleavage product, 6-MP. Many of the effects of Aza can be explained through the release of 6-MP, but it is clear that these two agents have different activities in vivo (MEDZIHRADSKY et al. 1981, 1982) and in vitro (BACH et al. 1969; ELION 1977; AL-SAFI and MADDOCKS 1984; DALKE et al. 1984). While Aza is consistently more active than 6-MP in vitro, it is rapidly converted to 6-MP in the presence of red blood cells (RBC) and some of the conflicting results which have been reported involving Aza activity in vitro may be explained by the presence of varying amounts of RBC contamination in the cell suspensions under study. Results from in vivo experiments comparing Aza and 6-MP are less clear, although the superior safety: efficacy ratio of Aza has led to its broader use.

Whether or not 6-MP is administered as such or is released in vivo from Aza by nucleophilic attack on the 5 position of the nitroimidazole ring (ELION and HITCHINGS 1975), its metabolism is qualitatively the same. 6-MP is an inhibitor as well as a substrate for hypoxanthine-guanine phosphoribosyl transferase (HGPRT), and is converted to its ribonucleotide, 6-thioinosinic acid, by this enzyme. This step appears to be essential for its action, since 6-MP is not inhibitory to cells that lack this enzyme (BROCKMAN 1960, 1965; ALLISON et al. 1975; DALKE et al. 1984). It has also been reported that Aza does not inhibit de novo purine biosynthesis in Lesch-Nyhan patients who lack HGPRT (KELLEY et al. 1967). 6-Thioinosinic acid is further metabolized to a number of other compounds, including 6-methylthioinosinic acid, 6-thioguanylic acid, 6-thioguanosine 5'-di and -triphosphates, 6-thioxanthylic acid, 6-thiouric acid, 6-methylthiouric acid, 6-thioxanthine, and 6-methylsulfinyl-8-hydroxypurine. 6-Thioinosinic acid has been shown to inhibit a number of enzymes involved in purine metabolism. These include phosphoribosylpyrophosphate amidotransferase, adenylosuccinic acid synthetase, adenylosuccinase, HGPRT, PNP, xanthine oxidase, glycinamide ribonucleotide transformylase, 5-amino-4-imidazolecarboximide ribonucleotide transformylase, and inosinic acid dehydrogenase (for references see KELLEY et al. 1967). Furthermore, metabolites of 6-MP may be incorporated into DNA (TIDD and PATERSON 1974), RNA (BRETER 1985), or bound to tissue proteins (HYSLOP and JARDINE 1981).

The metabolic disposition of the methylnitroimidazole (MNI) moiety of Aza has been studied extensively, using Aza labeled with ^{14}C at carbons 4 and 5 of the MNI ring, in humans (ELION et al. 1970), rats (DE MIRANDA et al. 1973), and dogs (DE MIRANDA et al. 1975). Beside 1-methyl-4-nitro-5-thioimidazole, which had previously been identified in the urine of Aza-treated patients (CHALMERS et al. 1967; ELION 1968), a number of other imidazole ring metabolites are formed. These include 1-methyl-4-nitro-5-(S-glutathionyl)imidazole, 1-methyl-4-nitro-5-(N-acetyl-S-cysteinyl)imidazole and N,N'-[5-(1-methyl-4-nitro)imidazolyl]cystine. The possible role of these imidazole metabolites in the pharmacologic effects of Aza is unknown, but they are especially interesting in light of a recent report (DALKE et al. 1984) of HGPRT-independent toxicity of Aza that was not reversed by supplementation with inosine or adenine. They found that the growth of two HGPRT-deficient B cell lines, one from a Lesch-Nyhan patient, was inhibited by 30 μM Aza, but not by 200 μM 6-MP. Purine supplementation did prevent the toxicity of both Aza and 6-MP in B lymphoblast lines that were normal for HGPRT.

III. Effects on Lymphocyte Subsets

1. T Lymphocytes

The comprehensive review by ELION and HITCHINGS (1975) covered the literature up to that time concerning the effects of Aza and 6-MP on the two major lymphocyte classes. They reported that these agents appeared to have a selective effect on T lymphocytes, as indicated by their ability to inhibit a number of T lymphocyte responses in vitro including rosette formation, mixed lymphocyte reaction, response to phytohemagglutinin (PHA), and lysis of specific target cells, as well as T cell responses in vivo, including those involving autoimmune diseases and graft rejections. They also pointed out that, although both Aza and 6-MP had been shown to inhibit antibody production by B lymphocytes maximally when given at the time of antigen challenge, patients receiving Aza treatment have not always shown a decrease in immunoglobulin levels. Also, specific suppression of cell-mediated immunity could be demonstrated in the absence of suppression of antibody to the same antigenic challenge. In their review, ELION and HITCHINGS (1975) also discussed the continuing controversy concerning the relative immunosuppressive activities of Aza and 6-MP, presenting evidence that Aza was generally more active than 6-MP in vitro, while differences in vivo were small, and suggested that the superiority of Aza as an immunosuppressive agent may depend on its better safety: efficacy ratio. These issues have been discussed previously, and for reasons of space, this chapter will be restricted generally to papers, especially recent ones, involving the effects of 6-MP and Aza on lymphocyte subsets.

2. B Lymphocytes

Although Aza and 6-MP have been shown to influence humoral as well as cell-mediated immunity, the effects of these agents on B lymphocytes themselves have been difficult to analyze. Most reports involve in vivo or in vitro situations (i.e., antibody formation or B lymphocyte activation) where the function of the B lymphocyte is dependent on regulatory T lymphocytes or their products. Also, many investigators have used much higher levels of these agents than those obtainable in vivo in the clinical setting. While the results of in vitro experiments may not always be directly comparable to those occurring in vivo, in part because of metabolic differences, recent work involving a number of in vitro models indicates that B lymphocytes are directly inhibited by Aza and 6-MP at very low concentrations. B lymphocyte responses have been broadly classified, on the basis of the requirement for T lymphocytes, into those that require T lymphocyte help (T-dependent) and those that do not (T-independent). In experiments comparing the effects of Aza, in vitro, on T lymphocyte-dependent and T lymphocyte-independent B lymphocyte responses, the former response was 100-fold (Galanaud et al. 1975) or 300-fold (Röllinghoff et al. 1973) more sensitive than the latter. Galanaud et al. (1976) further delineated the effect of Aza on B lymphocytes with two different T-independent antigens. The mouse spleen B lymphocyte response to trinitrophenol (TNP) coupled to a nonmitogenic carrier, polyacrylamide, was, like the T lymphocyte-dependent anti-TNP response (Galanaud et al. 1975), highly sensitive to Aza ($IC_{50} < 0.36 \ \mu M$). The response to TNP coupled to a mitogenic carrier, lipopolysaccharide, was much less sensitive to Aza ($IC_{50} = 3.6 \ \mu M$). In their detailed study of the Aza sensitivity of human lymphocytes involved in the pokeweed mitogen (PWM) induction of antibody responses in vitro, Dimitriu and Fauci (1978) found that the responding B cell was inhibited by $0.036 \ \mu M$ Aza while the regulatory cells involved in this response were much less sensitive. Human T and B lymphocyte cell lines were sensitive to 6-MP and Aza at $2.9–14 \ \mu M$ in vitro (Ohnuma et al. 1978; Kazmers et al. 1983), as were clonable murine B lymphocytes (Kincade et al. 1980). These findings that B and T lymphocytes are directly affected by Aza and 6-MP may provide further insight into the mechanism of action of these agents.

3. T Helper and T Suppressor Cells

T lymphocytes comprise a heterogeneous group of cells with important regulatory functions. These include T helper lymphocytes (Th), which are needed for the activation and differentiation of lymphocytes and other cells, and T suppressor lymphocytes (Ts), which are capable of suppressing the immune response through direct action on B cells or Th cells. The effects of Aza on Th and Ts cells have been studied with either specific mouse monoclonal antibody to characteristic surface antigens on these cells or assays that measure their helper or suppressor functions.

Lymphocytes with the Th-associated phenotype OKT4 (also termed Leu-3) or the Ts-associated phenotype OKT8 (also termed Leu-4) have been monitored in a number of patients with autoimmune diseases or renal transplants who were undergoing treatment with Aza, usually in combination with corticosteroids

(CS), to study changes in the absolute numbers and the Th:Ts ratios. A decrease in the Th:Ts ratio is thought to be associated with a diminished immune response, while an increase may be predictive of an enhanced immune status. In patients with chronic active hepatitis receiving Aza (plus CS) (FRAZER and MACKAY 1982), with chronic progressive multiple sclerosis receiving Aza (TROTTER et al. 1982), or with progressive relapsing multiple sclerosis receiving Aza (SPINA 1984), the percentage decrease in the OKT8$^+$ T cells was greater than the percentage decrease in the OKT4$^+$ T cells, thus resulting in increased OKT4:OKT8 ratios. The effect of Aza on these cells in renal transplant patients is less clear. A wide range of responses has been reported which possibly reflect the immune status of individual patients. No changes in the ratio were found, owing to equal decreases in the numbers (SWENY and TIDMAN 1982) or to no change in the numbers (VAN BUREN et al. 1982) of OKT4$^+$ T cells or OKT8$^+$ T cells. In other studies, COSIMI et al. (1981), CHATENOUD et al. (1981), and DUPONT et al. (1983) reported great variability in the levels of these cells in their Aza (plus CS)-treated patients with well-tolerated renal transplants; however, generally, a predominant decrease in the number of OKT4$^+$ T cells led to a decreased OKT4:OKT8 ratio. In the study reported by CHATENOUD et al. (1981), two patients who received Aza alone showed a marked reduction of OKT4$^+$ T cells, while the OKT8$^+$ T cells were reduced in a third patient.

There have been a number of reports concerning the effects of Aza and 6-MP on the actual functions of Th and Ts cells. In vitro assays of Th cell function have taken advantage of the requirement for these cells in the PWM stimulation of immunoglobulin synthesis by B cells. The effect of Aza has been studied on both naturally occurring and concanavalin A (Con A)-induced suppressor cell generation and on the ability of these Ts cells to inhibit various in vitro immune responses, such as the immunoglobulin response to specific antigens or PWM, or the inhibition of the mixed lymphocyte reaction. VAN BUREN et al. (1982) found that lymphocytes from renal transplant patients undergoing treatment with Aza (plus CS) showed increased Ts cell and normal Th cell activity, as assessed in vitro, even though there was no change in the OKT4:OKT8 ratio. Peripheral blood lymphocytes (PBL) from Aza (plus CS)-treated renal allograft recipients had a depressed capacity to generate Ts cells on Con A activation in vitro (DUCLOS et al. 1979). The in vitro generation of spontaneously induced, but not Con A-induced, Ts cells from mouse spleen was inhibited by the presence of 0.36 μM Aza (DUCLOS et al. 1982), while the Con A-induced generation of human peripheral blood Ts cells required ten times more Aza for inhibition (DIMITRIU and FAUCI 1978). The in vitro activity of Con A-generated human splenic Ts cells (SAMPSON et al. 1975) and human peripheral blood-Ts cells was inhibited by Aza, while human peripheral blood Th cells were resistant to Aza in vitro (DIMITRIU and FAUCI 1978), as measured by the inhibition of sheep red blood cell-specific antibody synthesis, and were inhibited by Aza (GÓRSKI et al. 1983), as measured by the inhibition of total immunoglobulin synthesis. Using in vivo models, SMITH et al. (1979) reported that Aza inhibited Ts generation, while MEDZIHRADSKY et al. (1981) found that 6-MP was a much more potent inhibitor of Ts cell generation than Aza.

Although few data are available concerning the effect of Aza on Th cell function taken as a whole, these data suggest that Ts cell function is more sensitive to Aza than is Th cell function. The relevance of this effect of Aza to its clinical use is unclear, and must await a more detailed understanding of the interactions involved within the various cells of the immune response.

4. Cytolytic Cells

Various lymphoid cell populations have been shown to be cytolytic to other cells in vitro. These include cytotoxic T lymphocytes (CTL), as well as natural killer (NK) and killer (K) cells, which are not readily classified as either T or B lymphocytes. Although the biologic significance of these cells is not completely clear, they appear to be important elements in the immune response and, as such, have been investigated as likely targets for the immunosuppressive effects of Aza and 6-MP.

a) Cytotoxic T Lymphocytes

CTL may be generated in vivo or in vitro and are capable of lysing antigen-specific cells independently of antibody and complement. Cell-to-cell contact between the CTL and the target cells is required, and lysis is usually measured in vitro after 1–48 h incubation with target cells. Cytolytic activity in humans is expressed by $OKT8^+$ lymphocytes.

The effects of Aza and 6-MP on the in vivo and in vitro generation of CTL, as well as the in vitro lympholysis of target cells by CTL, have been studied by a number of investigators. While the in vivo generation of mouse CTL (OTTERNESS and CHANG 1976) and the in vitro generation of mouse (RÖLLINGHOFF et al. 1973) or baboon CTL (BROWN et al. 1976) can be inhibited by Aza or 6-MP, PBL from renal transplant patients undergoing treatment with Aza (plus CS) were able to mount a cytotoxic T cell response to donor antigens (KEOWN et al. 1984) or autologous Epstein–Barr virus-infected B cells (CRAWFORD et al. 1981), as well as to generate CTL on in vitro induction in a mixed lymphocyte culture (TEN BERGE et al. 1981). In the studies by RÖLLINGHOFF et al. (1973) and BROWN et al. (1976), the cytolytic activity of mouse and baboon CTL were not inhibited by 72 and 225 μM Aza, respectively, present during the 3-h in vitro assay. WILSON (1965) had previously reported that rat CTL were inhibited by as little as 3.6 μM Aza in vitro when present throughout a 48-h culture period. In unpublished experiments in our laboratory with mouse CTL in an in vitro assay (previously described by WOLBERG et al. 1975), the inhibition by Aza increased dramatically with time of preincubation of CTL with Aza. The 50% inhibitory concentration decreased from 730 μM without preincubation to 130 μM after 6 h and < 50 μM after 23 h preincubation. 6-MP was much less inhibitory to CTL than Aza at all times, again showing the striking difference between these two thiopurines in vitro.

b) Natural Killer Cells

NK cells are large granular lymphocytes (LGL) that exist in the absence of any known immunization and have the ability to lyse an assortment of tumor cells and virus-infected cells. Since their description by HERBERMAN et al. (1975) and

KIESSLING et al. (1975), they have been found in peripheral blood as well as in spleens, lymph nodes, and the peritoneal cavity in a wide variety of species, including humans. They bear surface receptors for the Fc portion of immunoglobulins, but the killing mechanism is antibody independent and requires cell-to-cell contact. While the clinical relevance of these cells in unclear, it has been suggested that they are involved in "immune surveillance," which may play a vital role in preventing tumors (HERBERMAN 1982).

While no correlation between NK cell activity and transplant rejection or clinical disease has been firmly established, it has been reported that Aza treatment for inhibition of rejection (LIPINSKI et al. 1980; MOREAU et al. 1981, 1983; GUILLOU et al. 1982; WALTZER et al. 1984; PRINCE et al. 1984; DUPONT et al. 1984; RAMSEY et al. 1984), multiple sclerosis (SHIH et al. 1982), or rheumatoid arthritis (PEDERSEN et al. 1984), 6-MP treatment for Crohn's disease (BROGAN et al. 1985), or the treatment of acute lymphoblastic leukemia with a regimen of agents including 6-MP (MCGEORGE et al. 1982) lead to marked depression of NK cell activity and numbers of LGL (RAMSEY et al. 1984). This NK cell depression induced by Aza (plus CS) was evident in two kidney transplant patients as early as 2–4 days after beginning treatment, and almost total depression was seen by day 60, even though drug dosage was continually decreased (LIPINSKI et al. 1980). MOREAU et al. (1981, 1983) reported a progressive depression of NK cell activity as early as 3 months after transplantation and treatment with Aza (plus CS). This depression continued for 60 months, with NK cell activity falling to approximately 10% of normal. NK cell activity then tended to be restored in those patients. A similar return to normal was found by GUILLOU et al. (1982). While most of these patients received CS as well as Aza, a number of findings indicate that Aza induced the NK cell depression: (a) one patient received a graft from an HLA-identical sibling, was treated only with Aza, and showed a 24.6% depression of NK cell activity (LIPINSKI et al. 1980); (b) patients treated with CS alone did not show decreased NK cell activity (MOREAU et al. 1983; PRINCE et al. 1984); (c) one patient on Aza (plus CS) who had depressed NK cell activity returned to normal on discontinuing Aza, but not CS (PRINCE et al. 1984); (d) Aza alone induced suppression of NK cell activity during treatment for multiple sclerosis (SHIH et al. 1982) or rheumatoid arthritis (PEDERSEN et al. 1984). The clinical relevance of these Aza-induced NK cell depressions is not clear. LIPINSKI et al. (1980) found that acute rejection crisis was associated with a rise in NK cell activity, but WALTZER et al. (1984) and GUILLOU et al. (1982) reported that NK cell activity was not a reliable index of allograft rejection.

Aza or 6-MP may decrease NK cell activity by: (a) decreasing progenitor cells; (b) killing or inactivating NK cells directly; or (c) inducing inhibitory suppressor cells or soluble mediators. DUPONT et al. (1984) found that patients treated with Aza (plus CS) had decreased number of NK cells capable of binding and killing target cells, as well as decreases in the percentage and absolute numbers of LGL. SHIH et al. (1982) reported that patients treated with Aza had a reduction in the percentage of lymphocytes that could bind NK-sensitive target cells and also a decreased ability of these target-binding cells to lyse targets. Neither sera nor peripheral blood cells from patients receiving Aza (plus CS) were inhibitory to the activity of NK cells of normal individuals, and NK cell activity from patients were not more susceptible to Con A-induced suppression (Moreau et al. 1983). Also, no direct in vitro effects of 36 μM Aza (activated by 2-h incubation with RBC) (Moreau et al. 1983) or 66 μM 6-MP (Dupont et al. 1984) were found. Aza was inhibitory to NK cell activity in vitro only at concentrations above 100 μM (Moreau et al. 1983; Kelly et al. 1984).

Since interferon (IFN) has been shown to regulate NK cell activity (Minato et al. 1980; Chap. 9), a number of investigators have examined the ability of exogenous IFN preparations to enhance the activity of Aza-depressed NK cells in vitro and have reported varied results. IFN was able to augment the NK cell activity in two studies (Ramsey et al. 1984; Kelley et al. 1984), suggesting the presence of pre-NK cells. However, no significant augmentation was found in other studies (Moreau et al. 1983; Gui et al. 1983; Shih et al. 1982). Paradoxically, IFN-α-administered to renal transplant recipients receiving Aza (plus CS) led to greater decrease in NK activity, while it augmented the activity of NK cells from these patients in vitro (Kelley et al. 1984).

While there appears to be general agreement that Aza treatment decreases NK cell activity, some controversy exists concerning the kinetics of the decrease, the recovery of activity, and the augmentation of the depressed NK cell activity by IFN. These reported differences may reflect differences in: (a) dosage and timing of Aza; (b) combinations of drugs; (c) types of IFN; (d) the length of time the patients have been treated; or (e) the tests used for in vitro assessment of NK cell activity (differences here include types of target cell, length of incubation time, and different effector cell: target cell ratios).

The relationship of these findings to the efficacy or side effects of Aza or 6-MP is unclear. Immunosuppressed patients, as well as those with primary immunodeficiency diseases, have higher incidences of malignancies and infections. Whether or not this is related to decreased NK cell activity is not known, but it is interesting that there appears to be a recovery of the lost NK cell activity after 4–5 years when the risk of malignancy is still present. Also, one may postulate that loss of NK cell activity would benefit the prevention of allograft rejection and diseases that appear to involve immunopathogenesis, such as rheumatoid arthritis or multiple sclerosis, but proof of this awaits further work.

c) Killer Cells

K cells are lymphoid cells which have a membrane receptor for the Fc portion of IgG antibody and are cytolytic to antibody-coated target cells in vitro. This lytic process has been termed antibody-dependent cell-mediated cytotoxicity (ADCC), and requires cell-to-cell interaction. The K cells resemble NK cells, although it is controversial whether or not the NK and ADCC killing are properties of the same cells or of a heterogeneous group of Fc receptor-bearing cells with different abilities to express K or NK killing (Koren and Williams 1978; De Landazuri et al. 1979). The effect of Aza on ADCC is also controversial. A decrease in ADCC in patients undergoing treatment with Aza has been reported in a number of human studies (Campbell et al. 1976; Shih et al. 1982; Prince et al. 1984; Spina 1984), as well as in mice treated with Aza (Purves and Berenbaum 1975), but Descamps et al. (1977) and Lipinski et al. (1980) found normal K cell activity in their patients. It is especially interesting that K cell activity may remain normal while NK cell activity is greatly decreased (LIPINSKI et al. 1980) and that in vitro treatment of a K cell-enriched population with 1.8 mM Aza for 4 h did not alter the cytolytic capacity of these cells (DESCAMPS et al. 1977). DUMBLE et al. (1981) found that the survival of renal allografts in patients treated with Aza (plus CS) correlated with a suppression of ADCC effector cell function, and that the generation of ADCC preceded the onset of graft rejection. They concluded that ADCC was important in graft rejection.

C. Adenosine Deaminase and Purine Nucleoside Phosphorylase Deficiencies

A discussion of the importance of purines to lymphocyte function would be incomplete without at least a brief mention of two inherited immunodeficiency diseases that are associated with deficiencies of either ADA or PNP (for comprehensive reviews see HIRSCHHORN 1977; POLMAR 1980; EDWARDS and FOX 1984; EDWARDS 1985). ADA catalyzes the deamination of adenosine (Ado) and 2'-deoxyadenosine (dAdo) to inosine and 2'-deoxyinosine, respectively, while PNP catalyzes the phosphorolysis of inosine, 2'-deoxyinosine, guanosine, and 2'-deoxyguanosine (dGuo) to their corresponding free bases and ribose-(deoxyribose) 1-phosphate. The discovery of these inborn errors of metabolism has led to an explosion of information concerning the effects of purine derivatives on lymphocyte function, and has provided clues for the treatment of lymphoid cell malignancies and immune deficiencies as well as autoimmune diseases and transplant rejection.

ADA deficiency is found in approximately one-third to one-half of patients with autosomal recessive severe combined immunodeficiency disease, or SCID (HIRSCHHORN 1977; POLMAR 1980). SCID is characterized by a progressive reduction in numbers, and ultimate loss of T and B lymphocytes. The immune defects, which include hypogammaglobulinemia and absence of cutaneous delayed hypersensitivity, become more severe with age, and the children suffer from episodes of bacterial, viral, and fungal infections. In these respects, patients resemble those with non-ADA-related SCID. Without infusions of irradiated human erythrocytes (as a source of ADA), begun early in disease while T and B cells are still present (POLMAR et al. 1976), or bone marrow transplantation (CHEN et al. 1978), the disease is uniformly fatal.

There is some biochemical understanding of the basis of the SCID in these ADA-deficient patients. Patients have elevated levels of Ado and dAdo in their erythrocytes, plasma, and urine (HIRSCHHORN and RATECH 1983), as well as increased levels of 2'-deoxyadenosine 5'-triphosphate (dATP) in their erythrocytes, lymphocytes, and bone marrow (COLEMAN et al. 1978; COHEN et al. 1978 a; DONOFRIO et al. 1978; MILLS et al. 1978); and most laboratory investigations have been devoted to the potential role of these particular compounds in causing SCID. Owing to the paucity of lymphocytes obtainable from the ADA-deficient patients, most experiments have involved in vitro studies of transformed or freshly isolated lymphocytes. Potent inhibitors of ADA, such as erythro-9-(2-hydroxy-3-nonyl)adenine and 2'-deoxycoformycin, have allowed the development of in vivo (TEDDE et al. 1980) and in vitro (WOLBERG et al. 1975; HIRSCHHORN and SELA 1977) experimental models that appear to mimic pharmacologically the human disease associated with ADA deficiency.

A number of hypotheses have been proposed to explain the lymphocyte defect (or defects) associated with ADA deficiency. These include: (a) Ado nucleotide-induced pyrimidine starvation (GREEN and CHAN 1973) or inhibition of glycolysis (AGARWAL et al. 1976); (b) Ado-induced elevation of lymphocyte cAMP that inhibits cell function (WOLBERG et al. 1975); (c) condensation of Ado with L-homocysteine, catalyzed by S-adenosylhomocysteine (SAH) hydrolase, resulting in inhibition of S-adenosylmethionine-dependent methyltransferases by accumulated SAH (KREDICH and MARTIN 1977); (d) inactivation of SAH hydrolase by dAdo, resulting in elevated cellular SAH levels and inhibition of methyltransferases (HERSHFIELD 1979); (e) inhibition of ribonucleotide reductase by elevated dATP, causing inhibition of DNA synthesis (ULLMAN et al. 1978; CARSON et al. 1978); (f) inhibition of RNA synthesis by elevated dATP (MATSUMOTO et al. 1983); and (g) NAD and ATP depletion, owing to dATP-stimulated synthesis of poly(ADP-ribose) (SETO et al. 1985).

PNP deficiency is less common than ADA deficiency. Most PNP-deficient patients exhibit a marked reduction in T lymphocytes and a loss of the cellular immune function; however, unlike ADA-deficient SCID, PNP-deficient patients exhibit adequate (or even enhanced) humoral immune function with normal numbers of B cells (GIBLETT et al. 1975; HIRSCHHORN and RATECH 1983). Children with this disease first present with clinical signs (recurrent, predominantly viral infections) at any time from a few months to years after birth.

Experiments concerning the biochemical basis for PNP-associated T cell immunodeficiency have been focused on dGuo and its phosphorylated metabolite 2'-deoxyguanosine 5'-triphosphate (dGTP). Like the other nucleoside substrates (inosine, guanosine, and 2'-deoxyinosine) of PNP, dGuo is markedly elevated in the urine of these patients (COHEN et al. 1976). Moeover, dGTP was found to accumulate in patients' erythrocytes and lymphocytes (COHEN et al. 1976; GODAY et al. 1982). Like dATP, dGTP is an allosteric inhibitor of ribonucleotide reductase (MOORE and HURLBERT 1966), and it blocks the conversion of CDP and UDP to their respective deoxyribonucleotide forms (THELANDER and REICHARD 1979), and thus inhibits DNA synthesis. As was the case for studies on the mechanism (or mechanisms) involved in ADA-related SCID, the dGuo-induced toxicity has been studied with lymphoid cell lines and freshly isolated lymphocytes. Inhibitors of PNP, such as 8-aminoguanosine (KAZMERS et al. 1981; SIDI and MITCHELL 1984), formycin B (WILLEMOT et al. 1979), and allopurinol riboside (NISHIDA et al. 1979) have been used to mimic the human disease pharmacologically. The report by NISHIDA et al. (1979) is particularly intriguing since allopurinol riboside decreased the cellular response, but not the humoral response to sheep red blood cells. Unfortunately, no measurements of dGuo or dGTP were reported to validate the model. Also, very high levels of allopurinol riboside were needed to inhibit PNP.

The selective T cell toxicity associated with PNP deficiency appears to be due to differences in purine metabolism in the thymus, T cells, and B cells. It has been suggested that thymocytes and T cells, which have high levels of deoxycytidine kinase to phosphorylate dGuo, trap greater quantities of dGTP intracellularly, since they contain relatively lower levels of deoxynucleotidase than B cells (CARSON et al. 1977, 1979, 1981; Fox et al. 1981). dGuo has been found to be selectively toxic to T lymphoblasts (OCHS et al. 1979), presumably owing to the greater accumulation of dGTP in T cells than in B cells (CARSON et al. 1979; OSBORNE and SCOTT 1983). The possible role of increased guanine ribonucleotide (GTP) levels in this disease is unclear (SPAAPEN et al. 1984; SIDI and MITCHELL 1984).

The different immunologic phenotypes seen with ADA and PNP deficiencies may be due to a number of factors. While both diseases involve an allosteric inhibition of ribonucleotide reductase, inhibition by dATP in the ADA deficiency may be more profound, since the reduction of all four ribonucleoside diphosphates is affected, while inhibition by dGTP in the PNP deficiency only involves the pyrimidine nucleoside diphosphates. In both diseases, the lymphocyte functions requiring proliferation, such as the development of mature T cells from thymic T cell precursors and the development of suppressor/cytotoxic T cells, are markedly decreased as a consequence of the inhibition of DNA metabolism (MARTIN and GELFAND 1981), while the nonproliferation-dependent functions, such as those involving T helper cells, are inhibited only in the more severe ADA-associated disease.

D. Conclusions

In the review by ELION and HITCHINGS (1975), it was concluded that "a satisfactory rationalization of the immunosuppressive effects of azathioprine is at present beyond reach." They suggested, however, that the answer might lie in a better understanding of lymphocyte subsets, even though only data on T versus B lymphocytes were available at that time. In the last decade, a number of studies have shown that Aza and 6-MP do appear to have selective effects on the various lymphoid components involved in the immune response. The Aza-induced inhibition of NK and K cell cytotoxicity, Ts cell generation, and one pathway of B lymphocyte activation, demonstrates the many potential targets for Aza and, at the same time, the difficulty in identifying its predominant mechanism (or mechanisms) of action. Thus, it appears that this conclusion of ELION and HITCHINGS still holds more than a decade later and that further work is required to provide a clear understanding of the thiopurines.

The demonstration of two inherited enzyme deficiency-induced immunodeficiency diseases has further emphasized the crucial role of purine metabolism in lymphocyte function, and probably should not have been surprising in light of the known ability of the thiopurines to influence immune regulation. Further studies involving these so-called experiments of nature, as well as those involving exogenously supplied purines, promise to provide more detailed insights into normal and abnormal lymphocyte functions. Such investigations may provide clues for the use of purines in the therapy of immune disorders through highly selective modulation of lymphocyte subsets.

References

Agarwal RP, Crabtree GW, Parks RE Jr, Nelson JA, Keightley R, Parkman R, Rosen FS, Stern RC, Polmar SH (1976) Purine nucleoside metabolism in the erythrocytes of patients with adenosine deaminase deficiency and severe combined immunodeficiency. J Clin Invest 57:1025–1035

Allison AC, Hovi T, Watts RWE, Webster ADB (1975) Immunological observations on patients with Lesch-Nyhan syndrome and on the role of de-novo purine synthesis in lymphocyte transformation. Lancet II:1179–1183

Al-Safi SA, Maddocks JL (1984) Azathioprine and 6-mercaptopurine (6-MP) suppress the human mixed lymphocyte reaction (MLR) by different mechanisms. Br J Clin Pharmacol 17:417–422

Bach JF, Dardenne M, Fournier C (1969) In vitro evaluation of immunosuppressive drugs. Nature 222:998–999

Breter HJ (1985) The quantitative determination of metabolites of 6-mercaptopurine in biological materials. VI. Evidence for posttranscriptional modification of 6-thioguanosine residues in RNA from L5178Y cells treated with 6-mercaptopurine. Biochim Biophys Acta 825:39–44

Brockman RW (1960) A mechanism of resistance to 6-mercaptopurine: metabolism of hypoxanthine and 6-mercaptopurine by sensitive and resistant neoplasms. Cancer Res 20:643–653

Brockman RW (1965) Resistance to purine antagonists in experimental leukemia systems. Cancer Res 25:1596–1605

Brogan M, Hiserodt J, Oliver M, Stevens R, Korelitz B, Targon S (1985) The effect of 6-mercaptopurine on natural killer-cell activities in Crohn's disease. J Clin Immunol 5:204–211

Brown TE, Ahmed A, Filo RS, Knudsen RC, Sell KW (1976) The immunosuppressive mechanism of azathioprine. I. In vitro effect on lymphocyte function in the baboon. Transplantation 21:27–35

Campbell AC, Skinner JM, Maclennan ICM, Hersey P, Waller CA, Wood J, Jewell DP, Truelove SC (1976) Immunosuppression in the treatment of inflammatory bowel disease. II. The effects of azathioprine on lymphoid cell populations in a double blind trial in ulcerative colitis. Clin Exp Immunol 24:249–258

Calne RY, Alexandre GPJ, Murray JE (1962) A study of the effects of drugs in prolonging survival of homologous renal transplants in dogs. Ann NY Acad Sci 99:743–761

Carson DA, Kaye J, Seegmiller JE (1977) Lymphospecific toxicity in adenosine deaminase deficiency and purine nucleoside phosphorylase deficiency: possible role of nucleoside kinase(s). Proc Natl Acad Sci USA 74:5677–5681

Carson DA, Kaye J, Seegmiller JE (1978) Differential sensitivity of human leukemic T cell lines and B cell lines to growth inhibition by deoxyadenosine. J Immunol 121:1726–1731

Carson DA, Kaye J, Matsumoto S, Seegmiller JE, Thompson L (1979) Biochemical basis for the enhanced toxicity of deoxyribonucleosides toward malignant human T cell lines. Proc Natl Acad Sci USA 76:2430–2433

Carson DA, Kaye J, Wasson DB (1981) The potential importance of soluble deoxynucleotidase activity in mediating deoxyadenosine toxicity in human lymphoblasts. J Immunol 126:348–352

Chalmers AH, Knight PR, Atkinson MR (1967) Conversion of azathioprine into mercaptopurine and mercaptoimidazole derivatives in vitro and during immunosuppressive therapy. Aust J Exp Biol Med Sci 45:681–691

Chatenoud L, Kreis H, Jungers P, Bach JF (1981) The effect of immunosuppressive agents on T-cell subsets, as evaluated by use of monoclonal anti-T-cell antibodies. Transplant Proc 13:1651–1656

Chen SH, Ochs HD, Scott CR, Giblett ER, Tingle AJ (1978) Adenosine deaminase deficiency: disappearance of adenine deoxynucleotides from a patient's erythrocytes after successful marrow transplantation. J Clin Invest 62:1386–1389

Claman HN, Chaperon EA, Triplett RF (1966) Thymus-marrow cell combinations. Synergism in antibody production. Proc Soc Exp Biol Med 122:1167–1171

Cohen A, Doyle D, Martin DW Jr, Ammann AJ (1976) Abnormal purine metabolism and purine overproduction in a patient deficient in purine nucleoside phosphorylase. N Engl J Med 295:1449–1454

Cohen A, Gudas LJ, Ammann AJ, Staal GEJ, Martin DW Jr (1978a) Deoxyguanosine triphosphate as a possible toxic metabolite in the immunodeficiency associated with purine nucleoside phosphorylase deficiency. J Clin Invest 61:1405–1409

Cohen A, Hirschhorn R, Horowitz SD, Rubinstein A, Polmar SH, Hong R, Martin DW Jr (1978b) Deoxyadenosine triphosphate as a potentially toxic metabolite in adenosine deaminase deficiency. Proc Natl Acad Sci USA 75:472–476

Coleman MS, Donofrio J, Hutton JJ, Hahn L, Daoud A, Lampkin B, Dyminski J (1978) Identification and quantitation of adenine deoxynucleotides in erythrocytes of a patient with adenosine deaminase deficiency and severe combined immunodeficiency. J Biol Chem 253:1619–1626

Cosimi AB, Colvin RB, Burton RC, Rubin RH, Goldstein G, Kung PC, Hansen WP, Delmonico FL, Russell PS (1981) Use of monoclonal antibodies to T-cell subsets for immunologic monitoring and treatment in recipients of renal allografts. N Engl J Med 305:308–314

Crawford DH, Edwards JMB, Sweny P, Hoffbrand AV, Janossy G (1981) Studies on long-term T-cell-mediated immunity to Epstein-Barr virus in immunosuppressed renal allograft recipients. Int J Cancer 28:705–709

Dalke AP, Kazmers IS, Kelley WN (1984) Hypoxanthine-guanine phosphoribosyltransferase-independent toxicity of azathioprine in human lymphoblasts. Biochem Pharmacol 33:2692–2695

Davies AJS, Leuchars E, Wallis V, Marchant R, Elliott EV (1967) The failure of thymus-derived cells to produce antibody. Transplantation 5:222–231

De Landazuri MO, Silva A, Alvarez J, Herberman RB (1979) Evidence that natural cytotoxicity and antibody-dependent cellular cytotoxicity are mediated in humans by the same effector cell populations. J Immunol 123:252–258

De Miranda P, Beacham LM III, Creagh TH, Elion GB (1973) The metabolic fate of the methylnitroimidazole moiety of azathioprine in the rat. J Pharmacol Exp Ther 187:588–601

De Miranda P, Beacham LM III, Creagh TH, Elion GB (1975) The metabolic disposition of ^{14}C-azathioprine in the dog. J Pharmacol Exp Ther 195:50–57

Descamps B, Gagnon R, Van Der Gaag R, Meyer O, Crosnier J (1977) Influence of azathioprine and prednisone in vivo treatment on lymphocyte-dependent antibody-mediated cytotoxicity (LDAC) in 57 human renal allograft recipients. Transplant Proc 9:981–984

Dimitriu A, Fauci AS (1978) Activation of human B lymphocytes. XI. Differential effects of azathioprine on B lymphocytes and lymphocyte subpopulations regulating B cell function. J Immunol 121:2335–2339

Donofrio J, Coleman MS, Hutton JJ, Daoud A, Lampkin B, Dyminski J (1978) Overproduction of adenine deoxynucleosides and deoxynucleotides in adenosine deaminase deficiency with severe combined immunodeficiency disease. J Clin Invest 62:884–887

Duclos H, Maillat MC, Kreis H, Galanaud P (1979) T suppressor cell function impairment in peripheral blood lymphocytes from transplant recipients under azathioprine and corticosteroids. Transplantation 28:437–438

Duclos H, Maillot MC, Galanaud P (1982) Differential effects of azathioprine on T cells regulating murine B-cell function. Immunology 46:595–601

Dumble LJ, Macdonald IM, Kincaid-Smith P, Clunie GJ (1981) Enhanced renal allograft survival from azathioprine/steroid modified antibody-dependent cellular cytotoxicity. Proc Eur Dial Transplant Assoc 18:475–480

Dupont E, Schandene L, Devos R, Lambermont M, Wybran J (1983) Depletion of lymphocytes with membrane markers of helper phenotype: a feature of acute and chronic drug-induced immunosuppression. Clin Exp Immunol 51:345–350

Dupont E, Vandercruys M, Wybran J (1984) Deficient natural killer function in patients receiving immunosuppressive drugs: analysis at the cellular level. Cell Immunol 88:85–95

Edwards NL (1985) Immunodeficiencies associated with errors in purine metabolism. Med Clin North Am 69:505–518

Edwards NL, Fox IH (1984) Disorders associated with purine and pyrimidine metabolism. Spec Top Endocrinol Metab 6:95–140

Elion GB (1968) Discussion. In: Miescher PA, Grabar P (eds) 5th International symposium on immuno pathology. Grune and Stratton, NY, pp 399–401

Elion GB (1977) Immunosuppressive agents. Transplant Proc 9:975–979

Elion GB, Hitchings GH (1975) Azathioprine. In: Sartorelli AC, Johns DG (eds) Handbook of experimental pharmacology, vol 38. Springer, New York, pp 404–425

Elion GB, Benezra FM, Carrington LO, Strelitz RA (1970) Metabolic fate of ^{14}C-azathioprine. Fed Proc 29:607

Fox RM, Piddington SK, Tripp EH, Tattersall MHN (1981) Ecto-adenosine triphosphatase deficiency in cultured human T and null leukemic lymphocytes. A biochemical basis for thymidine sensitivity. J Clin Invest 68:544–552

Frazer IH, Mackay IR (1982) T lymphocyte subpopulations defined by two sets of monoclonal antibodies in chronic active hepatitis and systemic lupus erythematosus. Clin Exp Immunol 50:107–114

Galanaud P, Crevon MC, Dormont J (1975) Effect of azathioprine on in vitro antibody response. Differential effect of B cells involved in thymus-dependent and independent responses. Clin Exp Immunol 22:139–152

Galanaud P, Crevon MC, Erard D, Wallon C, Dormont J (1976) Two processes for B-cell triggering by T-independent antigens as evidenced by the effect of azathioprine. Cell Immunol 22:83–92

Gershon RK, Kondo K (1970) Cell interactions in the induction of tolerance: the role of thymic lymphocytes. Immunology 18:723–737

Giblett ER, Anderson JE, Cohen F, Pollara B, Meuwissen HJ (1972) Adenosine-deaminase deficiency in two patients with severely impaired cellular immunity. Lancet II:1067–1069

Giblett ER, Ammann AJ, Wara DW, Sandman R, Diamond LK (1975) Nucleoside-phosphorylase deficiency in a child with severely defective T-cell immunity and normal B-cell immunity. Lancet I:1010–1013

Glick B, Chang TS, Jaap RG (1956) The bursa of Fabricius and antibody production. Poult Sci 35:224–225

Goday A, Webster DR, Simmonds HA (1982) Nucleotide levels in peripheral blood mononuclear cells in immunodeficient children: problems of measurement. J Clin Chem Clin Biochem 20:370

Good RA, Dalmasso AP, Martinez C, Archer OK, Pierce JC, Papermaster BW (1962) The role of the thymus in development of immunologic capacity in rabbits and mice. J Exp Med 116:773–796

Górski A, Korczak-Kowalska G, Nowaczyk M, Paczek L, Gaciong Z (1983) The effect of azathioprine on terminal differentiation of human B lymphocytes. Immunopharmacology 6:259–266

Green H, Chan TS (1973) Pyrimidine starvation induced by adenosine in fibroblasts and lymphoid cells: role of adenosine deaminase. Science 182:836–837

Gui XE, Rinaldo CR Jr, Ho M (1983) Natural killer cell activity in renal transplant recipients receiving cyclosporine. Infect Immun 41:965–970

Guillou PJ, Hegarty J, Ramsden C, Davison AM, Will EJ, Giles GR (1982) Changes in human natural killer activity early and late after renal transplantation using conventional immunosuppression. Transplantation 33:414–421

Herberman RB (1982) Natural killer cells and their possible relevance to transplantation biology. Transplantation 34:1–7

Herberman RB, Nunn ME, Lavrin DH (1975) Natural cytotoxic reactivity of mouse lymphoid cells against syngeneic and allogeneic tumors. I. Distribution of reactivity and specificity. Int J Cancer 16:216–229

Hershfield MS (1979) Apparent suicide inactivation of human lymphoblast S-adenosylho-mocysteine hydrolase by 2′-deoxyadenosine and adenine arabinoside. J Biol Chem 254:22–25

Hirschhorn R (1977) Adenosine deaminase deficiency and immunodeficiencies. Fed Proc 36:2166–2170

Hirschhorn R, Ratech H (1983) Genetic deficiencies of adenosine deaminase and purine nucleoside phosphorylase and their implications for therapy of leukemias. Curr Top Hematol 4:1–35

Hirschhorn R, Sela E (1977) Adenosine deaminase and immunodeficiency: an in vitro model. Cell Immunol 32:350–360

Hyslop RM, Jardine I (1981) Metabolism of 6-thiopurines. II. Covalent binding of a 6-thio-purine metabolite to mammalian tissue protein in vivo. J Pharmacol Exp Ther 218:629–635

Kazmers IS, Mitchell BS, Dadonna PE, Wotring LL, Townsend LB, Kelley WN (1981) Inhibition of purine nucleoside phosphorylase by 8-aminoguanosine: selective toxicity for T lymphoblasts. Science 214:1137–1139

Kazmers IS, Daddona PE, Dalke AP, Kelley WN (1983) Effect of immunosuppressive agents on human T and B lymphoblasts. Biochem Pharmacol 32:805–810

Kelley WN, Rosenbloom FM, Seegmiller JE (1967) The effects of azathioprine (Imuran) on purine synthesis in clinical disorders of purine metabolism. J Clin Invest 46:1518–1529

Kelly AP, Schooley RT, Rubin RH, Hirsch MS (1984) Effect of interferon alpha on natural killer cell cytotoxicity in kidney transplant recipients. Clin Immunol Immunopathol 32:20–28

Keown PA, Stiller CR, Muirhead N, Hellstrom A, Coles R, Howson W (1984) Cyclosporine inhibits cytotoxic T lymphocyte generation in vivo in the naive and immunologically primed allograft recipient. Transplant Proc 16:1462–1463

Kiessling R, Klein E, Wigzell H (1975) Natural killer cells in the mouse I. Cytotoxic cells with specificity for mouse Moloney leukemia cells. Specificity and distribution according to genotype. Eur J Immunol 5:112–117

Kincade PW, Lee G, Scheid MP, Blum MD (1980) Characterization of murine colony-forming B cells. II. Limits to in vitro maturation, Lyb-2 expression, resolution of IgD$^+$ subsets, and further population analysis. J Immunol 124:947–953

Koren HS, Williams MS (1978) Natural killing and antibody-dependent cellular cytotoxicity are mediated by different mechanisms and by different cells. J Immunol 121:1956–1960

Kredich NM, Martin DW Jr (1977) Role of S-adenosylhomocysteine in adenosine-mediated toxicity in cultured mouse T lymphoma cells. Cell 12:931–938

Lipinski M, Tursz T, Kreis H, Finale Y, Amiel JL (1980) Dissociation of natural killer cell activity and antibody-dependent cell-mediated cytotoxicity in kidney allograft recipients receiving high-dose immunosuppressive therapy. Transplantation 29:214–218

Martin DW Jr, Gelfand EW (1981) Biochemistry of disease of immunodevelopment. Annu Rev Biochem 50:845–877

Matsumoto SS, Yu J, Yu AL (1983) Inhibition of RNA synthesis by deoxyadenosine plus deoxycoformycin in resting lymphocytes. J Immunol 131:2762–2766

McGeorge MB, Russell EC, Mohanakumar T (1982) Immunologic evaluation of long-term effects of childhood ALL chemotherapy: analysis of in vitro NK- and K-cell activities of peripheral blood lymphocytes. Am J Hematol 12:19–27

Medzihradsky JL, Hollowell RP, Elion GB (1981) Differential inhibition by azathioprine and 6-mercaptopurine of specific suppressor T cell generation in mice. J Immunopharmacol 3:1–16

Medzihradsky JL, Klein C, Elion GB (1982) Differential interference by azathioprine and 6-mercaptopurine with antibody-mediated immunoregulation: synergism of azathioprine and antibody in the control of an immune response. J Immunol 129:145–149

Miller JFAP (1961) Immunological function of the thymus. Lancet II:748–749

Mills GC, Goldblum RM, Newkirk KE, Schmalstieg FC (1978) Urinary excretion of purines, purine nucleosides, and pseudouridine in adenosine deaminase deficiency. Biochem Med 20:180–199

Minato N, Reid L, Cantor H, Lengyel P, Bloom BR (1980) Mode of regulation of natural killer cell activity by interferon. J Exp Med 152:124–137

Moore EC, Hurlbert RB (1966) Regulation of mammalian deoxyribonucleotide biosynthesis by nucleotides as activators and inhibitors. J Biol Chem 241:4802–4809

Moreau JF, Ythier A, Soulillou JP (1981) Natural killer activity in kidney allograft recipients. Transplant Proc 13:1610–1613

Moreau JF, Soulillou JP, Ythier A, Hegaret A, Fauconnier (1983) Decrease in natural killer cell activity in kidney allograft recipients. Ann Immunol (Inst Pasteur) 134C:191–205

Murray JE, Merrill JP, Harrison JH, Wilson RE, Dammin GJ (1963) Prolonged survival of human-kidney homografts by immunosuppressive drug therapy. N Engl J Med 268:1315–1323

Murray JE, Barnes BA, Atkinson J (1967) Fifth report of the human kidney transplant registry. Transplantation 5:752–774

Nishida Y, Kamatani N, Tanimoto K, Akaoka I (1979) Inhibition of purine nucleoside phosphorylase activity and of T-cell function with allopurinol-riboside. Agents Actions 9:549–552

Ochs UH, Chen SH, Ochs HD, Osborne WRA, Scott CR (1979) Purine nucleoside phosphorylase deficiency: a molecular model for selective loss of T cell function. J Immunol 122:2424–2429

Ohnuma T, Arkin H, Minowada J, Holland JF (1978) Differential chemotherapeutic susceptibility of human T-lymphocytes and B-lymphocytes in culture. J Natl Cancer Inst 60:749–752

Osborne WRA, Scott CR (1983) The metabolism of deoxyguanosine and guanosine in human B and T lymphoblasts. A role for deoxyguanosine kinase activity in the selective T-cell defect associated with purine nucleoside phosphorylase deficiency. Biochem J 214:711–718

Otterness IG, Chang YH (1976) Comparative study of cyclophosphamide, 6-mercaptopurine, azathioprine and methotrexate. Relative effects on the humoral and the cellular immune response in the mouse. Clin Exp Immunol 26:346–354

Pedersen BK, Beyer JM, Rasmussen A, Klarlund K, Horslev-Petersen K, Pedersen BN, Helin P (1984) Azathioprine as single drug in the treatment of rheumatoid arthritis induces complete suppression of natural killer cell activity. Acta Pathol Microbiol Immunol Scand [C] 92c:221–225

Polmar SH (1980) Metabolic aspects of immunodeficiency disease. Semin Hematol 17:30–43

Polmar SH, Stern RC, Schwartz AL, Wetzler EM, Chase PA, Hirschhorn R (1976) Enzyme replacement therapy for adenosine deaminase deficiency and severe combined immunodeficiency. N Engl J Med 295:1337–1343

Prince HE, Ettenger RB, Dorey FJ, Fine RN, Fahey JL (1984) Azathioprine suppression of natural killer activity and antibody-dependent cellular cytotoxicity in renal transplant recipients. J Clin Immunol 4:312–318

Purves EC, Berenbaum MC (1975) Selective suppression of murine antibody-dependent cell-mediated cytotoxicity by azathioprine. Transplantation 19:274–276

Ramsey KM, Djeu JY, Rook AH (1984) Decreased circulating large granular lymphocytes associated with depressed natural killer cell activity in renal transplant recipients. Transplantation 38:351–356

Reinherz EL, Kung PC, Goldstein G, Schlossman SF (1979) Separation of functional subsets of human T cells by a monoclonal antibody. Proc Natl Acad Sci USA 76:4061–4065

Röllinghoff M, Schrader J, Wagner H (1973) Effect of azathioprine and cytosine arabinoside on humoral and cellular immunity in vitro. Clin Exp Immunol 15:261–269

Sampson D, Grotelueschen C, Kauffman HM Jr (1975) The human splenic suppressor cell. Transplantation 20:362–367

Schwartz RS, Stack J, Dameshek W (1958) Effect of 6-mercaptopurine on antibody production. Proc Soc Exp Biol Med 99:164–167

Seto S, Carrera CJ, Kubota M, Wasson DB, Carson DA (1985) Mechanism of deoxy-adenosine and 2-chlorodeoxyadenosine toxicity to nondividing human lymphocytes. J Clin Invest 75:377–383

Shih WWH, Ellison GW, Myers LW, Durkos-Smith D, Fahey JL (1982) Locus of selective depression of human natural killer cells by azathioprine. Clin Immunol Immunopathol 23:672–681

Sidi Y, Mitchell BS (1984) 2'-Deoxyguanosine toxicity for B and mature T lymphoid cell lines is mediated by guanine ribonucleotide accumulation. J Clin Invest 74:1640–1648

Smith SR, Terminelli C, Kipilman CT, Smith Y (1979) Comparative effects of azathio-prine, cyclophosphamide and frentizole on humoral immunity in mice. J Immunopharmacol 1:455–481

Spaapen LJM, Rijkers GT, Staal GEJ, Rijksen G, Wadman SK, Stoop JW, Zegers BJM (1984) The effect of deoxyguanosine on human lymphocyte function. 1. Analysis of the interference with lymphocyte proliferation in vitro. J Immunol 132:2311–2317

Spina CA (1984) Azathioprine as an immune modulating drug: clinical applications. Clin Immunol Allergy 4:415–446

Sweny P, Tidman N (1982) The effect of cyclosporin A on peripheral blood T cell subpopulations in renal allografts. Clin Exp Immunol 47:445–448

Tedde A, Balis ME, Ikehara S, Pahwa R, Good RA, Trotta PP (1980) Animal model for immune dysfunction associated with adenosine deaminase deficiency. Proc Natl Acad Sci USA 77:4899–4903

Ten Berge RJ, Schellekens PT, Surachno S, The TH, ten Veen JH, Wilmink JM (1981) The influence of therapy with azathioprine and prednisone on the immune system of kidney transplant recipients. Clin Immunol Immunopathol 21:20–32

Thelander L, Reichard P (1979) Reduction of ribonucleotides. Annu Rev Biochem 48:133–158

Tidd DM, Paterson ARP (1974) A biochemical mechanism for the delayed cytotoxic reaction of 6-mercaptopurine. Cancer Res 34:738–746

Trotter JL, Rodey GE, Gebel HM (1982) Azathioprine decreases suppressor T cells in patients with multiple sclerosis. N Engl J Med 306:365–366

Ullman B, Gudas LJ, Cohen A, Martin DW Jr (1978) Deoxyadenosine metabolism and cytotoxicity in cultured mouse T lymphoma cells: a model for immunodeficiency disease. Cell 14:365–375

Van Buren CT, Kerman R, Agostino G, Payne W, Flechner S, Kahan BD (1982) The cellular target of cyclosporin A action in humans. Surgery 92:167–174

Waltzer WC, Bachvaroff RJ, Anaise D, Rapaport FT (1984) Natural killer activity after renal transplantation. Transplant Proc 16:1527–1529

Willemot J, Martineau R, DesRosiers C, Kelly S, Létourneau J, Lalanne M (1979) Inhibition of purine nucleoside phosphorylase and mitogen-stimulated transformation in immunocompetent murine spleen cells by formycin B. Life Sci 25:1215–1222

Wilson DB (1965) Quantitative studies on the behavior of sensitized lymphocytes in vitro II. Inhibitory influence of the immune suppressor, Imuran, on the destructive reaction of sensitized lymphoid cells against homologous target cells. J Exp Med 122:167–172

Wolberg G, Zimmerman TP, Hiemstra K, Winston M, Chu LC (1975) Adenosine inhibition of lymphocyte-mediated cytolysis: Possible role of cyclic adenosine monophosphate. Science 187:957–959

CHAPTER 24

Isoprinosine and NPT 15392:
Hypoxanthine-Containing Immunomodulators

J. GORDON and TH. GINSBERG

A. Isoprinosine

Isoprinosine (inosine pranobex, INPX) is an immunopharmacologic agent which has demonstrated an enhancing effect on the function and number of various cells of the immune system, particularly the T lymphocyte, in numerous in vitro and in vivo studies. These drug effects on the host immune response have been associated with clinical benefit to patients with seemingly unrelated conditions characterized by acquired immunodeficiency, such as viral infections, burns, surgery, recurrent infections, and pre-AIDS. This chapter will review the chemistry, toxicology, and pharmacology of INPX, and will discuss the in vitro animal and human studies that establish INPX as an immunomodulator of therapeutic importance.

I. Chemistry

INPX is a molecular complex of inosine and the p-acetamidobenzoic acid (PAcBA) salt of N,N-dimethylamino-2-propanol (DIP) in a 1:3 molar ratio (Fig. 1). Inosine is a naturally occurring substance found in the metabolic pathway of purines and in varying, but small, amounts in cells and tissue fluids. The PAcBA moiety is chemically related to p-aminobenzoic acid (PABA), a naturally occurring metabolite in human tissue.

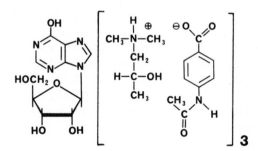

Fig. 1. Chemical structure of Isoprinosine (inosiplex, inosine pranobex, INPX)

II. Pharmacokinetics and Bioavailability

1. Inosine Pharmacokinetics and Metabolism

The metabolism of the inosine component of INPX was determined with 8-^{14}C-inosine-labeled INPX in cats and rhesus monkeys, both p.o. and i.v. (Ginsberg et al. 1978 a; Ginsberg 1972; Ginsberg et al. 1978 b). The resulting pattern of metabolite distribution revealed rapid catabolism and excretion to the purine end product, allantoin. In monkeys, INPX administration resulted in excretion of equal quantities of uric acid and allantoin. Of particular importance is the metabolic lability of the inosine moiety of INPX, which has a half-life of 3 min (following i.v. administration) and 50 min (following administration p.o.) in rhesus monkeys.

In humans, the major excretion product of inosine is uric acid. Because inosine is rapidly catabolized, and because endogenous plasma inosine levels are variable, human metabolism of inosine from INPX has been evaluated by examining urinary uric acid levels and pooled serum uric acid levels. This data has been derived from a number of clinical studies in which patients were administered various dosages of INPX (Salo and Lassus 1983; Pachuta et al. 1974; Waldman et al. 1977; Schiff et al. 1978; Tsang P et al. 1985 b). Uric acid accounts for 30%–70% of the administered inosine. At a therapeutic dose of 4 g/day, about 60% of the male subjects had serum uric acid levels in excess of 7 mg%. Female volunteers receiving 6 g/day INPX had a mean elevation in serum uric acid of only 0.9 mg%. Even at levels that could be considered hyperuricemic, no evidence of pathologic signs or symptoms was noted. These increased serum uric acid levels returned to normal within 1–3 days of cessation of INPX administration for most subjects.

2. N,N Dimethylamino-2-propanol p-Acetamidobenzoate (DIP-PAcBA) Pharmacokinetics and Metabolism

PAcBA is excreted in urine mainly as the o-acylglucuronide conjugate in both rhesus monkeys and humans, and partially as a glycine conjugate PAcHA (p-acetamidohippuric acid) in monkeys (Ginsberg et al. 1978 b; Ginsberg 1972; Streeter and Pfadenhauer 1984; Nielsen and Beckett 1981). DIP is oxidatively transformed to the extremely polar N-oxide, and excreted in the urine of both humans and monkeys. Absorption of both DIP and PAcBA from solution is extremely rapid. Peak blood levels of DIP and PAcBA reached approximately 4 and 7 µg/ml, respectively 1 h after administration of 1 g INPX tablets. Elimination is also relatively rapid, with an elimination half-life of 50 min for PAcBA and 3.5 h for DIP, as measured by excretion of the unchanged drug components in the urine (Nielsen and Beckett 1981).

3. Bioavailability

The human bioavailability of INPX formulations has been evaluated by radiotracer methods following the administration of a single oral dose of 1 g in solution and also utilizing a crossover design and various dosage forms, including solution, tablets, and syrup. Absorption of INPX from solution was nearly quantitative as measured by 24-h urinary recovery of DIP and PAcBA (Nielsen and Beckett 1981). Urine recoveries from the tablet and syrup formulations were 84% and 77% for DIP, and 90% and 92% for PAcBA respectively.

III. Pharmacology

The preclinical pharmacology of INPX has been evaluated in six animal species. Over a wide range of doses administered p.o., i.v., i.p. or intraduodenally, INPX has no major pharmacologic effects. No neuromuscular, analgesic, sedative, antipyretic, or anticonvulsive effects were observed. Slight CNS depression and cardiovascular effects were noted at very high doses (Hadden J and Giner-Sorolla 1981).

IV. Toxicology

Studies to establish the safety of INPX in animals include acute, subacute, and chronic toxicity, teratology, fertility, reproduction, and carcinogenicity (Simon and Glasky 1978; Hadden J and Giner-Sorolla 1981; Chang and Heel 1981).

1. Acute Toxicity

INPX has an extremely low level of single-dose acute toxicity. In certain cases, the LD_{50} had to be otherwise estimated because doses high enough to result in sufficient animal mortality could not be achieved. Table 1 illustrates the acute toxicity of INPX in four species of animals and via three routes of administration.

Toxicologic signals observed in surviving high dose mice included labored breathing, decreased motor activity, and postmortem congestion of the viscera. In rats, toxic signs included flaccidity, decreased motor activity, prostration, and paralysis. Ataxia, reduced locomotion, mydriasis, and reduced pupillary reflexes were observed in guinea pigs. Toxic signs seen in cats were mydriasis, emesis, and defecation.

Table 1. The acute toxicity of INPX in various species

Animal species	Route of administration	No. of animals	Dosage (mg/kg)	LD_{50} (mg/kg)
Mouse	p.o.	110	1000–20000	10000–15000
	i.v.	50	500– 2000	1850
	i.p.	110	1000– 8000	3900
Rat	p.o.	90	3000–20000	14700
	i.p.	99	1000– 8000	3500
Guinea pig	i.p.	40	1500–10000	6400
Cat	p.o.	8	5000	> 5000

2. Subacute Toxicity

Subacute toxicity studies were conducted in the rat, the dog, and the monkey with doses of INPX ranging from 125 to 3000 mg/kg. Minor toxic effects were noted only at doses greater than 500 mg/kg p.o. in the rat and the dog. No toxic effects were observed in monkeys receiving 125–500 mg/kg INPX.

3. Chronic Toxicity

In a 2-year chronic toxicity study, rats (CD-Sprague-Dawley) were given saline solution as a control, and saline solutions of INPX, 375, 750, or 1500 mg kg^{-1} day^{-1} in their food. Food consumption, mortality, hematology, clinical blood chemistry, urinalysis, organ weights and ratios, and gross and microscopic pathology revealed no differences between the control and drug-treated animals. The only statistically significant effect was a decreased tumor incidence in the low dose INPX group compared with the control group.

Chronic toxicity was also evaluated in rhesus monkeys, with animals receiving saline solution as a control, and saline solutions of INPX, 375, 750, or 1500 mg kg^{-1} day^{-1} p.o. After 12, 18, and 24 months, no abnormalities were found in body weight, mortality, ECG, clinical chemistry, hematologic profile, urinalysis, ophthalmologic examination, and gross or microscopic pathology of the major organs.

4. Reproduction, Fertility, and Teratology

The effect of INPX on fertility and reproduction was evaluated in male and female Charles River albino rats with a control group and two test groups (500 and 100 mg kg^{-1} day^{-1}). The results revealed normal growth, weight gain, and behavior for all animals. Lactation, survival, live birth incidence, and progeny body weights were normal for all groups throughout the study.

In a second study, female albino rats were treated with INPX at 1000 mg kg^{-1} day^{-1} throughout the gestation period and for 21 days postpartum. No statistically significant effects on length of gestation, litter size, litter weight, male:female offspring ratio, or rebreeding capacity were observed. No teratogenic effects were observed in mice, rats, or rabbits treated with INPX at doses of 500–2000 mg/kg p.o. from days 6 to 15 or 6 to 18 of gestation. Positive control animals treated with thalidomide did experience teratogenic abnormalities.

5. Carcinogenicity

Studies have been conducted in NMRI mice and in Sprague-Dawley rats to determine the possible carcinogenic effect of long-term oral administration of INPX. Behavior and external appearance of the animals, feces, food and water intake, hematology, eyesight, hearing, dentition, and both macroscopic and microscopic examination at autopsy did not indicate any side effects of INPX. Microscopic examination revealed a comparable tumor incidence between the control and INPX groups, with no drug effect on the nature or location of tumors. Thus, INPX did not display any neoplastigenic properties, even at the highest dose level of 1500 mg kg^{-1} day^{-1}.

V. Pharmacodynamics

1. In Vitro Studies

HADDEN JW et al. (1976) were the first to report that INPX could influence the activity of a cell type which is intrinsically involved in the immune processes of the mammalian host. They showed that INPX enhanced phytohemagglutinin (PHA)-induced human peripheral blood mononuclear cell (HPBMC) proliferation, but had no effect in the absence of mitogen. Numerous reports have since appeared in the literature which corroborate or amplify those early results pertaining to augmentation of mitogen-induced proliferation by INPX in vitro (MORIN et al. 1980; HADDEN JW et al. 1977; RENOUX et al. 1979 b; OHNISHI et al. 1983; IKEHARA et al. 1981; SIMON and GLASKY 1978; RENOUX et al. 1977). This significant body of work has firmly established immunopharmacodynamics as the primary basis for the mechanism of action of INPX.

Recent studies have focused on the fundamental nature of the cell type responsive to INPX in mitogen and other putative assays of T cell immune function. It has been shown that preincubation of human T cells or T and B cells, but not B cells alone, with INPX resulted in an increased responsiveness to PHA (PASINO et al. 1982). Both autorosettes (cells of the T helper population capable of forming rosettes with erythrocytes obtained from the original cell donor) and active rosettes (T cells which form stable rosettes with sheep erythrocytes, SRBC), are increased by INPX in vitro (REY et al. 1983; WYBRAN 1978; WYBRAN 1980a; DE SIMONE et al. 1982b). The autorosette-forming cell (ARFC) is a T cell subset which is generally reactive with OKT4 monoclonal antibody (see Chap. 6). ARFC are therefore probably part of the T helper population, and by inference INPX is a potentiator of the activity of this subset in vitro. INPX at 50–100 µg/ml also accelerates the rate at which SRBC receptors reappear on trypsin-treated lymphocytes (GOMEZ et al. 1981; NEKAM et al. 1981).

Murine T cell differentiation is similarly influenced by INPX in vitro. IKE-HARA et al. (1981) demonstrated that Thy-1 antigenic presentation on null cells from the spleens of nude mice was maximally enhanced at an INPX concentration of 1 µg/ml. INPX also increases the number of T cells which can react with 5/9 monoclonal antibody, an antibody capable of identifying effector cells in allogeneic mixed lymphocyte culture (MLC) (WYBRAN 1978; DE SIMONE et al. 1982a; PASINO et al. 1982).

Other T cell subsets are similarly modulated by INPX in vitro. The activity of natural killer (NK) cells has been potentiated by in vitro INPX. It has been shown that INPX is as effective as interferon in stimulating NK activity in HPBMC (BALESTRINO et al. 1983). This phenomenon was time dependent, with maximal stimulation seen after 4 h coincubation of HPBMC with INPX. Adherent cells, but not interferon induction mechanisms, were required for this augmentation of NK cytotoxicity. In vitro INPX enhanced NK cytotoxicity directed at K-562 and melanoma (MM200) target cells, but only if suppressor macrophages were first removed from the effector cell population obtained from either normal or melanoma patients (HERSEY and EDWARDS 1984). TSANG KY et al. (1983) reported that incubation with INPX could potentiate depressed NK-mediated cytotoxicity in 17 of 18 lung cancer patients, 10 of 10 patients with breast adenocarcinoma, and 3 of 4 patients with diagnosed malignant melanoma.

The influence of INPX on other immunologically active, non-T cell populations has also been studied. In vitro INPX increased both macrophage mitogenic factor (MMF)-induced guinea pig macrophage proliferation as well as macrophage phagocytosis of *Listeria monocytogenes* in the presence of macrophage-activating factor (MAF) (HADDEN JW et al. 1979). Macrophage phagocytosis of SRBC was also enhanced by INPX (ZERIAL and WERNER 1981), as was the lymphokine-mediated phagocytosis and killing of *Listeria monocytogenes* by oil-induced guinea pig peritoneal macrophages (HADDEN JW et al. 1979). INPX can also potentiate each of the eosinophil-mediated defense mechanisms considered important in resistance to parasitic infection, including eosinophil chemotaxis against zymozan-activated human serum, cytotoxicity directed toward ^{51}Cr chicken erythrocytes, and Fc and complement receptor display (DE SIMONE et al. 1984b).

The immunopotentiating effect of INPX has also been demonstrated in cells obtained from individuals with various pathologic conditions. In fact, CAMPO et al. (1982a,b) reported data which suggest that only depressed immunologic functions are positively influenced by in vitro INPX. While INPX had little effect on mitogen-induced proliferation or rosette formation by lymphocytes from normal subjects, these functions were significantly enhanced for lymphocytes obtained from patients with cerebral neoplasia, from patients with carcinoma of the breast, stomach, or colon, and from patients with chronic exposure to radiation. Similar data have been generated by incubating INPX with HPBMC from normal subjects and from those seropositive for Epstein–Barr virus (EBV) (SUNDAR et al. 1985). While INPX enhanced lymphocyte responses to PHA for both normal and EBV-positive (EBV$^+$) individuals, only lymphocytes from EBV$^+$ subjects displayed increased responsiveness to EBV antigens in the presence of INPX. In addition, IPNX potentiated the reponse of HPBMC from EBV$^+$ subjects to autologous EBV-transformed lymphocytes in a mixed lymphocyte reaction (MLR), which translated into the enhanced generation of cytotoxic T lymphocyte killing of MLR stimulator cells. TSANG KY et al. (1983) found that in vitro INPX restored depressed Con A responsiveness, NK cytotoxicity (as discussed previously), and monocyte chemotaxis of mononuclear cells from patients with cancer (lung, breast, melanoma) to normal or near-normal levels. In another study by TSANG KY et al. (1985b), INPX at 100 µg per 10^6 cells per milliliter restored Con A-induced lymphocyte proliferation, NK activity, neutrophil chemotaxis, and interleukin-2 (IL-2) production to normal or near-normal levels in most of the 64 elderly (>65 years) subjects in the study.

These findings on the in vitro influence of INPX on lymphocyte function and phenotypic surface marker presentation have been extended to male homosexual subjects with either acquired immunodeficiency syndrome (AIDS) or AIDS-related complex (pre-AIDS). The immunomodulating effect of INPX was evaluated in this patient population, characterized by reduced T helper cells and impaired proliferative responses (TSANG P et al. 1984, 1985a,b). Incubation of INPX at 100 µg/ml with HPBMC from these patients resulted in significant increases, and in some cases, normalization, of lymphocyte proliferation responses to PHA and PWM (Table 2). The greatest increases were seen in patients with pre-AIDS. These data support the probable effect of INPX on cell surface

Table 2. Effect of isoprinosine on lymphocyte functions

	PWM-induced response			PHA-induced response		
	Without ISO	With ISO	Upward modulation[a]	Without ISO	With ISO	Upward modulation[a]
	(cpm × 10³)		(%)	(cpm × 10³)		(%)
Heterosexual control (n=118)	92.6	116.0	25.3	96.3	123.5	28.2
Homosexual males						
-PWM (n=22)	70.8	93.5	32.1	93.8	146.2	55.9
-PWM (n=52)	44.5	65.3	46.7	74.9	108.2	44.5
AIDS patients (n=23)	17.4	26.1	50.0	28.8	41.5	44.1

Percentage modulation = [(cpm with ISO − cpm without ISO)/cpm without ISO] × 100.

markers in this patient population, i.e., at an earlier stage of disease. POMPIDOU et al. (1985a) found that incubation of HPBMC from pre-AIDS patients with Isoprinosine at 100 µg/ml resulted in a significant increase in both the percentage and absolute number of T4$^+$ (T helper) lymphocytes.

2. In Vivo Animal Studies

Data consistent with the results obtained by incubating INPX with HPBMC from immunodepressed individuals have been generated in animal models of immunodeficiency. Cells obtained from animals given INPX, particularly animals with a depressed immune response, display enhanced immunologic function, and this effect is often associated with clinical improvement. IKEHARA et al. (1981) showed that in vivo INPX had a greater potentiating effect on mitogen responses in aging mice than in younger mice. Similar results were noted in hamsters displaying an age-related decline in cellular immune function, as manifested by a significant decrease in PHA proliferative response, NK cytotoxicity and monocyte chemotaxis, and increased suppressor cell activity. Weekly administration of INPX (5 mg/kg, i.p.) restored each of these immunologic responses to normal or near normal levels (TSANG KY et al. 1983).

Positive data has also been generated following the administration of INPX to laboratory animals experimentally implanted with tumor cells. After a single i.p. dose of INPX (2 mg/kg), Con A-induced lymphoproliferation, monocyte chemotaxis, and NK cytotoxicity were all increased in human osteosarcoma-bearing hamsters (TSANG and FUDENBERG 1982). CERUTTI et al. (1978) showed that INPX could enhance the antitumor effect of low dose beta interferon in mice inoculated with 10⁶ sarcoma 180/T6 tumor cells, with significant increases in mean survival time and final survival rate, and decreased tumor incidence. A 7-

day injection schedule of INPX at 50 mg/kg in mice immunized with irradiated L1210 leukemia cells prior to viable cell challenge provided substantial protection to animals subsequently challenged with 10^5 or 10^6 leukemia cells (RENOUX et al. 1979 a). BINDERUP (1985) has also evaluated the influence of in vivo INPX in animal models of depressed immune function, including rats suppressed with cyclophosphamide. INPX administered at 50 mg kg^{-1} day^{-1} p.o. for 14 days increased Con A-induced spleen cell responses by 74% in comparison with the controls, while 7 days treatment with INPX had no effect on this immunologic parameter.

3. Mechanism of Action

While the precise biochemical mechanism through which INPX modulates immunologic functions is not entirely understood, the molecular events associated with the in vitro and in vivo activation of immunocompetent cells by INPX have been illuminated in several recent studies. Data that support the action of INPX on surface receptors of T lymphocytes have been provided by recent in vitro work (POMPIDOU et al. 1985 b) in which cells infected with human immunodeficiency virus (HIV), the etiologic agent of AIDS, exhibited a 48% decrease in reverse transcriptase activity in PBL when virus and cells were coincubated with INPX at a concentration of 200 μg/ml. POMPIDOU et al. (1985 b) concluded that INPX is active against HIV during the first steps of viral infection of T helper cells, either

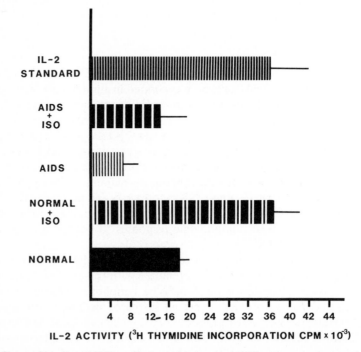

Fig. 2. Effects of in vitro INPX on IL-2 production in AIDS patients and normal controls ($n = 10$ for AIDS patients; $n = 30$ for normal controls). (TSANG KY et al. 1985 a)

at the stage of viral transduction through the cell membrane or by preventing incorporation of DNA in the nucleus. Data also indicate that HPBMC from normal subjects, the aged, patients with rheumatoid arthritis, systemic lupus erythematosus, or AIDS respond to in vitro INPX with increased production of interleukin 1 (IL-1) and/or interleukin 2 (IL-2) (NAKAMURA et al. 1983; HERSEY et al. 1984; TSANG KY et al. 1984a, 1985a,b, 1986a,b). LPS-stimulated adherent cells from the peripheral blood of normal humans have been shown by HERSEY et al. (1984) to produce increased quantities of IL-1 in the presence of INPX. Using a similar method, TSANG KY et al. (1986) have demonstrated that INPX potentiates IL-1 production by monocytes from both normal subjects and patients with AIDS.

These observations have been amplified by showing that Leu-3$^+$ T lymphocytes (helper/inducer) from both controls and AIDS patients absorbed more IL-1 and produced significantly greater quantities of IL-2 in the presence of INPX (TSANG KY 1984a, 1985a). In addition, Leu-2$^+$ cells (suppressor/cytotoxic T lymphocytes) responded to in vitro INPX with increased expression of Tac antigen, the putative IL-2 receptor on this T cell subset (see Chap. 2). The depressed production of IL-2 by lymphocytes from AIDS patients was nearly normalized in the presence of INPX (Fig. 2). It is therefore conceivable that these lymphokines, known to play a major role in immunoregulation and modulation, are responsible for triggering the molecular events that lead to the enhanced expression of immune function that has been observed in numerous in vitro and in vivo systems in which INPX has been studied.

VI. Clinical Efficacy and Safety

The immunopharmacologic effects of INPX on numerous cells of the immune system have found clinical application in the treatment of viral disease, particularly in the immunodeficient patient, and in conditions of diverse etiology characterized by an acquired immunodeficiency, such as severe burns, surgery, recurrent infections in the elderly, and pre-AIDS. The efficacy of INPX has been established in double-blind trials in herpes simplex virus infections (SALO and LASSUS 1983; BOUFFAUT and SAURAT 1980; BRADSHAW and SUMNER 1977), viral hepatitis (SCASSO et al. 1983), influenza (BETTS et al. 1978), and rhinovirus infection (WALDMAN and GANGULY 1978), as well as in subacute sclerosing panencephalitis (SSPE), a disease of the central nervous system associated with measles infection (JONES et al. 1982; HUTTENLOCHER and MATTSON 1979; MATTSON et al. 1975; DURANT and DYKEN 1983).

Of particular interest is a series of clinical trials which have demonstrated the efficacy of INPX as an immunomodulator in patients with acquired immunodeficiencies associated with HIV infection. A group of 157 male homosexual patients with pre-AIDS, or persistent generalized lymphadenopathy (PGL), were treated with INPX or placebo for 28 days and then followed clinically and immunologically for up to 1 year (TSANG P et al. 1985b; GLASKY et al. 1985). INPX-treated patients experienced significant enhancement of the initially depressed immunologic parameters, particularly NK cell activity, with drug effects persisting for up to 11 months after the cessation of treatment. Drug effects on total and

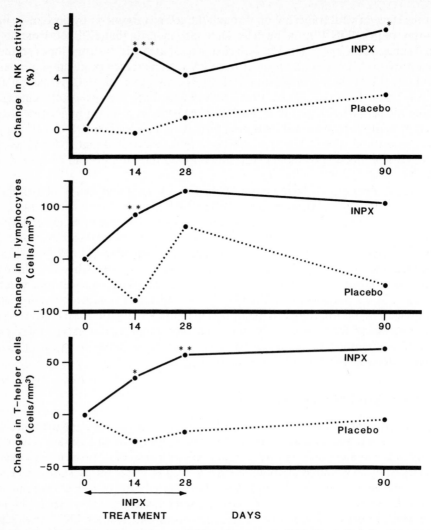

Fig. 3. Change in NK cell activitiy, total T lymphocytes, and T helper cells following treatment with INPX or placebo. *** $P<0.01$; ** $P<0.05$; * $P<0.10$

T helper lymphocytes, while of lesser magnitude and duration, support the concept that INPX is capable of promoting production of stem cells that can acquire the differentiated characteristics of one or more cell types, the first of which is the NK cell, followed by cells phenotypically identifiable as thymus derived (Fig. 3). Clinical benefit to the patients was associated with these immunorestorative effects, with fewer INPX-treated patients progressing to AIDS as compared with placebo-treated patients.

This correlation of enhanced immune response and clinical benefit has been demonstrated in other controlled trials in patients with different acquired immunodeficiencies. Severely burned patients, who typically experience an extremely

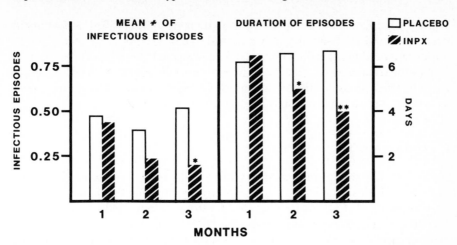

Fig. 4. Mean number and duration of urinary and respiratory infections in elderly subjects treated for 3 months with INPX ($n=25$) or placebo ($n=25$). * $P<0.005$; ** $P<0.001$. (MERONI et al. 1984)

high incidence of infection, when treated with INPX showed a reduction in mortality to 10%, as compared with 30% in the controls, and a reduction in septic complications to 40%, as compared with 90% in the controls (DONATI et al. 1983). This clinical improvement was associated with increased functional activity of polymorphonuclear leukocytes. CIRULLI and ROXAS (1980) and RONCONI et al. (1981) evaluated surgical patients immunologically by means of intradermal skin reactivity to a variety of antigens. Anergic/hypoergic patients were randomized to receive either INPX or placebo. The incidence of infection and mortality was significantly reduced by treatment with INPX, and the INPX-treated patients showed increased skin test responses. These findings were extended to a group of elderly patients suffering from recurrent upper respiratory infection (URI) or urinary tract infection (UTI) (MERONI et al. 1984). Both the frequency and the duration of URI and UTI were significantly reduced in the INPX-treated patients as compared with the placebo-treated patients, and skin test reactivity to *Candida* antigen increased in the INPX-treated patients (Fig. 4).

The only consistently reported side effect of INPX in humans is a mild and transient elevation of serum and urinary uric acid, owing to the conversion of the inosine moiety of INPX to uric acid through normal purine metabolic pathways. No clinical symptoms have been attributed to these increased uric acid levels. INPX has been administered continuously for periods of 2–14 years to seriously ill patients in relatively high doses: 3–4 g/day to patients with amyotrophic lateral sclerosis and 100 mg kg^{-1} day^{-1} to patients with SSPE (JONES et al. 1982). In these studies and in other long-term studies, a wide range of other drugs were used with no clinically significant side effects or drug interactions noted (GLASKY et al. 1975).

In conclusion, the enhancing effect of INPX on various cells involved in the host immune response, such as NK cells and T lymphocytes, has been associated with clinical benefit to patients with pre-AIDS, burns, recurrent infections, etc.

While the mechanism of action of the drug remains to be clarified, it possibly involves IL-1 and IL-2 and may play a central role in the molecular events that result in enhanced immune function. The data presented here support the use of an immunopharmacologic agent that affects some fundamental aspect of immunocompetent cells as an effective means of restoring immunity and controlling infection in a broad range of clinical indications.

B. NPT 15392

The purine-containing compound, erythro-9-(2-hydroxy, 3-nonyl)hypoxanthine (Fig. 5) is a 9-substituted hypoxanthine derivative in which the side chain is identical to that of EHNA (erythro-9-(2-hydroxy, 3-nonyl)adenine), a potent adenosine deaminase inhibitor. Although NPT 15392 is at a much earlier stage of development then Isoprinosine, there is sufficient information to warrant a discussion in this chapter. Several comprehensive reviews of the immunopharmacology of NPT 15392 have been published (HADDEN JW and WYBRAN 1981; HADDEN J and GINER-SOROLLA 1981; O'NEILL et al. 1984; TSANG KY et al. 1984b; SIMON et al. 1984).

I. Toxicology

Toxicity studies in mice and rats have shown a single-dose acute oral LD_{50} > 5000 mg/kg (HADDEN JW and WYBRAN 1981). Subacute toxicity was studied in rats and beagle dogs given 0.25, 1.0, and 2.5 mg/kg (up to 250 times the minimum effective dose) daily for 90 days. In rats, the only noticeable effect was a statistically significant increase in blood glucose after the highest dose. The elevated value was still within the normal range. Elevated bilirubin and total globulin were observed in female purebred beagles following the highest dose (SIMON et al. 1984).

Single-dose tolerance studies (0.7, 3.5, 7.0, 21, or 35 mg NPT 15392 per individual) have been conducted in human volunteers. The loss of small quantities of hair was the only reported effect possibly due to the drug, in some high dose subjects. No drug-related changes were seen in any clinical chemistry urinalysis or hematologic values, even at the highest dosage studied (HADDEN J and GINER-SOROLLA 1981). Volunteers in multiple dose tolerance trials, with 0.7 mg, 2.5 mg, and placebo on days 0, 3, 6, and 9 indicated no adverse effect and no changes in mean laboratory values outside normal limits (SIMON et al. 1984). A radioimmunoassay for NPT 15392 in blood and urine has been developed and used to eval-

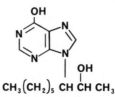

Fig. 5. Chemical structure of NPT 15392

uate samples from the multiple dose tolerance studies (PFADENHAUER et al. 1983). Values for 24-h urinary excretion following single oral administration of 0.7, 3.0, and 9.0 mg amounted to 28%, 9.6%, and 9.4% of the administered doses, respectively.

II. Immunopharmacology

1. Proliferative Response to Mitogens

SIMON et al. (1980) found that, in vitro, NPT 15392 consistently, but only moderately, augmented the Con A- and PHA-induced proliferation of mouse spleen cells. IKEHARA et al. (1981) established the optimal concentration range of NPT 15392 to be 0.1–1.0 μg/ml. HADDEN J et al. (1982) found that concentrations of NPT 15392 equal to or greater than 10 μg/ml resulted in inhibition of the proliferative responses of HPBMC, while lower concentrations had variable effects. The spleen cells of hamsters immunosuppressed with methotrexate showed an increased proliferative response to PHA following incubation with NPT 15392, while normal cells were not affected (TSANG KY and FUDENBERG 1982). DE SIMONE et al. (1984a) depleted HPBMC of $OKT4^+$, $OKT8^+$, and $OKM1^+$ cells by treatment with the respective monoclonal antibodies to these surface markers (see Chap. 6). They then studied the effect of NPT 15392 on the whole and on the depleted cell populations. On the basis of their results, they suggested that low doses of NPT 15392 principally affect the $OKT4^+$ cells, whereas relatively high doses act on a mixture of $OKT8^+$ and $OKM1^+$ cells.

In vivo administration of NPT 15392 to mice produced varied results, depending on the strain of mouse, conditions, and the status of the immune system in the animals. A single dose of 0.01 mg/kg resulted in significant augmentation of the Con A response of normal mice or mice immunosuppressed with Friend leukemia virus (SIMON et al. 1980). FLORENTIN et al. (1982a,b) found inconsistent effects on Con A responses and a consistent decrease of PHA responses following i.p. administration of NPT 15392 to BALB/c mice. TSANG KY et al. (1982) found that the proliferative responses of hamsters administered NPT 15392 varied according to the animals' initial immune status, with very young and aged animals (i.e., those initially immunodepressed) showing a greater increase in proliferative responses than mature animals.

Responses to the B cell mitogens, lipopolysaccharide (LPS) (IKEHARA et al. 1981) and dextran sulfate (FLORENTIN et al. 1982b) were also enhanced by in vivo NPT 15392. In these studies, immune status played a role in the magnitude of response to LPS: 18-month-old animals showed a 2.5-fold greater increase than 3-month-old animals. The effects of LPS were confirmed by VECCHI et al. (1980). Response to dextran sulfate was increased by as much as 100% following a single i.p. injection of NPT 15392. Adherent cells were necessary for the full drug effect (FLORENTIN et al. 1982b).

2. Effect on Suppressor Cells

In vitro incubation of human peripheral blood lymphocytes with NPT 15392 resulted in the induction of suppressor cells, as measured by responses to Con A or to allogeneic stimulation in a one-way mixed lymphocyte culture (HADDEN J et al. 1982). With NPT 15392 alone, maximal inhibition (30% suppression) occurred at 1 µg/ml. In combination with Con A or MLC, the respective suppression (41% and 61%) was enhanced by about 10%–20%, with maximal inhibition occurring at 0.1 µg/ml NPT 15392.

3. Effect on Plaque-Forming Cells

The augmentation of plaque formation by spleen cells (PFC) in the Mishel–Dutton or Jerne plaque assays (see Chap. 5) was demonstrated in vivo in mice receiving 0.3–3 mg/kg NPT 15392 (MERLUZZI et al. 1982). This T cell-dependent function was not observed when the T-independent antigen, TNP-LPS was used with similar dosage regimens, suggesting that the NPT 15392 effects on B cell activity are T cell mediated. FLORENTIN et al. (1982a) also used NPT 15392 in vivo in mice, and found maximum enhancement of PFC at 0.1 mg/kg NPT 15392, while higher or lower doses tended to suppress the PFC response.

4. Surface Marker Acquisition

The acquisition of the surface marker Thy-1 on immature T cells (prothymocytes) from the spleens of young athymic (nu/nu) mice was enhanced by incubation with NPT 15392 in vitro in the concentration range 0.1–10 µg/ml (IKEHARA et al. 1981). The acquisition of human T lymphocyte antigen (HTLA) by human prothymocytes was similarly enhanced by in vitro NPT 15392 (TOURAINE et al. 1982). NPT 15392 in vitro also increased the number of active rosettes formed with human T lymphocytes (HADDEN J et al. 1982). WYBRAN (1980b) reported augmentation of the percentage of active rosettes following in vivo administration of NPT 15392 to humans.

5. Cytotoxic Activity

FLORENTIN et al. (1982a,b) found that NPT 15392 increased the ability of spleen and peritoneal cells (NK cells) of mice to lyse YAC-4 tumor target cells. FAANES et al. (1980) confirmed in vivo enhancement of NK cell activity in mice, as did TSANG KY et al. (1982) in hamsters. MERLUZZI et al. (1982) demonstrated that NPT 15392 increased lymphocyte-mediated cytotoxicity by spleen cells immunized in vitro with allogeneic tumor cells. Combinations of NPT 15392 and interferon have at least an additive effect on NK cell activity (FLORENTIN 1982b).

6. Interleukin 2 (IL-2) Production

WIRONOWSKA-STEWART and HADDEN (1985) described the enhancement of PHA-induced IL-2 production by NPT 15392. DONNELY et al. (1986) have demonstrated the augmentation of Con A induction of IL-2 in vitro in human mononuclear cells. They suggest that this may be a central pathway by which NPT 15392 augments many lymphoid effector functions.

7. Autoimmunity

JONES et al. (1983) have shown that spontaneous development of autoimmune hemolytic anemia in New Zealand Black (NZB) mice is retarded in young mice administered NPT 15392. Levels of erythrocyte-specific antibody were reduced in older mice treated with NPT 15392. This suggests possible clinical utility of NPT 15392 in the treatment of autoimmune diseases.

III. Clinical Experience

Clinical experience with NPT 15392 is still limited. Patients with recently diagnosed cancer were treated with 0.4 or 0.7 mg NPT 15392 on days 0, 4, 7, and 10 of a phase II clinical study. Immune assays performed prior to, during, and following treatment showed that T lymphocyte counts, percentage of E rosettes, and autologous rosettes were augmented (WYBRAN 1982). MIKSCHE et al. (1982) found that NK cell activity was increased in patients in whom this parameter was initially depressed.

In summary, NPT 15392 has a number of properties similar to those of Isoprinosine, including a low degree of toxicity, yet its effects, in common with those of Isoprinosine, are produced by concentrations 10- to 100-fold lower. These effects occur over a narrower concentration range, with suppressive effects apparent at higher concentrations. The major cellular target of NPT 15392 appears to be the T cell, although indirect action has been demonstrated on B cells, macrophages, and granulocytes. It has been suggested that IL-2 induction may be connected with a number of lymphocyte effector functions of NPT 15392. COFFEY et al. (1984) have demonstrated that NPT 15392 is a potent and selective inhibitor of mouse lymphocyte cyclic GMP phosphodiesterase. They postulate that this property may be associated with its immunopharmacologic activities. Further clinical evaluation in human disease characterized by immunodepression or autoimmunity appears to be warranted.

References

Balestrino C, Montesoro E, Nocera A, Ferrarini M, Hoffman T (1983) Augmentation of human peripheral blood natural killer activity by methisoprinol. J Biol Response Mod 2:577–585

Betts R, Douglas JR R, George S, Rinehart C (1978) Isoprinosine in experimental influenza a infection in volunteers. 78th Annual meeting of American Society for Microbiology, 14--19 May 1978. Las Vegas, Nevada

Binderup L (1985) Effects of Isoprinosine on animal models of depressed T-cell function. Int J Immunopharmacol 7:93–101

Bouffaut P, Saurat J (1980) Isoprinosine as a therapeutic agent in recurrent mucocutaneous infections due to herpes virus. Int J Immunopharmacol 2:193

Bradshaw L, Summer H (1977) In vitro studies on cell-mediated immunity in patients treated with inosiplex for herpes virus infection. Ann NY Acad Sci 284:190–196

Campo M, Chiavaro I, Canfarotta C, Stivala F, Bernardini A (1982a) Effect of levamisole and methisoprinol on in vitro lymphocyte reactivity in chronically irradiated subjects and patients affected by neoplasias. J Immunopharmacol 4:127–137

Campo M, Chiavaro I, Petralia S, Bernardini A (1982b) In vitro lymphocyte sensitivity test to methisoprinol in different pathological conditions. J Immunopharmacol 4:109–126

Cerutti I, Chany C, Schlumberger JF (1978) Isoprinosine increases the antitumor action of interferon. Cancer Treat Rep 62:1971–1974

Chang T, Heel R (1981) Ribavirin and inosiplex: a review of their present status in viral diseases. Drugs 22:111–128

Cirulli G, Roxas MA (1980) Clinical evaluation of skin test responses in surgical patients treated with methisoprinol. Riv Gen Ital Chir 31:553–564

Coffey R, Hartley L, Hadden J (1984) Selective inhibition by NPT 15392 of lymphocyte cyclic GMP phosphodiesterase. Biochem Pharmacol 33:3411–3417

De Simone C, Canonica GW, Corte G, Meli D (1982a) Influence of methisoprinol on surface antigens of T lymphocytes. Curr Chemother Immunother 2:1161–1162

De Simone C, Meli D, Sbricoli M, Rebuzzi E, Koverech A (1982b) In vitro effect of inosiplex on T-lymphocytes. J Immunopharmacol 4:139–152

De Simone C, Cilli A, Zansoglu S, Pugnaloni I, De Santis S et al. (1984a) The effect of NPT 15392, 9-(erythro-2-hydroxy-3-nonyl)-6-hydroxypurine on the phytohemagglutinin of OKT3$^+$, OKT4$^+$, OKT8$^+$ and OKTM1$^+$ cell-depleted and undepleted peripheral blood mononuclear cells. Clin Immunol Immunopathol 33:191–198

De Simone C, Zansoglu S, Pugnaloni L, Sorice F (1984b) Role of methisoprinol in viral infection: influence of methisoprinol on eosinophilic granulocytes. In: Fudenberg HH, Whitten HD, Fabo A (eds) Immunomodulation: new frontiers and advances. Plenum, New York, pp 375–384

Donati L, Lazzarin A, Signorini M, Candiani P, Klinger M et al. (1983) Preliminary clinical experiences with the use of immunomodulators in burns. J Trauma 23:816–831

Donnely RP, Tsang KY, Bishop LR, Fudenberg HH (1986) Kinetic analysis of the immunopotentiating effect of the hypoxanthine analog, NPT 15392, on the interleukin-2 production potential of human lymphocytes. Int J Immunopharmacol 8:621

Durant RH, Dyken PR (1983) The effect of inosiplex on the survival of subacute sclerosing panencephalitis. Neurology 33:1053–1055

Faanes RB, Merluzzi VJ, Walker M, Williams N, Ralph P, Hadden J (1980) Immunoenhancing activity of NPT 15392: a potential immune response modifier. Int J Immunopharmacol 2:197

Florentin I, Kraus L, Mathe G, Hadden J (1982a) In vivo study in mice of the immunopharmacological properties of NPT 15392. In: Serrou B, Rosenfeld C, Daniels J (eds) Current concepts in human immunology and cancer immunomodulation. Elsevier, Amsterdam, pp 463–471

Florentin I, Taylor E, Davigny M, Mathe G, Hadden J (1982b) Kinetic studies of the immunopharmacologic effects of NPT 15392 in mice. Int J Immunopharmacol 4:225–234

Ginsberg T (1972) Urinary excretion of purine metabolites in *macaca mulatta* following administration of inosine and 1-(dimethylamino)-2-propanol, *p*-acetamidobenzoate. 5th International Congress of Pharmacology, 27 July 1972. San Francisco, CA

Ginsberg T, Simon LN, Glasky AJ (1978a) Isoprinosine: pharmacological and toxicological properties in animals. 7th International Congress of Pharmacology, 16 July 1978. Paris, France

Ginsberg T, Streeter D, Pfadenhauer E (1978b) Metabolism of the *N,N*-dimethylamino-2-propanol (DIP) and *p*-acetamidobenzoic acid (PAcBA) components of Isoprinosine in rhesus monkeys. 7th International Congress of Pharmacology, 16 July 1978. Paris, France

Glasky AJ, Pfadenhauer E, Settineri R, Ginsberg T (1975) A purine derivative: metabolic, immunological and antiviral effects. Combined immunodeficiency disease and adenosine deaminase deficiency, a molecular deficiency, a molecular defect. Academic, New York, pp 156–172

Glasky A, Gordon J, Hoehler F, Wallace J, Bekesi J (1985) Isoprinosine (INPX) in progressive generalized lymphadenopathy (PGL) – kinetics of action and clinical response. 3rd International Conference on Immunopharmacology, 6–9 May 1985. Florence, Italy

Gomez G, Lucivero G, Antonaci S (1981) Effect of methisoprinol on E-rosette formation by trypsin-treated lymphocytes. Boll 1st Sieroter (Milan) 60:302–306

Hadden J, Giner-Sorolla A (1981) Isoprinosine and NPT 15392: modulators of lymphocyte and macrophage development and function. In: Hersh EM, Chirigos MA, Mastangelo MJ (eds) Augmenting agents in cancer therapy. Raven, New York, pp 497–552

Hadden J, Hadden E, Spira T, Settineri R, Simon L, Giner-Sorolla A (1982) Effects of NPT 15392 in vitro on human leukocyte functions. Int J Immunopharmacol 4:235

Hadden JW, Wybran J (1981) Immunopotentiators. II. Isoprinosine, NPT 15392 and azimexone: modulators of lymphocyte and macrophage development and function. In: Hadden J, Chedid L, Mullen P, Spreafico F (eds) Advances in immunopharmacology. Pergamon, New York, pp 457–468

Hadden JW, Hadden EM, Coffey RG (1976) Isoprinosine augmentation of phytohemagglutinin-induced lymphocyte proliferation. Infect Immun 13:381–387

Hadden JW, Lopez C, O'Reilly, Hadden E (1977) Levamisole and inosiplex: antiviral agents with immunopotentiating action. Ann NY Acad Sci 284:139

Hadden JW, England A, Sadlik JR, Hadden EM (1979) The comparative effects of Isoprinosine, levamisole, muramyl dipeptide and SM1213 on lymphocyte and macrophage proliferation and activation in vitro. Int J Immunopharmacol 1:17–27

Hersey P, Edwards A (1984) Effect of Isoprinosine on natural killer cell activity of blood mononuclear cells in vitro and in vivo. Int J Immunopharmacol 4:315–320

Hersey P, Bindon C, Bradley M, Hasic E (1984) Effect of Isoprinosine on interleukin 1 and 2 production and on suppressor cell activity in pokeweed mitogen stimulated cultures of B and T cells. Int J Immunopharmacol 6:321–328

Huttenlocher PR, Mattson RH (1979) Isoprinosine in subacute sclerosing panencephalitis. Neurology 29:763–771

Ikehara S, Hadden JW, Good RA, Lunzer DG, Pahwa R (1981) In vitro effects of two immunopotentiators, Isoprinosine and NPT 15392, on murine T-cell differentiation and function. Thymus 3:87–95

Jones C, Dyken P, Huttenlocher P, Jabbour J, Maxwell K (1982) Inosiplex therapy in subacute sclerosing panencephalitis. Lancet II:1034–1037

Jones C, Lee C, Hoehler F, Koyama P, Skinner W, Lamott J (1983) Observations on the immunomodulator NPT 15392 in New Zealand black mice. Int J Immunopharmacol 5:85–90

Mattson RH, Lott T, Fink AJ (1975) Treatment of SSPE with inosiplex. Arch Neurol 32:503

Merluzzi V, Walker M, Williams N, Susskind B, Hadden J, Faanes R (1982) Immunoenhancing activity of NPT 15392: a potential immune response modifier. Int J Immunopharmacol 4:219

Meroni P, Palmieri R, Palmieri G, Froldi M, Zanussi C (1984) Effetto di un trattamento con methisoprinolo sulla frequenza e durata di episodi infettivi delle vie respiratorie ed urinarie in soggetti in età avanzata. Rec Prog Med 75:2–8

Miksche M, Kokoschka FM, Rainer H, Uchida A (1982) Augmentation of natural killer (NK) cell activity in cancer patients by NPT 15392. Int J Immunopharmacol 4:283

Morin A, Touraine JL, Renoux G, Hadden JW (1980) Isoprinosine as immunomodulating agent. Symposium of new trends in human immunology and cancer immunotherapy, 7 Nov 1980. Montpellier, France

Nakamura T, Miyasaka N, Pope RM, Talal N, Russell IJ (1983) Immunomodulation by Isoprinosine: effects on in vitro immune functions of lymphocytes from humans with autoimmune diseases. Clin Exp Immunol 52:67–74

Nekam K, Fudenberg HH, Mandi B, Lang I, Gergely P, et al. (1981) Resynthesis of trypsinized sheep red blood cell receptors on human lymphocytes: comparison of the effects of immunopotentiators of biological and synthetic origin in vitro. Immunopharmacology 3:31–39

Nielsen P, Beckett AH (1981) The metabolism and excretion in man of N,N-dimethyl-aminoisopropanol and p-actamidobenzoic acid after administration of Isoprinosine. J Pharm Pharmacol 33:549

Ohnishi H, Kosume H, Inaba H, Ohkura M, Shimada L et al. (1983) The immunomodulatory action of inosiplex in relation to its effects in experimental viral infections. Int J Immunopharmacol 5:181–196

O'Neill BB, Ginsberg T, Hadden J (1984) Immunopharmacology of the hypoxanthine-containing compounds Isoprinosine and NPT 15392. In: Kende M, Gainer J, Chirigos M (eds) Chemical regulation of immunity in veterinary medicine. Liss, New York, pp 525–541

Pachuta D, Togo Y, Hornick R, Schwartz A, Tominaga S (1974) Evaluation of Isoprinosine in experimental human rhinovirus infection. Antimicrob Agents Chemother 5:403–408

Pasino M, Bellone M, Cornaglia P, Tonini G, Massimo L (1982) Methisoprinol effect on enriched B and T lymphocyte populations stimulated with phytohemagglutinin. J Immunopharmacol 4:101–108

Pfadenhauer EH, Jones CE, Maxwell KW (1983) Radioimmunoassay of the immunomodulator erythro-9-(2-hydroxy-3-nonyl) hypoxanthine in human serum and urine. J Pharm Sci 72:914–917

Pompidou A, Delsaux MC, Telvi L, Mace F, Coutance F et al. (1985a) Isoprinosine and Imuthiol, two potentially active compounds in patients with AIDS-related complex symptoms. Cancer Res 45:4671–4673s

Pompidou A, Zaqury D, Gallo R, Sun D, Thornton A, Sarin P (1985b) In vitro inhibition of LAV/HTLV-III infected lymphocytes by dithiocarb and inosine pranobex. Lancet II:1423

Renoux G, Renoux JM, Guillaumin JM (1977) Un agent antiviral, l'Isoprinosine, stimule les responses immunes. Ann Immunol Inst Pasteur 128C:40

Renoux G, Renoux M, Guillaumin JM (1979a) Isoprinosine as an immunopotentiator. J Immunopharmacol 1:337–356

Renoux G, Renoux JM, Guillaumin JM, Gouzien C (1979b) Differentiation and regulation of lymphocyte population: evidence for immunopotentiator-induced T cell recruitment. J Immunopharmacol 1:415

Rey A, Cupissol D, Thierry C, Esteve C, Serrou B (1983) Modulation of human T-lymphocyte functions by Isoprinosine. Int J Immunopharmacol 5:99–103

Ronconi P, Bellantone R, Pittiruti M (1981) Treatment of anergy in the surgical patient using methisoprinol. Chir Patol Sperimentale 24:20–33

Salo O, Lassus A (1983) Treatment of recurrent genital herpes with Isoprinosine. Eur J Sex Trans Dis 1:101–105

Scasso A, Paladini A, Della Santa M (1983) Methisoprinol in the treatment of acute B viral hepatitis: controlled clinical study. Curr Ther Res 34:423–435

Schiff G, Roselle M, Young B, May D, Rolte T, Glasky A (1978) Clinical evaluation of Isoprinosine in artificially induced influenza in humans. Abstracts of the 78th annual meeting of the American Society for Microbiology, 14–19 May 1978. Las Vegas, Nevada

Simon L, Glasky A (1978) Isoprinosine: an overview. Cancer Treat Rep 62:1963–1969

Simon L, Settineri R, Pfadenhauer E, Jones C, Maxwell K, Glasky A (1980) NPT 15392: a pharmacological and toxicologic profile. Int J Immunopharmacol 2:200

Simon LN, Hoehler FK, Ginsberg T, Hadden JW (1984) NPT 15392, a new chemically defined biological response modifier. In: Fenichel RL, Chirigos MA (eds) Immune modulation agents and their mechanisms. Dekker, New York, pp 475–486

Streeter D, Pfadenhauer E (1984) Inosiplex: metabolism and excretion of the dimethylaminoisopropanol and p-acetamidobenzoic acid components in rhesus monkeys. Drug Metab Dispos 12:199–203

Sundar SK, Barile G, Menezes J (1985) Isoprinosine enhances the activation of sensitized lymphocytes by Epstein-Barr virus antigens. Int J Immunopharmacol 7:187–192

Touraine JL, Touraine F, Sanudji K, Ferrett G, Fournie G (1982) Isoprinosine and NPT 15392: effects on T-cell suppressor activity in vitro and in vivo. Int J Immunopharmacol 4:287

Tsang KY, Fudenberg HH (1981) Isoprinosine as an immunopotentiator in an animal model of human osteosarcoma. Int J Immunopharmacol 3:383–389

Tsang KY, Fudenberg HH (1982) In vitro modulation of virus susceptibility by Isoprinosine and NPT 15392. Clin Res 30:564A

Tsang KY, Phillips CB, Gnagy MJ, Fudenberg HH (1982) In vivo and in vitro effects of NPT 15392 on the immune response of hamsters. Fed Proc 41:812

Tsang KY, Fudenberg HH, Gnagy MJ (1983) Restoration of immune responses of aging hamsters by treatment with Isoprinosine. J Clin Invest 71:1750–1755

Tsang KY, Fudenberg HH, Galbraith GMP (1984a) In vitro augmentation of interleukin-2 production and lymphocytes with the Tac antigen marker in patients with AIDS. N Engl J Med 310:987

Tsang KY, Fudenberg HH, Hoehler FK, Hadden JW (1984b) Immunostimulating compounds; Isoprinosine and NPT 15392. In: Fenichel RL, Chirigos MA (eds) Immune modulation agents and their mechanisms. Dekker, New York, pp 79–95

Tsang KY, Fudenberg HH, Galbraith GMP, Donnelly RP, Bishop LR et al. (1985a) Partial restoration of impaired interleukin-2 production and Tac antigen (putative interleukin-2 receptor) expression in AIDS patients by Isoprinosine treatment in vitro. J Clin Invest 75:1538–1544

Tsang KY, Pan JF, Swanger DL, Fudenberg HH (1985b) In vitro restoration of immune responses in aging humans by Isoprinosine. Int J Immunopharm 7:199–206

Tsang KY, Boutin B, Pathak S, Donnelly R, Koopman W, Fleck R, Miribel L, Arnaud L (1986a) Effect of isoprinosine on sialylation of interleukin-2. Immunol Lett 12:195–200

Tsang KY, Donnelly RP, Galbraith GMP, Fudenberg HH (1986b) Isoprinosine effects on interleukin-1 production in acquired immune deficiency syndrome (AIDS). Int J Immunopharmacol 8:437–442

Tsang P, Tangnavard K, Solomon S, Bekesi G (1984) Modulation of T- and B-lymphocyte functions by Isoprinosine in homosexual subjects with prodromata and in patients with acquired immune deficiency syndrome (AIDS). J Clin Immunol 4:469–478

Tsang P, Lew F, O'Brien G, Selikoff IJ, Bekesi GJ (1985a) Immunopotentiation of impaired lymphocyte functions in vitro by Isoprinosine in prodromal subjects and AIDS patients. Int J Immunol 7:511–514

Tsang P, Warner M, Bekesi JG (1985b) Impaired B- and T-lymphocyte subsets and function restored by Isoprinosine in prodromal homosexuals and AIDS patients. Cancer Dectect Prev 8:580

Vecchi A, Sironi M, Serraglia N, Mantovani A, Spreafico F (1980) On the immunomodulatory activity of NPT 15392: in vitro effects on mouse and human cells. Int J Immunopharmacol 2:204

Waldman R, Ganguly R (1978) Therapeutic efficacy of inosiplex in rhinovirus infection. ORL Allergy Digest 84:153–160

Waldman RH, Khakoo RA, Watson G (1977) Isoprinosine: efficacy against influenza challenge infection in humans. Curr Chemother 1:368–370

Wironowska-Stewart M, Hadden JW (1985) Effects of Isoprinosine and NPT 15392 on interleukin-2 (IL-2) production. Int J Immunopharmacol 7:613

Wybran J (1978) Inosiplex, a stimulating agent for normal human T cells and human leukocytes. J Immunol 121:1184–1187

Wybran J (1980a) Immunomodulatory properties of Isoprinosine in man: in vitro and in vivo data. Presented at Symposium on new trends in human immunology and cancer immunotherapy, 17–19 Jan 1980. Montpellier, France

Wybran J (1980b) Immunomodulating properties of NPT 15392 in man: in vitro and in vivo. Int J Immunol 2:201

Wybran J (1982) Immunomodulation of T cell and NK function by NPT 15392 in cancer patients. In: Serrou B, Rosenfeld C, Daniels J (eds) Current concepts in human immunology and cancer immunomodulation. Elsevier, Amsterdam, pp 471–482

Zerial A, Werner G (1981) Effect of immunostimulating agents on viral infections. Acta Microbiol Acad Sci Hung 28:325–337

CHAPTER 25

Bacterial and Fungal Products

H. Takada, J. Hamuro, and S. Kotani

A. Bacterial Products as Mitogens and Immunomodulators

There are a number of immunomodulators of bacterial origin, most of which activate lymphocytes in a variety of ways (Table 1). Many bacterial cell surface components activate lymphocytes, but little is known about the ability of bacterial exotoxins to stimulate lymphocytes, probably because the extremely high cytotoxicity of typical exotoxins such as diphtheria make it technically difficult to examine their stimulatory effects on immunologically competent cells, including lymphocytes.

In this chapter we will review the lymphocyte-activating effects of immunomodulating cell surface components, with particular emphasis on chemically well-defined compounds and synthetic compounds, and only cite references on the exotoxins. We will also speculate about the involvement of stimulatory effects of bacterial cell surface components on immunocompetent cells, particularly lymphocytes and macrophages, in the development of host defense mechanisms.

I. Bacterial Peptidoglycans

Peptidoglycan is a ubiquitous structural component of the cell walls of all bacteria, except *Mycoplasma*, L-forms, and *Chlamydia* (Figs. 1 and 2). Damais et al. (1975) were the first to report that peptidoglycan isolated from *Escherichia coli* and *Bacillus megaterium* exhibits mitogenic effects on splenocytes from nude mice as well as normal mice, while peptidoglycan from *Micrococcus lysodeikticus* (bacteria which lack adjuvanticity by themselves) unlike the previously mentioned peptidoglycan, did not induce lymphoblast formation. While Damais et al. (1975) reported that the lysozyme digest of *E. coli* peptidoglycan, a monomer of the peptidoglycan subunit, was unable to activate lymphocytes, subsequent studies revealed that peptidoglycans retained their mitogenicity after being digested by a cross-bridge (between *N*-acetylmuramyl peptide subunits) cleaving enzyme to a "polymer" of peptidoglycan subunits (Ciorbaru et al. 1976; Takada et al. 1979, 1980a). The question whether peptidoglycan monomers are mitogenic or not was elucidated by using synthetic *N*-acetylmuramyl-L-alanyl-D-isoglutamine (muramyl dipeptide, MDP), the minimum structure responsible for the adjuvanticity and other bioactivities of peptidoglycan (Fig. 2) (Ellouz et al. 1974; Kotani et al. 1975), and its analogs. MDP and its adjuvant-active analogs were weakly but significantly mitogenic, while adjuvant-inactive analogs were not (Takada et al. 1977, 1979; Damais et al. 1977, 1978; see also Chap. 22). Another

Table 1. Bacterial mitogens

B cell mitogens

I. Peptidoglycans and related compounds
   Purified peptidoglycans (Damais et al. 1975; Dziarski and Dziarski 1979;
   Takada et al. 1980b)/Water-soluble peptidoglycan fragments (Ciorbaru et al.
   1976; Takada et al. 1979, 1980b)/MDP (Takada et al. 1977; Damais et al. 1977)
II. LPS and lipid A
   LPS (Peavy et al. 1970)/Lipid A (Andersson et al. 1973)/Synthetic lipid A
   (Galanos et al. 1985; Kotani et al. 1985; Homma et al. 1985)
III. Outer membrane proteins (OMP)
   Endotoxin protein (Sultzer and Goodman 1976)/Lipid A associated protein
   (Morrison et al. 1976)/Lipoprotein (Bessler and Ottenbreit 1977)/
   Porin (Chen et al. 1980; Mohri et al. 1982)
IV. Lipoteichoic acids (LTA) and related amphiphiles
   LTA prepared from *Streptococcus mutans, Streptococcus sanguis,* and
   Streptococcus pyogenes (Hamada et al. 1985)/Lipopeptidopolysaccharide (LPPS)
   complex prepared from *Listeria monocytogenes* (Hofman et al. 1985)/An amphiphile
   prepared from *S. sanguis* (Yamamoto et al. 1985b)/Amphiphiles prepared from
   Mycobacterium tuberculosis, Mycobacterium bovis (BCG), *Nocardia rubra, Gordona
   aurantiaca,* and *Rhodococcus terrae* (Ikeda-Fujita et al. 1987)
V. Others
   Nocardia water-soluble mitogen (Bona et al. 1974)/Protein A (Forsgren et al. 1976;
   Romagnani et al. 1978)/Cytoplasmic membrane of *Staphylococcus aureus* L-forms
   (Takada et al. 1980)/Carbohydrate antigen of *S. mutans* (Hamada et al. 1981)/
   A cell wall component of *Actinomyces viscosus* (Kimura et al. 1983)/Mycoplasma
   mitogen (Naot and Ginsburg 1978) Pertussis B mitogen (Ho et al. 1981)

T cell mitogens

I. Gram-positive bacteria
   Staphylococcal enterotoxin (Peavy et al. 1970; Archer et al. 1979)/
   Streptococcal pyrogenic exotoxin (Barsumian et al. 1978; Schlievert et al. 1979b)/
   Staphylococcal pyrogenic exotoxin (Schlievert et al. 1979a, b)/
   Protein A of *S. aureus* (Ringdén and Rynnel-Dagöö 1978; Nakao et al. 1980)
II. Gram-negative bacteria
   Pertussis toxin (Kong and Morse 1977a, b)
III. *Mycobacteriaceae*
   Trehalose dimycolate (TDM) (Kierszenbaum and Walz 1981)/
   Cell walls of mycobacteria, nocardia, corynebacteria (Azuma et al. 1976)/
   A mycolic acid (Azuma et al. 1977)

expression of stimulatory effects on B cells, polyclonal B cell-activating (PBA) effects of peptidoglycan in vivo as well as in vitro, were demonstrated by Dziarski (1980, 1982 a,b) by using peptidoglycan from *Staphylococcus aureus.* In vitro PBA activity was also observed with MDP (Specter et al. 1977, 1978).

Although there have been no reports that bacterial peptidoglycan or synthetic MDP is mitogenic on murine T lymphocytes, a cell transfer study in mice demonstrated that T cells were target cells in the antigen-specific immunopotentiation by MDP (Löwy et al. 1977; Sugimoto et al. 1978).

There have also been many studies indicating that MDP activates macrophages (for review see Leclerc and Chedid 1982; see also Chap. 22), and there

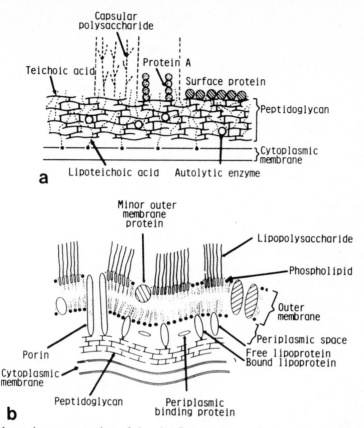

Fig. 1. Schematic representation of the ultrafine structure of cell surface layers of gram-positive (**a**) and gram-negative (**b**) bacteria. (HAMMON et al. 1984)

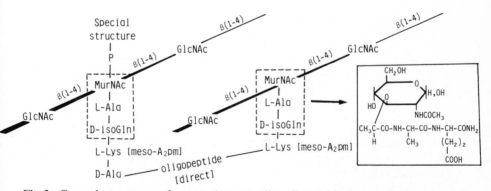

Fig. 2. General structures of group A type cell wall peptidoglycans (SCHLEIFER and KANDLER 1972) of the L-lysine type (*Staphylococcus aureus, Streptococcus pyogenes*, etc.) and those of 2,6-diaminopimelic acid type (*Escherichia coli, Mycobacterium tuberculosis, Lactobacillus plantarum*, etc.). *Boxes*, indicate *N*-acetylmuramyl-L-alanyl-D-isoglutamine (MDP) as the key component of peptidoglycans. MurNAc *N*-acetylmuramic acid; GlcNAc *N*-acetylglucosamine; L-Ala L-alanine; D-isoGln D-isoglutamine; L-Lys L-lysine; *meso*-A_2pm *meso*-2,6-diaminopimelic acid

seem to be agreement that macrophages play a more important role than lymphocytes in the various manifestations of the different bioactivities of MDP (and peptidoglycan) through generation of monokines such as interleukin-1 (IL-1)
(Chedid 1983; Leclerc and Chedid 1984).

II. Endotoxic Lipopolysaccharide and Lipid A

Lipopolysaccharide (LPS) is the ubiquitous component of the outer membrane
of gram-negative bacteria (see Fig. 1) and possesses endotoxic and numerous
other bioactivities (for review see Galanos et al. 1977). Since the in vivo study
of Takano and Mizuno (1968) and the in vitro study of Peavy et al. (1970), demonstrating the strong mitogenic effect of bacterial LPS on murine lymphocytes,
there have been a number of reports on the mitogenic effect of LPS. LPS is now
most frequently used as a standard B cell mitogen (Andersson et al. 1972). The
structure of the LPS molecule responsible for its mitogenicity has long been assumed to be located in the lipid A portion (Fig. 3; Andersson et al. 1973) where
most of the other bioactivities of LPS are located. However until recently, there
had been some ambiguity regarding the active bioprinciple of LPS because of its
complex molecular structure. The controversy was settled by studies with syn-

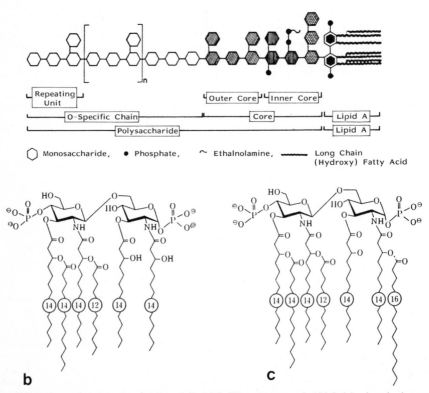

Fig. 3a–c. General structure of *Salmonella* LPS (Westphal et al. 1986) (**a**), chemical structure of *E. coli*-type (**b**) and *Salmonella minnesota*-type (**c**) lipid A, as verified by snythetic
and biologic studies

thetic lipid A preparations. *E. coli*-type synthetic lipid A (IMOTO et al. 1985) exerted full endotoxic and other bioactivities, including B cell mitogenicity and PBA activity, comparable to those of bacterial lipid A (GALANOS et al. 1985; KOTANI et al. 1985; HOMMA et al. 1985). LPS lacked the direct mitogenic effect on T cells (ANDERSSON et al. 1972), but much evidence suggests that LPS-T cell interaction plays an important role in the stimulation of antigen-specific immune responses (for review see MORRISON and RYAN 1979). The general view seems to be that the initial target cells for most, if not all, of the bioactivities of LPS and lipid A are macrophages (for reviews see MORRISON and RYAN 1979; RIETSCHEL et al. 1982).

III. Outer Membrane Protein

There are several reports on the powerful B cell mitogenicity of protein components associated with endotoxin, such as the endotoxin protein (SULTZER and GOODMAN 1976) and lipid A-associated protein (MORRISON et al. 1976). GOLDMAN et al. (1981) demonstrated that these proteins are identical to outer membrane protein (OMP) (see Fig. 1); that is, a mixture of porin, protein II, lipoprotein, and others. In fact, purified OMP fractions, including porin fractions, are mitogenic for murine B cells (BESSLER and OTTENBREIT 1977; CHEN et al. 1980; MOHRI et al. 1982). The porin fraction isolated from *Salmonella thyphimurium* G30/C21 (Re mutant) was also shown to enhance the cytocidal effect of macrophages from C3H/HeJ as well as C3H/HeN mice on the allogeneic sarcoma 3T12 cell line (WEINBERG et al. 1983). Recently, we have demonstrated that a porin fraction of *Fusobacterium nucleatum* ATCC 10953 exhibited various immunobiologic activities: B cell mitogenicity, PBA activity, and macrophage-activating effects (enhancement of superoxide anion generation and glucosamine incorporation), in vitro and the stimulation of antibody production in C3H/HeJ and C3H/HeN mice in vivo (TAKADA et al., in press). These findings clearly indicate that OMP, represented by porin, acts as a powerful immunomodulator of bacterial cell surface origin.

IV. Lipoteichoic Acids and Related Amphiphiles

Lipoteichoic acid (LTA) is an amphipathic compound extractable from a wide range, but not all, of gram-positive bacteria by Westphal's phenol-water method which is routinely used for the preparation of LPS. This amphiphile is a linear glycerophosphate polymer which consists of 25–30 residues linked 1–3 by phosphodiester bonds. The glycerol residues are substituted variously with sugars in a glycoside linkage and D-alanine in an ester linkage. The phosphomonoester end of the polymer is covalently linked to a lipid (Fig. 4). Similarities of their physical properties (such as the solubilitiy in the aqueous phase of phenol-water mixtures and the coexistence of lipophilic and hydrophobic moieties in the molecules) to those of LPS prompted us to study their bioactivity (WICKEN and KNOX 1980). Some controversy exists regarding their stimulatory effects on lymphocytes. MILLER et al. (1976), who were the first to report on the mitogenicity of LTA isolated from *Streptococcus pyogenes* 1-RP41, did not detect any stimulatory effect on splenocytes from C3H/He mice. BEACHEY et al. (1979), on the other hand, reported T cell mitogenicitiy of LTA isolated from the same strain, and HAMADA

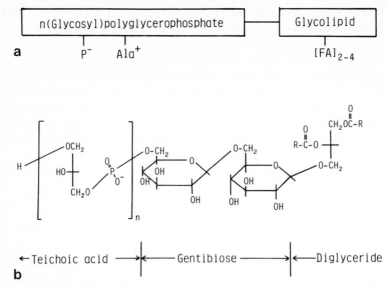

Fig. 4a,b. General structure of lipoteichoic acid (Wicken and Knox 1980) (a) and presumed chemical structure of the lipoteichoic acid of *S. pyogenes* (b). P phosphoric acid; Ala D-alanine; FA fatty acid

et al. (1985) reported the B cell mitogenicity of LTA from a different strain (Strain Sv). There are a few reports on immunomodulating activities of LTA. Friedman (1983) reported that streptococcal LTA enhanced antibody responses both in vivo and in vitro, and their activity was comparable to that of LPS. Yamamoto et al. (1985a) showed the ability of streptococcal LTA to induce tumor necrosis factor in *Propionibacterium acnes*-primed mice. Discrepancies among reported results on the mitogenicity of streptococcal LTA may partly be due to differences in chemical composition or molecular structure, which tend to change depending on growth conditions of the bacteria (Wicken et al. 1982), in view of the physiologic functions of LTA to control the autolytic processes of bacterial cells by acylation and deacylation (Cleveland et al. 1975).

With regard to biologically active amphiphiles other than LTA, Ikeda-Fujita et al. (1987) recently demonstrated that an aqueous phase fraction obtained from the phenol-water extracts of *Mycobacteriaceae* had remarkable bioactivities, partly similar to those of LPS, including strong mitogenicity and PBA activity on B cells. The chemical entity responsible for the bioactivities of this fraction has not yet been identified, but chemical analyses clearly show that the active agent is a novel amphiphile, consisting of a polysaccharide mainly composed of mannose and arabinose, a lipid made up of palmitic, stearic, and tuberculostearic (10-methylstearic) acid, and smaller amounts of glycopeptides, but containing neither 3-hydroxymyristic acid characteristic of LPS, nor muramic acid and 2,6-diaminopimelic acid peculiar to peptidoglycan. The latter finding makes this substance totally different from the previously described immunomodulators of bacterial origin. There is a possibility that the B cell mitogenicity of nocardia watersoluble mitogen (NWSM) reported by Bona et al. (1974) is at least partly due to the amphiphiles described here. The existence of a similar biologically active amphiphile (lipopeptidopolysaccharide complex) in *Listeria monocytogenes* has been reported by MÁRA et al. (1980) and HOFMAN et al. (1985).

V. Others

Cord factor or trehalose diesters, represented by α,α-D-trehalose 6,6′-dimycolate (TDM) (Fig. 5), is a toxic glycolipid located on cell surface layers of mycobacteria, nocardia, and corynebacteria. TDM is a powerful immunomodulator activating host defense mechanisms against tumor and microbial infections, and the target cells of the immunostimulating activities are assumed to be macrophages (LE-MAIRE et al. 1986). But there are only a few reports of its direct action on lymphocytes, probably because its high hydrophobicity makes it difficult to examine its bioactivity in vitro. KIERSZENBAUM and WALZ (1981) reported the mitogenicity of homogeneous suspensions (particle diameter 0.7–6.0 μm) in a cell culture medium on rat thymocytes and lymph node cells. This finding suggests the interaction of TDM and T cells. In this context, AZUMA et al. (1976) found that the cell walls of mycobacteria, nocardia, corynebacteria, and anaerobic coryneforms

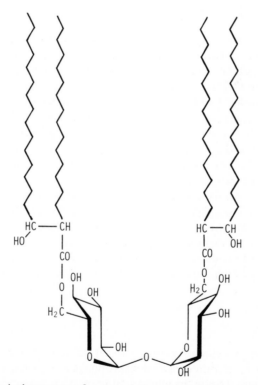

Fig. 5. General chemical structure of α,α-D-trehalose-λ-6,6′-λ-dimycolate (TDM) (LEMAIRE et al. 1986). Numbers of carbon atoms of mycolic acid residues are 30–38 for corynebacteria, 40–60 for nocardia, and 80–90 for mycobacteria

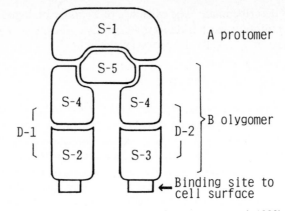

Fig. 6. Schematic structure of pertussis toxin. (After TAMURA et al. 1982)

were mitogenic for murine thymocytes. They also showed that the T cell mitogenicity of mycobacterial cell walls was carried by a mycolic acid moiety, not by peptidoglycan (AZUMA et al. 1977). SUGIMURA et al. (1977) further demonstrated that the T cell mitogenicity of *Nocardia rubra* cell walls required the presence of macrophages.

Pertussis toxin (pertussigen), which is a product of phase I (virulent) *Bordetella pertussis*, and probably originates in cell surface layers (MUNOZ and BERGMAN 1979), unlike other typical bacterial exotoxins, exhibits various unique pharmacologic activities which are described as follows: (a) sensitization of animals to histamine and other stresses (histamine-sensitizing factor, HSF); (b) induction of leukocytosis, especially lymphocytosis (leukocytosis- or lymphocytosis-promoting factor, LPF); and (c) increase of serum insulin level (activity as an islet-activating protein, IAP) (for reviews see MUNOZ and BERGMAN 1977; WARDLAY and PARTON 1983). This toxin, unlike the bacterial immunomodulators already described, is not a B cell mitogen, but a strong T cell mitogen (KONG and MORSE 1977 a,b). This mitogenicity is known to depend on the presence of mature B cells and to be suppressed by thymic T cells (Thy-1[+]) (HO et al. 1979, 1980). TAMURA et al. (1982) demonstrated that pertussis toxin is a hexamer, consisting of five types of protein subunit (Fig. 6). They demonstrated that the B oligomer moiety of the toxin was responsible for T cell mitogenicity (TAMURA et al. 1983). Pertussis toxin is also a powerful immunopotentiator (for review see MUNOZ and BERGMAN 1977).

VI. Speculation

A described in the preceding sections, a variety of cell surface components have been shown to be B cell mitogens and macrophage activators, and thus powerful immunomodulators, despite the marked differences in chemical composition and molecular structure. This tempts us to make the following speculation. Extremely long-range interactions between parasitic bacteria and host should have a major influence on the evolution of defense mechanisms of the host in two different ways. One is via the antigen-specific system (acquired immunity) which is carried by specialized immunocompetent cells, namely lymphocytes and macrophages. In this system, numerous fine, complex structures of bacterial cell surfaces, such as polysaccharide portions (0 antigens) of LPS from *Enterobacteriaceae* and type-specific M proteins of *S. pyogenes* are specifically recognized by antibodies and antibody-like molecules on lymphocyte surfaces, and the lymphocytes respond "monoclonally." A second system, probably older in evolutionary terms, and more primitive than the first, is antigen-nonspecific and is carried by almost all the host cells. These cells might recognize ubiquitous structures of bacterial cell surfaces, such as lipid A and peptidoglycan (MDP), and should respond "polyclonally." Consequently, the ubiquitous bacterial cell surface components not only activate lymphocytes polyclonally, but also stimulate the functions of almost every type of host cell, irrespective of their immunocompetence. Indeed, the pyrogenic (FELDBERG 1975; KOTANI et al. 1976; RIVEAU et al. 1980) and somniferous (KRUEGER et al. 1982 a,b; KRUEGER et al. 1987) activity of MDP and lipid A suggest that the central nervous system is capable of responding to these bacterial components. Moreover, as pointed out by LEDERER (1982) and CHEDID (1983), there is the possibility that these bacterial components are "digested" to appropriate structures and are used as "vitamins" or "endogenous immunomodulators" by mammals.

B. Fungal Polysaccharides as Immunopotentiators Against Cancer

There is reliable clinical evidence of the presence of intrinsic resistance of the human body to cancer, and experimental evidence indicates that the host possesses the ability to attack even autologous cancer through cell-mediated immune reactions. To clarify the mechanisms of this resistance and to find a substance that will increase it seems to be the most important means to develop new possibilities for immunotherapy in the treatment of cancer. Fungal polysaccharides from folk remedies said to be effective against cancer in Asian countries have been widely investigated in Japan. We found that lentinan, a polysaccharide extracted and isolated from *Lentinus edodes* (Berk.) Sing., a popular edible mushroom in Japan, exerted a strong growth inhibitory effect on sarcoma 180 transplanted into ICR or Swiss mice, resulting in almost complete regression of this tumor. Krestin, a glycoprotein extracted and semipurified from *Coriolus versicolor (Fr.) Quél*, which contains 36% protein as a component beside its β(1-4)glucosidic skeletal structure, is another such substance. Schizophyllan (SPG) is another active low molecular weight polysaccharide obtained by ultrasonication of the high molecular weight polysaccharide extracted from the culture broth of *Schizophyllum commune (Fr.)*. Among these three polysaccharides, krestin and lentinan have recently been approved as anticancer chemotherapeutic and immunotherapeutic agents by the Japanese Ministry of Health.

I. Lentinan

1. Antitumor Effects

In contrast to BCG, *Corynebacterium parvum*, and many other immunostimulants of polyanionic nature, lentinan is distinct: (a) in that it is a strictly chemically
defined polysaccharide sufficiently purified after extraction, and (b) in that its
physical and chemical characteristics have been completely clarified (Chihara et
al. 1970). Therefore, the biologic activity of lentinan is reproducible and no differences are observed from batch to batch.

Lentinan is a β(1-3)glucan with an average molecular weight of 500 000; its re-
peat unit is composed of five β(1-3)glucopyroside-linked branches (Chihara et
al. 1970; Sasaki et al. 1976). Thus, lentinan is composed solely of glucose with
no other sugar components. Elemental analysis verified the molecular formula as
$(C_6H_{10}O_5)_n$ consistent with structural elucidation, and no nitrogen, phosphorus,
or sulfur was detected. According to X-ray analysis, lentinan has a triple-helical
structure. The higher order structure or micelle formation in polysaccharide solution seems to have an important role in the biologic activity.

Lentinan exerts prominent antitumor effects on various allogeneic tumors in
animal models, and is devoid of direct cytocidal effects on these tumors when
tested in cell culture systems. Specifically, lentinan does not have any direct effects
on tumor cells in terms of their growth rate and DNA synthesis.

Table 2 shows the growth inhibitory effects of lentinan on syngeneic P815,
L5178Y, MM46, and MM102 tumors. The time of injection of lentinan seems to
be critical for significant antitumor activity in the MM10-C3H/He system, suggesting that the action of lentinan as an immunologic adjuvant depends on the
host-tumor immunologic status. In contrast, the activity of lentinan on the P815-
DBA/2 system is remarkable, regardless of the timing of administration. Interestingly, the later the injection of lentinan at the same dose and frequency, the
stronger is the growth inhibition of the P815 tumor. Optimal timing of administration appears to be 2–3 weeks after P815 transplantation. Results showing the
same tendency were also obtained in the L5178Y-DBA/2 and MM46-C3H/He
syngeneic systems. Why administration of lentinan at this period causes the
strong growth inhibition is at present unclear (Hamuro and Chihara 1985a).

Lentinan also showed growth inhibitory activity against other tumors such as
the Lewis lung carcinoma, B16 melanoma, SR-C3H/He sarcoma, and colon 26
in syngeneic murine systems, as well as the A/Ph,MC.SI fibrosarcoma produced
by methylcholanthrene in A/Ph(A/J) mice. Thus, immunogenetic analysis of the
hosts as well as of the common basis of host response to transplantation antigens
and tumor antigens should provide valuable information.

Lentinan, when administered together with cyclophosphamide, has also been
found to prolong by more than twofold the survival of C3H/HeN mice bearing
primary autologous tumors induced by methylcholanthrene. In this context, it
might be worthwhile to mention that lentinan prevents methylcholanthrene-induced carcinogenesis when it is administered before, or within 3 weeks after,
methylcholanthrene inoculation (83%–33%) (Shiio and Yugari 1980). Table 2
shows the antitumor and preventive effects of carcinogenesis by lentinan.

Table 2. The antitumor effects of lentinan in allogeneic, syngeneic, and autochthonous hosts and the prevention of carcinogenesis

Tumors[a]	Mice	Dose of lentinan (mg/kg)	Days of lentinan injection[b]	Tumor inhibition ratio (%)	Ref.
Allogeneic					
Sarcoma 180	ICR	1×10	1–11	100	CHIHARA et al. (1970)
CCM adenocarcinoma	SWM/Ms	1×10	1–11	65.3	MAEDA et al. (1973)
MM102 carcinoma	C3H/Arima	1×10	1–11	40.3	MAEDA et al. (1973)
NTF reticulum cell sarcoma	SWM/Ms	1×10	1–11	27.3	MAEDA et al. (1973)
Syngeneic					
A/Ph, MC.S1 sarcoma	A/Ph(A/J)	1×10	1–11	100	ZÁKÁNY et al. (1980)
Lewis lung carcinoma	C57BL/6	1×6	1– 7	59.3	SHIIO and YUGARI (1980)
EL4 lymphoma	C57BL/6	10×1	1	72	HAMURO and CHIAHARA (1984)
B16 melanoma	BDF$_1$	1×5	1– 6	50.7	SHIIO and YUGARI (1980)
MM46 carcinoma	C3H/HeN	5×2	13, 15	100	HAMURO and CHIAHARA (1984)
MM102 carcinoma	C3H/HeN	10×1	7	60	HAMURO and CHIAHARA (1984)
SR-C3H/He sarcoma	C3H/He	1×10	1–11	47.5	MAEDA et al. (1973)
P815 mastocytoma	DBA/2	5×4	8, 10, 15, 17	82	HAMURO and CHIAHARA (1984)
L5178Y lymphoma	DBA/2	10×3	7, 14, 21	89	HAMURO and CHIAHARA (1984)
Autochthonous					
MC-induced primary tumor	C3H/HeN	1×20	21–41[c]	>200% survival	SHIIO and YUGARI (1980)
Prevention of carcinogenesis		1×10	21–31	83–33[d]	SHIIO and YUGARI (1980)

[a] All tumors were solid forms implanted s. c.
[b] Tumors were implanted on day 0.
[c] 8-mm tumor diameter on day 0, when 100 mg/kg cyclophosphamide was injected.
[d] Determination at 30 weeks after methylcholanthrene treatment.

2. Antibacterial, Antiviral, and Antiparasitic Effects

When lentinan was administered to normal mice by i.p. injection, conspicuously enlarged lung granulomas were formed in response to either *Schistosoma mansoni* or *S. japonicum* eggs, or to antigen-coated polyacrylamide beads. Liver granulomas around cercariae of *S. mansoni* infections were augmented up to eightfold in volume. In contrast, athymic nude mice showed a complete absence of hypersensitivity granulomas. Lentinan-potentiated granulomas show a distinct histopathologic picture, characterized by frequent, extensive central necrosis, uncommon in unpotentiated schistosome foci (Byrum et al. 1979).

Recent studies have indicated that lentinan reduces the frequency of postchemotherapy relapse in experimental tuberculosis (Kanai et al. 1980). After termination of 5 months intensive chemotherapy (streptomycin, isoniazid, rifampicin), one group of mice received lentinan for 4 weeks and again for 4 weeks after a 1-month interval. The results indicate that the later multiplication of the latent bacilli was strongly reduced by lentinan treatment during the postchemotherapy period. Prophylactic effects of lentinan to prolong survival in vesicular stomatitis, virus encephalitis and Abelson virus infection have been reported (Chang 1981). Preventive effects on viral tumorigenesis by adenovirus type 12 have also been reported (Hamada 1981).

3. Immunologic Properties

In vivo application of lentinan causes increases in the levels of certain types of serum proteins, both acutely and subacutely (Maeda et al. 1974). One of the increased serum proteins is the functionally designated colony-stimulating factor (CSF) (Hamuro et al. 1982). On in vitro incubation of nylon wood column-purified splenic T cells with lentinan, CSF is released into the supernatant in amounts five times greater than the control. This CSF may then act on immunoregulatory Ia^+ macrophages to produce increased amounts of IL-1. The augmented production of IL-1 was also observed when peritoneal macrophages were incubated in vitro with lentinan, as assessed by the increased production of a factor mitogenic for thymocytes (see Chap. 7).

Recent studies clearly indicate that lentinan augments the generation of antigen-specific cytotoxic T lymphocytes (CTL) against alloantigen and hapten-conjugated syngeneic cells in vivo and in vitro (Hamuro et al. 1978 a,b). Thus, lentinan is an effective immunoadjuvant for both alloreactive CTL responses and H-2-restricted CTL responses specific to foreign antigens. As is well known, IL-1 can differentiate premature T cells into immunocompetent mature T cells (IL-2-producing and IL-2-responding T cells). From these results, it is suggested that lentinan augments the production of IL-1 by Ia^+ immunoregulatory macrophages directly and/or indirectly via CSF production from T cells.

Lentinan not only augments antigen-specific cellular immune responses, but can also trigger antigen-nonspecific immune responses against neoplastic cells. Lentinan and related substances with antitumor activity can induce cytotoxic peritoneal macrophages after intraperitoneal injection. In contrast, inactive polysaccharides show only a weak ability to induce cytotoxic macrophages (Hamuro et al. 1980). In spite of many experiments, all attempts to render normal or thio-glycolate-induced peritoneal exudate cells cytotoxic by the in vitro addition of lentinan have failed. Thus, lentinan is capable of rendering peritoneal exudate cells cytotoxic only under in vivo conditions, in contrast to most other immuno-adjuvants, which can render peritoneal exudate cells cytotoxic on in vitro incuba-tion. Lentinan does not cause elevated release of lysosomal enzymes from cul-tured macrophages, whereas most immunopotentiators do. The functions of lentinan-induced macrophages are thus distinct in many respects from macro-phages induced by other means.

Interestingly, lentinan augmented the reactivity of macrophages to one or more macrophage-activating factors (MAF), generated from activated T cells, re-sulting in the augmented generation of cytostatic and cytotoxic macrophages against tumor cells. In this context, macrophages stimulated by lentinan in vitro are neither cytotoxic nor cytostatic, but they possess elevated reactivity to MAF, one of the T cell-derived lymphokines relevant to the induction of effector mac-rophages.

As already mentioned, lentinan cannot render resident or stimulated macro-phages cytotoxic under in vivo conditions, so we suggest that the capacity of lenti-nan to induce in vivo cytotoxic macrophages is related to the ability of lentinan to activate the alternative complement pathway to produce C3b (which may then be the component required to render macrophages cytotoxic), or to the ability of lentinan to augment the reactivity of macrophages to activated T cell-derived MAF.

To elucidate the mechanism of action of lentinan to augment antitumor de-layed-type hypersensitivity reaction (DTH), we examined whether antitumor DTH was adoptively transferred into normal syngeneic C3H/He mice. Intrader-mal injection of tumor antigens with sensitized lymph node cells showed a signifi-cantly positive DTH only when recipient mice were injected with lentinan. Also, the results are consistent with the previously described interpretation that lenti-nan stimulates effector macrophages to show augmented reactivity to activated T cell-derived lymphokines (MAF) (HAMURO and CHIHARA 1985 b).

Lentinan-induced peritoneal macrophages showed no elevation of phagocytic activity compared with controls when harvested 7 days after injection of 0.1 mg lentinan. In contrast, the injection of zymosan or LPS markedly increased phago-cytosis by macrophages within 2 days of injection.

Thus, lentinan seems to be distinct from zymosan, LPS, and most other im-munoadjuvants, which act as reticuloendothelial system stimulants. Intravenous injection of lentinan at a dose of 10 mg/kg, at which dose lentinan exerted strong growth inhibitory actions against syngeneic murine tumors, did not increase car-bon clearance of macrophages harvested 2–7 days after injection in inbred mice (C3H/HeN, BALB/c, DAB/2, and C57BL/6). These findings indicate the absence of direct participation of the phagocytic function of macrophages in the appear-ance of the antitumor activity of lentinan.

It is well known that LPS, zymosan, poly(I:C), pyran copolymer, C. parvum, BCG, and most known immunoadjuvants cause elevated release of lysosomal en-zymes from macrophages when cocultured in vitro. However, lentinan is com-pletely devoid of this effect when tested on cultured macrophages.

When peritoneal macrophages were harvested from mice that had received intraperitonealy lentinan 4 days before, the spontaneous release of prostaglandin E and F (PGE, PGF) was strikingly reduced in resident macrophages (Hamuro et al. 1979). The diminished spontaneous release of both PGE and PGF was still apparent when macrophages were examined from mice that had received lentinan 8 days before. This effect is in contrast to that of *C. parvum* and BCG, which have been shown to induce a high spontaneous release of prostaglandins from spleen cells and peritoneal macrophages. This finding indicates a possible inverse correlation between the depression of prostaglandin release by lentinan-induced macrophages and augmentation by lentinan of T cell functions. Thus, it is possible that a decrease in inhibitory activities of prostaglandins may facilitate the cytotoxic action of T cells and/or macrophages in cell-mediated immune responses (see Chap. 15).

Recently, other antitumor immune effector cells, lymphokine activated killer (LAK) cells, have attracted attention. Lentinan administration (intraperitoneal, intravenous) synergizes with IL-2 in LAK generation. Thus, 10 mg/kg lentinan injected 1 day before lymphocyte harvesting prominently augmented the LAK generation measured by killing of EL4 and P815 tumor cells, as well as NK generation measured by cytolysis of YAC-1 and RL♂-1. Furthermore, a combination of lentinan with the chemotherapeutic agents, cyclophosphamide or tegafur (FT207) caused more efficient generation of LAK on in vitro exposure to IL-2 (Hamuro and Taki, unpublished).

4. Mode of Action

Lentinan augments the reactivity of precursor effector cells reponding to major lymphokines, such as IL-2, MAF, and B-cell growth factor (BCGF), and the generation of CTL, NK cells, LAK, activated macrophages, and antibody. Thus, lentinan exerts its effect on T cell-dependent immune responses by augmenting the generation of tumor-specific and tumor-nonspecific but selective effector cells triggered by T cell activation.

Lentinan triggers increased production of IL-1, either by direct actions on immune regulatory macrophages, or indirectly via augmented CSF production (e.g., from lentinan-stimulated alveolar macrophages). Thus, increased production of IL-1 results in the augmented maturation of premature lymphoid cells into mature cells capable of responding to lymphokines. Then, on stimulation by lentinan, mature cells are differentiated into effector CTL, NK cells, LAK, activated macrophages, and plasma cells in the presence of IL-2, to form an amplification loop to produce IL-1 (Fig. 7). Thus IL-1 generation may play a central role in increasing acute phase proteins or in increasing a unique class of serum proteins (see Chap. 7). Some of these increased serum proteins may then trigger or modulate the specific or nonspecific immune response.

In summary, lentinan is a neutral, well-characterized, purified, and nontoxic immunotherapeutic agent capable of positively influencing the immunologically specific limb of T cell-mediated cytotoxic immune responses, as well as the nonspecific limb of macrophage-, NK cell-, and LAK-mediated responses.

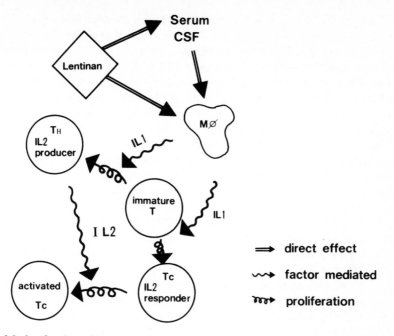

Fig. 7. Mode of action of lentinan. CSF colony-stimulating factor; Mφ macrophages; *IL-1* interleukin 1; *IL-2* interleukin 2; *T* T lymphocytes; *Tc* cytotoxic T cells; T_H helper T cells

II. Krestin and Schizophyllan

Krestin is now widely used clinically against cancer. One of the characteristics of krestin resides in the possibility of peroral administration to restore the suppressed cellular immune responses of tumor-bearing hosts to the level of normal hosts. When compared with the ineffectiveness of peroral administration of lentinan and schizophyllan, this distinct feature of krestin may be due to the presence of a large amount of protein in the compound. The other characteristics of krestin are that it shows direct cytocidal effects against neoplastic cells (rat hepatoma AH-13). In this context, it is noteworthy that krestin showed prominent, direct inhibitory effects against DNA and RNA synthesis of Ehrlich, sarcoma 180, EL4, P815, L5178Y, and other human transformed cell lines. It is still not certain whether the reported antitumor effects of krestin against murine allogeneic and syngeneic tumors are dependent on its immunorestorative activities, as the detailed studies on the immunologic activities of krestin are limited (e.g., when compared with studies on lentinan). Krestin suppresses the augmented suppressor T cell function during tumor progression, restores the depressed resistance against tumor-bearing hosts, and augments the production of interferon and IL-2 (TSU-KAGOSHI et al. 1984). Consequently, it is possible to imagine that the antitumor effects of krestin may be mediated by both direct cytocidal and immunorestorative activities.

Schizophyllan (SPG) is a β(1–3)glucan with an average molecular weight of 450 000; it also has β(1–6)glucosidic linkages, as does lentinan. In this context, SPG is physicochemically similar to lentinan, althouth its quaternary structure in solution is strikingly different. Antitumor effects of SPG have also been verified against various transplantable allogeneic and syngeneic tumors in animal models. Its tumor growth inhibitory and life span prolongation effects were mainly observed after subcutaneous and intramuscular injection. Similar to lentinan, SPG synergizes with other antitumor chemotherapeutic drugs, such as mitomycin C and 5-fluorouracil, and it prevents the carcinogenesis induced by chemical carcinogens such as mitomycin C and N-ethyl-N'-nitro-N-nitrosoguanidine.

The mechanism of action of SPG seems to be similar to that of lentinan, although there exist quite distinct differences between them. For example, as mentioned previously, lentinan does not augment the phagocytic activity of macrophages, whereas SPG does. In this context, SPG belongs to the family of reticuloendothelial system stimulants, such as BCG and zymosan. SPG does not elicit direct cytocidal effects against various neoplastic cells, and its antitumor effects are considered to be mediated by host immune surveillance mechanisms, because manipulations such as neonatal thymectomy, anti-lymphocyte serum treatment, and macrophage inhibitor treatment diminish the effects of SPG. However, it is not clear which effector cells may be driven by SPG.

References

Andersson J, Möller G, Sjöberg O (1972) Selective induction of DNA synthesis in T and B lymphocytes. Cell Immunol 4:381–393

Andersson J, Melchers F, Galanos C, Lüderitz O (1973) The mitogenic effect of lipopolysaccharide on bone marrow-derived mouse lymphocytes. Lipid A as the mitogenic part of the molecules. J Exp Med 137:943–953

Archer DL, Smith BG, Ulrich JT, Johnson HM (1979) Immune interferon induction by T-cell mitogens involves different T-cell subpopulations. Cell Immunol 48:420–426

Azuma I, Taniyama T, Sugimura K, Aladin AA, Yamamura Y (1976) Mitogenic activity of the cell walls of mycobacteria, nocardia, corynebacteria and anaerobic coryneforms. Jpn J Microbiol 20:263–271

Azuma I, Sugimura K, Yamawaki M, Uemiya M, Yamamura Y (1977) Mitogenic activity of cell-wall components in mouse spleen cells. Microbiol Immunol 21:111–115

Barsumian EL, Schlievert PM, Watson DW (1978) Nonspecific and specific immunological mitogenicitiy by group A streptococcal pyrogenic exotoxins. Infect Immun 22:681–688

Beachey EH, Dale JB, Grebe S, Ahmed A, Simpson WA, Ofek I (1979) Lymphocyte binding and T cell mitogenic properties of group A streptococcal lipoteichoic acid. J Immunol 122:189–195

Bessler WG, Ottenbreit BP (1977) Studies of the mitogenic principle of the lioprotein from the outer membrane of Escherichia coli. Biochem Biophys Res Commun 76:239–246

Bona C, Damais C, Chedid L (1974) Blastic transformation of mouse spleen lymphocytes by a water-soluble mitogen extracted from Nocardia. Proc Natl Acad Sci USA 71:1602–1606

Byrum JE, Sher A, DiPietro J, von Lichtenberg F (1979) Potentiation of schistosome granuloma by lentinan, a T-cell adjuvant. Am J Pathol 94:201–222

Changs KSS (1981) Lentinan-mediated resistance against VSV-encephalitis, Abelson virus induced tumor, and trophoblast tumor in mice. In: Aoki T, Urushizaki I, Tsubura E (eds) Manipulation of host defense mechanisms. Excerpta Medica, Amsterdam pp 88–103

Chedid L (1983) Muramyl peptides as possible endogenous immunopharmacological mediators. Microbiol Immunol 27:723–732

Chen YU, Hancock REW, Mischell RI (1980) Mitogenic effects of purified outer membrane proteins from *Pseudomonas aeruginosa*. Infect Immun 28:178–184

Chihara G, Hamuro J, Maeda YY, Arai Y, Fukuoka (1970) Fractionation and purification of the polysaccharides with marked antitumor activity, especially lentinan, from *Lentinus edodes* (Berk.) Sing. (an edibile mushroom). Cancer Res 30:2776–2781

Ciorbaru R, Petit JF, Lederer E, Zissman E, Bona C, Chedid L (1976) Presence and subcullular localization of two distinct mitogenic fractions in the cells of *Nocardia rubra* and *Nocardia opaca*: preparation of soluble mitogenic peptidoglycan fractions. Infect Immun 13:1084–1090

Cleveland RF, Holtje JV, Wicken AJ, Tomasz A, Daneo-Moore L, Shockman GD (1975) Inhibition of bacterial wall lysins by lipoteichoic acids and related compounds. Biochem Biophys Res Commun 67:1128–1135

Damais C, Bona C, Chedid L, Fleck J, Nauciel C, Martin JP (1975) Mitogenic effect of bacterial peptidoglycans possessing adjuvant activity. J Immunol 115:268–271

Damais C, Parant M, Chedid L (1977) Nonspecific activation of mouse spleen cells in vitro by a synthetic immunoadjuvant (*N*-acetyl-muramyl-L-alanyl-D-isoglutamine). Cell Immunol 34:49–56

Damais C, Parant M, Chedid L, Lefrancier P, Choay J (1978) In vitro spleen cell responsiveness to various analogs of MDP (*N*-acetylmuramyl-L-alanyl-D-isoglutamine), a synthetic immunoadjuvant, in MDP high-responder mice. Cell Immunol 35:173–179

Dziarski R (1980) Polyclonal activation of immunoglobulin secretion in B lymphocytes induced by staphylococcal peptidoglycan. J Immunol 125:2478–2483

Dziarski R (1982a) Preferential induction of autoantibody secretion in polyclonal activation by peptidoglycan and lipopolysaccharide. I. In vitro studies. J Immunol 128:1018–1025

Dziarski R (1982b) Preferential induction of autoantibody secretion in polyclonal activation by peptidoglycan and lipopolysaccharide. II. In vivo studies. J Immunol 128:1026–1030

Dziarski R, Dziarski A (1979) Mitogenic activity of staphylococcal peptidoglycan. Infect Immun 23:706–710

Ellouz F, Adam A, Ciorbaru R, Lederer E (1974) Minimal structural requirement activity of bacterial peptidoglycan derivatives. Biochem Biophys Res Commun 59:1317–1325

Feldberg W (1975) Body temperature and fever: changes in our views during the last decade. Proc R Soc Lond [Biol] 191:199–229

Forsgren A, Svedjelund A, Wigzell H (1976) Lymphocyte stimulation by protein A of *Staphylococcus aureus*. Eur J Immunol 6:207–213

Friedman H (1983) Immunomodulation by small molecular weight bacterial products. Adv Exp Med Biol 166:199–214

Galanos C, Lüderitz O, Rietschel ET, Westphal O (1977) Newer aspects of the chemistry and biology of bacterial lipopolysaccharides, with special reference to their lipid A component. Int Rev Biochem 14:239–335

Galanos C, Lüderitz O, Rietschel ET, Westphal O, Brade H, Brade L, Freudenberg M, Schade U, Imoto M, Yoshimura H, Kusumoto S, Shiba T (1985) Synthetic and natural *Escherichia coli* free lipid A express identical endotoxic activities. Eur J Immunol 148:1–5

Goldman RC, White D, Leive L (1981) Identification of outer membrane proteins, including known lymphocyte mitogens, as the endotoxin protein of *Escherichia coli* O111. J Immunol 127:1290–1294

Hamada C (1981) Inhibitory effect of lentinan on the tumorigenesis of adenovirus type 12 in mice. In: Aoki T, Urushizaki I, Tsubura E (eds) Manipulation of host defense mechanisms. Excerpta Medica, Amsterdam, pp 76–87

Hamada S, McGhee JR, Kiyono H, Torii M, Michalek SM (1981) Lymphoid cell responses to bacterial cell wall components: mitogenic responses of murine B cells to *Streptococcus mutans* carbohydrate antigens. J Immunol 126:2279–2283

Hamada S, Yamamoto T, Koga T, McGhee JR, Michalek SM, Yamamoto S (1985) Chemical properties and immunobiological activities of streptococcal lipoteichoic acids. Zentralbl Bakteriol Mikrobiol Hyg [A] 259:228–243

Hammond SM, Lambert PA, Rycroft AN (1984) The bacterial cell surface. Croom Helm, London

Hamuro J, Chihara G (1984) Lentinan, a T cell-oriented immunopotentiator – its experimental and clinical applications and possible mechanism of immune modulation. In: Fennichel RL, Chirigos MA (eds) Immune modulation agents and their mechanism. Dekker, New York, pp 409–435

Hamuro J, Chihara G (1985 a) Immunopotentiation by the antitumor polysaccharide lentinan. In: Hadden JW, Szentivanyi A (eds) The reticuloendothelial system, vol 8. Plenum, New York, pp 285–307

Hamuro J, Chihara G (1985 b) Lentinan, a T-cell-oriented immunopotentiator: its experimental and clinical applications and possible mechanism of immune modulation. In: Fenichel RL, Chirigos MA (eds) Immune modulation agents and their mechanisms. Dekker, New York, pp 409–436

Hamuro J, Röfflinghoff M, Wagner H (1978 a) β-1,3-Glucan mediated augmentation of alloreactive murine cytotoxic T-lymphocytes in vivo. Cancer Res 38:3080–3085

Hamuro J, Wagner H, Röllinghoff M (1978 b) β-1,3-Glucans as a probe for T-cell specific immune adjuvants: enhanced in vitro generation of cytotoxic T-lymphocytes. Cell Immunol 38:328–335

Hamuro J, Röllinghoff M, Wagner H, Seitz M, Grimm W, Gemsa D (1979) Depressed prostaglandin release from peritoneal cells induced by a T-cell adjuvant, lentinan. Z Immunitätsforsch 155:248–254

Hamuro J, Röllinghoff M, Wagner H (1980) Induction of cytotoxic peritoneal exudate cells by T-cell immune adjuvants of the β-1,3-glucan type lentinan and its analogues. Immunology 39:551–559

Hamuro J, Akiyama Y, Iguchi Y, Izawa N, Matsuo T (1982) Distinct roles of serum factor induced by T cell specific immune adjuvant lentinan in cellular immune responses. Int J Immunopharmacol 4:268

Ho M, Kong AS, Morse SI (1979) The in vitro effects of Bordetella pertussis lymphocytosis-promoting factor on murine lymphocytes. III. B-cell dependence for T-cell proliferation. J Exp Med 149:1001–1017

Ho M, Kong AS, Morse SI (1980) The in vitro effects of Bordetella pertussis lymphocytosis-promoting factor on murine lymphocytes. V. Modulation of T cell proliferation by helper and suppressor lymphocytes. J Immunol 124:362–369

Ho MK, Morse SI, Kong AS (1981) Studies on a new lymphocyte mitogen from Bordetella pertussis. I. Identification and polyclonal antibody formation. J Exp Med 153:75–88

Hofman J, Pospísil M, Mára M, Hříbalová (1985) Phenol-water extracts of gram-positive Listeria monocytogenes and gram-negative Salmonella typhimurium. Comparison of biological activities. Folia Microbiol 30:231–236

Homma JY, Matsuura M, Kanegasaki S, Kawakubo Y, Kojima Y, Shibukawa N, Kumazawa Y, Yamamoto A, Tanamoto K, Yasuda T, Imoto M, Yoshimura H, Kusumoto S, Shiba T (1985) Structural requirements of lipid A responsible for the functions: a study with chemically synthesized lipid A and its analogues. J Biochem 98:395–406

Ikeda-Fujita T, Kotani S, Tsujimoto M, Ogawa T, Takahashi I, Takada H, Shimauchi H, Nagao S, Kokeguchi S, Kato K, Yano I, Okamura H, Tamura T, Harada K, Usami H, Yamamoto A, Tanaka S, Kato Y (1987) Possible existence of a novel amphipathic immunostimulator in the phenol-water extracts of Mycobacteriaceae. Microbiol Immunol 31:289–311

Imoto M, Yoshimura H, Sakaguchi N, Kusumoto S, Shiba T (1985) Total synthesis of Escherichia coli lipid A. Tetrahedron Lett 26:1545–1548

Kanai K, Kondo E, Jacques PJ, Chihara G (1980) Immunopotentiating effect of fungal glucans as related by frequency limitation of post chemotherapy relapse in experimental mouse tuberculosis. Jpn J Med Sci Biol 33:283–293

Kierazenbaum F, Walz DR (1981) Proliferative responses of central and peripheral rat lymphocytes elicited by cord factor (trehalose 6,6'-dimycolate). Infect Immun 33:115–119

Kimura S, Hamada S, Torii M, Morisaki I, Koopman WJ, Okada H, Michalek SM, McGhee JR (1983) Lymphoid cell responses to bacterial cell wall components: murine B-cell responses to a purified cell wall moiety of *Actinomyces*. Scand J Immunol 17:313–322

Kong AS, Morse SI (1977 a) The in vitro effects of *Bordetella pertussis* lymphocytosis-promoting factor on murine lymphocytes. I. Proliferative response. J Exp Med 145:151–162

Kong AS, Morse SI (1977 b) The in vitro effects of *Bordetella pertussis* lymphocytosis-promoting factor on murine lymphocytes. II. Nature of the responding cells. J Exp Med 145:163–174

Kotani S, Watanabe Y, Kinoshita F, Shimono T, Morisaki I, Shiba T, Kusumoto S, Tarumi Y, Ikenaka K (1975) Immunoadjuvant activities of synthetic *N*-acetylmuramyl-peptides or -amino acids. Biken J 18:105–111

Kotani S, Watanabe Y, Shimono T, Harada K, Shiba T, Kusumoto S, Yokogawa K, Taniguchi M (1976) Correlation between the immunoadjuvant activities and pyrogenicities of synthetic *N*-acetylmuramyl-peptides or -amino acids. Biken J 19:9–13

Kotani S, Takada H, Tsujimoto M, Ogawa T, Takahashi I, Ikeda T, Otsuka K, Shimauchi H, Kasai N, Mashimo J, Nagao S, Tanaka A, Tanaka S, Harada K, Nagaki K, Kitamura H, Shiba T, Kusumoto S, Imoto M, Yoshimura H (1985) Synthetic lipid A with endotoxic and related biological activities comparable to those of a natural lipid A from an *Escherichia coli* Re-mutant. Infect Immun 49:225–237

Krueger JM, Pappenheimer JR, Karnovsky ML (1982 a) The composition of sleep-promoting factor isolated from human urine. J Biol Chem 257:1664–1669

Krueger JM, Pappenheimer JR, Karnovsky ML (1982 b) Sleep-promoting effects of muramyl peptides. Proc Natl Acad Sci USA 79:6102–6106

Krueger JM, Kubillus S, Shoham S, Davenne D (1987) Enhancement of slow-wave sleep by endotoxin and lipid A. Am J Phsyiol 251:R591–R597

Leclerc C, Chedid L (1982) Macrophage activation by synthetic muramyl peptides. Lymphokines 7:1–21

Leclerc C, Chedid L (1984) Immunomodulation of macrophages by muramyl peptides: recent findings concerning somnogenic activity of muramyl peptides and monokine. Int J Tissue React 6:213–218

Lederer E (1982) Immunomodulation by muramyl peptides: recent developments. Clin Immunol Newslett 3:83–86

Lemaire G, Tenu JP, Petit JF (1986) Natural and synthetic trehalose diesters as immunomodulators. Med Res Rev 6:243–274

Löwy I, Bona C, Chedid L (1977) Target cells for the activity of a synthetic adjuvant: muramyl dipeptide. Cell Immunol 29:195–199

Maeda YY, Hamuro J, Yamada YO, Ishimura K, Chihara G (1973) The nature of immunopotentiation by the antitumor polysaccharide lentinan and the significance of biogenic amines in its action. Ciba Found Symp 18:259–286

Maeda YY, Chihara G, Ishimura K (1974) Unique increase of serum proteins and action of antitumor polysaccharides. Nature 252:250–252

Mára M, Lurák J, Kotelko K, Hofman J, Veselská H (1980) Phenol-extracted lipopeptidopolysaccharide (LPPS) complex from *Listeria monocytogenes*. J Hyg Epidemiol Microbiol Immunol 24:164–176

Miller GA, Urban J, Hackson RW (1976) Effects of a streptococcal lipoteichoic acid on host responses in mice. Infect Immun 13:1408–1417

Mohri S, Watanabe T, Nariuchi J (1982) Studies of the immunological activities of the outer membrane protein from *Escherichia coli*. Immunology 46:271–280

Morrison DC, Ryan JL (1979) Bacterial endotoxins and host immune responses. Adv Immunol 28:293–450

Morrison DC, Betz SJ, Jacobs DM (1976) Isolation of a lipid A bound polypeptide responsible for "LPS-initiated" mitogenesis of C3H/HeJ spleen cells. J Exp Med 144:840–846

Munoz JJ, Bergman RK (1977) *Bordetella pertussis*. Dekker, New York

Munoz JJ, Bergman RK (1979) Mechanism of action of pertussigen, a substance from *Bordetella pertussis*. In: Schlessinger D (ed) Microbiology 1979. American Society for Microbiology, Washington, DC, pp 193–197

Nakao Y, Kishihara M, Baba Y, Fujita T, Fujiwara K (1980) Mitogenic response of human and murine T lymphocytes to staphylococcal protein A: not mediated by binding to cell surface immunoglobulins. Cell Immunol 50:361–368

Naot Y, Ginsburg H (1978) Activation of B lymphocytes by mycoplasma mitogen(s). Immunoloy 34:715–720

Peavy DL, Adler WH, Smith RT (1970) The mitogenic effects of endotoxin and staphylococcal enterotoxin B on mouse spleen cells and human peripheral lymphocytes. J Immunol 105:1453–1458

Rietschel ET, Schade U, Jensen M, Wollenweber HW, Lüderitz O, Greisman SG (1982) Bacterial endotoxins: chemical structure, biological activity and role in septicaemia. Scand J Infect Dis 31 [Suppl]:8–21

Ringdén O, Rynnel-Dagöö B (1978) Activation of human B and T lymphocytes by protein A of *Staphylococcus aureus*. Eur J Immunol 8:47–52

Riveau G, Mašek K, Parant M, Chedid L (1980) Central pyrogenic activity of muramyl dipeptide. J Exp Med 152:869–877

Romagnani S, Amadori A, Guidizi MG, Biagiotti R, Maggi E, Ricci M (1978) Different mitogenic activity of soluble and insoluble staphylococcal protein A (SpA). Immunology 35:471–478

Sasaki T, Takasuka N, Chihara G, Maeda YY (1976) Antitumor activity of degraded products of lentinan: its correlation with molecular weight. Gann 67:191–195

Schlievert PM, Schoettle DJ, Watson DW (1979a) Purification and physicochemical and biological characterization of a staphylococcal pyrogenic exotoxin. Infect Immun 23:609–617

Schlievert PM, Schoettle DJ, Watson DW (1979b) Nonspecific T-lymphocyte mitogenesis by pyrogenic exotoxins from group A streptococci and *Staphylococcus aureus*. Infect Immun 25:1075–1077

Shiio T, Yugari Y (1980) Antitumor effect of lentinan on syngeneic and autologous tumor-host systems, and suppression of chemical carcinogenesis. Int J Immunopharmacol 2:172

Shleifer KH, Kandler O (1972) Peptidoglycan types of bacterial cell walls and their taxonomic implications. Bacteriol Rev 36:407–477

Specter S, Friedman H, Chedid L (1977) Dissociation between the adjuvant vs mitogenic activity of a synthetic muramyl dipeptide for murine splenocytes. Proc Soc Exp Biol Med 155:349–352

Spector S, Cimprich R, Friedman H, Chedid L (1978) Stimulation of an enhanced in vitro immune response by a synthetic adjuvant, muramyl dipeptide. J Immunol 120:487–491

Sugimoto M, Germain RN, Chedid L, Benacerraf B (1978) Enhancement of carrier-specific helper T cell function by the synthetic adjuvant, *N*-acetyl muramyl-L-alanyl-D-isoglutamine (MDP). J Immunol 120:980–982

Sugimura K, Uemiya M, Azuma I, Yamawaki M, Yamamura Y (1977) Macrophage dependency of T-lymphocyte mitogenesis by *Nocardia rubra* cell-wall skeleton. Microbiol Immunol 21:525–530

Sultzer BM, Goodman GW (1976) Endotoxin protein: a B-cell mitogen and polyclonal activator of C3H/HeJ lymphocytes. J Exp Med 144:821–827

Takada H, Kotani S, Kusumoto S, Tarumi Y, Ikenaka K, Shiba T (1977) Mitogenic activity of adjuvant-active *N*-acetyl muramyl-L-alanyl-D-isoglutamine and its analogues. Biken J 20:81–85

Takada H, Tsujimoto M, Kotani S, Kusumoto S, Inage M, Shiba T, Nagao S, Yano I, Kawata S, Yokogawa K (1979) Mitogenic effects of bacterial cell walls, their fragments, and related synthetic compounds on thymocytes and splenocytes of guinea pigs. Infect Immun 25:645–652

Takada H, Hirachi Y, Hashizume H, Kotani S (1980a) Mitogenic activity of cytoplasmic membranes isolated from L-forms of *Staphylococcus aureus*. Microbiol Immunol 24:1079–1090

Takada H, Nagao S, Kotani S, Kawata S, Yokogawa K, Kusumoto S, Shiba T, Yano I (1980b) Mitogenic effects of bacterial cell walls and their components on murine splenocytes. Biken J 23:61–68

Takada H, Ogawa T, Yoshimura F, Otsuka K, Kokeguchi S, Kato K, Umemoto T, Kotani S (1988) Immunobiological activities of a porin fraction isolated from *Fusobacterium nucleatum* ATCC 10953. Infect Immun 56 (in press)

Takano T, Mizuno D (1968) Dynamic state of the spleen cells of mice after administration of the endotoxin of *Proteus vulgaris*. I. Cellular proliferation after administration of the endotoxin. Jpn J Exp Med 38:171–183

Tamura M, Nogimori K, Murai S, Yajima M, Ito K, Katada T, Ui M, Ishii S (1982) Subunit structure of islet-activating protein, pertussis toxin, in conformity with the A-B model. Biochem 21:5516–5522

Tamura M, Nogimori K, Yajima M, Ase K, Ui M (1983) A role of the B-oligomer moiety of islet-activating protein, pertussis toxin, in development of the biological effects on intact cells. J Biol Chem 258:6756–6761

Tsukagoshi S, Hashimoto Y, Fujii G, Kobayashi H, Nomoto K, Osita K (1984) Overview on the experimental studies of a polysaccharide preparation; krestin obtained from *Coriolus versicolor (Fr.) Quél.* with special reference to its clinical application. Cancer Treat Rev 11:131–136

Wardlaw AC, Parton R (1983) *Bordetella pertussis* toxins. Phramacotherapy 19:1–53

Weinberg JB, Ribi E, Wheat RW (1983) Enhancement of macrophage-mediated tumor cell killing by bacterial outer membrane proteins (porins). Infect Immun 42:219–223

Westphal O, Lüderitz O, Galanos C, Mayer H, Rietschel ET (1986) The story of bacterial endotoxin. Adv Immunopharmacol 3:13–34

Wicken AJ, Knox KW (1980) Bacterial cell surface amphiphiles. Biochim Biophys Acta 604:1–26

Wicken AJ, Broady KW, Ayres A, Knox KW (1982) Production of lipoteichoic acid by lactobacilli and streptococci grown in different environments. Infect Immun 36:864–869

Yamamoto A, Usami H, Nagamuta M, Sugawara Y, Hamada S, Yamamoto T, Kato K, Kokeguchi S, Kotani S (1985a) The use of lipoteichoic acid (LTA) from *Streptococcus pyogens* to induce a serum factor causing tumour necrosis. Br J Cancer 51:739–742

Yamamoto T, Koga T, Mizuno J, Hamada S (1985b) Chemical and immunological characterization of a novel amphipathic antigen from biotype B *Streptococcus sanguis*. J Gen Microbiol 131:1981–1988

Zákány J, Chihara G, Fachet (1980) Effect of lentinan on tumor growth in murine allogeneic and syngeneic hosts. Int J Cancer 25:371–376

CHAPTER 26

Nonsteroidal Anti-inflammatory Drugs: Effects on Lymphocyte Function

K. BRUNE

A. Introduction

The pioneering work of MORLEY (for review see MORLEY 1978) has indicated that prostaglandins (PG) are regulators of immune functions in vivo (see Chap. 16); nonsteroidal anti-inflammatory drugs (NSAID), on the other hand, are known to interfere with PG synthesis (VANE 1971). Consequently, experimental and clinical effects of NSAID on immune functions in vivo and in vitro have been postulated for more than a decade (for reviews see BRAY 1980; GOODWIN and WEBB 1980; GOODWIN and CEUPPENS 1983). Nevertheless, a clear-cut definition of the impact of NSAID at clinical dosage on immune functions is still lacking, and the contribution of these putative effects to therapeutic results remains elusive. Moreover, the experimental basis of assumptions about possible clinical effects remains meagre. The situation is very well described by GOODWIN and CEUPPENS (1983). They state in their review on *Regulation of the Immune Response by Prostaglandins* (p. 304):

By far, the most confusing area of research on PGE and immunity is comprised of those experiments dealing with the regulation of immunoglobulin production and suppressor-cell function by PGE. Not only are seemingly conflicting results reported by different groups using different assay systems, but directly contradictory results have been reported by different groups using the same assay system. In some instances both sets of contradictory data have been reproduced by yet other groups.

The pharmacologist is tempted to relate this apparent confusion, despite intensive experimental work, to two rather trivial aspects of NSAID (and consequently PG synthesis inhibition in the body) which are often not adequately taken into account – their typical pharmacodynamics, and their specific pharmacokinetics.

B. Principal Effects of Nonsteroidal Anti-inflammatory Drugs

NSAIDs are known to interfere with PG production (VANE 1971; FERREIRA and VANE 1978). It is less widely recognized, however, that these substances are by no means acting in well-defined ways on well-characterized receptors, but by more or less non-specific interactions with macromolecular structures (FLOWER 1974; BRUNE et al. 1976; HUMES et al. 1981; BRUNE and LANZ 1984). Consequently, these compounds interfere not only with the enzyme cyclooxygenase, but with the function of many other systems as well, as discussed by FLOWER (1974). Moreover, recent publications indicate that, for example, indomethacin, apart from blocking cyclooxygenase in inflammatory cells at concentrations of approximately 10^{-9} mol/l (BRUNE et al. 1981), interferes with cyclic AMP-dependent protein kinase at 10^{-8} mol/l (KANTOR and HAMPTON 1978), inhibits phosphodiesterase at 10^{-6} mol/l (CIOSEK et al. 1974a,b), and phospholipase A_2 at a similar concentration (ETIENNE and POLONOVSKI 1984). At the latter concentration, more effects are likely to be discovered. Knowing this, one is surprised that almost all experiments in vitro employ, for example, indomethacin at 10^{-6} mol/l or higher (e.g., EMERY et al. 1984; EZDINLI et al. 1986; GARIN and BARRATT 1982; GARIN et al. 1983; GOODACRE and BIENENSTOCK 1982; GREENE et al. 1983; HASLER et al. 1983; JOHNSEN et al. 1982; LECLERC et al. 1984; MACA and PANJE 1982; TILDEN and BALCH 1982). All of these papers have been published since 1980, when many workers had realized that PGs and NSAIDs may cause surprising effects, depending on the dose or concentration used (GOODWIN and WEBB 1980). Only a few publications report experiments in which non-specific effects of indomethacin due to too high concentrations ($> 10^6$ mol/l) were avoided (e.g., LAMMIE and KATZ 1983; DROLLER and GOMOLKA 1983), both these groups reported little or no effect of indomethacin on lymphocyte functions. In conclusion, it may be stated that most of the work on the effects of NSAID on lymphocyte functions in vitro employed concentrations at which no valid conclusion can be reached about the events observed. On the basis of these results extrapolations about clinical effects are not permissible because, while the peak concentrations of indomethacin observed in plasma are around 10^{-6} mol/l, these concentrations last only for short periods of time. In addition, the (active) free fraction of indomethacin in plasma or blood, i.e., at 100% serum concentration, is certainly lower (indomethacin is 99% bound to serum protein in vivo, HELLEBERG 1981) than under tissue culture conditions where such concentrations are likely to exceed the binding capacity of the small amounts of serum in the culture medium (BRUNE et al. 1981). In other words, 10^{-6} mol/l indomethacin in tissue culture is by no means comparable to 10^{-6} mol/l in vivo.

On the other hand, one central aspect of the pharmacology of NSAID, namely their pharmacokinetic behavior (BRUNE and LANZ 1985), is often overlooked. These compounds achieve comparatively high concentrations in certain body compartments, and consequently are likely to cause close to 100% inhibition of cyclooxygenase activity in these compartments only. These compartments are some areas of the gastrointestinal tract, the blood, the liver, the kidney, and inflamed tissue. This unequal distribution is likely to explain some organ-specific effects of NSAID on lymphocyte functions in vivo.

C. Effects on Nonsteroidal Anti-inflammatory Drugs on Lymphocytes

I. Clinical Observations

Some clinical effects on the immune system, believed to have resulted from the use of NSAID, are compiled in Table 1, together with comments (see also

Table 1. Clinical evidence attributing effects on lymphocytes to NSAID use

Effect observed	Drug used	Comments
Human, in vivo		
Reduction of RF concentration[a, b]	NSAID	No effect on NK cells and $T_4:T_8$ lymphocyte ratio[a, c]
Hampered delayed sensitivity reaction, improved[d]	Indomethacin	Effect not seen in healthy humans[e]
Enhanced titer after vaccination[e]	Indomethacin	Effect seen only with certain antigens[e]
Regression of cancer[f, g]	NSAID	Little evidence for specific effect on lymphocytes[h, i]
Human, ex vivo		
Enhancement of mitogen response of lymphocytes from aged[j, k], RA[m, n], Bartter Syndrome[o], or AIDS[p] patients	NSAID	Effect not observed[l] in RA patients
Suppression of the proliferation of maternal lymphocytes by newborn PBMC[q]	Indomethacin	NSAID do not cause fetus rejection
Animal, in vivo		
Enhancement of delayed hypersensitivity reactions[r, s]	Indomethacin	Effect not seen in healthy humans[e]
Allograft survival shortened[t]	Indomethacin	Not seen by other authors[u]
Enhancement of antitumor therapy[v]	Indomethacin	Indomethacin reduces effect of chemotherapy[w]
Animal, ex vivo		
Enhancement of NK activity[v]	Indomethacin	Acetyl salicylic Acid reduces NK activity in humans[x]
Enhanced number of PFC after SRBC[y]	Indomethacin	Opposite effect also reported[z]

FORRE et al. (1984)
GOODWIN et al. (1984)
SALMON et al. (1984)
GOODWIN et al. (1978a)
GOODWIN et al. (1978b)
PANJE (1981)
KARIM and RAO (1976)
LYNCH et al. (1978)
BRUNE (1985)

[j] HALLGREN and YUNIS (1977)
[k] HASLER et al. (1983)
[l] PALMER et al. (1982)
[m] PALMER et al. (1981)
[n] CEUPPENS et al. (1982)
[o] GARIN and BARRATT (1982)
[p] REDDY et al. (1985)
[q] JOHNSON et al. (1982)
[r] MUSCOPLAT et al. (1978)

[s] LIPSMEYER (1982)
[t] ANDERSON et al. (1977)
[u] FLOERSHEIM (1965)
[v] TRACEY and ADKINSON (1980)
[w] HOFER et al. (1980)
[x] GROHMANN et al. (1981)
[y] WEBB and OSHEROFF (1976)
[z] ROJO et al. (1981)

Chap. 16). As a whole, these observations indicate that under normal conditions, i.e., in healthy human beings or animals, the effects of NSAID on immune functions are very limited or not measurable at all (BACON 1984). This conclusion is in line with the clinical impression that there is no major impact of these drugs on the immune system in healthy humans. However, from these data, one also gets the impression that NSAID are contributing to an enhanced immune response in compromised patients or animals, i.e., patients treated with cytotoxic drugs, patients suffering from rheumatoid arthritis (RA), Bartter syndrome, or AIDS, and possibly many others. It may be speculated that this effect is related to reduced Ts cell function, owing to enhanced phagocyte activity leading to increased PG release (Morley 1978). Under these conditions, therapeutic doses of NSAID may not only improve the well-being of patients, but also slightly add to their immune functions. In addition, it appears that there is indeed a direct effect of NSAID on the production of rheumatoid factor (RF). If we accept that a major source of RF in rheumatoid patients is the enlarged pannus tissue (Smiley et al. 1968), and if, in addition, we take into consideration the unequal distribution of NSAID in the human body, leading to high drug concentrations in inflamed tissue (Brune and Lanz 1985), then it may be speculated that the local effects of high NSAID concentrations on T and B cell proliferation and activity in the inflamed joints of RA patients (compare Tables 2 and 3) may be the reason for the frequently described reduction of RF concentration owing to NSAID use. These clinical observations are paralleled by effects seen in experimental animals (see also Table 1).

Whether the anti-tumor effects of NSAID (Karim and Rao 1976; Lynch and Salomon 1979; Panje 1981), observed in humans and animals, are related to improved lymphocyte functions, or whether there are direct effects of high NSAID concentrations on the invasive growth of the tumor (Brune 1985) remains a matter of speculation (Goodwin and Ceuppens 1983).

II. T Cell Effects

Some of the many effects of NSAID on T lymphocyte functions, reported in the literature, are compiled in Table 2. Obviously, very high indomethacin concentrations have been employed, and some effects observed are not completely compatible with others reported in the literature. The picture that emerges, however, is that, at high concentrations, T cell activity may be enhanced by NSAID, possibly owing to a reduced production of inhibitory PG by adherent mononuclear cells in the lymphocyte population investigated (for review see Morley 1978; Goodwin and Webb 1980; Goodwin and Ceuppens 1983). Further experiments should try to dissect this indirect effect from the direct effects on the T cell which have also been claimed (Tilden and Balch 1982). A very detailed analysis of the indirect, i.e., eicosanoid-mediated effects, is to be found in Chap. 15.

III. B Cell Effects

From the experimental data compiled in Table 3, it becomes evident that in contrast to T cell functions, B cell functions (e.g., production of antibodies and RF are only indirectly interfered with by NSAID, if at all. It is obvious that lack of suppression of Ts cells by reduced PG concentrations may lead to an enhanced B cell proliferation and antibody production (Table 3; Kurland et al. 1977). As discussed already, owing to the specific pharmacokinetics of NSAID, these indirect effects are particularly likely to occur in the pannus of inflamed joints in RA patients because inflammation will lead to NSAID accumulation and, as outlined by Ziff's group (Smiley et al. 1968) and others, the enlarged pannus of RA

Table 2. NSAID effects on T lymphocyte functions

Function measured	Drug, concentration	Effect	Comments
T cell proliferation	Indomethacin $\geqq 10^{-6}$ mol/l	Increased response to PHA[a]	PWM effect was not altered[b]
Lymphokine production	Indomethacin $\geqq 10^{-6}$ mol/l	Drug enhances lymphokine production[c,d]	Cultures contained macrophages[c,d]
Ts activity	Indomethacin $\geqq 10^{-6}$ mol/l	Reduces inhibition by MPH[e], restores proliferation to PWM, PHA[e,f,g]	Indirect effect likely[c,d] not in cells of peripheral lymphnodes[h]
NK cells	Indomethacin $\geqq 10^{-6}$ mol/l	Enhances NK activity[i,j]	Effect not observed[i,k]
ADCC	Indomethacin $\geqq 10^{-6}$ mol/l	Enhances ADCC[l]	Effect MPH dependent[l]

a GOODWIN et al. (1978)
b STAITE and PANAYI (1982)
c GORDON et al. (1976)
d RAPPAPORT and DODGE (1982)

e BINDERUP (1983)
f EZDINLI et al. (1986)
g TILDEN and BALCH (1982)
h GOODACRE and BIENENSTOCK (1982)

i TRACEY and ADKINSON (1980)
j GROHMANN et al. (1981)
k DROLLER and GOMOLKA (1983)
l MAHOWALD et al. (1983)

Table 3. NSAID effects on B lymphocyte functions

Function measured	Drug, concentration	Effect	Comments
B activation by Epstein-Barr virus	Indomethacin ($\geqq 10^{-6}$ mol/l)	Enhanced activity in RA patients corrected by indomethacin[a,b]	Effect probably due to insufficient Ts number[c]
Ig synthesis in tissue culture	Indomethacin (10^{-6}–10^{-8} mol/l)	Suppression in PWM-stimulated cultures[d,e,f]	Effect due to lack of Ts[e]
Antigen-specific antibody production in tissue culture	Indomethacin (10^{-6}–10^{-8} mol/l)	Suppression of antigen-specific antibody production[g,h]	Indomethacin enhances PFC when given together with T-independent antigen[i]

a TOSATO et al. (1981)
b HASLER et al. (1983)
c GOODWIN et al. (1984)

d CEUPPENS and GOODWIN (1982)
e PANAYI et al. (1981)
f STAITE and PANAYI (1982)

g COOK (1978)
h WIEDNER and WEBB (1981)
i ZIMECKI and WEBB (1976)

patients comprises a major lymphoid organ likely to produce large quantities of antibodies, including RF. If the physicochemical characteristics of NSAID are likely to cause their specific accumulation in the inflamed tissue (BRUNE and WHITEHOUSE 1978), perhaps this knowledge should be used in the future for targeting other drugs toward the pannus which directly inhibit or regulate lymphocyte functions.

D. Conclusion and Outlook

One may safely assume that NSAID cause only minor effects on immune functions of the human body. There is some evidence that these widely-used drugs may indirectly (via inhibition of PG release) exert some second-line modulation of immune responses (BRAY 1980). This effect may be mediated by eicosanoid-modulated IL-1 (KUNKEL and CHENSUE 1985) and IL-2 (RAPPAPORT and DODGE 1982) release. In this context, it appears to be of major importance to learn more about drugs which directly interfere with IL-1 or IL-2. The remarkable effects of glucocorticoids, which were recently found to inhibit IL-1 production from mouse macrophages at nanomolar concentrations (OTTERNESS, to be published) indicates new lines of research (see also Chap. 17).

On the one hand, experimental and clinical evidence suggests that NSAID, possibly by suppressing the release of immune regulatory PG, may ameliorate symptoms of comprised lymphocyte function under clinical conditions. On the other hand, the view that NSAID may lead to exacerbation of RA is also held (LEWIS and BARRETT 1986). Further work should help to define distinct clinical disease entities in which the patient may benefit from NSAID, i.e.not only from the analgesic and anti-inflammatory action, but also from improvement of the disordered immune functions.

References

Anderson CB, Jaffee BM, Graff RJ (1977) Prolongation of murine skin allografts by prostaglandin El. Transplantation 23:444–449
Bacon PA (1984) Nonsteroidal anti-inflammatory drugs and immunologic function. Overview of the European experience. Am J Med 77:26–31
Binderup L (1983) Lymphocyte-macrophage co-operation during induction of T-suppressor cell activity in rats with adjuvant arthritis. Ann Rheum Dis 42:687–692
Bray MA (1980) Prostaglandins: fine tuning the immune system? Immunol Today 9:65–69
Brune K (1985) Tissue accumulation of non-steroidal anti-inflammatory drugs. In: Nilsen OG (ed) Tiaprofenic acid. Pharmacology and pharmacokinetics communications. Excerpta Medica, Amsterdam, pp 31–37
Brune K, Lanz R (1984) Nonopioid analgesics. In: Kuhar M, Pasternak G (eds) Analgesics: neurochemical, behavioral and clinical perspectives. Raven, New York, pp 149–173
Brune K, Lanz R (1985) Pharmacokinetics of non-steroidal anti-inflammatory drugs. In: Bonta IL, Bray MA, Parnham MJ (eds) Handbook of inflammation, vol 5. Elsevier, Amsterdam, pp 413–449
Brune K, Whitehouse MW (1978) Cytostats with effects in chronic inflammation. In: Vane JR, Ferreira SH (eds) Handbook of experimental pharmacology, vol 50/II. Springer, Berlin Heidelberg New York, pp 531–578

Brune K, Glatt M, Graf P (1976) Mechanisms of action of anti-inflammatory drugs. Gen Pharmacol 7:27–33

Brune K, Rainsford KD, Wagner K, Peskar A (1981) Inhibition by anti-inflammatory drugs of prostaglandin production in cultures macrophages. Naunyn-Schmiedebergs Arch Pharmacol 315:269–276

Ceuppens J, Goodwin JS (1982) Endogenous prostaglandin E enhances polyclonal immunoglobulin production by tonically inhibiting T suppressor cell activity. Cell Immunol 70:41–54

Ceuppens JL, Rodriguez MA, Goodwin JS (1982) Non-steroidal anti-inflammatory agents inhibit the synthesis of IgM rheumatoid factor in vitro.

Ciosek CP, Ortel RW, Thanassi NM, Newcombe DS (1974a) Indomethacin potentiates PGEl stimulated cyclic AMP accumulation in human synoviocytes. Nature 251:148–150

Ciosek CP, Ortel RW, Thanassi NM, Newcombe DS (1974b) Inhibition of phosphodiesterase by non steroidal anti-inflammatory drugs. Nature 251:148–150

Cook R (1978) Regulation of the in vitro anamnestic antibody response by cyclic AMP. II. Prostaglandins of the E series. Cell Immunol 40:128–133

Droller MJ, Gomolka D (1983) Enhancement of natural cytotoxicity in lymphocytes from animals with carcinogen-induced bladder cancer. J Urol 129:625–629

Emery P, Panayi GS, Nouri ME (1984) Interleukin-2 reverses deficient cell-mediated immune responses in rheumatoid arthritis. Clin Exp Immunol 57:123–129

Etienne J, Polonovski J (1984) Phospholipase A2 activity in rat and human lymphocytes. Biochem Biophys Res Com 125:719–727

Ezdinli EZ, Kucuk O et al. (1986) Hypogammaglobulinemia and hemophagocytic syndrome associated with lymphoproliferative disorders. Cancer 57:1024–1037

Ferreira SH, Vane JR (1978) Mode of action of anti-inflammatory agents which are prostaglandin synthetase inhibitors. In: Vane JR, Ferreira SH (eds) Handbook of experimental pharmacology, vol 50/II. Springer, Berlin Heidelberg New York, pp 348–398

Floersheim GL (1965) Pharmakologische Beeinflußbarkeit cellulärer Immunität. Z Naturwiss Med Grundlagenforsch 2:307–365

Flower RJ (1974) Drugs which inhibit prostaglandin biosynthesis. Pharmacol Rev 26:33–67

Forre O, Thoen J, Helgetveit K, Haile Y (1984) Nonsteroidal anti-inflammatory drugs in rheumatoid arthritis. Inflammation [Suppl] 9:109–113

Garin EH, Barratt TM (1982) Effects of indomethacin on lymphocyte response to mitogens in puromycin aminonucleoside nephrosis in the rat. Clin Exp Immunol 49:639–644

Garin EH, Sausville PJ, Richard GA (1983) Serum inhibitor of phytohemagglutinin-induced lymphocyte proliferation in Bartter syndrome. J Pediatr 102:569–572

Goodacre RL, Bienenstock J (1982) Reduced suppressor cell activity in intestinal lymphocytes from patients with Crohn's disease. Gastroenterology 82:653–658

Goodwin JS, Ceuppens J (1983) Regulation of the immune response by prostaglandins. J Clin Immunol 3:295–315

Goodwin JS, Webb DR (1980) Regulation of the immune response by prostaglandins. Clin Immunol Immunopathol 15:106–122

Goodwin JS, Bankhurst AD, Murphy S, Selinger DS, Messner RP, Williams RC jr (1978) Partial reversal of the cellular immune defect in common variable immunodeficiency with indomethacin. J Clin Lab Immunol 1:197–204

Goodwin JS, Messner RP, Peake GT (1978a) Prostaglandin suppression of mitogen-stimulated lymphocytes in vitro. Changes with mitogen dose and preincubation. J Clin Invest 62:753–760

Goodwin JS, Selinger DS, Messner RP, Reed WP (1978b) Effect of indomethacin in vivo on humoral and cellular immunity in humans. Infect Immun 19:430–433

Goodwin JS, Ceuppens JL, Rodriguez MA (1984) Effect of non-steroidal anti-inflammatory agents on immunologic function in patients with rheumatoid arthritis. Inflammation [Suppl] 8:49–55

Gordon D, Bray MA, Morley J (1976) Control of lymphokine secretion by prostaglandins. Nature 262:401–402

Greene BM, Fanning MM, Ellner JJ (1983) Non-specific suppression of antigen-induced lymphocyte blastogenesis in *Onchocerca volvulus* infection in man. Clin Exp Immunol 52:259–265

Grohmann P, Porzsolt F, Quirt I, Miller R, Phillips R (1981) Stimulation of human NK cell activity by cultured cells. Clin Exp Immunol 44:611–614

Hallgren HM, Yunis EJ (1977) Suppressor lymphocytes in young and aged humans. J Immunol 118:1004–1009

Hasler F, Bluestein HG, Zvaifler NJ, Epstein LB (1983) Analysis of the defects responsible for the impaired regulation of EBV-induced B cell proliferation by rheumatoid arthritis lymphocytes. II. Role of monocytes and the increased sensitivity of rheumatoid arthritis lymphocytes to prostaglandin El. J Immunol 131:768–772

Helleberg L (1981) Clinical pharmacokinetics of indomethacin. Clin Pharmacol 6:245–258

Hofer D, Duibitsky AM, Reilly P, Santoro MG, Jaffee BM (1980) The interactions between indomethacin and cytotoxic drugs in mice bearing B-16 melanomas. Prostaglandins 20:1033–1039

Humes JL, Winter CA, Sadowski SJ, Kuehl FA (1981) Multiple sites on prostaglandin cyclooxygenase are determinants in the action of nonsteroidal antiinflammatory agents. Proc Natl Acad Sci USA 78:2053–2056

Johnsen S, Olding LB, Westberg NG, Wilhelmsson L (1982) Strong suppression by mononuclear leukocytes from human newborns on maternal leukocytes: mediation by prostaglandins. Clin Immunol Immunopathol 23:606–615

Kantor HS, Hampton M (1978) Indomethacin in submicromolar concentrations inhibits cyclic AMP-dependent protein kinase. Nature 276:841–842

Karim SMM, Rao B (1976) Prostaglandins and tumors. In: Karim SMM (ed) Prostaglandins: physiological, pharmacological and pathological aspects. MTP Press, Lancaster, pp 303–325

Kunkel SB, Chensue SW (1985) Arachidonic acid metabolites regulate interleukin-1 production. Biochem Biophys Res Commun 128:892–897

Kurland JI, Kincade PW, Moore MAS (1977) Regulation of B-lymphocyte clonal proliferation by stimulatory and inhibitory macrophage-derived factors. J Exp Med 146:1420–1435

Lammie PJ, Katz SP (1983) Immunoregulation in experimental filariasis. I. In vitro suppression of mitogen-induced blastogenesis by adherent cells from jirds chronically infected with brugia pahangi. J Immunol 130:1381–1385

Leclerc C, Morin A, Deriaud E, Chedid L (1984) Inhibition of human IL 2 production by MDP and derivates. J Immunol 133:1996–2000

Lewis GP, Barrett ML (1986) Immunosuppressive actions of prostaglandins and the possible increase in chronic inflammation after cyclooxygenase inhibitors. Agents Actions 19:59–65

Lipsmeyer E (1982) Effect of cimetidine and indomethacin on delayed hypersensitivity. Transplantation 33:107–113

Lynch NR, Salomon J (1979) Tumor growth inhibition and potentiation of immunotherapy by indomethacin in mice. J Natl Cancer Inst 62:117–121

Lynch NR, Casatles M, Astonin M, Salomon JC (1978) Mechanism of inhibition of tumor growth by aspirin and indomethacin. Br J Cancer 38:503–509

Maca RD, Panje WR (1982) Indomethacin sensitive suppressor cell activity in head and neck cancer patients pre- and postirradiation therapy. Cancer 50:483–489

Mahowald ML, Dalmasso AP, Messner RP (1983) Endogenous inhibition of autologous lymphocyte antibody-dependent cellular cytotoxicity. Clin Immunol Immunopathol 29:211–222

Morley J (1978) Lymphokines. In: Vane JR, Ferreira SH (eds) Handbook of experimental pharmacology, vol 50/I. Springer, Berlin Heidelberg New York, pp 314–342

Muscoplat CC, Rakich PM, Thoen CO, Johnson DW (1978) Enhancement of lymphocyte blastogenic and delayed hypersensitivity skin responses by indomethacin. Infect Immun 20:627–632

Palmer DG, Barbezat GO, Gibbins BL, Grennan DM, Lum J, Myers DB, Wilson K (1981) A single-blind crossover trial of the anti-inflammatory drug sodium meclofenamate and placebo, including an evaluation of hand grip and of lymphocyte responsiveness. Curr Med Res Opin 7:359–367

Palmer DG, Ferry DG, Gibbins DL, Hall SM, Grennan DM, Lum J, Myers DB (1982) Ibuprofen and diflunisal in rheumatoid arthritis: a double blind comparative trial. NZ Med J 2:45–48

Panayi GS, Staite ND, Unger A (1981) Indomethacin inhibits in vitro immunoglobulin production by human B lymphocytes. Agents Actions 11:608–610

Panje WR (1981) Regression of head and neck carcinoma with a prostaglandin synthesis inhibitor. Arch Otolaryngol 107:658–663

Rappaport RS, Dodge GR (1982) Prostaglandins E inhibits the production of human interleukin 2. J Exp Med 155:943–948

Reddy MM, Manvar D, Ahuja KK, Moriarty ML, Grieco MH (1985) Augmentation of mitogen-induced proliferative reponses by in vitro indomethacin in patients with acquired immune deficiency syndrome and AIDS-related complex. Int J Immunopharmacol 7:917–921

Rojo JM, Barasoain I, Portoles A (1981) Further studies on the immunosuppressive effects of indomethacin. Int J Clin Pharmacol Ther Toxicol 19:220–222

Salmon M, Bacon PA, Johnson GD, Walton KW (1984) The use of cytocentrifuge preparations for the demonstration of T cell surface antigens. J Immunol Methods 66:327–330

Smiley J, Sachs C, Ziff M (1968) In vitro synthesis of immunoglobulin by rheumatoid synovial membrane. J Clin Invest 47:624–632

Staite ND, Panayi GS (1982) Regulation of human immunoglobulin production in vitro by prostaglandin E2. Clin Exp Immunol 49:115–122

Tilden AB, Balch CM (1982) Immune modulatory effects of indomethacin in melanoma patients are not related to prostaglandin E2-mediated suppression. Surgery 92:528–532

Tosato G, Steinberg AD, Blaese RM (1981) Defective EB virus-specific suppressor cell function in rheumatoid arthritis. N Engl J Med 305:1238–1244

Tracey DE, Adkinson NF (1980) Prostaglandin synthesis inhibitors potentiate the BCG-induced augmentation of natural killer cell activity. J Immunol 125:136–141

Vane JR (1971) Inhibition of prostaglandin synthesis as a mechanism of action for aspirin-like drugs. Nature New Biol 231:232–235

Webb DR, Osheroff PK (1976) Antigen stimulation of prostaglandin synthesis and control of immune responses. Proc Natl Acad Sci USA 73:1300–1309

Wiedner KJ, Webb DR (1981) The effect of prostaglandin metabolism on immunoglobulin and antibody production in naive and educated whole spleen cells. Prostaglandins Leukotrienes Med 7:79–90

Zimecki M, Webb DR (1976) The regulation of the immune response to T-independent antigens by prostaglandins and B cells. J Immunol 117:2158–2164

CHAPTER 27

Future Prospects for Drug Design of Lymphocyte Modulators

J. Drews and W. Haas

A. Introduction

There are well-established procedures for the design and presentation of scientific reviews. Unfortunately, all of the conventions and rules developed in this context are quite useless when it comes to writing a scientific preview, or to put it more bluntly, to predicting the future of a given area of research. By its very nature, scientific progress is unpredictable. We are entitled to assume that progress will continue in the future as it has in the past, but we know nothing about its quality, and we can only guess at which point in time a particular scientific question can be answered. The task of designing future therapy in any area of pharmacology is therefore a rather futile one, and is more likely to contribute to the amusement of future generations of scientists than to the enlightenment of the present one. However, drug therapy is not only a matter of research, but also a matter of applying the results of basic research to a particular therapeutic purpose, a process which we may call development.

In contrast to progress in basic research, developmental progress can be predicted to a considerable extent. In other words: therapeutic modalities that already exist as experimental models can be qualified according to their clinical potential, and to their probability of being developed into viable, clinically useful drugs or procedures. The average time span which can be assigned to the development of a new drug from its first chemical and biologic conceptualization to the completion of clinical studies amounts to 10 years. This period of time, therefore, sets the limits within which reasonable predictions can be attempted: all drugs which will enter the therapeutic arena by the middle of the next decade must be known today, either as therapeutic concepts based on established scientific facts or merely as chemical entities. Describing future prospects for the design of lymphocyte modulators, therefore, can be reduced to the task of selecting those concepts and compounds from today's experimental scene which are most likely to stand the test of the next 10 years – in pharmacologic, toxicologic, and, most importantly, in clinical terms.

B. Potential Targets for Lymphocyte Modulators

There are two major classes of lymphocytes, B cells and T cells. The prominent role of T cells in practically every immune response makes them the major targets for immunomodulators. There are two major T cell subsets. T cells with the T4 marker recognize antigens in conjunction with class II Mhc (major histocompatibility complex) antigens and are mostly helper cells. T cells with the T8 marker recognize antigens in conjunction with class I Mhc antigens and are mostly killer cells (Chap. 1). The functions of the T4 and T8 plasma membrane proteins are not known. There are some indications that these molecules somehow increase the strength of the T cell interaction with antigen-presenting cells by attaching to nonpolymorphic regions of class I, or class II Mhc proteins (MacDonald et al. 1982; Marrack et al. 1983; Swain 1983; Biddison et al. 1984; Greenstein et al. 1985).

The Mhc-restricted antigen specificity of both classes of T cells resides in a heterodimer consisting of α and β chains which resemble immunoglobulins (Dembic et al. 1986). These "receptors" are associated with the T3 complex which in turn is made up of three invariant chains T3γ, T3δ, and T3ε (Borst et al. 1983, 1984). In some minor subsets of T cells, the T3 complex is associated with other less well-defined receptor molecules (Brenner et al. 1986; Moingeon et al. 1986). With the aid of antibodies which activate or inhibit lymphocyte functions, a variety of other plasma membrane proteins have been identified. Examples are the B cell differentiation antigens Bp 35 (CD22), Bp 140 (C3d receptor, CD21), Bp 150, Bp 135 (CD22), and Bp 45 (CD23) or the T cell differentiation antigens Tp 150 (sheep red blood cell receptor, CD2). Tp 67 (CD5), Tp44 and Lp 220 (for references see Clark and Ledbetter 1986 and Chap. 2). Virtually nothing is known about the physiologic role of these molecules.

The interaction of external ligands with surface receptors can induce a cascade of biochemical events which eventually lead to proliferation and/or differentiation (Haas and von Boehmer 1985). As an example, the interaction of T cells with antigen-presenting cells first leads to the expression of receptors for interleukin 1 (IL-1) which bind IL-1 produced by the antigen-presenting cells. Subsequently, interleukin 2 (IL-2) receptors are expressed. Their association with an unknown plasma membrane component leads to the expression of "high affinity" IL-2-binding sites. IL-2 is secreted and binds to the receptors of the same or other cells. This is followed by the expression of transferrin receptors which are endocytosed after binding the iron carrier transferrin. Only after this does DNA synthesis commence, and the cell divides. The binding of external ligands to T cells can also induce T cell effector functions such as help for B cells, cytolytic activity, or secretion of factors acting on lymphocytes, other hematopoietic cells, or non-hematopoietic cells. Very little is known about the different signals which are required for the activation of distinct genetic programs in the various lymphocyte subpopulations (see Chaps. 1–4).

Considerable progress has recently been made in the elucidation of biochemical pathways by which signals are transduced in lymphocytes from the surface membrane into the cytoplasm and eventually into the nucleus (for review see Isakov et al. 1986 and Chaps. 2–4). The interaction of external ligands with T cell surface proteins stimulates (probably via GTP-binding transducer proteins) phospholipase C, to hydrolyze phosphatidylinositol-4,5-bisphosphate (PIP_2), which is normally present in the lipid bilayer in minute quantities only. As a result of this reaction, two second messengers are formed: diacylglycerol (DAG) and inositol-1,4,5-trisphosphate (IP_3), which trigger two synergistic pathways of signal transduction. DAG activates protein kinase C (PKC) by increasing the affinity of this enzyme for Ca^{2+}. Activated PKC is then translocated from the cytosol to the plasma membrane and catalyzes the phosphorylation of several proteins, including the $T3\gamma$ and $T3\delta$ chains, the IL-2 receptor, and probably an Na^+/H^+ exchanger. IP_3 on the other hand releases Ca^{2+} from intracellular stores. EGTA added to lymphocyte cultures blocks lymphocyte activation. This indicates that the entry of extracellular Ca^{2+} is also required, probably to sustain elevated Ca^{2+} levels. The two signal pathways initiated by DAG and IP_3 can be studied separately by the use of tumor promoters which mimic the effect of DAG, and of calcium ionophores which mimic the signals normally provided by IP_3 and Ca^{2+} increase. All lymphocytes, as well as many nonlymphoid cells, appear to use similar, if not identical signal transduction pathways (BERRIDGE and IRVINE 1984; NISHIZUKA 1984; CAMBIER et al. 1985; BIJSTERBOSCH et al. 1985). Lymphocyte-specific molecules involved in signal transduction have not yet been identified. Thus, the structures which can currently be considered as targets for selective lymphocyte modulators reside: (a) in the plasma membrane; (b) in products secreted by lymphocytes, and (c) in target cells or target molecules of the secreted lymphocyte products. Other target structures must, of course, reside in the nucleus. However, more than 10 years will probably elapse before lymphocyte modulators can be designed which are addressed to these specific targets.

C. Lymphocyte Modulators

The term "lymphocyte modulators" comprises all compounds which can somehow alter lymphocyte function – irrespective of the pharmacologic mechanisms or the lymphocyte subsets involved and also irrespective of the in vivo effects which result from lymphocyte modulation. In fact, however, lymphocyte modulators can only be of interest to the immunopharmacologist if they can serve clearly defined therapeutic purposes. This means that the effects elicited by these compounds at the molecular and cellular levels must translate at the level of the human organism into reproducible actions which can be used to treat diseases or to manipulate the immune system in a clinically desirable way. Therefore, we will discuss lymphocyte modulators according to clinical requirements. We need lymphocyte modulators to prevent or inhibit: (a) immune responses leading to graft rejection, graft-versus-host disease, or autoimmunity; (b) chronic tissue damage and inflammation in patients with rheumatoid arthritis or related chronic inflammatory conditions; and (c) acute hypersensitivity reactions in patients with atopic or allergic conditions. In addition, lymphocyte modulators could be used to substitute or enhance lymphocyte functions in immunocompromised patients with infections or cancer.

I. Transplantation and Autoimmunity

1. Cyclosporin (see also Chap. 21)

The fungal metabolite cyclosporin (CSA), which is the most selective immunosuppressive drug discovered so far, blocks the activation of lymphocytes at a very early stage (for review see HESS et al. 1986). It inhibits, by an unknown mechanism, the accumulation of mRNAs coding for IL-2 and other lymphokines without interfering with the transcription of other genes (Krönke et al. 1984). At higher doses, CSA also appears to interfere with the expression of IL-2 receptors and the function of antigen-presenting cells. CSA binds to calmodulin and to cyclophilins. However, this can hardly explain the selectivity of its action since these proteins are present in all cells. The use of CSA as an immunosuppressive drug is limited by its nephrotoxicity. The chance, however, that improved, less nephrotoxic cyclosporins may become available is high when one considers that many cyclosporins other than CSA have already been discovered (Traber et al. 1977a,b). Promising results have already been obtained with cyclosporin G and dehydrocyclosporin C.

Most interestingly, in many animal experiments, a specific long-lasting tolerance could be induced to antigens, which were present in the animals at the time when CSA was given. Immunosuppression by CSA appears to facilitate the generation of suppressor cells (for review see Hess et al. 1986). Unfortunately, induction of tolerance has not yet been achieved in patients. The in vivo effects of CSA on the various lymphocyte subpopulations are still poorly understood. Recent animal experiments suggest that CSA not only interferes with T cell activation, but also with normal T cell development in the thymus. CSA inhibits the production of IFN-γ which appears to be required to sustain high levels of class II Mhc antigen expression by epithelial cells in the cortex and dendritic cells in the medulla of the thymus. In the absence of a high expression of these Mhc-encoded proteins, self-reactive lymphocytes are apparently not eliminated and appear in the periphery where they respond to self-antigens when CSA treatment is interrupted (Hess et al. 1985). However, no autoimmune responses were observed in patients who were treated with CSA for a period of 50 days after reconstitution with allogeneic bone marrow (Storb et al. 1986). Probably, the dose of CSA normally given to patients is lower than that required to interfere with normal T cell development.

2. Interleukin 2 Antagonists (see also Chap. 8)

The dominant strategy in the search for new immunosuppressive agents is directed at the action of IL-2, since this glycoprotein has a pivotal role in the amplification and regulation of all immune responses. The genes encoding human IL-2 and IL-2 receptors have been cloned and the structure-function relationships of these molecules are being studied in many laboratories with a variety of methods involving monoclonal antibodies, X-ray crystallography, recombinant DNA technology, in vitro mutagenesis, and computer-assisted predictive methods (Wang et al. 1984; Kuo and Robb 1986; Kuo et al. 1986; Shu-mei Liang et al. 1986; Cohen et al. 1986). These studies are well advanced and there is no doubt that IL-2 antagonists will soon become available for preclinical tests.

An interesting hypothesis published recently suggests a less cumbersome and more general approach to the design of receptor-blocking agents. The hypothesis says that complementary strands of DNA often encode proteins which interact with each other. The available experimental evidence supporting this prediction, which has little appeal at first glance, has been extended recently by the correctly predicted IL-2 receptor blocking activity of a synthetic hexapeptide (WEIGENT et al. 1986) which corresponds to the NH_2 terminal portion of the envelope protein of the HTLV-III virus. Unfortunately our recent attempts to reproduce these findings (F. SINIGAGLIA, unpublished observation) were unsuccessful.

Peptides found in one way or the other, which inhibit IL-2 binding could serve as lead structures for the design of nonpeptidic compounds which act similarly, but have the advantage of displaying more favorable pharmakokinetic parameters, such as oral bioavailability and a long biologic half-life.

3. Antibodies

Xenogeneic anti-lymphocyte globulin (ALG) or anti-thymocyte globulin (ATG) have been widely used to treat aplastic anemia or graft rejection episodes with some success (NYDEGGER 1985). The poor reproducibility of the effects of these antisera is probably largely due to variations between batches, particularly with ALGs (RAEFSKY et al. 1986). More reproducible results were obtained with the murine anti-T3 IgG antibodies OKT3. Such antibodies have been used successfully to reverse kidney graft rejection episodes in more than 90% of 150 patients (GOLDSTEIN et al. 1985; Ortho Multicenter Transplant Group 1985). However, the OKT3 treatment was effective only in combination with low doses of azathioprine and steroids, caused a variety of side effects, and induced a humoral immune response against isotypic and idiotypic OKT3 epitopes which prevented the treatment of subsequent rejection episodes with the same antibodies (CHATENOUD et al. 1985, 1986).

A more selective immunosuppression might be achieved by using antibodies which are specifically directed against antigens expressed by T cell subsets only. In mice, rats, and monkeys, autoimmunity as well as delayed-type hypersensitivity and transplantation reactions, could be inhibited by the administration of antibodies against IL-2 receptors (KIRKMAN et al. 1985; KUPIEC-WEGLINSKI et al. 1986; KELLEY et al. 1986; FERRARA et al. 1986), or antibodies against the animal's T4 antigens (BROSTOFF and MASON 1984; WOFSY and SEAMAN 1985; WALDOR et al. 1985), or antibodies against a surface antigen of natural killer (NK) cells (LIKE et al. 1986).

Ideally, the unwanted immune responses should remain absent or suppressed after the recovery of the immune system from transient suppression. It has been shown by several investigators that a long-lasting, specific nonresponsiveness can be induced by the application of antigens in mice which were transiently depleted of T4 cells by the administration of appropriate antibodies (WOFSY et al. 1985; BENJAMIN et al. 1986; COBBOLT et al. 1986; BENJAMIN and WALDMANN 1986; GORONZY et al. 1986). However, this treatment protocol allowed the induction of nonresponsiveness to some antigens only. It was insufficient to induce tolerance either to highly immunogenic proteins, including xenogeneic antibodies binding to recipient cells (BENJAMIN et al. 1986), or to allogeneic bone marrow or skin grafts (COBBOLT et al. 1986). In order to induce specific tolerance to minor or major transplantation antigens, the recipients had to be irradiated sublethally and to be depleted of both major classes of T cells by the in vivo administration of appropriate monoclonal antibodies (COBBOLT et al. 1986).

Although antibodies against T3, T4, T8, or IL-2 receptors can inhibit T cell functions in vitro, the mechanism of their immunosuppressive activity in vivo remains unclear. In most treatment protocols in animals and humans T cell-specific antibodies caused an almost complete, but transient, elimination of their target cells from the circulation and most lymphoid organs. The degree of elimination depends on the dose and the class of antibodies used. However, in some studies immunosuppression could also be achieved with very low doses of antibodies or with (Fab')$_2$ fragments which did not eliminate the target cells (H. WALDMANN 1986, personal communication; GORONZY et al. 1986).

Antibodies against class II Mhc antigens have also been used for the suppression of immune responses. Since T cells which play a role in the pathogenesis of autoimmune diseases appear sometimes to be restricted to particular Mhc alleles (i.e., they are controlled by *Ir* genes in the Mhc) it should be possible to prevent or inhibit the pathologic immune response by interfering with the responses of those T cells only. This strategy has been applied successfully in mice and in rats (STEINMAN et al. 1981; ADELMAN et al. 1983; WALDOR et al. 1983; BOITARD et al. 1985). However, the price to be paid for the selective inhibition of T cells was a severe depletion of B cells which express class II Mhc antigens (WALDOR et al. 1984). Furthermore, application of antibodies against class II Mhc antigens in monkeys was sometimes associated with severe side effects and even death. The reasons for these reactions are unknown.

In summary, treatment with T cell-specific monoclonal antibodies has already been proven to reverse acute rejection episodes in transplanted patients, and will probably be done with increasing frequency. It remains to be seen, however, whether any of the more complex strategies of immunosuppression which have been developed in animal models will be applicable to humans.

A more general comment on possible future developments which could emerge from the work with monoclonal antibodies might be in order at this point. Genetic engineering allows the production of new molecules. Murine antibodies can be "humanized," e.g., by replacing the constant parts or even the framework regions of the variable parts with those of human antibodies. The variable regions of antibodies have also been combined with proteins other than immunoglobulins, and it is conceivable that new, specific, and therapeutically useful molecules will soon be constructed (NEUBERGER et al. 1984; MORRISON 1985; JONES et al. 1986). Eventually, the variable parts of antibodies could be replaced by nonpeptidic molecules which share with the antibody nothing but the affinity for the antigen. Such compounds could perhaps be selected with the aid of idiotype-specific antibodies. Developments along these lines must, however, be viewed as long-term goals.

4. Endogenous Immunosuppressive Factors

Various normal and/or neoplastic cells produce factors which inhibit the activation or growth of lymphocytes or other hematopoietic cells. Some of these factors appear to act mainly or exclusively on lymphocytes (HARDT et al. 1981; KRAMER and KOSINOWSKI 1982; LOU et al. 1985; KAWANO et al. 1985; HONDA et al. 1985; SHIRAKAWA et al. 1986; CHIAO et al. 1986; MEDOFF et al. 1986). The elucidation of the structure and mode of action of such factors might eventually lead to the development of novel immunosuppressive agents, which can be used therapeutically. Again, the 10-year time span selected for this "preview" appears too short for these prospects to materialize.

II. Chronic Inflammatory Processes

1. Cyclooxygenase Inhibitors (see also Chap. 26)

Treatment of chronic inflammatory processes with nonsteroidal anti-inflammatory drugs, such as indomethacin, ibuprofen, mefenamic acid, or piroxicam has reached its limits. All of these substances act by inhibiting cyclooxygenase and subsequently the synthesis of prostaglandins. This intervention leads to symptomatic relief. But at least in the case of chronic polyarthritis there is no indication that nonsteroidal anti-inflammatory agents have any effect on the progression of bone and cartilage damage which is the hallmark of this disease (WARD and SAMUELSON 1982). It is well known that prostaglandin E_2 (PGE_2), one of the most important products of the cyclooxygenase pathway, exerts immune regulatory functions, many of which are anti-inflammatory and "anti-tissue-destructive." PGE_2 inhibits the synthesis of lymphokines in activated lymphocytes (WALKER et al. 1983; RAPPAPORT and DODGE 1982), the generation of oxygen radicals, of IL-1 (CAHILL and HOPPER 1984), and of lysosomal enzymes from granulocytes, the degranulation of mast cells (TRANG 1980), and many other functions which contribute to tissue damage and chronic inflammation (GOODWIN and CEUPPENS 1983; Chaps. 14, 15). Inhibitors of prostaglandin synthesis prevent the direct acute inflammatory reactions which are generated by these compounds, but at the same time they eliminate a very important regulatory element which is capable of preventing excessive tissue destruction (GEMSA et al. 1982). In view of this negative feedback control of chronic inflammatory reactions through PGE_2 (MORLEY 1979), one would assume that stable analogs of this prostaglandin might be of value in the suppression of chronic inflammatory reactions. Experimental evidence supporting this proposition is available. The hydantoin derivatives of PGE_2 as well as the prostacyclin derivative carbacyclin, which are more stable than their natural analogs, are capable of inhibiting mitogen-induced lymphocyte transformation in concentrations ranging between 10^{-9} and 10^{-5} M (KINGSTON et al. 1985). The efficacy of existing PGE_2 and PGI_2 analogs is probably not yet sufficient to warrant their development as novel anti-inflammatory agents. In principle, however, this line of research appears to be feasible, and may well lead (or may even have led already) to the discovery of agents which are truly novel in their anti-inflammatory mode of action.

2. Interleukin 1 Antagonists

The second important approach in the search for a new anti-inflammatory agent centers around interleukin 1 (IL-1). In addition to its crucial role in T cell activation IL-1 exerts a large number of additional functions: it stimulates chondrocytes and synovial cells to produce and secrete collagenase and other neutral proteases

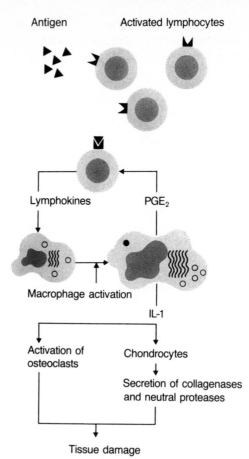

Fig. 1. Potential roles of PGE_2 and IL-1 in chronic inflammation. Antigen induces lymphocytes to secrete lymphokines which in turn activate macrophages. In rheumatoid arthritis and other chronic inflammatory reactions, PGE_2 fails to exert negative feedback control of lymphocyte function. IL-1 also secreted by activated macrophages causes tissue damage through various mechanisms

which degrade cartilage and cause tissue damage. It activates osteoclasts, thereby initiating the resorption of bone, and it causes fever (DUFF and DURUM 1983; DUFF 1985; OPPENHEIM et al. 1986; DINARELLO 1986). All these effects as well as the fact that IL-1 is secreted by activated macrophages and other antigen-presenting cells, make this lymphokine a central element in inflammatory reactions and a primary target for pharmacologic intervention aimed at the abrogation of chronic inflammation (Chap. 7). The potential roles of PGE_2 and IL-1 in chronic inflammatory reactions are shown in Fig. 1. There are at least two different species of human IL-1, both of which have been cloned recently (LOMEDICO et al. 1984; DINARELLO 1986). Although IL-1-α (p17) and IL-1-β (p15) have only 26% amino acid sequence homology, they appear to bind to the same receptors. One can now look for antagonists of these lymphokines in very much the same way as that briefly described for the search of IL-2 antagonists. If such compounds can be identified, they can be expected to represent a totally new approach to the treatment of chronic inflammatory reactions.

III. Acute Hypersensitivity Reactions

IgE represents a minor class of antibodies that is largely responsible for human immediate hypersensitivity disease states. IgE binds to high affinity receptors of basophils and mast cells. Cross-linking of cell-bound IgE leads to the release of various mediators of acute hypersensitivity reactions such as histamine, leukotrienes, or platelet-activating factor (PAF). Thus, anti-allergic drugs could either interfere with the IgE synthesis, or IgE binding to mast cells, or with the release or action of mediators.

1. Inhibition of IgE Synthesis (see also Chap. 10)

The ideal treatment of allergy would be the selective inhibition of the "pathologic" IgE response to the allergen. Despite improved methods using polymerized antigen, desensitization is successful in only some cases. Many investigators have therefore studied the regulation of IgE synthesis with the aim of finding compounds or treatment modalitites which would interfere with the production of

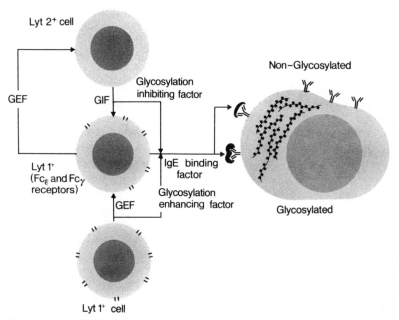

Fig. 2. Regulation of IgE synthesis. T helper lymphocytes carrying Fc_y and Fc_ε receptors secrete IgE-binding factor. Cells of the same subset produce a factor (lipomodulin-related) which enhances glycosylation. The glycosylated factor stimulates IgE synthesis in specialized B cells. At the same time, the lipomodulin-related GEF stimulates T suppressor cells (Lyt-2⁺) to secrete a kallikrein-related peptide which inhibits glycosylation. The nonglycosylated IgE-binding factor inhibits IgE synthesis and secretion by B cells

this class of antibodies, regardless of their specificity. Katz and collaborators described at least six distinct factors which regulate the expression of low affinity Fc_ε receptors by B and T cells and the synthesis or secretion of IgE by B cells (MARCELETTI and KATZ 1984; KATZ 1984). Two of these factors which bind to the Fc region of IgE might be identical with the IgE-binding factors (IgE-BF) described by ISHIZAKA et al. (1983). IgE-BF has a molecular weight of 15 000 dalton and is secreted by Fc_ε receptor-carrying T cells on stimulation with antigen or in the presence of aggregated IgE. When heavily glycosylated with oligosaccharides rich in mannose residues, the factor enhances the formation of IgE antibodies (YODOI et al. 1982; IWATA et al. 1984). In the presence of lipomodulin (also called lipocortin) or fragments of lipomodulin, which is a strong inhibitor of phospholipase A_2, glycosylation of IgE-BF is suppressed (UEDE et al. 1983, 1984). The nonglycosylated factor selectively suppresses IgE secretion without interfering with the production of other Ig classes (JARDIEU et al. 1984). The main features of this regulatory scheme are shown in Fig. 2. Since lipomodulin belongs to a group of proteins which are synthesized in response to glucocorticoids (BLACKWELL et al. 1980; HIRATA et al. 1980; CLOIX et al. 1983; ROTHHUT et al. 1983; Chap. 17), some of the beneficial actions of these substances on allergic reactions could perhaps be attributed to the inhibition of the glycosylation of IgE-BF. Human IgE-BF (KUFF et al. 1986) as well as lipomodulin (WALLNER et al. 1986) have been cloned recently. Information on the structure and the availability of these molecules in pure form will greatly facilitate the analysis of the regulation of IgE synthesis and could lead to the development of a therapeutically useful compound.

2. Inhibition of the Activation of Basophils and Mast Cells

Basophils and mast cells express high affinity receptors for the constant region of IgE. These receptors consists of α subunits (55 kdalton), β subunits (30–33 kdalton) and γ subunits (10 kdalton). Cloning of the genes encoding these proteins is in progress (LIU et al. 1985). The binding of IgE to the receptor can be blocked by monoclonal antibodies (BASCIANO et al. 1986) or by cloned fragments of IgE (GEHA et al. 1985). Preliminary in vivo experiments suggest that allergic reactions could be inhibited by the cloned Fc_ε receptor antagonist (GEHA et al. 1985). However, considering the high turnover rate of Fc_ε receptors, it is unlikely that this approach will lead to the development of a therapeutically useful drug. The signal transduction from cross-linked Fc_ε receptors into the mast cells appears to follow pathways very similar to those already described for lymphocyte activation. A selective inhibition of mast cell activation would become feasible only if mast cell-specific transducer proteins could be identified.

3. Mediator Antagonists

New concepts regarding the pathophysiology of bronchial asthma have moved three substances to the center stage of scientific attention: slow reacting substance of anaphylaxis (which comprises the leukotrienes C4, D4, and E4), prostaglandin D2, and most prominently platelet-activating factor (PAF) (MORLEY 1982). Antagonists against all of these compounds are being looked for in many laboratories. Since some of the antagonists effective in vitro can also be shown to exert antagonistic effects in animal experiments, the prospects for novel drugs interfering with allergic reactions are good. In particular, this seems to be true for antagonists of leukotrienes and PAF. PAF and leukotriene antagonists are compounds which interfere with the functions of these mediators at their peripheral targets, e.g., at the smooth muscle cells of the bronchioli or the endothelial cells of blood capillaries.

IV. Infections and Cancer

1. Synthetic Compounds

Synthetic compounds, such as isoprinosine and cimetidine, which have clearly defined effects on lymphocytes and on the immune system as a whole, have not yet made an important impact on the treatment of viral infections or tumors. Isoprinosine stimulates RNA synthesis in activated lymphocytes and exerts a number of additional effects in lymphocyte cultures (HERSEY et al. 1984). This is probably accomplished through an increased availability of inosine to the activated cells. Under certain conditions, activated lymphocytes appear to depend on the utilization of salvage pathways of purine biosynthesis (HIRSCHHORN 1983; GOODMAN 1984). Inosine, which, in the form of its complex with p-aminobenzoate of N_1,N-dimethylamino-2-propanol, is taken up by lymphocytes three times more efficiently than in its uncomplexed form, is phosphorylated within the cell, and utilized for the synthesis of AMP and GMP. Thus, isoprinosine appears to amplify events which are triggered by other specific signals (Chap. 24). If this currently accepted interpretation turns out to be correct, an extension of this line of investigation is unlikely to result in much further progress (PASINO et al. 1982; DE SIMONE et al. 1982; NAKAMURA et al. 1983).

Cimetidine is an antagonist of histamine which has been shown to play a role in the induction of T suppressor lymphocytes via H_2 receptors on the surface of these cells (SUZUKI and HUCHET 1981; Chap. 14). Cimetidine as an H_2 antagonist reverses this process and can by this mechanism enhance humoral as well as T cell-mediated immune responses (VAN DIJK et al. 1980). There are reports, both experimental and clinical, which seem to illustrate that a pharmacologic intervention with the formation of T suppressor cells can reduce the number of metastases in experimental tumors (GIFFORD et al. 1981; BENNETT et al. 1982), and can also restore weak or absent delayed-type hypersensitivity skin reactions against microbial antigens to a normal level in patients (AVELLA et al. 1978; JORIZZO et al. 1980). The clinical relevance of these findings is not yet clear. However, the existing body of evidence might well warrant a more detailed investigation of H_2 receptors on T lymphocytes, the function of histamine in T suppressor cell induction, and the potential of H_2 antagonists to inhibit this process. More potent and clinically useful compounds could be the result of such studies.

2. Agents of Microbial Origin

Agents of microbial origin, in particular cell wall constituents, exert pleiotropic effects, characterized mainly by the activation of macrophages, B cells, and T cells. These compounds, when used in well-defined experimental situations, can be shown to be capable of eradicating experimental bacterial and fungal infections, and reducing the number of tumor metastases (for review see Drews 1984, 1986). However, the large spectrum of side effects, which is typical of these compounds, has so far precluded any broad clinical application. The muramyl dipeptides came closest to becoming clinically useful since a separation of macrophage-activating and pyrogenic effects was achieved in at least a few derivatives (Chedid et al. 1982; Chap. 22). However, even with these compounds, galenical targeting to macrophages via liposomes may be necessary in order to achieve an acceptable degree of selectivity (Fraser-Smith and Matthews 1981; Fraser-Smith et al. 1983; Talmadge et al. 1986; Tandom et al. 1986).

3. Interferons (see also Chap. 9)

Many human interferon (IFN) genes (14 IFN-αs, 1 IFN-β, 1 IFN-γ) have been cloned and expressed in bacteria or other heterologous hosts (Pestka 1986). Information on the amino acid sequences and the availability of pure IFNs have provided a great impetus to IFN research which will probably soon lead to a better understanding of the mechanisms underlying the antiviral, antiproliferative, and other biologic effects of IFNs. IFNs can enhance a variety of host defense mechanisms (Nathan et al. 1983). It is, however, not clear to what extent these effects contribute to the therapeutic properties of IFNs. Purified natural IFNs and more recently various recombinant IFNs have been applied to several thousand patients with infectious or malignant diseases (Goldstein and Laszlo 1986). IFN-α-2 was found to be effective in the treatment of lymphoid malignancies, in particular hairy cell leukemia and perhaps chronic myeloid leukemias and myelomas. Some encouraging results were also reported for papilloma and condyloma, Kaposi sarcoma, renal cell carcinoma, melanoma, and glioma. More recently, IFN-γ has been claimed to be effective in patients with rheumatoid arthritis (Obert and Brzoska 1986). Various interferons have been used with some success to treat chronic hepatitis or other viral infections. Many clinical trials are in progress to test the usefulness of IFNs alone or in combination with other lymphokines or with chemotherapy. The development of IFNs as therapeutic agents on a more rational basis largely depends on further progress in basic IFN research.

4. Hematopoietic Growth Factors (see also Chap. 8)

The recent cloning of the four human hematopoietic growth factors multi-CFS or IL-3 (Yu-Chung Yang et al. 1986), GMF-CSF (Cantrell et al. 1985), G-CSF or CSF-β (Souza et al. 1986), and M-CSF or CSF-1 (Kawasaki et al. 1985) greatly facilitates the analysis of their structures and biologic activities. These factors are produced by a variety of cell types, such as hematopoietic cells, endothelial cells, or fibroblasts. GM-CSF, which can be produced by T cells, enhances the recruitment of granulocytes and monocytes and activates these cells to express a variety of effector functions (Metcalf 1985). These effects could be very useful after the aggressive cytostatic treatment of malignancies. Granulocytes and the intactness of mucosal surfaces appear to be the most crucial elements in warding off bacterial septic infections in such patients, and any measure providing one or the other is likely to permit more aggressive tumor treatment. Preclinical studies with GM-CSF in monkey have provided very encouraging results (DONAHUE et al. 1986). Because of its differentiation-inducing capacity, G-CSF has been considered for the treatment of patients with myeloid leukemias (NICOLA et al. 1985; SOUZA et al. 1986). GM-CSF and various other hematopoietic growth and differentiation factors alone or in combination will probably become useful therapeutic agents in the near future.

5. Interleukin 2 (see also Chap. 8)

Presently, there is a considerable interest in interleukin 2 (IL-2) as a new cancer drug. Therefore, we will discuss the potential applications of this lymphokine in greater detail. With the aid of IL-2, T cell lines and clones can be maintained and expanded in long-term cultures (Chap. 12), which opens up the possibility of adoptive immunotherapy with T cell populations. Various strategies for adoptive immunotherapy have been tested in animal experiments with tumor cell-specific T cell lines and clones or T cell populations activated by allogeneic cells or by lectins. In the course of these studies, the surprising finding was made that the short-term incubation of murine spleen cells with IL-2 led to the proliferation of some lymphoid cells, which acquired in culture the ability to lyse a wide variety of tumor cells. Apart from IL-2, this "activation" does not require any more stimuli.

The adoptive transfer of such lymphokine-activated killer (LAK) cells was found to produce a drastic reduction in the number of pulmonary and hepatic metastases in various animal tumor models. The efficiency of the treatment was enhanced further by the repeated i.v. or i.p. administration of IL-2, beginning shortly after LAK cell infusion (for review see ROSENBERG 1984; MERLUZZI and LAST-BARNEY 1985). Human LAK cells could be generated in a similar way by short incubation of mononuclear cells derived from the blood of tumor patients or healthy individuals. The nature of these human LAK cells has been studied extensively in several laboratories (ITOH et al. 1985; PHILLIPS and LANIER 1986; LANIER et al. 1986; HOYER et al. 1986; ORTALDO et al. 1986). There seems to be no single unique progenitor of cells with LAK activity. However, at least in blood, the majority of the LAK cells appear to be derived from natural killer (NK) cells. These NK cells comprise 5%–10% of total peripheral blood lymphocytes. They are large granular lymphocytes and express Leu-19 (or NKH-1, a marker for NK cells also present on a subset of T cells), the sheep red blood cell receptor (CD2, a pan-T cell marker) and, with the exception of a small subset, they express Fc receptors for IgG (CD16 or Leu-11). Freshly explanted NK cells lyse a restricted number of tumor cells (hence the name natural killer cells). Within a 1–2 day culture period in IL-2-conditioned medium, they acquire the ability to lyse cells from a wide variety of freshly explanted malignant tumors, including leukemias and lymphomas (OSHIMI et al. 1986). LAK cells appear to have the capacity to distinguish malignant from normal cells. However, this distinction is not absolute: low but significant levels of lysis of some nonmalignant target cells were recently observed with in vitro activated LAK cells (OSHIMI et al. 1986; ITO et al. 1986) as well as with LAK cells isolated from the blood of patients treated with high doses of IL-2 (SONDEL et al. 1986). LAK cells are not Mhc restricted, i.e., they kill autologous as well as allogeneic or xenogeneic tumor targets. They do not express the T3/T cell receptor complex and show no rearrangement of the T cell receptor β genes. However, some cells with "NK-like-activity" from human blood or thymus and some NK cell clones derived from human fetal blood do show β gene (but not α gene) transcription. They also express T3 molecules which appear to be associated with a novel 85 kdalton T cell receptor protein (YANAGI et al. 1985; MOINEGEON et al. 1986; Chap. 2).

A 4-day culture initially containing about 10^6/ml human mononuclear blood cells and about $1-2 \times 10^3$ units/ml IL-2 (which is almost ten times the dose needed for the growth of activated T cells) appears to be optimal for LAK cell generation. LAK cell induction appears to be enhanced by depletion of monocytes, but also by the addition of IL-1 to the culture medium. IFN-α and IFN-β were reported to inhibit LAK cell proliferation, but not LAK cell activation (HOYER et al. 1986).

The findings made with LAK cells in vitro suggested the possibility that LAK cells could also be induced in vivo in cancer patients. Indeed, the intraperitoneal application of high doses of IL-2 has been shown to induce tumor regressions in mice. Unfortunately, however, the IL-2 dose used in these experiments was 200-fold higher than that tolerated in human phase I trials. Several hundred cancer patients have been treated with varying doses of IL-2 which was administered either by continuous i.v. or i.p. infusions or by bolus injections via various routes (s.c., i.m., i.p., i.v., or locally into tumor lesions) (PIZZA et al. 1984; ATKINS et al. 1986; KONRAD and BRADLEY 1986). When applied by continuous i.v. or i.p. infusion, $1-3 \times 10^3$ units per kilogram body weight per hour appears to be the highest tolerated dose in humans while IL-2 administered i.v. as a bolus injection of $1-3 \times 10^4$ units/kg every 8 h was tolerated well by most patients (ROSENBERG 1985). Higher doses induce severe side effects, including a drastic weight gain due to fluid retention. LAK cell activity in the blood of patients treated with IL-2 was very variable and in only a few cases were objective tumor regression observed.

For these reasons, several physicians, in particular the group at the NIH (ROSENBERG 1985), began to investigate the potential therapeutic use of LAK cells activated ex vivo. As expected from the results of animal experiments, no clinical responses were observed in any patients treated with LAK cells alone (ROSENBERG 1985). However, in 11 of 25 patients with various types of advanced cancers, tumor regressions of at least 50% of the initial tumor volume and one complete remission were observed after treatment with a combination of LAK cells activated ex vivo and i.v. bolus injections of IL-2 every 8 h at doses of up to 10^5 units/kg (ROSENBERG et al. 1985). These encouraging results suggest that tolerable doses of IL-2 are sufficient to maintain in vivo the cytolytic activity of LAK cells which were induced ex vivo in the presence of IL-2. It remains to be seen whether this new approach to cancer therapy will eventually become an accepted procedure which might even be curative when applied to patients at earlier stages of the disease and in combination with other cytoreductive measures such a chemotherapy, radiation, and surgery.

In animal experiments, encouraging results have also been obtained by the transfer of tumor-specific, Mhc-restricted cytolytic T lymphocytes (CTL) expanded ex vivo in conjunction with in vivo administration of IL-2 and cyclophosphamide (CHEEVER et al. 1984; GREENBERG et al. 1985; ROSENBERG et al. 1986). Tumor-specific CTL isolated from tumors in mice and transferred to tumor-bearing mice after expansion in vitro were shown to induce regressions of metastases much more efficiently than LAK cells, when compared on a numerical basis. This was particularly true if the mice also received IL-2 in addition to cyclophosphamide (ROSENBERG et al. 1986). Thus, one could envisage a new treatment strategy for human cancer patients comprising the removal of the primary tumor by surgery, the isolation and in vitro expansion of tumor-infiltrating CTL or LAK cells, and the adoptive transfer of those cells in conjunction with the administration of IL-2 and cyclophosphamide. These are encouraging prospects. However, it is questionable whether this strategy will be successful in patients with advanced cancers, since, in such patients, the lymphocytes infiltrating the tumors have been found to lack the expression of activation markers (i.e., appear not to be activated by the tumor cells) and, like the peripheral blood cells of the same patients, showed a drastically reduced proliferative response to lectins (WHITESIDE et al. 1986a,b).

As has often been the case in the past, a promising new treatment modality has been introduced which is based on the pragmatic application of a poorly understood phenomenon – in the present case the LAK phenomenon. Much basic research is required to elucidate the molecular and cellular details of the LAK phenomenon, and many clinical trials are needed to determine the conditions for its optimal therapeutic use. One important first step is the identification of the most useful IL-2 species and the elaboration of the conditions for its mass production and purification. Six IL-2 species derived from eukaryotic cells and six recombinant IL-2 species derived from bacteria showed considerable variability in their biologic activity and purity (THURMAN et al. 1986; Chap. 8).

6. Antibodies

Polyclonal γ-globulins which can be applied intravenously are used for the treatment of microbial infections in immunocompromised patients with increasing frequency (SCHULTE-WISSERMANN et al. 1982; SIDIROPOULOS et al. 1981; JESDINSKY 1983). Monoclonal antibodies to bacterial antigens can act synergistically with antibiotics in the treatment of experimental bacterial infections and are promising candidates for the treatment of endotoxin shock (YOUNG 1985).

Very intensive efforts are being made at present to develop more selective treatment modalities in cancer patients with the aid of monoclonal antibodies against tumor-associated antigens (BALDWIN and BYERS 1985; SELL and REISFELD 1985; ALUM et al. 1986; STEVENSON 1986). Unmodified antibodies can inhibit tumor cell growth, or eliminate tumor cells by antibody-dependent cell-mediated cytotoxicity (ADCC), complement-mediated lysis, or the promotion of tumor cell phagocytosis by macrophages. Antibodies can also serve as carriers for toxins, drugs, isotopes, other biologically active factors, or as targeting devices for drug-containing liposomes. While each of these strategies has its specific problems, there are three major difficulties:

1. Practically all tumor-associated antigens which have so far been identified are also expressed by normal cells.
2. Tumor cell populations are genetically unstable and show considerable heterogeneity with respect to the expression of cell surface antigens.
3. Murine monoclonal antibodies induce strong humoral immune responses in most patients. These responses are undesirable because the Ig-specific antibodies can cause anaphylactic shock and because idiotyp-specific antibodies which are produced as a primary response can neutralize the therapeutic effect of antibodies which are applied on subsequent occasions.

Until now, most clinical trials have been performed with unmodified murine monoclonal antibodies, which were infused into the bloodstream either directly or after adsorption onto mononuclear cells obtained from the patients by leukopheresis. Tumor regressions have been observed in some cases, but no definitive conclusions can be drawn, since results of controlled clinical trials are not yet available.

At least some leukemias and a few solid tumors are considered to be curable by high doses of radiotherapy and chemotherapy, followed by autologous or allogeneic bone marrow tranplantation. Monoclonal antibodies have been used in attempts to improve this approach by depleting allogeneic bone marrow grafts of T cells to prevent graft-versus-host disease (BORTIN 1986) or by freeing autologous grafts from tumor cells in order to prevent recurrences originating from reinfused tumor cells (JANSEN et al. 1984). There is no doubt that the use of antibodies in bone marrow transplantation could make a major contribution to the treatment of some malignancies. However, the following three prerequisites will have to be fulfilled before this can happen:

1. More efficient treatment protocols must be developed for the elimination of the tumor cells in vivo.
2. The rejection rate of allogeneic bone marrow grafts must be further reduced by a more rigorous immunosuppression of the recipient (for example, by total lymphoid irradiation or in vivo application of antibodies).
3. More effective measures for the prevention of infections must be developed, perhaps by the administration of antibodies against gram-negative bacteria or by the application of hematopoietic factors such as GM-CSF or G-CSF.

D. Conclusions

In spite of some almost inevitable shortcomings which are represented in a lack of completeness on one hand and in a certain subjectiveness in the selection of topics on the other hand, this short "preview" may be able to convey one fact: the manipulation of lymphocyte functions by substances which can be microbial, synthetic, or mammalian in origin is a rather well-established field of immunologic experimentation, and to some extent even an area of therapeutic utilization. While, 10–15 years ago, serious doubts concerning the scientific soundness of all attempts to modulate lymphocyte function pharmacologically could still be raised, the field has now become scientifically acceptable and, in a few cases, has even gained clinical credibility. There are two main reasons which seem to support the contention that both scientific acceptance and therapeutic utilization will grow rapidly: the first reason refers to the rapid rate of progress in immunology, driven by molecular biology, while the second argument is based on the immense medical needs represented by those diseases which seem to be amenable to the pharmacologic modulation of lymphocyte function. However, despite much progress, particularly at the molecular level, we still have only a very fragmentary picture of the immune system. Virtually nothing is known about the regulation of lymphopoiesis and the mechanisms underlying immunologic memory or tolerance. It is therefore conceivable that, in addition to the rational approaches being taken, serendipity will be required to find novel lymphocyte modulators which can be used for therapy. Such compounds will also serve as investigative tools and will thus help to further our understanding of the immune system.

References

Adelman NE, Watling DL, McDevitt HO (1983) Treatment of (NZB × NZW) F_1 disease with anti-IA monoclonal antibodies. J Exp Med 158:1350–1355

Allum WH, Macdonald F, Fielding JW (1986) Monoclonal antibodies in the diagnosis and treatment of malignant conditions. Surg Annu 18:41–64

Atkins MB, Gould JA, Allegretta M, Li JJ, Dempsey RA, Rudders RA, Parkinson DR, Reichlin S, Mier JW (1986) Phase I evaluation of a recombinant interleukin-2 in patients with advanced malignant disease. J Clin Oncol 4:1380–1391

Avella J, Binder HJ, Madsen JE, Askenase PhW (1978) Effect of histamine H_2 receptor antagonists on delayed hypersensitivity. Lancet I:624–626

Baldwin RW, Byers VS (1985) Monoclonal antibodies for cancer detection and therapy. Academic, London

Basciano L-AK, Berenstein EH, Kmak L, Siraganian RP (1986) Monoclonal antibodies that inhibit IgE binding. J Biol Chem 261:11823–11831

Benjamin RJ, Waldmann H (1986) Induction of tolerance by monoclonal antibody therapy. Nature 320:449–451

Benjamin RH, Cobbolt SP, Clark MR, Waldmann H (1986) Tolerance to rat monoclonal antibodies. Implications for serotherapy. J Exp Med 163:1539–1552

Bennett J, Zloty P, McKneally M (1982) Cimetidine blocks the development of tumor-induced suppressor T-cell activity. Int J Immunopharmacol 4:280 abstr

Berridge MJ, Irvine RF (1984) Inositol triphosphate, a novel second messenger in cellular signal-transduction. Nature 312:315–321

Biddison WE, Rao PE, Talle MA, Goldstein G, Shaw S (1984) Possible involvement of the T4 molecules in T cell recognition of class II HLA antigens: evidence from studies of CTL-target cell binding. J Exp Med 159:783–797

Bijsterbosch MK, Meade ChJ, Turner GA, Klaus GGB (1985) B lymphocyte receptors and polyphosphoinositide degradation. Cell 41:999–1006

Blackwell GJ, Carnuccio R, DiRosa M, Flower RJ, Parente L, Persico P (1980) Macrocortin: a polypeptide causing the anti-phospholipase effect of glucocorticoids. Nature 287:147–149

Boitard C, Mishic S, Serrurier P, Butcher GW, Larkins AP, McDevitt HO (1985) In vivo prevention of thyroid and pancreatic autoimmunity in the BB rat by antibody to class II major histocompatibility gene products. Proc Natl Acad Sci USA 82:6627–6632

Borst J, Alexander S, Elder J, Terhorst C (1983) The T3 complex on human T lymphocytes involves four structurally distinct glycoproteins. J Biol Chem 258:5135–5141

Borst J, Coligan JE, Oettgen H, Pessano S, Malin R, Terhorst C (1984) The δ and ε-chains of the human T3/T-cell receptor complex are distinct polypeptides. Nature 312:455–458

Bortin MM (1986) Allogeneic bone marrow transplantation in leukemia patients. Curr Probl Cancer 10:1–52

Brenner MB, McLean J, Dialynas DP, et al. (1986) Identification of a putative second T cell receptor. Nature 322:145–149

Brostoff SW, Mason DW (1984) Experimental allergic encephalomyelitis: successful treatment in vivo with a monoclonal antibody that recognizes T helper cells. J Immunol 133:1938–1943

Cahill J, Hopper KE (1984) Immunoregulation by macrophages III. Prostaglandin E suppresses lymphocyte activation but not macrophage effector function during *Salmonella enteritidis* infection. Int J Immunopharmacol 6:9–17

Cambier JC, Monroe JG, Coggeshall KM, et al. (1985) The biochemical basis of transmembrane signalling by B lymphocyte surface immunoglobulin. Immunol Today 6:218–222

Cantrell MA, Anderson D, Cerretti DP, et al. (1985) Cloning sequence and expression of a human granulocyte/macrophage colony-stimulating factor. Proc Natl Acad Sci USA 82:6250–6254

Chatenoud L, Baudrihaye MF, Kreis H, Goldstein G, Bach JF (1985) The restricted immune response to the murine monoclonal OKT3 antibody. Transplant Proc 17:558–559

Chatenoud L, Jonker M, Villemain G, Goldstein G, Bach JF (1986) The human immune response to the OKT3 monoclonal antibody is oligoclonal. Science 232:1406–1408

Chedid LA, Parant MA, Audibert FM, Riveau GJ, Parant FJ, Lederer E, Choay JP, Lefrancier PL (1982) Biological activity of a new synthetic muramyl peptide adjuvant devoid of pyrogenicity. Infect Immun 35:417–424

Cheever MA, Greenberg PD, Fefer A (1984) Potential for specific cancer therapy with immune T lymphocytes. J Biol Response Mod 3:113–127

Chiao JW, Heil M, Arlin Z, Lutton JD, Choi JS, Leung K (1986) Suppression of lymphocyte activation and functions by a leukemia cell-derived inhibitor. Proc Natl Acad Sci USA 83:3432–3436

Clark EA, Ledbetter JA (1986) Amplification of the immune response by agonistic antibodies. Immunol Today 7:267–270

Cloix JF, Colard O, Rothut B, Russo-Marie F (1983) Characterization and partial purification of "renocortins": two polypeptides formed in renal cells causing the anti-phospholipase-like action of glucocorticoids. Br J Pharmacol 79:313–321

Cobbolt SP, Martin G, Ain S, Waldmann H (1986) Monoclonal antibodies to promote marrow engraftment and tissue graft tolerance. Nature 323:164–166

Cohen FE, Kosen PA, Kuntz ID, Eppstein LB, Ciardelli TL, Smith KA (1986) Structure-activity studies of interleukin-2. Science 234:349–352

De Simone C, Meli D, Sbricoli M, Rebuzzi E, Koverech A (1982) In vitro effect of inosiplex on T lymphocytes. J Immunopharmacol 4:139–152

Dembic Z, Haas W, Weiss S, McCurbey J, Kiefer H, v. Boehmer H, Steinmetz M (1986) Transfer of specificity by murine α and β T cell receptor genes. Nature 320:232–238

Dijk H van, Rademaker PM, Kerkhofs JP, Willers JMN (1980) Histamine 2-receptor-mediated immunomodulation in the mouse. II. Immunomodulation by the H_2 antagonist metiamide. Int J Immunopharmacol 2:345–352

Dinarello CA (1986) Interleukin-1: amino acid sequences, multiple biological activities and comparison with tumor necrosis factor (cachectin). In: Cruse M, Lewis RE (eds) The Year in Immunology, vol 2. Karger, Basel, pp 68–89

Donahue RE, Wang EA, Stone DK, Kamen R, Wong GG, Sehgal PK, Nathan DG, Clark SC (1986) Stimulation of hematopoiesis in primates by continuous infusion of recombinant human GM-CFS. Nature 321:872–875

Drews J (1984) The experimental and clinical use of immune-modulating drugs in the prophylaxis and treatment of infections. Infection 13:241–250

Drews J (1986) Immunpharmakologie, Grundlagen, Perspektiven. Springer, Berlin Heidelberg New York Tokyo

Duff G (1985) Many roles for interleukin-1. Nature 313:352–353

Duff GW, Durum SK (1983) The pyrogenic and mitogenic actions of interleukin-1 are related. Nature 304:449–451

Ferrara JLM, Marion A, McIntyre JF, Murphy GF, Burakoff SJ (1986) Amelioration of acute graft versus host disease due to minor histocompatibility antigens by in vivo administration of anti-interleukin-2 receptor antibody. J Immunol 137:1874–1877

Fraser-Smith EB, Matthews TR (1981) Protective effect of muramyl dipeptide analogs against infections of *Pseudomonas aeruginosa* or *Candida ablicans*. Infect Immun 34:676–683

Fraser-Smith EB, Eppstein DA, Larsen MA, Matthews TR (1983) Protective effect of a muramyl dipeptide analog encapsulated in or mixed with liposomes against *Candida albicans* infection. Infect Immun 39:172–178

Geha RS, Helm B, Gould H (1985) Inhibition of the Prausnitz-Küstner reaction by an immunoglobulin E-chain synthesized by *E. coli*. Nature 315:577–578

Gemsa D, Deimann W, Bärlin E, Seitz M, Leser HG (1982) Die Rolle von Prostaglandinen aus Makrophagen bei Regulation und Suppression der Immunantwort. Allergologie 5:142–150

Gifford RRM, Ferguson RM, Voss BV (1981) Cimetidine reduction of tumor formation in mice. Lancet I:638–639

Goldstein D, Laszlo J (1986) Perspectives in cancer research: interferon therapy in cancer: from imagination to interferon. Rev Cancer Res 46:4315–4329

Goldstein G, Schindler J, Sheahan M, Barnes L, Tsai H (1985) Orthoclone OKT3 treatment of acute renal allograft rejection. Transplant Proc 17:129–130

Goodman MG (1984) Inductive and differentiative signals delivered by C8-substituted guanine ribonucleosides. Immunol Today 5:319–324

Goodwin JS, Ceuppens J (1983) Regulation of the immune response by prostaglandins. J Clin Immunol 3:295–315

Goronzy J, Weyand CM, Fathman CG (1986) Long-term humoral unresponsiveness in vivo induced by treatment with monoclonal antibody against L3T4. J Exp Med 164:911–925

Greenberg PD, Kern DE, Cheever MA (1985) Therapy of disseminated murine leukemia with cyclophosphamide and immune Lyt 1^+2^- T cells. Tumor eradication does not require participation of cytotoxic T cells. J Exp Med 161:1122–1134

Greenstein JL, Malissen B, Burakoff SJ (1985) Role of L3T4 in antigen-driven activation of a class I-specific T cell hybridoma. J Exp Med 162:369–374

Haas W, von Boehmer J (1985) T cell proliferation and differentiation. In: Weissman I (ed) Leukemia. Springer, Berlin Heidelberg New York, pp 21–30

Hardt C, Röllinghoff M, Pfizenmaier K, Mosmann H, Wagner H (1981) Lyt-23$^+$ cyclophosphamide-sensitive T cells regulate the activity of an interleukin-2 inhibitor in vivo. J Exp Med 154:262–274

Hersey P, Bindon C, Bradley M, Hasic E (1984) Effect of isoprinosine on interleukin 1 and 2 production and on suppressor cell activity in poke-weed mitogen stimulated cultures of B and T cells. Int J Immunopharmacol 6:321–328

Hess AD, Horwitz L, Beschorner WE, Santos GW (1985) Development of graft versus host disease like syndrome in cyclosporine treated rats after syngeneic bone marrow transplantation. I. Development of cytotoxic T lymphocytes with apparent polyclonal anti-Ia specificity including autoreactivity. J Exp Med 161:718–730

Hess AD, Colombani PM, Esa AH (1986) Cyclosporine and the immune response: basic aspects. Crit Rev Immunol 6:123–149

Hirata F, Schiffmann E, Venkatasubramamian K, Salomon D, Axelrod J (1980) A phospholipase A$_2$ inhibitory protein in rabbit neutrophils induced by glucocorticoids. Proc Natl Acad Sci USA 77:2533–2536

Hirschhorn R (1983) Metabolic defects and immunodeficiency disorders. N Eng J Med 308:714–716

Honda M, Chan Ch, Shevach EM (1985) Characterization and partial purification of a specific interleukin-2 inhibitor. J Immunol 135:1834–1839

Hoyer M, Meinecke T, Lewis W, Zwilling B, Rinehart J (1986) Characterization and modulation of human lymphokine (interleukin-2) activated killer cell induction. Cancer Res 46:2834–2838

Isakov N, Scholz W, Altman A (1986) Signal transduction and intracellular events in T lymphocyte activation. Immunol Today 7:271–277

Ishizaka K, Yodoi J, Suemura M, Hirashima M (1983) Isotype specific regulation of the IgE response by IgE binding factors. Immunol Today 4:192–194

Ito M, Bandyopadhyay S, Matsumoto-Kobayashi M, Clark SC, Miller D, Starr SE (1986) Interleukin-2 enhances natural killing of varicella-zoster virus infected targets. Clin Exp Immunol 65:182–189

Itoh K, Tilden AB, Kumagai K, Balch ChM (1985) Leu-11 + lymphocytes with natural killer (NK) activity are precursors of recombinant interleukin-2 (rIL-2)-induced activated killer (AK) cells. J Immunol 134:802–807

Iwata M, Huff TF, Ishizaka K (1984) Modulation of the biologic activities of IgE-binding factor. V. The role of glycosylation-enhancing factor and glycosylation-inhibiting factor determining the nature of IgE-binding factors. J Immunol 132:1286–1293

Jansen J, Falkenberg JHF, Stepan DE, LeBien TW (1984) Removal of neoplastic cells from autologous bone marrow grafts with monoclonal antibodies. Semin Hematol 21:164–181

Jardieu P, Uede T, Ishizaka K (1984) IgE-binding factor from mouse T lymphocytes. III. Role of antigen-specific suppressor T cells in the formation of IgE-suppressive factor. J Immunol 133:3266–3273

Jesdinsky HJ (1983) Cooperative group of additional immunoglobulin therapy in severe bacterial infections: multicenter randomized controlled trial on the efficacy of additional immunoglobulin therapy in cases of diffuse fibrino-purulent peritonitis – study design. Klin Wochenschr 61:445–450

Jones PT, Dear PH, Foote J, Neuberger MS, Winter G (1986) Replacing the complementarity-determining regions in a human antibody with those from a mouse. Nature 321:522–525

Jorizzo JL, Sams MW, Jegasothy BV, Olansky AJ (1980) Cimetidine as an immunomodulator: chronic mucocutaneous candidiasis as a model. Ann Intern Med 92 (1):192–195

Katz DH (1984) Regulation of the IgE system: experimental and clinical aspects. Allergy 39:81–106

Kawano M, Iwato K, Kuramoto A (1985) Identification and characterization of a B cell growth inhibitory factor (BIF) on BCGF-dependent B cell proliferation. J Immunol 134:375–381

Kawasaki ES, Ladner MB, Wang AM, et al. (1985) Molecular cloning of a complementary DNA encoding human macrophage-specific colony-stimulating factor (CSF-1). Science 230:291–296

Kelley VE, Noar D, Tarcic N, Gaulton GN, Strom TB (1986) Anti-interleukin-2 receptor antibody suppresses delayed-type hypersensitivity to foreign and syngeneic antigens. J Immunol 137:2122–2124

Kingston AE, Kay JE, Ivanyi J (1985) The effects of prostaglandin E and I analogues on lymphocyte stimulation. Int J Immunopharmacol 7:57–64

Kirkman RL, Barrett LV, Gaulton GN, Kelley VE, Ythier A, Strom TB (1985) Administration of anti-interleukin-2 receptor monoclonal antibody prolongs cardiac allograft survival in mice. J Exp Med 162:358–362

Konrad MW, Bradley EC (1986) The pharmacokinetics of a recombinant IL-2 muteine given by five routes in a number of phase I trials (abstract). Proc Am Soc Clin Oncol 5:235

Kramer M, Koszinowski U (1982) T cell-specific suppressor factor(s) with regulatory influence on interleukin-2 production and function. J Immunol 128:784–790

Krönke M, Leonard WJ, Depper JM, Arya SK, Wong-Staal F, Gallo RC, Waldmann TA, Greene WC (1984) Cyclosporine A inhibits T-cell growth factor gene expression at the level of mRNA transcription. Proc Natl Acad Sci USA 81:5214–5218

Kuff EL, Mietz JA, Troustine ML, Moore KW, Martens CL (1986) cDNA clones encoding murine IgE-binding factors represent multiple structural variants of intracisternal A-particle genes. Proc Natl Acad Sci USA 83:6583–6587

Kuo LM, Robb RJ (1986) Structure function relationships for the IL-2 receptor system. 1. Localization of a receptor binding site on IL-2. J Immunol 137:1538–1543

Kuo LM, Rusk CM, Robb RJ (1986) Structure function relationship for the IL-2 receptor system. II. Localization of an IL-2 binding site on high and low affinity receptors. J Immunol 137:1544–1551

Kupiec-Weglinski JW, Diamantstein T, Tilney NL, Strom TB (1986) Therapy with mono-clonal antibody to interleukin-2 receptors spares suppressor T cells and prevents or re-verses acute allograft rejection in rats. Proc Natl Acad Sci USA 83:2624–2627

Lanier LL, Le AM, Civin CI, Loken MR, Phillips JH (1986) The relationship of CD/6 (Leu 11), Leu 19 (NKH-1) antigen expression on human peripheral blood NK cells and cy-totoxic T lymphocytes. J Immunol 136:4480–4485

Like AA, Biron CA, Weringer EJ, Byman K, Sroczynski E, Guberski DL (1986) Preven-tion of diabetes in biobreeding/Worcester rats with monoclonal antibodies that recog-nize T lymphocytes or natural killer cells. J Exp Med 164:1145–1159

Liu FT, Albrand K, Mendel E, Kulczycki, Orida NK (1985) Identification of an IgE-bind-ing protein by molecular cloning. Proc Natl Acad Sci USA 82:4100–4104

Lomedico PT, Gubler U, Hellmann CP, Dukovich M, Giri JG, Pan Y-CE, Collier K, Semionow R, Chua AO, Mizel SB (1984) Cloning and expression of murine interleu-kin-1 cDNA in *Escherichia coli*. Nature 312:458–462

Lou CY, Wang EY, Li D, Budz-Tymkewycz S, Visconti V, Ishague A (1985) Mechanism of action of a suppressor-activating factor (SAF) produced by a human T cell line. J Immunol 134:3155–3162

MacDonald HR, Glasebrook AL, Bron C, Kelso A, Cerottini JC (1982) Clonal heteroge-neity in the functional requirement for Lyt-2/3 molecules on cytolytic T lymphocytes (CTL): possible implications for the affinity of CTL antigen receptors. Immunol Rev 68:89–115

Marceletti JF, Katz DH (1984) FcRε⁺ lymphocytes and regulation of the IgE antibody sys-tem. IV Delineation of target cells and mechanism of action of SFA and EFA in inhib-iting in vitro induction of FcRε expression. J Immunol 133:2845–2851

Marrack P, Endrew R, Shimonkevitz R, Zlotnik A, Dialynas D, Fitch F, Kappler J (1983) The major histocompatibility complex-restricted antigen receptor on T cells. II. Role of the L3T4 product. J Exp Med 158:1077–1091

Medoff JR, Clack VD, Roche JK (1986) Characterization of an immunosuppressive factor from malignant ascites that resembles a factor induced in vitro by carcinoembryonic antigen. J Immunol 137:2057–2064

Merluzzi VJ, Last-Barney K (1985) Potential use of human interleukin-2 as an adjunct for the therapy of neoplasia, immunodeficiency and infectious disease. Int J Immunophar-macol 7:31–39

Metcalf D (1985) The granulocyte-macrophage colony-stimulating factors. Science 229:16–22

Moingeon M, Ythier A, Goubin G, Faure F, Nowill A, Delmon L, Rainaud M, Forestier F, Daffos F, Bohuon C, Hercend T (1986) A unique T cell receptor complex expressed on human fetal lymphocytes displaying natural killer like activity. Nature 323:638–640

Morley J (1979) Prostaglandins and chronic inflammation. In: Rainsford KD, Ford-Hutchinson AW (eds) Prostaglandins and inflammation. Birkhäuser, Basel, pp 133–141

Morley J (ed) (1982) Bronchial hyperreactivity. Academic, London

Morrison SL (1985) Transfectomas provide novel chimeric antibodies. Science 229:1202–1207

Nakamura T, Miyasaka N, Pope RM, Talal N, Russel IJ (1983) Immunomodulation by isoprinosine: effects on in vitro immune functions of lymphocytes from humans with autoimmune diseases. Clin Exp Immunol 52:67–74

Nathan CF, Murray HW, Wiebe ME, Rubin BY (1983) Identification of interferon-γ as the lymphokine that activates human macrophage oxidative metabolism and antimi-crobial activity. J Exp Med 158:670–689

Neuberger MS, Williams GT, Fox RO (1984) Recombinant antibodies possessing novel ef-fector functions. Nature 312:604–608

Nicola NA, Begley CG, Metcalf D (1985) Identification of the human analogue of a regu-lator that induces differentiation in murine leukemic cells. Nature 314:625–628

Nishizuka Y (1984) Turnover of inositol phospholipids and signal transduction. Science 225:1365–1370

Nydegger UE (1985) Suppressive and substitutive immunotherapy: an essay with a review of recent literature. Immunol Lett 9:185–190

Obert HJ, Brzoska J (1986) Interferon-γ in therapy of rheumatoid arthritis. Drug Res 36:1557–1560

Oppenheim JJ, Kovacs EJ, Matsushima K, Durum SK (1986) There is more than one interleukin-1. Immunol Today 7:45–56

Ortaldo JR, Mason A, Overton R (1986) Lymphokine-associated killer cells. Analysis of progenitors and effectors. J Exp Med 164:1193–1205

Ortho Multicenter Tranplant Group (1985) A randomized clinical trial OKT3 monoclonal antibody for acute rejection of cadaveric renal transplants. N Engl J Med 313:337–342

Oshimi K, Oshimi Y, Akutsu M, Takei Y, Saito H, Okada M, Mizoguchi H (1986) Cytotoxicity of interleukin activated lymphocytes for leukemia and lymphoma. Blood 68:938–948

Pasino M, Bellone M, Cornaglia P, Tonini GP, Massimo L (1982) Methisoprinol effect on enriched B and T lymphocyte populations stimulated with phytohemagglutinin. J Immunopharmacol 4:101–108

Pestka S (1986) Interferons from 1981–1986. Methods Enzymol 119:3–14

Phillips JH, Lanier LL (1986) Dissection of the lymphokine-activated killer phenomenon. Relative contribution of peripheral blood natural killer cells and T lymphocytes to cytolysis. J Exp Med 164:814–825

Pizza G, Severini G, Menniti D, DeVinci C, Corrado F (1984) Tumor regressions after intralesional injection of interleukin-2 (IL-2) in bladder cancer: preliminary report. Int J Cancer 34:359–367

Raefsky EL, Gascon P, Gratwohl A, Speck B, Young NS (1986) Biological and immunological characterization of ATG and ALG. Blood 68:712–719

Rappaport RS, Dodge GR (1982) Prostaglandin E inhibits the production of human interleukin-2. J Exp Med 155:943–948

Rosenberg SA (1984) Adoptive immunotherapy of cancer: accomplishments and prospects. Cancer Treat Rep 68:233–255

Rosenberg SA (1985) Lymphokine-activated killer cells: a new approach to immunotherapy of cancer. J Natl Cancer Inst 75:595–603

Rosenberg SA, Lotze MT, Muul LM, et al. (1985) Observations on the systemic administration of autologous lymphokine-activated killer cells and recombinant interleukin-2 to patients with metastatic cancer. N Engl J Med 313:1485–1492

Rosenberg SA, Spiess P, Lafreniere R (1986) A new approach to the adoptive immunotherapy of cancer with tumor-infiltrating lymphocytes. Science 233:1318–1321

Rothhut B, Russo-Marie F, Wood J, DiRosa M, Flower RJ (1983) Further characterization of the glucocorticoid-induced antiphospholipase protein "Renocortin". Biochem Biophys Res Commun 117:878–884

Schulte-Wissermann H, Schofer O, Dinkel E (1982) Die Therapie mit γ-Globulin. Struktur, Wirkungsweise und Einsatzmöglichkeiten intravenös applizierbarer γ-Globulinpräparate. Immun Infekt 10:98–109

Sell S, Reisfeld RA (1985) Monoclonal antibodies in cancer. Human Press, Clifton, New Jersey

Shirakawa F, Tanaka Y, Oda S, Chiba S, Suzuki H, Eto S, Yamashita U (1986) Immunosuppressive factors from adult T cell leukemia cells. Cancer Res 46:4458–4462

Shu-Mei Liang, Thatcher DR, Chi-Ming Liang, Allet B (1986) Studies of structure-activity relationship of human interleukin-2. J Immunol 261:334–337

Sidiropoulos D, Böhme U, von Muralt G, Morell A, Barandun S (1981) Immunglobulin-substitution bei der Behandlung der neonatalen Sepsis. Schweiz Med Wochenschr 111:1649–1655

Sondel MP, Hank JA, Kohler PC, Chen BP, Minkoff DZ, Molenda JA (1986) Destruction of autologous human lymphocytes by interleukin-2 activated cytotoxic cells. J Immunol 137:502–511

Souza LM, Boone TC, Gabrilove A, et al. (1986) Recombinant human granulocyte colony-stimulating factor: effects on normal and leukemic myeloid cells. Science 232:61–65

Steinman L, Rosenbaum J, Sriram S, McDevitt HO (1981) In vivo effects of antibodies to immune response gene products: prevention of experimental allergic encephalitis. Proc Natl Acad Sci USA 78:7111–7114

Stevenson GT (1986) The prospect for treating cancer with antibody. Sci Prog 70:505–519

Storb R, Deeg HJ, Whitehead J, et al. (1986) Methotrexate and cyclosporine compared with cyclosporine alone for prophylaxis of acute graft versus host disease after marrow transplantation for leukemia. N Eng J Med 314:729–735

Suzuki S, Huchet R (1981) Mechanism of histamine-induced inhibition of lymphocyte response to mitogens in mice. Cell Immunol 62:396–405

Swain SL (1983) T cell subsets and the recognition of MHC class. Immunol Rev 74:129–142

Talmadge JE, Lenz BF, Klabonsky R, Simon R, Rigg C, Guo S, Oldham RK, Fidler IJ (1986) Therapy of autochthonous skin cancers in mice with intravenously injected liposomes containing muramyltripeptide. Cancer Res 46:1160–1163

Tandom P, Utsugi T, Sone S (1986) Lack of production of interleukin-1 by human blood monocytes activated to the antitumor state by liposome-encapsulated muramyl tripeptide. Cancer Res 46:5039–5044

Thurman GB, Maluish AE, Rossio JL et al. (1986) Comparative evaluation of multiple lymphoid and recombinant human interleukin-2 preparations. J Biol Response Mod 5:85–107

Traber R, Kuhn M, Rüegger A, Lichti H, Loosli HR, von Wartburg A (1977a) Die Struktur von Cyclosporin C. Helv Chim Acta 60:1247–1255

Traber R, Kuhn M, Loosli HR, Pache W, von Wartburg A (1977b) Neue Cyclopeptide aus *Trichoderma polysporum* (Link ex Pers.) Rifai: die Cyclosporine B, D und E. Helv Chim Acta 60:1568–1578

Trang LE (1980) Prostaglandins and inflammation. Semin Arthritis Rheum 9:153–159

Uede T, Hirata F, Hirashima M, Ishizaka K (1983) Modulation of the biologic activities of IgE-binding factors. I. Identification of glycosylation-inhibiting factor as a fragment of lipomodulin. J Immunol 130:878–884

Uede T, Huff TF, Ishizaka K (1984) Suppression of IgE synthesis in mouse plasma cells and B cells by rat IgE-suppressive factor. J Immunol 133:803–808

Waldor MK, Sriram S, McDevitt HO, Steinman L (1983) In vivo therapy with monoclonal anti-I-A antibody suppresses immune responses to acetylcholine receptor. Proc Natl Acad Sci USA 80:2713–2717

Waldor MK, Hardy RR, Hayakawa K, Steinman L, Herzenberg LA, Herzenberg LA (1984) Disappearance and reappearance of B cells after in vivo treatment with monoclonal anti-I-A antibodies. Proc Natl Acad Sci USA 81:2855–2858

Waldor MK, Sriram S, Hardy R, Herzenberg LA, Herzenberg LA, Lanier L, Lim M, Steinman L (1985) Reversal of experimental allergic encephalomyelitis with monoclonal antibody to a T cell subset marker. Science 227:415–419

Walker C, Kristensen F, Bettens F, deWeck AL (1983) Lymphokine regulation of activated (G_1) lymphocytes. I. Prostaglandin E_2-induced inhibition of interleukin-2 production. J Immunol 130:1770–1773

Wallner BP, Mattaliano RJ, Hession C, Cate RL, Tizard R, Sinclair LK, Foeller C, Pingchang Chow E, Browning JL, Ramachandran KL, Pepinsky RB (1986) Cloning and expression of human lipocortin, a phospholipase A_2 inhibitor with potential anti-inflammatory activity. Nature 320:77–81

Wang A, Shi-Da Lu, Mark DF (1984) Site specific mutagenesis of the human interleukin-2 gene: structure-function analysis of the cysteine residues. Science 224:1431–1433

Ward JR, Samuelson CO (1982) Nonsteroidal antiinflammatory drugs. In: Isselbacher KJ (ed) Update II. Harrison's principles of internal medicine. McGraw Hill, New York, pp 91–110

Weigent DA, Hoeprich PD, Bost KL, Brunck TK, Reiher WE, Blalock JE (1986) The HTLV-III envelope protein contains a hexapeptide homologous to a region of interleukin-2 that binds to the interleukin-2 receptor. Biochem Biophys Res Commun 139:367–374

Whiteside TL, Miescher S, Hürlimann J, Moretta L, von Fliedner V (1986 a) Separation, phenotyping and limiting dilution analysis of T-lymphocytes infiltrating human solid tumors. Int J Cancer 37:803–811

Whiteside TL, Miescher S, MacDonald HR, von Fliedner V (1986 b) Separation of tumor-infiltrating lymphocytes from tumor cells in human solid tumors. A comparison between velocity sedimentation and discontinuous density gradients. J Immunol Methods 90:221–233

Wofsy D, Seaman WE (1985) Successful treatment of autoimmunity in NZB/NZW F 1 mice with monoclonal antibody L3T4. J Exp Med 161:378–391

Wofsy D, Mayes DC, Woodcook J, Seaman WE (1985) Inhibition of humoral immunity in vivo by monoclonal antibody to L3T4: studies with soluble antigens in intact mice. J Immunol 135:1698–1703

Yanagi Y, Caccia N, Kronenberg M, et al. (1985) Gene rearrangement in cells with natural killer activity and expression of the β-chain of the T cell antigen receptor. Nature 314:631–633

Yodoi J, Hirashima M, Ishizaka K (1982) Regulatory role of IgE-binding factors from rat T lymphocytes. V. Carbohydrate moieties in IgE-potentiating factors and IgE-suppressive factor. J Immunol 128:289–295

Young LS (1985) Monoclonal antibodies: technology and application to gram-negative infections. Infection 13:224–228

Yu-Chung Yang, Ciarletta AB, Temple PA, Chung MP, Kovacic S, Witek-Giannotti JAS, Leary AC, Kriz R, Clark SC (1986) Human IL-3 (multi CSF): identification by expression cloning of a novel hematopoietic growth factor related to murine IL-3. Cell 47:3–10

Subject Index

A cells 275, 281
A23187 see calcium ionophore
Abelson virus 335, 566
accessory cells (AC) see also antigen
  presenting cells 1, 40–44, 321, 398,
  429, 446, 448, 503, 504, 507, 510, 511
AC-conditioned medium 40–42
p-acetamidobenzoic acid 535–537
acetylcholine 497
acquired immunodeficiency diseases
  (AIDS) 347, 393, 535, 540–545, 580
  pre-AIDS 535, 541, 545
actin 86, 87
actinomycin D 105, 260, 299, 301, 304
activation antigens (T cells) see also T cell
  surface receptors 37, 38, 40, 42
acute phase responses 226, 227, 568
acylCoA: lysophosphatide
  acyltransferase 387
acyltransferase 93, 94, 100
adenine 454, 519
adenocarcinoma 539
adenosine 107, 108, 525
  receptors (A2) 106
adenosine 3′, 5′ cyclic monophosphate
  (cAMP) 54, 57, 87, 93, 106, 108–113,
  115, 219, 366–370, 372–374, 376, 391,
  394, 401, 417, 419, 526
  8-bromo cAMP 55, 108
  cAMP dependent protein kinase 57,
    112, 113
  dibutyryl cAMP 54, 57, 108, 109, 112,
    368, 370
  specific antibodies 108
denosine deaminase 517, 525–527, 546
adenosine triphosphatase (ATPase) see
  also Na$^+$,H$^+$ ATPase; Mg^{++} ATPase
  69, 74, 86, 100, 101, 104, 107–109
adenosine triphosphate (ATP) 68, 72, 86,
  96, 107, 526
adenylate cyclase 54, 57, 87, 92, 107–109,
  115, 366, 369, 373
adjuvants see also individual adjuvants
  1, 148, 503, 507, 511, 512, 555
adjuvant arthritis 461, 475–477, 487, 495,
  499, 509

adrenaline 107, 108, 363, 373, 375
α-adrenoceptors 107, 373, 374
β-adrenoceptors 107, 108, 373, 374
  agonists 352, 364, 374, 375
affinity chromatography 368, 387
aging 148–150, 347, 392, 475, 541
agglutination 167
alkaline phosphatase 163, 269, 278, 279
alkylating agents 453, 454, 458, 464
allantoin 536
allele 1, 13, 29, 30
allergens see antigens
allergic rhinitis 283
alloantigen 40, 323
allograft see graft
allomorph 26, 30
alprenolol 374
aluminium hydroxide (alum) 148, 276,
  283, 492
alveolar cells 220, 568
amiloride 72, 73, 101, 102
amino acids 97, 105–107
p-aminobenzoic acid 535
2-aminoisobutyric acid 105, 106
aminopterin 190, 330
4-aminopyridine 60–62, 65
amphiphiles 559–561
analgesics 441, 582
antibiotics 320
antibodies (polyclonal) (Ab) see also
  monoclonal antibodies;
  immunoglobulins 1–5, 7, 8, 32, 109,
  141–175, 291, 338, 398, 504, 507, 591,
  592, 601
  Ab linked enzymes 170, 172, 175
  generation 21, 109, 141–158, 161–164,
    188, 191, 193, 200, 205, 276, 283, 319,
    329, 335, 353, 368, 369, 373, 374, 398,
    399, 404, 416, 418, 426, 427, 430, 434,
    443, 456, 472, 492, 499, 504, 505, 508–
    511, 519–521, 577, 580, 596
  high affinity 162, 173
  low affinity 162, 166, 173
  measurement 156–175
  polyclonal Ab (serum) 169, 172, 173

Handbook of Experimental Pharmacology

Editorial Board
G. V. R. Born, P. Cuatrecasas,
H. Herken, A. Schwarz

Springer-Verlag
Berlin Heidelberg New York
London Paris Tokyo

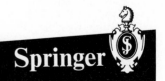

Handbook of Experimental Pharmacology

Editorial Board
G.V.R.Born, P.Cuatrecasas,
H.Herken, A.Schwarz

Springer-Verlag
Berlin Heidelberg New York
London Paris Tokyo

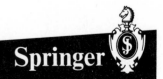

Springer